ADVANCING YOUR CAREER

FOURTH EDITION

ADVANCING YOUR CAREER

Concepts of Professional Nursing

Rose Kearney-Nunnery, RN, PhD, CNE
Member and Past President
South Carolina Board of Nursing

 F. A. DAVIS COMPANY • Philadelphia

F. A. Davis Company
1915 Arch Street
Philadelphia, PA 19103

Printed in the United States of America

Last digit indicates print number: 10 9 8 7 6 5 4 3 2 1

Acquisitions Editor: Joanne P. DaCunha, RN, MSN
Developmental Editor: Caryn Abramowitz
Project Editor: Kristin L. Kern

As new scientific information becomes available through basic and clinical research, recommended treatments and drug therapies undergo changes. The author and publisher have done everything possible to make this book accurate, up to date, and in accord with accepted standards at the time of publication. The author, editors, and publisher are not responsible for errors or omissions or for consequences from application of the book, and make no warranty, expressed or implied, in regard to the contents of the book. Any practice described in this book should be applied by the reader in accordance with professional standards of care used in regard to the unique circumstances that may apply in each situation. The reader is advised always to check product information (package inserts) for changes and new information regarding dose and contraindications before administering any drug. Caution is especially urged when using new or infrequently ordered drugs.

Library of Congress Cataloging-in-Publication Data

Kearney-Nunnery, Rose.
    Advancing your career: concepts of professional nursing/Rose Kearney-Nunnery.—4th ed.
    p. ; cm.
    Includes bibliographical references and index.

    ISBN-13: 978-0-8036-1827-5
    ISBN-10: 0-8036-1827-1

    1. Nursing—Vocational guidance. 2. Nursing—Vocational guidance—United States. 3. Nursing—Philosophy.
4. Career development. I. Title.
    [DNLM: 1. Nursing. 2. Career Mobility. WY 16 K24aa 2008]
    RT82.N85 2008
    610.7306' 9—dc22

                                2007046908

dedicated to
Jimmie E. Nunnery

Preface

The nursing profession has undergone major changes in the past decades, and the pace of change seems to accelerate daily. We are firmly in the new millennium while moving from our former role of defending nursing as a profession to our present pivotal role in health care despite the shortages. Focusing on human beings in their respective environments with their unique health-care needs that are addressed through nursing care is vitally important with our rapidly expanding knowledge base and the dynamic changes continually occurring in health care. In essence, our quest in our respective nursing roles is to expand knowledge, become involved within the profession and in interdisciplinary health care, utilize evidence-based practice and expanding technologies, and broaden the vision of professional practice.

This book is directed to the RN student returning to school. The intent is to provide you, the practicing RN, with professional concepts to advance your practice. These concepts build on your prior nursing education, and their application will greatly enhance your professional practice and growth. The aim is to engage you intellectually in an ongoing professional dialogue and journey with your peers, colleagues, and instructors; broaden your professional development; and build on your preexisting knowledge and experiences. You, the RN student, are challenged to delve further into professional education and conceptual practice. The book is written for the adult learner with the characteristics of self-direction, prior experiences, applicability to practice, and motivation to meet the challenge to expand his or her knowledge base.

The fourth edition has been updated but is still divided into five sections. As with the previous editions, each chapter contains chapter objectives, key terms, key points, chapter exercises to assist in meeting each of the chapter objectives, references, online resources, and bibliographical sources. Interactive exercises have been extended from the third edition and are provided on an Intranet site to truly engage the adult learner progressing through the content. The book's Intranet site also houses a, thorough glossary of terms, important Internet links, discussion sections, and bonus information as Web lessons in presentation graphics with interactive challenges and Web links.

Section I introduces the concepts of professional nursing practice. Chapter 1 focuses on the characteristics of professional nursing as a profession and as a unique professional discipline. Included in this updated chapter is a focus on the core competencies for all health-care professionals. Readers are challenged to develop personal perspectives of professional nursing as a philosophy statement. The associated Web lesson looks at competencies for genetics and genomics in current practice. Coping with returning to school is the theme of Chapter 2. Dr. Bernadette Dorsch Curry's presentation highlights strategies for success in the arduous process of returning to the student role.

Section II addresses the theoretical bases of nursing practice. First, Chapter 3 presents theory development, description, and use. Terminology is applied to theories from other disciplines and those successfully applied in professional nursing, including Maslow's hierarchy of basic needs, developmental theories, and systems theory. New content includes the challenges with quantum theory and the issue of conventional wisdom. The associated Web lesson applies developmental theories to nursing of children. In Chapter 4, Dr. Jacqueline Fawcett and Barbara Swoyer address the evolution of nursing theory. In addition to a discussion of the evolution, vocabulary, and advantages of these nursing models, the chapter and the Web lesson present applications for selecting and using the models as a guide for practice. The bases of nursing theories are followed by discussion of health and illness models that have been successfully used to guide nursing practice (Chapter 5). The theories of health and illness presented include Dunn's high-level wellness, the health belief model, a health promotion model, and a chronic illness model. Focusing on health, the chapter includes issues with levels of prevention and an expanded focus on transcultural models and cultural competence. The Web lesson for this chapter is on Complementary and Alternative Medicine (CAM). Section II concludes with a focus on evidence-based nursing in Chapter 6, with the view of the research process and the use of evidence of efficacy as a basis for practice. Legal and ethical considerations and utilization and critique of research are highlighted. The associated Web lesson focuses on locating information for evidence-based practice. A new feature on thinking about evidence-based practice begins with Chapter 6.

Section III features critical components of professional nursing practice. Eight critical components of professional nursing are reviewed: communication, working with groups, critical thinking, teaching and learning, leadership, management in organizations, change, and professional ethics. The first of these critical components is presented by Jacqueline Owers

Favret in Chapter 7, with a discussion of communication models, essential ingredients of effective communication, nonverbal communication forms, and specific communication techniques, including communication skills for interdisciplinary practice. The associated Web lesson looks at the issues with communication breakdowns that can occur with a disaster, as with Hurricane Katrina in 2005. Effective communication is broadened in Chapter 8 for use in groups including the characteristics and roles of groups and group leaders and the skills needed for collaboration, coordination, negotiation, and dealing with conflict and difficult people. In the associated Web lesson, readers are challenged to set up a virtual group.

Critical thinking is essential to professional nursing practice. In Chapter 9, Dr. Genevieve M. Bartol traces the historical aspects of critical thinking in nursing, along with the characteristics, measurement, and further development of critical thinking and analysis skills.

Chapter 10 has been updated and focuses on the teaching and learning process, learning theories including transformational learning, and learning readiness. Included in this chapter is a discussion on writing behavioral objectives, teaching skills and methods, and outcome evaluations while the Web lesson focuses on helping clients to locate reliable Web sources.

Drs. Theresa M. Valiga and Sheila C. Grossman address leadership as a critical component of professional nursing practice in Chapter 11. Along with definitions, theories, and styles of leadership, the chapter contains a description of the components of effective leadership.

Understanding organizations and effective management in organizational settings are essential parts of professional practice, as described in Chapter 12. Organizational theory focusing on systems theory, structure and function, culture, and communication skills is applied to a variety of organizational designs with a discussion of selected management theories, delegation principles, and strategies for management situations. Practice with delegation principles is the topic of the Web lesson for this chapter. Organizations have redefined themselves radically during the past decade. Dealing with change is an involved process. Chapter 13 has been updated with classic and recent theories on change, the characteristics of change agents, and change in individuals, families, groups, and organizations. Readers are challenged to determine their *change quotient* in the associated Web lesson.

Section III concludes with Chapter 14, "Professional Ethics" by Dr. Joseph T. Catalano. This chapter focuses on basic human rights, the right to privacy and dignity, access to care, informed consent, advance directives, organ transplantation, euthanasia, delegation, genetic manipulation, and workplace hazards.

Section IV delves into the concepts needed to provide care as a major activity in professional nursing practice, especially with the emphasis on safety and effective client outcomes. In Chapter 15. Vicki Budka has provided an update on the issues with managing and providing professional nursing care including a focus on the role of the work environment, differentiated practice, and models of care delivery for client-focused care. Included in the chapter is a presentation of issues related to documentation and the use of standardized nomenclatures and taxonomies. Providing care is challenging as we address at-risk populations and elimination of health disparities in Chapter 16. National strategies for improving health and eliminating health disparities for at-risk population groups are highlighted, including a focus on select populations, like the aging population with quality of healthy life considerations, minority health with identified health disparities, and rural health considerations. In the associated Web lesson, readers are challenged to investigate current progress on *Healthy People 2010.*

Providing care includes a necessary focus on quality. Quality care is discussed in Chapter 17 by Francoise Dunefsky, who highlights the issues of theoretical models for quality, quality improvement, continuous quality improvement, and quality management. These are presented as important considerations with the accreditation of health-care organizations. The use of informatics as one of the core competencies for health-care professionals is addressed in Chapter 18 by Dr. Julia Aucoin. Health-care information management systems and careers in informatics are discussed along with additional computer applications in professional practice. In Chapter 19, Drs. Cyril F. Chang and Susan K. Pfoutz address one of the major issues driving today's health-care system: economics. They discuss issues related to types of payers, effectiveness, system reforms, and marketplace considerations. Current information on drug plans is the focus for the Web lesson with this chapter.

In response to chemical and biologic terrorism and issues we have faced in this decade, Dr. Robin Vogt describes recent issues relating to protecting the populace including information on the various methods and agents along with issues and protections in different bioterrorism threat situations including the threats with Bird Flu in Chapter 20. The associated Web lesson looks at resources available online at the Centers for Disease Control and Prevention (CDC).

This section concludes with a presentation of the imperative for nursing to develop political efficacy. Chapter 21 includes a broad perspective on the political process as well as resources to assist nurses in developing internal political efficacy, which will help the profession in the demonstration of its external efficacy as the political imperative. The steps in contacting your congressperson are the focus of the associated Web lesson.

Section V confronts the reality of health care and the nursing profession. In Chapter 22, Sister Rosemary Donley addresses the health-care agenda and issues debated in both legislative and professional areas that have major implications for the health care of the nation and initiatives for the profession. The final chapter discusses challenges for the future. Topics include driving forces that demand change throughout the health professions and the call for action in the environment with a focus on safety and effective client outcomes.

This book is intended to enhance your professional practice and continued professional development through further education. Your personal characteristics of self-motivation, a thirst for information, and commitment to your clients and the profession will be enhanced as you develop a more conceptual and visionary approach to professional nursing practice. Advance your practice through ongoing education and the concepts basic to professional nursing practice.

Rose Kearney-Nunnery

Acknowledgments

Numerous people have been a large part of this process. Family members, friends, and colleagues have more than tolerated my preoccupation with the profession. My respect is extended to all my professional colleagues across the country for the opportunities they provided for reflection, discussion, and debate. My particular thanks are extended to all the contributors who have shared their expertise and insights in these pages. Joanne DaCunha, Caryn Abramowitz, and Kristin L. Kern merit particular credit for the completion of this project through their endless encouragement, assistance, enthusiasm, and belief in the potential for our profession. My thanks to my husband, Jimmie E. Nunnery, to whom this edition is dedicated, for his tolerance with my dedication to our profession and with his political background that contributed to the chapter on politics.

As a final note, I cannot describe the endless encouragement from my professional colleagues, friends, and students, all of whom added to this challenge for the nursing profession to focus on change in the future. And to all who give to clients of nursing, my endless and enduring respect!

Rose Kearney-Nunnery

Contributors

Julia W. Aucoin, DNS, RN, BC
Assistant Professor
University of North Carolina at Greensboro
Greensboro, North Carolina

Genevieve M. Bartol, RN, EdD
Professor Emeritus
The University of North Carolina at Greensboro
School of Nursing
Greensboro, North Carolina

Vicki L. Buchda, RN, MS
Director, Patient Care Resources
Mayo Arizona
Scottsdale, Arizona

Joseph T. Catalano, RN, PhD
Professor
East Central University
Ada, Oklahoma

Cyril F. Chang, PhD
Professor of Economics
Department of Economics
The University of Memphis
Memphis, Tennessee

Bernadette Dorsch Curry, RN, PhD
Chairperson
Mollory College
Rockville Center, New York

Sister Rosemary Donley, SC, PhD, APRN, BC, C–ANP, FAAN
Ordinary Professor, Chair Community/Public Health
    Nursing Graduate Program
The Catholic University of America
Washington, DC

Francoise Dunefsky, RN, MS, CNAA
Chief Executive Officer
Gateway Community Industries, Inc.
Kingston, New York

Jacqueline Owers Favret, RN, MPH
Assistant Professor of Clinical Nursing
Louisiana State University Health Science Center
School of Nursing
New Orleans, Louisiana

Jacqueline Fawcett, PhD, FAAN
Professor
University of Massachusetts
College of Nursing
Boston, Massachusetts

Sheila C. Grossman, RN, PhD
Associate Professor
School of Nursing
Fairfield University
Fairfield, Connecticut

Jimmie E. Nunnery, MA
Distinguished Professor Emeritus
University of South Carolina
Former Member of the South Carolina House of
    Representatives
Member/Secretary of the Medical Military, Public &
    Municipal Affairs Committee
Former Judge, Magistrate Court
Chester County, South Carolina

Susan K. Pfoutz, RN, PhD
Professor
Department of Nursing
Eastern Michigan University
Ypsilanti, Michigan

Barbara Swoyer, MSN, CRNP
Family Nurse Practitioner
Emkey Arthritis and Osteoporosis Clinic, Inc.
Wyomissing, Pennsylvania

Theresa M. Valiga, RN, EdD
Director of Research
National League for Nursing
New York, New York

Robin S. Vogt, RN, FNP-C, PhD
Medical Staff
Royal Oaks Hospital
Windsor, Missouri
President, Missouri State Board of Nursing
Jefferson City, Missouri

Consultants

Pamela S. Brown, RN, PhD
President
Blessing-Rieman College of Nursing
Quincy, Illinois

Mary J. Donnelly, RN, MSN, PhD(C)
Associate Professor
St. Francis Medical Center College of Nursing
Peoria, Illinois

Laurie A. Downes, RN, PhD
Associate Professor
Elms College
Chicopee, Massachusetts

Stacie Elder, RN, PhD
Assistant Professor
Northern Illinois University
DeKalb, Illinois

Joanne C. Langan, RN, PhD
Chair, Division of Mental Health
St. Louis University
Doisy College of Health Science
School of Nursing
St. Louis, Missouri

Robin S. Vogt, RN, PhD, FNP-C
Director of Medical Services
Royal Oaks Hospital
Windsor, Missouri

Contents

■ *Rose* **Kearney-Nunnery**

Your Professional Identity

> *" The past cannot be changed. The future is yet in your power. "*
>
> Mary Pickford, 1893–1979

Chapter Objectives

On completion of this chapter, the reader will be able to:

1. Relate the attributes of a profession to professional nursing practice.
2. Relate the core competencies for health professionals to professional nursing practice.
3. Describe clients of professional nursing practice.
4. Discuss responsibility and accountability in professional nursing practice.
5. Describe ethical responsibilities in professional nursing practice.
6. Discuss the formal and informal educational expectations for professional nursing practice.
7. Develop a personal philosophy of professional nursing.

Key Terms

Theory
Paradigm
Metaparadigm
Human Beings
Environment
Health
Nursing
Authority
Community Sanction
Code of Ethics

Professional Culture
Professional Development
Professional Organizations
Educational Background
Core Competencies
Continuing Education
Continued Competency
Communication and
  Publication

Autonomy and Self-
  Regulation
Responsibility
Accountability
Community Service
Theory Use, Development,
  and Evaluation
Evidence-Based Practice
Philosophy

As a registered nurse (RN) student pursuing an advanced degree in nursing, you must reevaluate personal and collegial perspectives on what truly constitutes professional practice. You are at a gateway for advancing your nursing practice and the profession. To advance in your professional career, you must broaden and build on your knowledge base. This involves Mezirow's (1991, 2000) theory of adult development and education as transformative learning. This theory proposes that the adult learns in one of four ways:

- By elaborating existing frames of reference
- By learning new frames of reference
- By transforming points of view
- By transforming habits of mind. (Mezirow, 2000, p. 19)

Building on your knowledge base and your personal *frame of reference*, you will be adding and learning new perspectives. This process will allow you as the adult learner to transform your views in new ways, and create new ways of approaching the world and professional practice. Learning occurs through reflection and interpretation to understand perceptions of the self and the world. Callin (1996) describes this "perspective transformation" in nursing as requiring the opportunity for reflection, review, and critical thinking. This concept of perspective transformation is an ongoing process in both personal and professional development.

From the professional standpoint, armed with technical skills and expertise in the practice setting, we chart a course into the conceptual components that embody and expand professional practice. These conceptual tools allow for creativity and refinement within the paradigm of professional nursing practice. As a start, consider the concepts that characterize both a profession in general and professional nursing practice specifically.

CHARACTERISTICS OF A PROFESSION

Greenwood (1957) developed a classic work on professionalism in which he proposed five characteristics of a profession. These attributes (Box 1–1) were then applied to the social work discipline to defend its professional status, but they are applicable to any profession, including professional nursing practice.

Systematic Theory and Knowledge Base

Each profession is guided by systematic theory, on which its knowledge base is built. As Greenwood (1957) noted, "The skills that characterize a profession flow

Box 1.1 Characteristics of a Profession

- Systematic Theory
- Authority
- Community Sanction
- Ethical Codes
- Professional Culture

Source: Greenwood, E. (1957). Attributes of a profession. *Social Work*, 2(3).

from and are supported by a fund of knowledge that has been organized into an internally consistent system called a body of theory" (p. 46). This system includes theoretical foundations unique to the profession as well as those adapted from other scientific disciplines.

Kerlinger and Lee (2000) define a **theory** as "a set of interrelated constructs (concepts), definitions, and propositions that present a systematic view of phenomena by specifying relations among variables, with the purpose of explaining and predicting the phenomena" (p. 11). This theory base is also referred to as the paradigm used by professionals or the practitioners in a particular scientific community.

Kuhn (1970) has provided us with the well-established definition of a **paradigm** as "universally recognized scientific achievements that, for a time, provide model problems and solutions to a community of practitioners" (p. vii). The paradigm consists of the beliefs and the belief system shared by members of a particular scientific community. When the paradigm is no longer useful in explaining, practicing, and conducting research in that community, the paradigm shifts and a new belief structure is promoted, adopted, and used by its members.

The paradigm is merely the phenomenon of concern that guides nursing practice. In Chapter 4, Fawcett proposes that *conceptual model* and *paradigm* are interchangeable terms relative to the phenomena of nursing. Various nursing paradigms or conceptual models are currently used in practice. The selection is based on the belief structure of the particular nursing community, such as care of people who are chronically ill and need major assistance with health needs versus the wellness initiatives applicable in occupational settings. The paradigm is determined by the type of nursing because it meets the health needs of a particular client group in a certain environment or setting.

The **metaparadigm** is the overall concern of nursing common to each nursing model, whether a conceptual model/paradigm or formal theory. Fawcett (1995, 2000, 2005) has described the four requirements for a discipline's metaparadigm: identity, inclusiveness, neutrality, and internationality. First, the metaparadigm must provide an identity for the profession that is distinctly different from that of others. Second, the metaparadigm must address all phenomena of interest to the profession in a manageable and understandable manner. Third, the metaparadigm must be neutral, so that all smaller practice paradigms can fit under the umbrella metaparadigm. And finally, the metaparadigm must be "international in scope and substance" (Fawcett, 2005, p. 5) to represent the profession across national, social, cultural, and ethnic boundaries. With that in mind, the metaparadigm of professional nursing incorporates four concepts:

- **Human being** represents the individual, family, group, or community receiving care, each with unique characteristics.
- The **environment** comprises the physical, social, cultural, spiritual, and emotional climate or setting(s) in which the person lives, works, plays, and interacts.
- **Health** is the focus for the particular type of nursing and specific care provisions needed.
- **Nursing** is defined by its activities, goals, and services.

In any area of professional nursing practice, we can evaluate who the person is as the client or recipient of nursing care, where the person and the caregiver are seen and are influenced by others, why the person needs professional nursing care, and how the professional nurse functions as a provider of care. These concepts are present whether the client is the frail elder in an acute-care setting, the expanding family in a birthing center, or an employee group in an occupational setting. Interestingly, Fawcett (2005) has provided a critique of various proposals for specifying the metaparadigm concepts of nursing. In her original work, the four concepts included person, environment, health, and nursing. She has since revised the four concepts, changing person to human beings to meet the requirement that the metaparadigm must be international in scope and substance, thus relative transculturally (Fawcett, 2005). Investigate these concepts specific to your own practice setting for an initial view of the systematic theory and knowledge base of your disciplinary paradigm.

Authority

The next characteristic of a professional is authority, as viewed by the client. This **authority** occurs through education and experience, which give the professional the knowledge and skills to make professional judgments. The client perceives the professional as having the knowledge and expertise to assist the client in meeting some need. The professional is therefore viewed as an authority in the area, and his judgments are trusted. Authority is the basis for the competence the client perceives and the client-professional relationship.

In the client-nurse relationship, the nurse is perceived as the authority figure whether providing a selected care technique or filling an informational need. The competence and skill demonstrated justify the client's trust in the professional nurse. Benner (1984) has described five levels of competency in clinical nursing practice: novice, advanced beginner, competent, proficient, and expert (p. xvii). The higher the levels of competence or expertise clients perceive in any profession, the greater trust or authority they place in the practitioners of that profession. Clients who see nurses as experts in providing needed health care view the profession as having more authority in health-care judgments. On the basis of this perception of authority, society grants the profession and its practitioners certain rights, privileges, and responsibilities.

Community Sanction

Society grants the profession certain powers and obligations to practice the specific profession. Nursing's Social Policy Statement (American Nurses Association [ANA], Nursing's, 2003) attributes professional nursing's authority to a social contract with the community. The professional community is responsible for ensuring safe and effective practice within the discipline. Professional and legal regulation of nursing practice as a **community sanction** occurs through statutes, rules and regulations, definition of practice, and expectations for practitioners. Powers for entry and continuity in the profession are granted through licensure and professional practice parameters dictated in the state practice acts. These laws define a specific practice and provide regulatory powers at the state level for the board, licensing of professionals and protection of title (e.g., RN), general practice standards, approvals for educational programs, and disciplinary procedures.

Definition of practice and specific practice standards are further specified within the professional community through major nursing associations. The American Nurses Association (ANA) has specified a variety of practice standards for the profession, both general and specific to certain practice areas. The ANA has prepared several specialty standards documents jointly with the particular specialty organization to reflect the expectations for specialized professional practice. These standards, which signify the sanction by the community of the nursing profession, are described as "authoritative statements by which the nursing profession describes the responsibilities for which its practitioners are accountable. . . . [S]tandards also define the nursing profession's accountability to the public and the outcomes for which registered nurses are responsible" (ANA, 2004, p. 1).

ANA Social Policy Statement Table of Contents at
**www.nursingworld.org/books/tocs/
socialpolicy.pdf**

The publication *Nursing: Scope and Standards of Practice* (ANA, 2004), for example, prescribes standards of practice and standards of professional performance. Standards of practice address safe practice and use of the nursing process with the actions of assessment, diagnosis, outcome identification, planning, implementation, and evaluation (ANA, 2004). Standards of professional performance are expected professional roles and behaviors, including quality of practice, education, professional practice evaluation, collegiality, collaboration, ethics, research, resource utilization, and leadership (ANA, 2004, p. 3).

Further standards of specialty practice are provided through the certification process with specialized education, testing, and ongoing learning requirements. Practice standards and expectations have also been developed by the applicable specialty organization.

Another area in which the community grants a profession certain privileges on the basis of professional knowledge and expertise is the education process. Educational programs are both approved at the individual state level, as by the Board of Nursing, and accredited at the national level by the National League for Nursing Accrediting Commission (NLNAC) and the Commission on Collegiate Nursing Education (CCNE). Development, implementation, and evaluation of the organization, curriculum, faculty, students, graduates, facilities, and program resources are important considerations within the accreditation and reaccreditation process. The job of establishing and evaluating these standards is granted to the professional accrediting groups. Here again, the profession is granted the power by the community and has the responsibility to provide the community with practitioners who are appropriately educated for safe and effective practice.

Greenwood (1957) identified confidentiality as one of the most important professional privileges. Professional nursing enjoys this privilege and conscientiously guards the confidentiality of client information. As discussed in relation to ethical codes, confidentiality is a major consideration in professional nursing practice.

Code of Ethics

A professional abides by a certain **code of ethics** applicable to the practice area. Developed within the profession, the code addresses general ethical practice issues. As Greenwood (1957) explains, although ethical codes vary among professions, they are uniform in describing client-professional and colleague-colleague relationships (p. 50). The ANA code embodies both the formal and informal ethical codes referred to by Greenwood. The ANA's *Code of Ethics for Nurses* is an ethical standard for professional nursing practice. As the ANA states, the "code makes explicit the primary goals, values, and obligations of the profession" through nine "nonnegotiable" provisions (Box 1–2) with interpretive statements (ANA, 2001, p. 5). The interpretive statements promote understanding for appropriate application of the code of ethics in professional practice. Adherence to this specific code may be regulated in your state's practice act. There are also other ethical codes, including the International Council of Nurses (ICN) *Code of Ethics for Nurses (ICN, 2006),* which presents four elements associated with nurses: people, practice, the profession, and coworkers. In addition, it illustrates, for each of the elements, the roles of practitioners and managers, educators and researchers, and national nursing associations. Achieving professional status requires ethical standards for expected behaviors with clients, colleagues, and other professionals.

Professional Culture

The fifth characteristic of a profession is a professional culture. Greenwood (1957) described **professional culture** as the formal and informal groups represented in the profession. *Formal groups* refer to the organizational systems in which the professionals practice, the educational institutions that provide for basic and continued learning, and the professional associations. *Informal groups* are the collegial settings that provide for collaboration, stimulation, and sharing of mutual values. These informal groups exist within each formal group, providing further professional, collegial inclusiveness. These groups and the unique culture of nursing are reinforced in the ANA *Code of Ethics for Nurses.*

Organizational systems in which professional nursing is practiced are diverse and multidimensional. As you will see in later chapters, hospital and home health-agency settings are complex parts of a larger system. Professional nursing practice provides a unique culture

ANA *Code of Ethics for Nurses with Interpretive Statements* at
**http://nursingworld.org/ethics/code/
protected_nwcoe813.htm**

ICN Code of Ethics for Nurses at
http://www.icn.ch/icncode.pdf

BOX 1.2 The Code of Ethics for Nurses

1. The nurse, in all professional relationships, practices with compassion and respect for the inherent dignity, worth, and uniqueness of every individual, unrestricted by consideration of social or economic status, personal attributes, or the nature of health problems.
2. The nurse's primary commitment is to the patient, whether an individual, family, group, or community.
3. The nurse promotes, advocates for, and strives to protect the health, safety, and rights of the patient.
4. The nurse is responsible and accountable for individual nursing practice and determines the appropriate delegation of tasks consistent with the nurse's obligation to provide optimum patient care.
5. The nurse owes the same duties to self as to others, including the responsibility to preserve integrity and safety, to maintain competence, and to continue personal and professional growth.
6. The nurse participates in establishing, maintaining, and improving health-care environments and conditions of employment conducive to the provision of quality health care and consistent with the values of the profession through individual and collective action.
7. The nurse participates in the advancement of the profession through contributions to practice, education, administration, and knowledge development.
8. The nurse collaborates with other health professionals and the public in promoting community, national, and international efforts to meet health needs.
9. The profession of nursing, as represented by associations and their members, is responsible for articulating nursing values, for maintaining the integrity of the profession and its practice, and for shaping social policy.

Source: Reprinted with permission from the American Nurses Association, *Code of Ethics for Nurses with Interpretive Statements*, ©2001 Nursebooks.org, Washington, DC.

with the values and norms expected of its practitioners. Organizational philosophies and mission statements provide information on the expressed culture of these settings. Further expression of the professional culture is apparent in the behaviors of professional nurses who practice in these settings.

Formal educational settings for professional nursing practice occur in institutions of higher learning with liberal and specialized learning requirements. In addition, values and norms for continued learning and competency in practice are transmitted as expectations for professional practice. Beyond basic educational practice, **professional development** is provided through continuing education and specialty preparation and continual competency as a professional.

Professional organizations or associations are a major component of the culture of professional nursing practice, but they vary in purpose or mission and membership. The purpose of some professional organizations, such as the ANA, is to represent the profession on a national basis. Specialty groups, with a more specific focus, promote education, skills, standards, and perhaps certification opportunities for a particular segment of the profession, such as the American Association of Critical-Care Nurses. Each organization has a unique philosophy or mission directed at professional nursing practice.

Professional organizations communicate values and norms in official publications, position statements, and specified practice standards. These organizations promote professional parameters for clinical practice,

education, administration, and research. They provide educational opportunities and foster expansion of the knowledge base of individual professionals and the discipline in general. Some organizations focus specifically on the science of the profession. Their purpose is to promote the scholarly aspects of the profession and to build professional skills through education, publications, and conferences. A more global view of practice can be seen in many professional organizations as they reach out to influence public policy.

Consider the organizations that represent professional nursing practice and education listed in Table 1–1. ANA and its state and territorial associations focus mainly on the profession as an entity, with concern for the health of society as well as the welfare of professional nurses through standards, official position statements, political action initiatives, and certification options for specialty practice. Specific to an area of specialty practice, the American Association of Critical-Care Nurses, with its worldwide membership, is the largest specialty organization. Also more globally, the International Council of Nurses (ICN) is composed of professional associations from more than 128 countries, including the American Nurses Association. The National League for Nursing (NLN) has two types of membership, individual and agency, with initiatives related to accreditation of nursing education programs. The American Association of Colleges of Nursing focuses on collegiate education, serving member schools with baccalaureate and higher degree programs

Table 1.1

Characteristics of Selected Professional Organizations

Organization	Focus, Mission, & Membership
American Nurses Association (ANA) and associated constituent state associations and organizational affiliate members Founded 1897 **http://www.nursingworld.org**	*Focus:* Professional nursing *Mission:* "...Advances the nursing profession by fostering high standards of nursing practice, promoting the economic and general welfare of nurses in the workplace, projecting a positive and realistic view of nursing, and by lobbying the Congress and regulatory agencies on health-care issues affecting nurses and the public" (ANA, 2003, p. 1) *Membership:* Individual membership; professional nurses at the state level obtain national and district membership
American Association of Colleges of Nursing (AACN) Founded 1969 **http://www.aacn.nche.edu**	*Focus:* Collegiate nursing education *Mission:* "...Serves the public interest by providing standards and resources, and by fostering innovation to advance professional nursing education, research, and practice" (AACN, 2004, p. 1) *Membership:* Deans and directors of member schools with baccalaureate and higher-degree nursing programs
American Association of Critical-Care Nurses (AACN) Founded 1969 **http://www.aacn.org**	*Focus:* Specialty care *Mission:* "...Patients and their families rely on nurses at the most vulnerable times of their lives. Acute and critical care nurses rely on AACN for expert knowledge and the influence to fulfill their promise to patients and their families. AACN drives excellence because nothing less is acceptable." (AACN, 2007, p. 1). *Membership:* Individual membership
International Council of Nurses (ICN) Founded 1899 **http://www.icn.ch**	*Focus:* Nursing internationally *Mission:* "To represent nursing worldwide, advancing the profession and influencing health policy" (ICN, 2006, p. 1) *Membership:* National nurses' associations representing nurses in more than 128 countries
National Council of State Boards of Nursing (NCSBN) Founded 1978 (previously a component of ANA) **http://www.ncsbn.org**	*Focus:* Nursing regulation and public protection *Mission:* "...Composed of Member Boards, provides leadership to advance regulatory excellence for public protection" (NCSBN, 2006, p. 1) *Membership:* All state boards of nursing in the 50 states, the District of Columbia, and four United States territories—American Samoa, Guam, Northern Mariana Islands, and the Virgin Islands
National League for Nursing (NLN) and associated constituent leagues Founded 1952 **http://www.nln.org**	*Focus:* Nursing education and community health *Mission:* "...Advances excellence in nursing education that prepares the nursing workforce to meet the needs of diverse populations in an ever-changing health-care environment" (NLN, 2006, p. 1) *Membership:* Individual and agency (diploma programs, associate degree programs, baccalaureate and higher degree programs) membership
Sigma Theta Tau International Honor Society of Nursing and member chapters Founded 1922 **http://nursingsociety.org**	*Focus:* Nursing scholarship (international) *Mission:* "...To support the learning, knowledge, and professional development of nurses committed to making a difference in health worldwide" (Sigma Theta Tau, 2006, p. 1) *Membership:* Individuals are invited to membership in chartered chapters with selection criteria as baccalaureate or higher degree students, faculty members, or community leaders.

Note: Reference citations in table are excerpts from online resources of the respective nursing organizations.

through educational standards, programs, policies, research, accreditation, and legislative initiatives directed at high-quality professional education. Sigma Theta Tau, the international honor society for nursing, has a distinctly scientific focus. This organization promotes knowledge development through research, dissemination of scientific information, technology, education, interdisciplinary collaboration, and adaptability for the improvement of the health of people worldwide.

A comprehensive listing of professional organizations and their Web site addresses is located on the book's Intranet site. In addition, useful links to additional resources may be discovered within these sites. Just one word of caution: Web site addresses change, as do physical addresses. Try to update your computer browser's address book and "favorites" listing continually with any changes and add new sites that you have found.

PROFESSIONALISM IN NURSING

The nursing profession is characterized by Greenwood's attributes of a profession. But what of its uniqueness? Miller and associates (1993) have proposed that "nurses must disclaim the traditional analysis of professional and professionalism by other disciplines as the only method to determine definitions and characteristics of professionalism in nursing" (p. 290). They proposed the use of a behavioral inventory to assist nurses in attaining higher degrees of professionalism (Miller, Adams, & Beck, 1993, p. 294). This behavioral inventory consists of nine categories of professional nursing characteristics that merit your consideration (Box 1–3). Think about each of these criteria for professionalism in nursing.

Box 1.3 Characteristics of Professional Nursing

- Educational background
- Adherence to the code of ethics
- Participation in the professional organization
- Continuing education and competency
- Communication and publication
- Autonomy and self-regulation
- Community service
- Use, development, and evaluation of theory
- Research involvement

Source: Miller, B. K., Adams, D., & Beck, L. (1993). A behavioral inventory for professionalism in nursing. *Journal of Professional Nursing, 9*, 290–295.

Educational Background

The **educational background** required for professional practice is specified to ensure safe and effective practice. In nursing, the basic education required for entry into the profession varies, with differences among baccalaureate, associate degree, diploma education, and even some entry-level graduate programs. But within each type of educational program, curricula and requirements are guided by general standards.

Although a school's curriculum is developed by its faculty members, certain standards are required for an educational program. Nursing curricula must contain essential content and hours as required by state boards of nursing, higher education boards, professional associations, and national accrediting bodies. Consumers of nursing care can be confused by the different educational routes leading to the title of registered nurse. The Pew Health Professions Commission critically reviewed the various health professions, their regulatory bodies, educational program requirements, and workforce needs to address the changing healthcare system. The Commission (1995) then made the following recommendations relative to basic nursing education:

- Recognize value of multiple entry points to professional practice.
- Consolidate professional nomenclature, such as a single title for each level of nursing preparation/service.
- Differentiate practice responsibilities among levels and strengthen existing career ladder programs:
  - Associate Degree in Nursing (A.D.N.): entry hospital and nursing home
  - Bachelor of Science in Nursing (B.S.N.): hospital care management and community practice
  - Master of Science in Nursing (M.S.N.): specialty practice in hospital and independent practice (p. 34).

Ongoing clarification of these areas among professionals and consumers of nursing will have a beneficial effect on the view of nursing as a profession and of individual nurses as true professionals.

As a follow-up to the work of the Pew Commission, two reports from the Institute of Medicine called for changes in education of health professionals. The 2001 report from the Institute of Medicine, *Crossing the Quality Chasm*, proposed 10 rules (Box 1–4) for the health system in the 21st century (Corrigan, Donaldson, Kohn, Maguire, & Pike, 2001, p. 48). A further report following a Health Professions Education Summit led to the identification of five **core competencies** (Box 1–5) for all health professionals to advance the 10 rules with an "overarching vision" that

Box 1.4 Rules for the 21st Century Health System

- Care is based on continuous healing relationships.
- Care is customized according to patient needs and values.
- The patient is the source of control.
- Knowledge is shared and information flows freely.
- Decision making is evidence-based.
- Safety is a system property.
- Transparency is necessary.
- Needs are anticipated.
- Waste is continuously decreased.
- Cooperation among clinicians is a priority.

Source: Greiner, A. C., & Knebel, E. (eds.). (2003). *Health professions education: A bridge to quality*. Washington, DC: Institute of Medicine. (p. 48)

Box 1.5 Core Competencies For Health Professionals

- Provide patient-centered care.
- Work in interdisciplinary teams.
- Employ evidence-based practice.
- Apply quality improvement.
- Utilize informatics.

Source: Greiner, A.C., & Knebel, E. (eds.). (2003). *Health professions education: A bridge to quality*. Washington, DC: Institute of Medicine.

"all health professionals should be educated to deliver patient-centered care as members of an interdisciplinary team, emphasizing evidence-based practice, quality improvement approaches, and informatics" (Greiner & Knebel, 2003, p. 45). To address these competencies in nursing education programs, curriculum must be constantly evaluated for currency, content, and practice opportunities. For example, most nurses will agree that providing patient-centered care is a component of our nursing programs. We need to assess carefully, however, whether all programs foster interdisciplinary and evidence-based practice focused on quality improvement and the use of informatics.

Adherence to a Code of Ethics

Adherence to a code of ethics is expected in any profession. As illustrated previously, the *Code of Ethics for Nurses with Interpretive Statements* (ANA, 2001) provides the broad guidelines. It is the responsibility of the practicing professional to know these guidelines and practice in accordance with the code. As Miller and associates (1993) reported, most professional nurse respondents did not have a copy of the ethical code, and many were unfamiliar with the document (p. 293). This problem occurred with the 1985 *Code of Ethics*. The question then becomes: how many nurses are aware of the 2001 revision that occurred several years ago? To meet this criterion of professionalism, nursing professionals need to demonstrate greater knowledge and understanding of the official ethical code. Periodic review of the nine ethical provisions and their interpretive statements is an important responsibility for all professional nurses. This is especially true when the roles of nurses or clients change, but it is also important for nurses to appreciate fully their professional responsibilities, challenges, and talents when roles are stable.

Participation in Professional Organizations

Participation in the professional organization is an important criterion for a profession. Unfortunately, in nursing this is quite a broad area, as is evident from the listing of professional organizations located on the Intranet site. Less than 10 percent of the almost 3 million nurses in the United States belong to the major professional group ANA. Many nurses prefer to associate with specialty groups that they believe better meet their educational and practice needs.

This brings us to two critical considerations: multiple memberships and activity. Professionals are not limited to membership in one professional association. If all nurses belonged to one official organization representing professional nurses, that organization would have an enormous influence on health care by virtue of the numbers. But because of different disciplinary paradigms, this is not the case. Professionals associate with organizations they view as most appropriate to their belief systems and practice, rather than with organizations they do not perceive as matching their professional practice needs. Yet ANA does represent all nurses in the United States and its territories. The ANA describes its role as follows:

> The American Nurses Association is the only full-service professional organization representing the nation's 2.9 million registered nurses (RNs) through its 54 constituent member associations. The ANA advances the nursing profession by fostering high standards of nursing practice, promoting the economic and general welfare of nurses in the workplace, projecting a positive and realistic view of nursing, and by lobbying the Congress and regulatory agencies on health-care issues affecting nurses and the public. (ANA, 2006)

For example, in response to the Institute of Medicine's published report, *Crossing the Quality*

Chasm: A New Health System for the 21st Century in 2001, the ANA (2005) identified a commitment to the principle that all persons are entitled to ready access to affordable, quality health care services. These areas of concern were incorporated into the ANA *Agenda for the Future* with specific action strategies.

We are beginning to see more collaboration among organizations on key issues. There are now a growing number of organizations that officially affiliate with the ANA, and others are members of a liaison forum (check the ANA Web site for a current listing of the affiliates). This movement will further strengthen the profession and create a sense of professional community among nurses. Membership and participation in a major nursing organization are important traits of professionalism for the professional nurse. Active involvement means more than paying dues; it consists of active support of and involvement in the issues addressed by the organization and the profession to promote high-quality health care for the consumer.

One example of an association's efforts to influence the professional culture occurred in 2005 in Michigan. The State Nurses Association Congress on Nursing Practice developed a list of 101 ways for nurses to improve the nursing culture and highlighted these ways in its newsletter (Evans, 2006). The listing included the categories of communication, respect, support, education, conflict management, collegiality, leadership, diversity, development of others, and professionalism. Each of these categories contained 10 suggestions for improvements in the work culture of nurses with the exception of the last one on professionalism, which contained 11. Think about these suggestions presented in Box 1–6.

Box 1.6 Eleven Ways to Improve the Nursing Culture: Professionalism

- Invest and value nursing to improve patient safety and quality of care.
- Separate personal from professional problems.
- Leave personal problems at home.
- Present a positive image of the nursing profession.
- Be a model for work ethics.
- Model professionalism on and off the job.
- Prohibit non-RNs from doing RN work.
- Be a peacemaker.
- Create team spirit.
- Be proud to be a Registered Nurse!
- Participate in professional organizations.

Source: Evans, N. (2006). 101 ways to improve nursing culture. Michigan Nurses Association. Retrieved July 4, 2006 from http://www.minurses.org/prac/101ways.htm

Continuing Education

The fourth characteristic of professionalism in nursing involves **continuing education** and **continued competency.** These attributes are crucial to safe, effective, and ethical professional practice. Ongoing improvement and knowledge are the goals of continuing education, which is required for relicensure in some states and recertification in specialty areas. A slowly increasing number of nurses are completing additional education beyond their basic nursing education. But continuing education is more than obtaining required credits, in-service hours, and formal degrees. Remaining current with ideas presented in the nursing and scientific literature is an important component of continued competency as a professional and to incorporate evidence-based practice.

The Internet has made remaining current on issues of concern to the profession more convenient. Yet, a word of caution is in order: It is important to evaluate the source of information and its validity. Consider whether the information is provided by an organization, an agency, or an individual's own Web site and personal perspective.

Identifying your own learning and developmental needs is an expectation and a continual process for competent professional practice. In essence, continuing education for competency involves self-assessment, ongoing learning, and self-evaluation. The focus is on discovery, as in baccalaureate and graduate education. Ongoing learning means that your mind is challenged every day with new ideas, building on a professional knowledge base and skills.

Opportunities for continuing education abound through a variety of formal programs as well as through professional journals and online resources. Many professional organizations have special online services for their members, such as reviews of current literature and care products, bookstores, continuing education programs, e-mail lists, and online discussion forums. Access the resources readily available at *nursingworld.org, medscape.com/nurses,* and *nurses.com*, to mention only a few. Look at resources provided online at Web sites of individual specialty groups such as AACN and the many others listed on the Intranet site. Publishers also have online resources with special discounts, e-mail updates, associated Web sites, discussion groups, and interactive continuing education offerings.

Communication and Publication

Communication and publication were identified as the fifth characteristic of professional nursing. Although Miller and colleagues (1993) reported limited involvement in this area from the subjects in their research study, they did stress that "scholarly writing for publication and communication to others must become a requisite for the professional nurse to maintain and promote professionalism in nursing" (p. 294). This does not necessarily mean that every nurse needs to publish a scholarly article each year. Innovative ideas are communicated in a variety of ways, both within the practice setting and worldwide through publications or on the Internet. Communication among professionals through well-developed and presented memoranda, proposed institutional policies and practices, and reports at the agency level is important and shows professionalism. Sharing with colleagues through specialty, district, or state nurses association newsletters or publications further promotes professionalism. Consider collaborating with colleagues from other health professions. It is the responsibility of the professional to share innovative ideas that can benefit other professionals. Ideas can be shared though interdisciplinary practice and professional organizations and communicated in professional journals, other publications, and through telecommunications.

Autonomy and Self-Regulation

Autonomy involves independent judgment and self-governing within the scope of one's practice, which changes in response to people's health-care needs. As key professionals in organizational settings, nurses make the time and commitment to ensure that high-quality care and standards are present and upheld. This involves critical thinking, communication, collaboration, and leadership. Important concepts in this area are professional **responsibility** and **accountability.** In the *Code of Ethics for Nurses*, responsibility is defined as accountability for performance of the duties associated with the professional role, and accountability as being answerable to oneself and others for one's judgments and actions in the course of nursing practice, irrespective of health-care organization policies or provider directives (ANA, 2001, pp. 16–17). Nurses are accountable to both themselves and their clients for good clinical judgment and clinical care. As we will see in later chapters, however, accountability is also extended to the broader population as the profession demonstrates involvement in social policy.

The ANA's *Nursing's Social Policy Statement* (2003) describes **self-regulation** as both personal accountability for the knowledge base for practice and participation in the peer review process (p. 11). Professional responsibility and accountability involve upholding quality standards as well as developing and critically analyzing those standards and the outcomes.

Professionals are responsible and answerable to clients for nursing care outcomes. Nurses are actively involved in supervising, delegating, and evaluating others. But their professional status can take the expectations of critical thinking, clinical judgment, expertise, and advocacy beyond a narrowly defined job description or institutional procedure manual. The regulation of nursing practice includes self-regulation expected of the professional as well as professional regulation through the defined scope of practice, further education, certification, and adherence to the code of ethics. An important component is the peer review process, whether through an annual performance evaluation or of a particular activity or contribution to the literature.

The profession is also regulated through licensure to enter the profession, continuing competency requirements, national certification, and the charge of each state board of nursing to protect the health and safety of the clients of nursing. An important note here is the focus of the state licensing board versus the state nurses association. The state nurses association is the advocate for the professionals providing care to clients, as long as the care is provided skillfully, professionally, and ethically. The licensing authority focuses on safe provision of nursing care to the public. This safety is addressed through a defined scope of professional practice, requirements for entry in and continuation in the profession, and disciplinary action in the cases posing danger to clients.

Community Service

Community service was proposed as the seventh characteristic of professionalism in nursing. Nurses are well equipped and talented in this area because of their orientation of service to clients and society at large. Nurses frequently lead health-promoting activities in their employment role, their professional community, and among their families and acquaintances. Consider how residents in a defined community always seem to know who the nurses in the area are and how frequently those nurses are approached with questions or requests to become involved in projects or serve on committees. Also consider how nurses reach out to others with information on health or means to foster wellness in their communities. All of these activities constitute community service.

Theory

Although all professions have systematic theory and knowledge on which to base their practice, the eighth characteristic of professionalism in nursing involves greater activity in this process: **theory use, development, and evaluation.** Theory is essential to guiding the practice and research of a profession. Nursing, as an evolving and dynamic profession, demands that its professionals develop, refine, and evaluate theory. We not only use theory but are constantly involved in critical analysis of the theory as clients, health care, and environments change. We are consistently expanding and refining our knowledge base. The challenge is to collect, analyze, and report data on efficacy related to trends in clients' outcomes. These trends, rather than individual cases, provide information that expands and refines the profession's knowledge base. The need for data collection and analysis leads to research, the final characteristic of professional nursing proposed.

Evidence-Based Practice

Nursing research is much more than leading or participating in a research study. We now look to the core competency of evidence-based practice to guide the way we practice. Greiner and Knebel (2003) define evidence-based practice as the integration of the best research with clinical expertise and the client's values for optimum care as well as participation in learning and research activities (pp. 45–46). As found in the interpretive statements of the *Code for Nurses*, "All nurses working alone or in collaboration with others can participate in the advancement of the profession through the development, evaluation, and application of knowledge in practice" (ANA, 2001, p. 23). Involvement in research, whether by using findings, participating in an investigation, or protecting human subjects, is a characteristic of professionalism in nursing. It adds to our knowledge base, enhances our practice, promotes improved outcomes for our clients, and fosters practice based on evidence of efficacy rather than the tradition of trial and error.

Fulfilling the characteristics described in the nine categories just discussed is the challenge to professionalism in nursing. Professionalism is an attribute in constant refinement.

Research adds to our knowledge base, enhances our practice, promotes improved outcomes for our clients, and fosters practice based on evidence of efficacy rather than the tradition of trial and error.

YOUR PHILOSOPHY OF NURSING

Virginia Henderson (1897–1996) was an outstanding leader in nursing. Her classic definition of nursing embodied her view of the unique role of the professional nurse as:

> Assisting the individual, sick or well, in the performance of those activities contributing to health or its recovery (or to a peaceful death) that he would perform unaided if he had the necessary strength, will, or knowledge. And to do this in such a way as to help him gain independence as rapidly as possible. (Henderson, 1966, p. 15)

This concrete definition was expanded and applied to nursing practice, education, and research. Henderson's philosophy of nursing was one of caring, assisting, and supporting the person. In her writings, she encouraged every nurse to develop a personal concept of nursing—in essence, one's philosophy of nursing.

A **philosophy** of nursing presents a particular professional nurse's belief system or worldview of nursing—the nurse's personal definition of nursing. Alligood (2006) describes a philosophy as providing a unique view of nursing practice with broad statements of beliefs and values that propose the nature and concerns of nursing and its moral obligation to society (p. 45). As we will see in Chapter 3, the first component on the structural hierarchy of contemporary nursing knowledge is the metaparadigm followed by the influence of the belief system or philosophy. Fawcett (2005) describes the function of a philosophy as directed at discovery of knowledge and truth for communication of one's beliefs and values in the practice discipline (p. 12).

As discussed previously, the metaparadigm concept of human beings relates to the people of concern for nursing. Nurses in different settings define clients uniquely within their practice (for example, as individuals versus families). The nurse's practice area and client populations also influence the environment, such as an intensive care unit in an acute care setting or a rural health-care clinic located in a community school or modular building. The concept of health also varies, being different for the professional who provides care for trauma victims and the nurse involved with health initiatives in an employee group. Specific nursing roles and the services provided influence the concept of nursing. In addition to the metaparadigm concepts in a personal philosophy of nursing, certain other values and beliefs are generally apparent as one's beliefs about nursing are illustrated.

Consider the following six essential features of professional nursing definitions identified in the ANA's *Nursing's Social Policy Statement* (2003):

1. Provision of a caring relationship that facilitates health and healing
2. Attention to the range of human experiences and responses to health and illness within the physical and social environments

3. Integration of objective data with knowledge gained from an appreciation of the patient or group's subjective experience
4. Application of scientific knowledge to the processes of diagnosis and treatment through the use of judgment and critical thinking
5. Advancement of professional nursing knowledge through scholarly inquiry
6. Influence on social and public policy to promote social justice. (p. 5)

Along with these criteria are interwoven ethical principles, standards of practice, and professional performance expectations. These are your values and beliefs.

At this point, you should critically analyze your belief system and express your views of nursing. We all have prior experiences that influence our thinking and actions. Try to place those aside and begin to craft your philosophy of nursing. Using these definitions and criteria, develop your views into a personal philosophy of nursing. Periodically reflect on your philosophy to analyze how your professional practice is enhanced in your ongoing quest for knowledge and expertise in your profession. This is your professional identity.

INTERACTIVE EXERCISES

Go to the Intranet and complete the interactive exercises provided for this Chapter.

K E Y   P O I N T S

■ The following are characteristics of a profession: (1) systematic theory and knowledge base, (2) authority, (3) community sanction, (4) an ethical code, and (5) a professional culture.

■ Kerlinger and Lee (2000) define a theory as "a set of interrelated constructs (concepts), definitions, and propositions that present a systematic view of phenomena by specifying relations among variables, with the purpose of explaining and predicting the phenomena" (p. 11).

■ A paradigm used by professionals in a scientific community consists of the beliefs and the belief system shared by members of that particular community to explain phenomena, practice the profession, and conduct research.

■ The metaparadigm of nursing is the overall concern of nursing common to each nursing model, whether a conceptual model/paradigm or formal theory, and it includes the concepts of human beings, environment, health, and nursing.

■ The *Code of Ethics for Nurses* (ANA, 2001) is the ethical standard for professional nursing practice. It identifies expected professional practice behaviors with clients, colleagues, and other professionals within nine provisions with interpretive statements.

■ *Autonomy* involves judgment and self-governing within one's scope of practice. This self-governing requires ongoing evaluation of both responsibility and accountability in professional practice. In the ANA's *Code of Ethics for Nurses, responsibility* is defined as accountability for performance of the duties associated with the professional role, and *accountability* is being answerable to oneself and others for one's judgments and actions in the course of nursing practice, irrespective of health-care organization policies and provider directives (ANA, 2001, pp. 16–17).

■ Miller and associates (1993) have proposed the use of a behavioral inventory to assist nurses in attaining higher levels of professionalism. The following characteristics of professionalism are listed in this inventory: educational background; adherence to the code of ethics; participation in the professional organization; continuing education and competency; communication and publication; autonomy and self-regulation; community service; theory use, development, and evaluation; and involvement in research.

■ The five competencies for health professionals are: providing patient-centered care, working in interdisciplinary teams, employing evidence-based practice, applying quality improvement, and using informatics (Greiner & Knebel, 2003).

■ A personal philosophy of nursing presents the belief system or worldview of nursing for a particular professional nurse. Incorporated into such a philosophy are definitions, values, and assumptions about the metaparadigm concepts of human beings, environment, health, and nursing.

Thought and Discussion Questions

1. Miller and associates (1993) have proposed that "nurses must disclaim the traditional analysis of professional and professionalism by other disciplines as the only method to determine definitions and characteristics of professionalism in nursing" (p. 290). From what you have read in this chapter and on what you know from the practice setting, can you explain why they would make such a statement? Propose another way to determine the definitions and characteristics of the profession of nursing.

2. Be prepared to participate in a discussion to be scheduled by your instructor on how you demonstrate the five core competencies of health professionals.

3. Explain your views on responsibility and accountability.

4. Describe how you demonstrate continued competency.

5. Review the Chapter Thought located on the first page of the chapter, and discuss it in the context of this chapter.

☐ REFERENCES

Alligood, M. R. (2006). Philosophies, models and theories: Critical thinking structures. In M. R. Alligood and A. M. Toomey, *Nursing theory: Utilization and application* (3rd ed., pp. 43–65). St. Louis: Mosby.

American Association of Colleges of Nursing. (2004). *Mission.* Retrieved July 4, 2006 from http://www.aacn .nche.edu/ContactUs/strtplan_mission.htm

American Association of Critical-Care Nurses. (2007). *Mission.* Retrieved September 22, 2007 from http://www.aacn.org/AACN/aacnhome.nsf/vwdoc/AACN Information

American Nurses Association. (2001). *Code of ethics for nurses with interpretive statements* (Publication No. CEN21 10M 08/01). Washington, DC: American Nurses Publishing.

American Nurses Association. (2005). *ANA's health care agenda 2005.* Retrieved September 22, 2007 from https://nursingworld.org/mainMenuCategories/Healthcara ndpolicyIssues/HSR.aspx

American Nurses Association. (2003). *Nursing's social policy statement* (2nd ed.) (Publication No. 03NSPS15M 09/03). Washington, DC: American Nurses Publishing.

American Nurses Association. (2004). *Nursing: Scope and standards of practice* (Publication No. 03SSNP). Washington, DC: American Nurses Publishing.

American Nurses Association. (2006). *About the American Nurses Association.* Retrieved July 1, 2006 from http://www.nursingworld.org/about/

Benner, P. (1984). *From novice to expert: Excellence and power in clinical nursing practice.* Menlo Park, CA: Addison-Wesley.

Callin, M. (1996). From RN to BSN: Seeing familiar situations in different ways. *Journal of Continuing Education in Nursing, 27,* 28–33.

Corrigan, M. S., Donaldson, M. S., Kohn, L. T., Maguire, S. K., & Pike, K. C. (2001). *Crossing the quality chasm: A new health system for the 21st century.* Washington, DC: National Academy Press.

Erwin, N. *(2006).* Practice: 101 ways to improve nursing culture. *Michigan Nurses Association News.* Retrieved July 4, 2006 from http://www.minurses.org/prac/101ways.htm

Fawcett, J. (1995). *Analysis and evaluation of conceptual models of nursing* (3rd ed.). Philadelphia: F. A. Davis.

Fawcett, J. (2000). *Analysis and evaluation of contemporary nursing knowledge: Nursing models and theories.* Philadelphia: F. A. Davis.

Fawcett, J. (2005). *Contemporary nursing knowledge: Analysis and evaluation of nursing models and theories* (2nd ed.). Philadelphia: F. A. Davis.

Greenwood, E. (1957). Attributes of a profession. *Social Work, 2*(3), 45–55.

Greiner, A. C., & Knebel, E. (Eds.). (2003). *Health professions education: A bridge to quality.* Washington, DC: Institute of Medicine.

Henderson, V. (1966). *The nature of nursing: A definition and its implications for practice, education, and research.* New York: Macmillan.

International Council of Nurses (ICN) (2006). About ICN. Retrieved June 29, 2006 from http://www.icn.ch/abouticn.htm

International Council of Nurses (2006). The ICN code of ethics for nurses. Retrieved July 4, 2006 from http://www.icn.ch/icncode.pdf

Kerlinger, F. N., & Lee, H. B. (2000). *Foundations of behavioral research* (4th ed.). Belmont, CA: Wadsworth Thompson Learning.

Kuhn, T. S. (1970). *The structure of scientific revolutions* (2nd ed.). Chicago: University of Chicago Press.

Mezirow, J. (1991). *Transformative dimensions of adult learning.* San Francisco: Jossey-Bass.

Mezirow, J. (2000). Learning to think like an adult: Core concepts of transformation theory. In J. Mezirow and Associates, *Learning as transformation: Critical perspectives on a theory in progress* (pp. 3–33). San Francisco: Jossey-Bass.

Miller, B. K., Adams, D., & Beck, L. (1993). A behavioral inventory for professionalism in nursing. *Journal of Professional Nursing, 9,* 290–295.

National Council of State Boards of Nursing (2006). About NCSBN. Retrieved June 29, 2006 from http://www.ncsbn.org/about.htm

National League for Nursing. (2006). *The NLN mission: Our purpose*. Retrieved June 29, 2006 from http://www.nln.org/aboutnln/ourmission.htm

Pew Health Professions Commission. (1995). *Critical challenges: Revitalizing the health professions for the twenty-first century*. San Francisco: USCF Center for the Health Professions.

Sigma Theta Tau. (2006). The society's vision and mission. Retrieved June 29, 2006 from http://www.nursingsociety. org/about/overview.html

BIBLIOGRAPHY

American Nurses Association. (1997). *Scope and standards of college health nursing practice* (Publication No. ST-1). Washington, DC: American Nurses Publishing.

American Nurses Association. (1997). *Scope and standards of forensic nursing practice* (Publication No. ST-4). Washington, DC: American Nurses Publishing.

American Nurses Association. (1999). *Scope and standards of public health nursing practice* (Publication No. 9910PH). Washington, DC: American Nurses Publishing.

American Nurses Association. (1999). *Scope and standards of home health nursing practice* (Publication No. 9905HH). Washington, DC: American Nurses Publishing.

American Nurses Association. (2000). *Scope and standards of pediatric oncology nursing* (Publication No. PONP20). Washington, DC: American Nurses Publishing.

American Nurses Association. (2000). *Scope and standards of practice for nursing professional development* (Publication No. NPD-20). Washington, DC: American Nurses Publishing.

American Nurses Association. (2000). *Scope and standards of psychiatric–mental health nursing practice* (Publication No. PMH-20). Washington, DC: American Nurses Publishing.

American Nurses Association. (2001). *Scope and standards of gerontological nursing practice* (2nd ed.) (Publication No. GNP21). Washington, DC: American Nurses Publishing.

American Nurses Association. (2001). *Scope and standards of nursing informatics practice* (Publication No. NIP21). Washington, DC: American Nurses Publishing.

American Nurses Association. (2002). *Scope and standards of hospice and palliative nursing practice* (Publication No. HPN22). Washington, DC: American Nurses Publishing.

American Nurses Association. (2002). *Scope and standards of neuroscience nursing practice* (Publication No. NNS22). Washington, DC: American Nurses Publishing.

American Nurses Association. (2003). *Scope and standards of diabetes nursing* (2nd ed.) (Publication No. 9808ST). Washington, DC: American Nurses Publishing.

American Nurses Association. (2003). *Scope and standards of pediatric nursing practice* (Publication No. PNP23). Washington, DC: American Nurses Publishing.

American Nurses Association. (2004). *Intellectual and developmental disabilities nursing: Scope and standards of practice* (Publication No. 04SSID). Washington, DC: American Nurses Publishing.

American Nurses Association. (2004). *Neonatal nursing: Scope and standards of practice* (Publication No. 04SSNN). Washington, DC: American Nurses Publishing.

American Nurses Association. (2004). *Scope and standards for nurse administrators* (2nd ed.) (Publication No. 03SSNA). Washington, DC: American Nurses Publishing.

American Nurses Association. (2004). *Scope and standards of addictions nursing practice* (Publication No. 04SSAN). Washington, DC: American Nurses Publishing.

American Nurses Association. (2004). *Scope and standards of vascular nursing practice* (Publication No. 04SSVN). Washington, DC: American Nurses Publishing.

American Nurses Association. (2005). *Faith community nursing: Scope and standards of practice* (Publication No. 05SSFC). Washington, DC: American Nurses Publishing.

American Nurses Association. (2005). *Pain management nursing: Scope and standards practice* (Publication No. 05SSPM). Washington, DC: American Nurses Publishing.

American Nurses Association. (2005). *Plastic surgery nursing: Scope and standards of practice* (Publication No. 05SSPS). Washington, DC: American Nurses Publishing.

American Nurses Association. (2005). *School nursing: Scope and standards of practice* (Publication No. 05SSSN). Washington, DC: American Nurses Publishing.

Kohn, L. T., Corrigan, M. S., & Donaldson, M. S. (1999). *To err is human: Building a safer health system*. Washington, DC: National Academy Press.

National League for Nursing. (2005). *The scope of practice for academic nurse educators*. New York: Author.

O'Neil, E. H. (1998). *Recreating health professional practice for a new century*. San Francisco: Pew Health Professions Commission.

ONLINE RESOURCES

ANA Code of Ethics for Nurses.
To view go to the ANA home page at **www.nursingworld.org** and the drop down menus for Professional Nursing Practice and Ethics and Standards

ICN Code of Ethics for Nurses **http://www.icn.ch/icncode.pdf**

■ *Bernadette* **Dorsch Curry**

Coping with Returning to School

> 66 *Change is an opportunity—an opportunity to grow, to discover, to risk, to thrive, to make a difference.* 99

Chapter Objectives

On completion of this chapter, the reader will be able to:

1. Evaluate personal and professional goals.
2. Identify personal and professional role conflicts and stressors.
3. Develop time management strategies for family, work, and educational demands.
4. Assemble resources to help meet family, work, and educational demands.
5. Develop a personalized study environment and study strategies.

Key Terms

Goals
Role Transition
Resources
Streamlining

Returning to school for an advanced degree in nursing may begin as an academic and professional goal. As the fullness of the experience unfolds, however, you will come to realize that education is more than academic exercises and credits. It is an intellectual pursuit that leads to personal growth in many areas. You have chosen the challenge and made the personal and professional commitment to goals. By adopting a positive attitude and using a variety of available resources, you can experience the exhilaration of success and the satisfaction of accomplishment.

WHAT TO EXPECT

Expectations can set the tone and influence behaviors. When you are returning to school, it is important to have valid and realistic expectations of the experience and of yourself—to be informed, committed, and confident in your desire and ability to succeed. On the basis of experiences with registered nurse (RN) students in a baccalaureate nursing program, Donea Shane (1980) described observations and set forth what is known as the *returning to school syndrome*. She characterized emotional responses and captured the essence of the process. In addition to identifying and documenting the behaviors, she wanted to alert RN students to prepare for the challenges. Though the health-care system changes over time, the responses of students returning to academic situations tend to be similar and reflect human nature.

Returning to School Syndrome

The syndrome has three phases. In the first phase, called the "honeymoon," fascination with the new and different activities associated with academe casts a positive glow on the experience, and a strong sense of satisfaction can be derived from embarking on the journey.

In phase two, called "conflict," new and different perspectives of nursing are presented, and students experience a growing discomfort with previous knowledge and familiar concepts, often accompanied by waning confidence. Insecurity and self-doubt can cause students to question their capabilities or blame others for perceived unsatisfactory achievement in the program. RN students may have had minimal or no experience with nursing theory (Fawcett, 1995), for instance, and the abstract nature of theory may elicit anxiety in students who previously learned in concrete and structured educational modes and functioned professionally with technical expertise.

"Biculturalism," the third phase, is described as the "ability to be as comfortable and effective in one culture (school) as in another (work)." This is the phase in which students learn that growth does not require destroying strong foundations, but does require building on them. Students realize that their past education and professional experiences serve as rich resources for professional development.

SETTING PERSONAL GOALS

Deciding to return to school is a major lifetime decision and the beginning of a new phase of goal setting. **Goals** are powerful entities that can provide a focus, sustain commitment, reinforce priorities, and provide a framework for current and future decisions. Goals help keep the decision maker focused by addressing both the time needed and the scope of the task. It is easy to overlook the power of goals if they are considered simply an end point of a process.

Remember the following points when setting your goals:

- You alone are the goal maker and in command of your personal quest.
- You alone create the goal, establish the plan, and accomplish the task.
- You can expect to invest considerable time and attention in developing your goals and their accompanying plans.
- Forethought, motivation, and creativity transform goals from ideas into reality.
- Personal goals are born of individual values, ambition, and abilities and are the result of introspective and selective processes.
- Genuine personal goals are holistic and help you to maintain perspective and respect priorities.

Both long- and short-term goals, and the means to achieve them, must be realistic and must acknowledge individual strengths and limitations, available resources, and personal flexibility. Capitalize on your strengths, and use available resources to overcome your limitations.

Flexibility is particularly important. Change is to be expected and may require adjustments to your original plans. Consider revising your goals or readjusting your plans as a positive response to the new developments. When establishing your goals and plans, be sure to develop a "plan B," to increase your ability to adapt quickly to a new situation.

Consider achieving an advanced degree as a long-term goal, for example. It requires patience, time, and energy to succeed. Building in short-term goals helps keep your achievements and remaining goals in perspective. Achieving these short-term goals provides a sense of satisfaction, which can energize and increase motivation. View each educational phase as a milestone and each course or semester completed as an accomplishment and progress toward the ultimate goal.

No matter how well you have set your goals, made realistic plans, or chose appropriate actions, you will face occasional stress, frustration, discouragement, and low motivation. Achievement rarely occurs without challenge. During these times, it helps to recall your reasons for setting the goal and to review the potential benefits. Achieving a goal is fulfilling a commitment to yourself. It is by working through challenges and succeeding that you grow. Being true to yourself when setting and living out goals is vital.

REFINING PROFESSIONAL IDENTITY

Neither personal nor professional growth occurs without individual energy and creativity. The purposeful decision to return to school begins an ongoing series of transitions leading to the goal. Each of those transitions requires the thought, attention, and action of the individual and contributes to professional change and personal growth.

Change can be an uncomfortable and negative experience, especially when it disrupts a well-established routine. It can also be invigorating and challenging and can have many positive results. Change is a fact of life; it is a constant to be anticipated. Returning to a student role opens the door for personal and professional growth and brings about changes that create pathways to potential. Curry (1994) found that the opportunity for career and educational mobility was the most influential factor for RNs deciding to pursue a baccalaureate degree. Personal desire to possess a bachelor's degree was the second. These motivators play an important part in the active roles expected of a student.

From the outset, you will have the opportunity to chart your own course of action, resulting in a change in professional identity. Planning is important because it allows time to develop a mind-set, a time frame, and methods for the journey. Participating in educational decisions sets the tone for establishing a new professional identity. In **role transition**, you not only assume but develop the new role (Strader & Decker, 1995); it is the opportunity for you to individualize educational and professional experiences and to use education as a vehicle for true change in your professional role.

Nursing education is designed to develop professionals who think critically and to provide the principles and guidelines for the myriad of diverse situations they encounter. Contemporary nursing education is not the simple acquisition of information. It is the building of knowledge in concert with expansion of thought and processes and with development of inquiry methods.

The fullness of your nursing role is limited only by your own imagination, creativity, and ability. During this transitional period, remember that health care is also in transition. As a student, you can craft a professional identity in tune with contemporary nursing, as well as with your personal interests and professional talents. As you progress, the change and personal growth in your professional persona will enrich your experience and serve as an impetus for lifelong learning.

CONFLICTS AND STRESSORS

As in any new experience, it can be expected that nurses returning to school may encounter a variety of new conflicts and stressors. It is the individual's ability to anticipate, understand, and address the situation with a positive attitude that can make a difference.

Nontraditional students come to the educational arena with a repertoire of life events that can ease adapting to new situations. In addition, those mature students who perceive themselves as "hardy" tend to experience less anxiety adjusting to school (Patton & Goldenberg, 1999). Stress can result from almost any type of change, even positive change. The happiest and most desirable things in life can take a physical and mental toll on the individual. Holmes and Rahe (1967) showed that both positive and negative life events can have a negative effect on health. It would be unrealistic to expect balance and harmony among all life roles during coursework. Significant numbers of students enter baccalaureate education with a wealth of life experience, and a sense of focus, motivation and readiness to succeed.

Role Conflicts and Stressors

Returning to school creates a new role for the nurse, and the time, attention, and energy it requires must be unearthed from a finite supply. Rearranging an established lifestyle and pattern of daily activities to accommodate the additional workload is often a necessary and thought-provoking challenge. The overall balance of life activities and parts of life roles can be affected and must be addressed.

ⓞ N L I N E Ⓒ O N S U L T

Information on the Holmes and Rahe (1967) Social Readjustment Rating Scale can be found at the following sites:
http://www.bhicares.org/pdf/manual/indepth assessment/homesrahestressinventory.pdf
http://www.geocities.com/beyond_stretched/ holmes.htm

Many nurses who return to school are employed, balancing roles of parent, nurse, and student. Though they may be challenging, multiple roles can yield a number of rewards and pleasures, providing a positive synergy the individual might not experience from only one role. Functioning in multiple roles can be instrumental in redefining your identity, goal setting, and personal achievement. Negative consequences, however, can also occur, particularly role conflict.

Educational Conflicts and Stressors

Being an adult learner may present a challenge. For some, the label itself elicits a sense of not belonging, of not "fitting in," or of lagging behind the traditional education schedule. In most disciplines, however, adult learners currently constitute a significant percentage of college students. You will not be the lone adult in nursing courses, on campus, or in an online chat room. Some degree of anxiety is to be expected with any new experience. Bear in mind that as a nurse you are normally engaged in anxiety ridden situations. Rubenfeld & Scheffer (2006) note the anxiety involved in the day-to-day reality of nursing. Give yourself credit for what you already do well, especially the challenge of being an adult learner.

Initial selection of courses presents a maze of choices and possibilities, which may seem overwhelming and strange. Keep in mind that the goal of the institution is to promote the success of each student. Faculty members are available to inform, support, and advise you. Be prepared to seek out your faculty advisor and to participate actively in your education. You have both a right and a responsibility to ask for guidance. Effective education includes two-way communication, and you will be both encouraged and expected to be an active student. Active participation in the student role and college activities is widely recognized as a positive factor leading to student success and satisfaction.

Grades

Most educational endeavors involve criteria and some form of evaluation. Grades are the most common format. Although grades are usually important to all students, the mature student may place undue emphasis on them. Some students may assume that previous professional experience or age requires them to excel in their courses. This assumption is both unrealistic and an unnecessary burden. Concern for grades can lead to a mental battle for self-esteem that focuses more on getting good grades than on assimilating information. A grade less than an "A" should not be perceived as a threat to your identity. It is also important to realize that grades do not automatically equal the time or money invested. Academic achievement evolves from effort

and understanding. Communication with professors about course objectives, policies, and specifics of assignments can facilitate achievement. Faculty members are eager for students to succeed and can clarify course criteria, content, and test modalities.

Contracting for a grade is an alternative that allows the student to select a grade and an accompanying level of performance criteria. The selected grade ("A" through "C") is agreed upon by student and professor via a contract at the beginning of the course and is awarded upon successful completion of the required elements for the specific grade level. Contracting permits the student to be independent and take ownership of planning and implementing objectives for the assignment. Malcom Knowles (1988), who has written extensively about adult learners, noted the specific fears and needs of nontraditional students.

Test Anxiety

Test anxiety is common among all learners and can be a major problem. Remember that some degree of anxiety is expected. Excessive anxiety before and during examinations, however, can interfere with thinking. Adequate preparation, understanding of the material, and a positive, self-confident attitude can control test anxiety. Keep in mind that "tests measure performance not personal value" (Katz, Carter, Bishop, & Kravits, 2000, p. 246).

Some basic tips to reduce test anxiety are as follows:

- Plan and use adequate time for study.
- Do not cram.
- Study with others after you have studied alone.
- Take control.
- Think positively.
- Keep your normal, reasonable routine.
- Use stress-reducing tapes.
- Pace your time to answer the questions.
- Do not be afraid to ask the professor for clarification.

Writing Papers

Assembling the material and thoughts to write a paper may seem overwhelming at first. But every college uses a format that can guide you through the process. Your course professor will provide direction and will be available to explain expectations. Plan sufficient time to research and develop the topic. Ask the professor for feedback as you proceed, and use the library staff to help acquire the appropriate references. Make sure you have a home copy of the writing format, such as American Psychological Assocation (APA) or Modern Language Association (MLA). Computer software for the APA format is available and can save considerable time and effort. Once you have the first draft written, put it aside and review it with an objective eye the next day. Pay attention to grammar and flow to convey thoughts accurately. Most colleges have a writing center with experienced staff to assist in development of writing skills.

Active Classroom-Active Learner

Today's classroom may vary significantly from your previous experiences. Note taking and passive learning have been replaced by group work, presentations, simulations, distance learning, and many other creative and dynamic educational strategies. Be an active listener—learn to sense the entire message, then interpret, evaluate, and react (Katz et al., 2000). Active listening paves the way for relevant logical questions and cues critical thinking processes. Be active and vocal, and realize that your point of view is respected. Often, there are many answers and no wrong answers. Multiple views can enliven the discussion and expand perspectives for all involved. Active participation can be a distinct advantage in learning. It can clarify thoughts and observations, prompt interactions, and lead to insights.

> Tell me and I'll forget. Show me and I may remember. Involve me and I'll understand.
> Chinese Proverb

To be fully engaged, both mind and body, often facilitates comprehension. Simulations have added a new dimension to learning and allow the learner to become involved in cognitive and tactile processes, including decision making, without the risk of untoward consequences. Computer simulations present situations to elicit critical thinking. Human simulators bring realistic clinical scenarios into the learning environment and challenge the student to synthesize knowledge, thought processes, and physical response. These situations feature practice, evaluation, reflection, and modification from a very dynamic perspective. Jeffries (2005) views simulators as a demonstration of technological advances in education, an effective vehicle for instruction of the realities of health care, and a means of emphasizing critical thinking.

Computer Anxiety

Developing computer skills while taking courses can be time-consuming and is not necessarily a confidence booster at the start. However, computers can produce a high-quality, finished document, and allow you to edit and duplicate readily. The computer is also an excellent tool to use to search for and print material for papers, saving time and trips to campus. College librarians frequently offer workshops that feature access and use of databases via computer and application to course objectives. Many professors communicate with students via e-mail, and most colleges require students to maintain an e-mail account for campus-wide and course-specific information. At the onset, assess your skills and areas where enhancements would be helpful.

Work-Related Problems

Working while attending school presents a host of stressors. Although scheduling classes around professional responsibilities may create some problems, it can also provide wonderful opportunities to implement concepts newly learned. Speak with your immediate supervisor and the human resources department about your decision, and emphasize that you intend to honor your responsibilities at work but want to explore time flexibility and any possibility for funding of courses. Some coworkers may be interested in sharing flexible time schedules. Many nurses are returning to the academic arena, and health-care institutions are usually supportive because both the individual and the agency benefit from additional education. Many employers will subsidize a portion of tuition to encourage advancement. Be proactive and try to develop support, understanding, and alternative plans in the workplace before complications arise.

Family Complications

The biggest conflicts or stressors may arise from situations involving those people closest to the student, especially family. Reorganizing responsibilities during school sessions can help, but continuing an education should never require the student to choose sides against family. In fact, family support and understanding of the experience are essential from both practical and emotional standpoints.

A supportive partner can be the most important asset in your education experience. Do not expect a partner to understand immediately and completely the expectations and pressures of the process, however. You will need to talk about the pressures of your new role if you expect your partner to understand and support your endeavor. Bear in mind that even with detailed conversation you cannot expect family members to see and understand from the same perspective as you and your academic peers. Accurate and adequate communication is essential to formulating new expectations within the family. When time with your family is curtailed to accommodate the demands of a course, you may experience considerable role strain and question the decisions and compromises you must make to pursue a degree.

The characteristically nurturing roles of wife and mother in U.S. society have been compatible with nursing, a traditionally gendered profession, for many decades. Currently, a significant percentage of nurses report that clinical responsibilites at work interfere with family (Grzywacz, Frone, Brewer, & Kovner, 2006). Initially, education may be viewed as an additional distraction. Nevertheless, increased organization frequently emerges with increased challenge. It follows from the old adage: if you want something done, ask a busy person.

Certainly, the parental role should not be taken lightly, and the addition of school-related activities to an already busy schedule can prompt feelings of guilt and anxiety. These feelings may be more intense for a single parent. In addition, the need for competent child care frequently extends beyond day care to evening care. Reliable supervision for school-age and teenage children is an equally important issue that may require much more coordination than the care of younger, less mobile children. It can be extremely difficult for a student to concentrate in class knowing that a teenage son with a new driver's license is driving home from school.

Students who are part of the "sandwich generation" may bear responsibility for both parents and children. Even though the parents do not live in the student's home, they may require additional time, attention, and emotional support.

Single students without children may have fewer family responsibilities but also fewer resources and support to draw on while still being responsible for the multiple functions of a single-person household. Few people experience a totally uncomplicated return to school.

The number of men in nursing schools is growing. Besides the increasing percentage of young men who enter nursing programs, there is a noticeable increase in the number of men choosing nursing as a second career (Curry, 1994). Men can be subjected to societal stressors and experience role conflict when they enter a primarily female profession. Returning to school may cause similar stressors when the male student is questioned about his continuing education or his career choice. The conventional roles of husband, father, and breadwinner are not often linked with nursing. Exposure to such narrow thinking can affect the many dedicated men striving to advance both themselves and the profession of nursing. The situation can be compounded when male mentors, role models, and peer support are not readily accessible. It is important to note that men have played a significant role in the history of nursing, and they bring a valuable perspective to the profession.

Multiple family roles added to the roles of nurse and student create a challenging combination. Yet multiple roles can have positive aspects, such as improvements in confidence, satisfaction, and perspective. Adding or modifying roles does not necessarily have negative consequences.

Personal Stressors

The most intense stress or conflicts students experience may be the pressures that come from within. Doubt, insecurity, and discouragement can become overwhelming enemies. Strive to be faithful to the commitment to yourself, and have trust in yourself, faith in your decisions, and courage to continue. To ensure success, embark on a plan of organization that will streamline activities, use resources, delegate tasks, and maximize results of efforts, and will not create unnecessary stress. Remember that you are the master of your own attitude. A positive attitude will allow you to enjoy the academic journey, not simply endure it.

TIME MANAGEMENT

Time is a precious, intangible commodity that cannot be stored, stopped, or renewed. It is invisible yet constantly makes its presence known. It can hang heavily on the hands of some and quickly fly by for others. Contemporary society is fascinated by time and ways to save it. *Time management* is a popular but inappropriate term. People do not manage the clock but, rather, organize their activities within the framework of time. The returning student has considerable experience with time from both personal and professional perspectives, but the student role can present new and different challenges. Returning students should approach time organization with a positive attitude rather than a stopwatch mentality and view it as an opportunity to plan and use time to their advantage.

Learning to allot sufficient time allows the opportunity to concentrate, develop and nurture thoughts, and provide for critical review. Allowing adequate time for an activity is especially crucial when other people, discussion, and coordination are involved. In addition, it is essential to plan well in advance to allow your potential to emerge. Ironically, the word "holiday" may take on a totally new and different meaning to the student; any opportunity for additional time may be viewed as a gift.

Practical Planning and Organization

Students benefit greatly when they take inventory of daily activities and develop a time plan that realistically addresses personal needs, family and professional responsibilities, and academic goals and expectations. The value of a schedule cannot be overrated. To be effective, it must be realistic and consider the time frame and the importance of other people and things involved. When you develop and use your plan for time management, you should keep in mind some key elements:

- The plan is simply a blueprint and can be modified.
- Its purpose is to assist in, not hinder, the use of time.
- Periodic reassessment and necessary modification are wise.
- The semester system provides an automatic time frame for reassessment in educational matters.
- Feasibility of the plan is essential.

Neither the most worthy goal nor unbounded motivation can turn an unrealistic plan into reality. A poignant example of realistic timing, given by Covey, Merrill, and Merrill (1994), is referred to as the "law of the farm." They observe that to have a crop in the fall, the farmer must plant seeds in the spring. You cannot "cram" on the farm. They also note that shortcuts and cramming in education are not effective. The knowledge acquired by these means is often temporary and does not serve the student well.

Time Plans

Realistic, individualized time plans cannot be purchased at the campus bookstore. But many time management methods and aids are available and can be used to meet individual student needs. Various forms of calendars and schedules can help you arrange activities into a reasonable time frame. Recording your schedule or list in writing is an important part of the time management process; it can serve as a point of direction, a reminder, and a visual commitment to the task. The written schedule tends to carry more importance and to improve organization.

It is important to organize from both short- and long-term perspectives. Within the framework of an academic year or semester, the student can plan according to monthly, weekly, and daily calendars. Meltzer and Palau (1993) state that the following three time-planning segments have slightly different functions:

- Monthly calendars assist students in arranging activities for long-term projects.
- Weekly calendars help with developing consistency.
- Daily calendars aid in prioritizing (p. 5).

To implement effective daily planning, set aside a few minutes each night to determine and list things to do the next day. Priorities can then be identified by ranking each item from 1 to 10 or by assigning items a level of importance (A, B, or C). The list should be very specific regarding the activity and the time allotted. Crossing off accomplished items can give the student satisfaction and motivation to continue. When items are still on the list at the end of the day, there are three choices: (1) do the task then and be done with it; (2) plan it for the next day; or (3) eliminate it because it was not important. Covey and associates (1994) suggest that organizing a weekly rather than daily plan helps reduce the problem of operating on a crisis basis. It allows the individual more flexibility without the pressure of a fixed daily schedule.

It is advisable to "frontload" whenever possible, accomplishing partial or complete assignments at the earliest opportunity. This eliminates working under increasing pressure when unanticipated complications arise. All too often, students take time, health, and necessary people and things for granted. Try to leave a buffer zone in time plans. Your mind might be ready to work when your body needs to rest, or your child is ill, or an elderly relative asks for help. Always plan to complete assignments before their due dates. Although some people claim to work better under pressure, working up to the last minute of a deadline on a regular basis is physically and emotionally exhausting, and the possibility always exists that circumstances will arise to prevent you from completing the task.

Barriers to Time Management

Watch out for the following barriers, any of which can be the downfall of an effective time management plan.

Procrastination

Delaying the inevitable can increase the emotional pressure attached to accomplishing a task or meeting a deadline. Procrastination creates a domino effect, pushing the task into a time slotted for other activities. Guilt often accompanies the delays, adding even more pressure, which interferes with your concentration when you finally address the task. Procrastinating in family responsibilities in order to meet academic requirements can elicit enormous self-imposed guilt when families are understanding and cooperative.

If you find you are procrastinating, look for the core reason for the delaying tactic, and act on it. If the task seems overwhelming, seek advice, break it down into smaller parts, and get started with one simple aspect. Simply thinking about a project does not accomplish the work, and perfection is not expected on the first attempt. Getting started can easily consume the most time and energy of a project, especially when the people involved allow themselves to be controlled by the situation rather than controlling it.

Interruptions

Interruptions can easily derail the most well-planned schedule. The lost time can range from minutes to months, and the impact can be monumental. Some interruptions are caused by other people or the environment, and others come from within. One of the most common forms of interruption was invented by Alexander Graham Bell. The ring of the telephone arrives without permission and often at inopportune times. A well-intentioned friend or relative who calls to say hello not only takes precious time but disrupts a line of thought that may never be retrieved again. At times you can feel victimized by the telephone because it seems impolite to keep the call brief. Conversely, the telephone may seem like a welcome distraction when you are involved in a difficult or unpleasant task. In either case, it takes time from the original plan. Either arrange for other family members to answer the telephone or screen calls and leave them for voice mail.

Artifical Urgency

Currently, we live in an era of artificial urgency. Advances in technology have brought an accessibility and perceived immediacy to communication and information. These developments can be extraordinarily helpful to students. At the same time, it becomes imperative that students determine what truly is urgent, important, or incidental. The lure of readily visible e-mail can entice an already busy student to engage in less than necessary messages that can drain valuable time. Likewise, text messaging and and an explosion of cell phone use for nonurgent communication can provide a sense of artificial urgency. Access to the flow of constant communication and a public tendency to (and an expectation of) immediate response does not necessarily confer valid urgency or importance to every item.

Time Savers

There are many ways to manage time and activities successfully. As you use time more effectively, you may develop new and different strategies specific to your individual situation. Follow these time management methods to experience more productive and enjoyable days:

- *Assess yourself.* When are you best able to concentrate? When are you most energetic? Many people are most productive in the early morning, when the world is very quiet, the mind clear, and the body refreshed.
- *Avoid the marathon approach.* Eight consecutive hours is a long time to focus on any one task, whether it is writing a paper or washing floors. The productivity level increases if activities are varied and performed in smaller blocks of time.
- *Allow for time spillovers.* Try to plan time with leeway between activities, to accommodate meetings that run late, unexpected appointments, or simply losing track of time.

- *Plan adequate travel time.* Not all trips from work to campus to home have to resemble an Indianapolis 500 race. Checking the most time-efficient routes, and having a back-up plan for heavy traffic or inclement weather, can save valuable time and anxiety. Familiarize yourself with school policy regarding communication of closings due to weather conditions. Allow sufficient time to find a parking space and walk to buildings.
- *Use five-minute fillers.* While waiting for a meeting or class to start, use the five- or 10-minute time slot to make a telephone call, photocopy an article, or review a study question with another student.
- *Make a "waiting room" portfolio.* Keep a portfolio of portable tasks that can be accomplished in the 20 or 30 minutes you spend in a dentist's or doctor's waiting room, or in the car during practice before a youngster's soccer game, or when a class or meeting is canceled. Keep a supply of notepads and pencils to make "to do" lists, outline projects, or write overdue letters. Thirty minutes can make a visible difference on a piece of needlework planned as a gift.
- *Keep a PDA or pocket calendar.* Combine family, work, school, and social events on the calendar to give yourself an overview and enable you to arrange appointments or meetings on the spot.
- *Do "double work" activities.* Always have some type of task ready to be done during telephone conversations. While conversing with a colleague about work or school, you can perform simple tasks, such as folding the laundry, washing dishes, polishing furniture, and sorting papers.
- *Use travel time.* Public transportation is a waiting room in motion and provides hands-free time for reading texts, reviewing policies for work, or keeping current with professional journals. Travel time in a car can be valuable time with yourself. It can be used to gear up mentally for, or wind down from, a busy day. Newscasts and informational talk shows capsulize current issues, and keep you in touch with the world. Listening to audiotapes for course review, relaxation, or motivation is an especially good way to pass this time. Listening to your favorite music can provide a brief oasis in a complicated schedule.
- *Make calls.* Telephone calls made "on the go" can open time slots in a busy schedule and accomplish personal business calls in privacy.
- *Leave open time.* Schedule times for nothing. An occasional blank space in a busy week can be a welcome event to be used as you choose.

Time management involves developing a respect for the clock, because time continues even when your energy and ideas are diminishing or depleted.

Setting Limits and Achieving Balance

Setting limits is not intended to create a restrictive environment or mind-set. In fact, it encourages you to focus on goals and to be proactive rather than reactive. Setting limits involves responsible assessment and recognition of boundaries. It requires being aware of capabilities and acknowledging limitations. Setting limits puts you in control. It allows you to be the decision maker and determine what is realistic and beneficial. The words *realistic* and *beneficial* are key elements in limits, and students can become painfully aware that things that could be helpful or desirable are not always possible.

Setting limits is not confined to time. Many aspects of daily life, including energy, money, and activities of all types, can be subject to limits. Effective limit setting involves balancing the various facets of life as well as the demands within each facet (social, professional, intellectual, physical, and so on). *Balancing* does not mean designating a time slot for everything each day but addressing your needs and goals weekly and monthly.

Balance requires firsthand knowledge of priorities and respect for individual needs, abilities, and interests. It means that you identify the minimum and maximum efforts required to meet your goals. Contemporary society often seems committed to the concept of maximum, sometimes to the point of excess. But less is sometimes better. Use your judgment to determine these circumstances.

> Setting limits involves responsible assessment and recognition of boundaries. It requires being aware of capabilities and acknowledging limitations.

A prime principle of limit setting is learning to say "No." This two-letter, one-syllable word is often the most difficult word to articulate. The desire to participate, to please, and to be viewed as cooperative and competent is very human. The altruistic nature common among nurses adds to their difficulty in limiting time and efforts, resulting in time binds and exhaustion. Responsibility to oneself is an important part of setting limits. Strive to know yourself well. Porter-O'Grady & Malloch (2003) note that "self knowledge is the beginning point of self direction."

Pace

A positive attitude, motivation, and zeal for knowledge enhance learning; however, unbridled enthusiasm can also lead you to push yourself beyond reasonable expectations. Overextending yourself at school can seriously limit the time and attention you have to devote to other responsibilities and can also lead to academic burnout. Remember that achieving a degree is a growth process—not a race, but a process of completion. Pace yourself so that you devote adequate time to all of your work activities.

Lack of pacing can result in frustration, diminished quality of effort and work, depletion of physical and mental resources, or abandonment of your goal. Set and abide by speed limits. Take advantage of opportunities and address unanticipated events, but always keep your set point at a realistic level. Reasonable pacing allows you to complete academic assignments, courses, and curricula and to participate in other life activities.

ASSEMBLING RESOURCES

Before embarking on a new venture, thoroughly assess the situation and take inventory of your available resources. These **resources** usually fall into three basic categories—educational, professional, and family. Each category offers a variety of opportunities for assistance, and students are encouraged to take advantage of all types (Table 2–1).

Assess all aspects of life to develop a comprehensive picture and identify resources that are currently accessible. Create a plan to determine how to use existing resources to meet your goal. Then be on the alert for new and additional sources of help. Just as new and different needs can emerge, so can resources. It is your responsibility to seek out and negotiate for resources and to know when and how to use them appropriately.

Educational Resources

The college campus, the very setting that facilitates achievement of the desired degree, is often the resource with which students are least familiar. Make an all-out effort to become aware of all the services and opportunities that are connected with the institution, both physically and online. Some resources may be apparent or mentioned in the application and admission process. Once you are enrolled, however, become familiar with the academic expectations and the people, methods, and activities to help meet those expectations. College offers many forms of assistance, but you must spend time and energy to become knowledgeable about them.

Campus Communication

A number of college resources are designed to distribute information. A brief review of your college's literature, such as the website, the catalog, view book, and department brochures, can provide an overview of its program, policies, and services. A campus map is extremely helpful to orient you to the physical layout and enable you to identify key locations and services quickly. Semester schedules and an array of weekly announcements are posted to inform students of current

Table 2.1

Examples of Where to Find Resources

Educational	Department chair
	Faculty
	Academic advisor
	Course professor
	Student orientation programs
	Adult and continuing education department
	Learning centers
	Library
	Financial aid office
	Bulletin boards
	Special-interest student groups
	Other students
Professional	Professional organizations
	Employer
	Mentor
Family/Friends	Available babysitters
	Family or friends with special talents, such as a computer whiz
	Neighbor willing to carpool
	Someone with library privileges at a nearby university
	Local groups that offer educational funding
	Access to computer or photocopying

curricular and extracurricular activities. Routine review of bulletin boards informs you of upcoming events that are beneficial or required.

Student orientation programs, especially those designed for mature students, are extremely helpful. These sessions capsulize the information in the institution's literature and focus on the practical aspects of the college experience. Orientation usually provides answers to commonly asked questions and alleviates some anxiety. Besides imparting information, the programs provide opportunity for interaction with key college personnel. Department chairs, faculty, and students are usually present and interested in talking with incoming students. An added benefit of attending orientation is meeting other incoming students—your academic peers.

Academic Advisor

One key resource in the educational setting is the faculty member who serves as your academic advisor. The importance of an advisor cannot be overestimated. Plan to meet with her at the beginning of the first semester and regularly throughout the experience. The advisor will assist you with course selection and will monitor your academic progress, but the role entails much more. You can expect your advisor to help you assess strengths and weaknesses, maintain focus, and to serve as a source of encouragement and information. By serving as a sounding board, the advisor can help you develop independence and critical thinking. An advisor guides each student through the education process in an individualized manner to meet specific learning needs and the criteria of a program. You must be a willing and active participant, however, and understand that the advisor's role is to guide and facilitate, not to handle your responsibilities or errands. The advisor can serve as a role model and an ongoing source of guidance and information for the process of socialization into academe.

Campus Services and Personnel

An advisor may direct the student to a variety of resources on the campus. Many institutions have a specific department or office that works with adult learners. This unit is often known as the Lifelong Learning, Adult Education, or Nontraditional division. It provides information on issues relevant to mature students, including transfer, life-experience credit, and financial opportunities for older students.

Every college also has a division that focuses on improving specific learning skills. Personnel with varied educational backgrounds work with students individually or in small groups to enhance abilities. Services can range from remediation in a specific learning area, such as mathematics, to supplemental instruction in sciences, to assistance in developing and writing papers. A variety of technological devices and methods may be available for educational goals, such as increasing reading rate. These learning centers are designed for students who desire to improve their methods and abilities. Study groups in subject areas and tutors can be arranged through the center. Students can be referred by a professor or an advisor or can seek assistance on their own. International or culturally diverse students can expect to find an office on campus dedicated to bridging cultural variation in the educational setting. Courses in English as a second language may come under the direction of this office.

One of the most traditional educational resources is the campus library. Students benefit from a formal orientation to the facility or an individual appointment with a librarian to learn about the reference services available and the computerized catalog- and information-search operations. Libraries often have individual study carrels and document-preparation equipment for the convenience of students. Some college libraries provide free photocopying service. Looking through copies of daily newspapers, weekly journals, and past issues bound in the stacks can help students develop current and historical perspectives for various courses. Also be aware of other libraries, public or university affiliated, that offer different or additional holdings. Some health-care institutions have libraries and librarians at the worksite. Collections in these libraries often reflect the focus of the hospital or agency. The library can also be a very convenient, quiet, and efficient place for a busy student to work.

Financial aid is available for all students, not just those coming directly from high school. The nursing department and financial aid office can apprise students of their eligibility for public funding. Employee benefit programs are another possible source of funding. A variety of state and federal assistance programs exist for students associated with the military. RNs can also benefit from scholarships and stipends offered by professional and civic groups exclusively for adult students. Diligent monitoring of announcements can be financially advantageous.

The course professor is an often overlooked resource. He is your first point of communication and usually welcomes the opportunity to clarify or expand topics. The professor can provide the course perspective, clarify criteria, and evaluate progress as well as refer students to other valuable resources as needed. Faculty members maintain office hours designated exclusively for interacting with students. Meetings with the course professor can correct assumptions, dispel rumors, and assist you in understanding the material. Students whose work and family schedules prevent them from meeting with professors during office hours can often arrange a telephone discussion or e-mail contact.

Student Peers

One of the most valuable educational resources for the student is the student peer. Sharing the common educational experience can forge an intellectual and emotional bond. Student peers offer information, understanding, and support. Fellow students have similar goals and circumstances. They can comprehend the pressures of your return to school in a way that no family member does, and they can offer creative solutions that have worked for them.

Study groups also can be helpful for reviewing course content, preparing for examinations, or developing projects. Discussion and exchange of ideas in a group can energize individuals and the whole. Group interaction creates a network of additional eyes and ears to garner information for a course assignment. The interplay of common goals and varied experiences can expand perspectives, broaden understanding, and make the task more enjoyable. The student peer study group can also provide immeasurable personal support. The camaraderie can help keep motivation at a productive level or assist in overcoming disappointment. Some students act as role models and serve as sources of encouragement, whereas others provide information or support. Each student brings unique characteristics, talents, and abilities that can be shared. Interaction as brief as a conversation during a class break may still be supportive. Students who choose not to belong to a student study group should make a point of interacting with some students individually. Exchanging e-mail addresses or telephone numbers helps, especially when students are on campus only one or two days a week.

It is widely recognized that students who are involved in campus associations and activities express more satisfaction with the experience, and Astin (2005-2006) notes that higher engagement with the campus is related to increased program completion. Student organizations connected with the academic major can provide access to professional information and networks. Campus organizations offer community service, athletic, artistic, and social opportunities.

Occasional student social gatherings add pleasure and balance to a goal-oriented schedule. Incorporating a lunch or dinner with other students into your campus or study regimen can be both pleasurable and productive.

Academic Items and Technology

Educational pursuits cannot take place in a vacuum, and certain items can be helpful in accomplishing academic tasks. Besides the required textbooks for each course, the student should have a current-edition dictionary, a thesaurus, and a copy of the format for writing papers preferred by the college.

A computer—either at home or conveniently available for use—is an efficient tool for developing, storing, and retrieving information. Depending on the capability of the computer and the student, information can be accessed from libraries and many other locations. As Catalano (2003) notes, a myriad of Web sites can provide a wealth of information about nursing. A sample of popular Web sites is listed in Table 2–2. Owning a computer and acquiring computer skills can be an integral part of the college experience. Computer use can both expand the depth and breadth of the experience and shorten the work and time of the task.

Professional Resources

The professional arena holds many resources. The cooperation of your immediate superior in the workplace is pivotal in facilitating the integration of professional responsibilities and educational goals. When you decide to return to school, you should schedule a meeting to notify your superior of your decision. Be prepared to present a well-defined plan, including how it will benefit the nurse, the unit, and the institution. It is important for the superior who is responsible for assignments, schedules, and evaluations to understand your circumstances and potential. The meeting may be an appropriate time to ask about adjusting your workload and schedule in the future and to note any precedent. It is primarily your role to devise viable possibilities and options compatible with the function of the unit. Supervising personnel can provide additional input and insight into constraints for plans you present. Enlist the cooperation of clinical colleagues to serve as interim backups or resources.

Many health-care agencies recognize the value of continued education and subsidize personnel for a portion of or the full cost of a course. Some institutions require that a specific grade be achieved for reimbursement. Such policies provide both financial and academic motivation for education.

Professional nursing organizations are resources in many ways. The continual dissemination of materials through such associations provides students with a conduit of professional information and issues. Conferences and workshops sponsored by nursing organizations give students the opportunity to listen to and possibly interact with leaders in the profession. Organization workshops or panels allow students to participate as presenters. Local and state chapters of many groups may have funds available for student education. Sigma Theta Tau, the international nursing honor society, fosters student achievement and rewards it with induction into the membership. State nurse and student nurse associations provide a stream of information and give members an opportunity to speak on contemporary issues of the profession.

Within the professional milieu, you may discover a person to serve as your mentor. Developing a relationship with a mentor is especially beneficial. A mentor is more than a role model and can offer much more than intellectual substance. A prime example is the development of

Table 2.2	
Popular Nursing Web Sites	
American Association of Colleges of Nursing	**http://www.aacn.nche.edu/**
American Association of Nurse Attorneys	**http://www.taana.org**
American College of Nurse Practitioners	**http://www.acnpweb.org**
American Nurses Association	**http://www.nursingworld.org**
Association of Perioperative Registered Nurses	**http://www.aorn.org**
Association of Women's Health, Obstetric, and Neonatal Nurses	**http://www.awhonn.org**
National Association of Pediatric Nurses Associates & Practitioners	**http://www.napnap.org**
National Association of School Nurses	**http://www.nasn.org**
National Institute of Nursing Research	**http://www.nih.gov/ninr**
National League for Nursing	**http://www.nln.org/**
Sigma Theta Tau International Honor Society of Nursing	**http://www.nursingsociety.org**

increased insight into critical thinking processes (Jackson, Ignatavicuis, & Case, 2006). You can expect to receive support and guidance from a person attuned to the politics, power, and processes of career paths. Mentors characteristically assist in the development of personal and professional growth. Although adult learners are self-directed, seeking a mentor is tied to the desire to obtain the expertise and resources to meet practical needs (Knowles, 1988). Having a mentor is not essential, but it can be a positive experience and often improves your success potential, leading to your own service as a mentor in the future. This chain of mentoring constitutes an ongoing form of repayment to the profession.

Participating in a professional position concurrently with college studies places the student in regular touch with contemporary care. The clinical experiences put real faces on the pages of textbooks and make the lessons relevant. Involvement in the workplace maintains access to an interdisciplinary network, which is necessary given a health-care system in transition.

Family Resources

Even your most devoted family and friends can never share your perspective about returning to school. Most families are eager, however, to encourage and support you, despite a limited understanding of the total picture. The encouragement and admiration of your family can help sustain your motivation throughout the semesters. Likewise, you can readily serve as a role model for both children and adults and can gain self-esteem and confidence from the experience. Additionally, the family can provide assistance in practical ways that save you time and energy. Some family and household responsibilities can be adjusted to accommodate your schedule or workload without overlooking the responsibilities and interests of other family members. The experience can benefit individual members in many practical ways, perhaps enhancing the sense of family for the group.

Negotiate and delegate with partner, children, or parents according to the needs of the family. Develop each individual's talents and abilities so there is opportunity for others to share or take on new responsibilities. Appreciate their help, no matter how small, and be sure to show your appreciation. Ease your standards. For instance, do not redo a task because the outcome does not meet your standards. It does not matter whether the towels are not folded and stacked the way you would do it. Students who are parents should keep in mind that they can learn from how a child approaches a project. A child who is computer literate can help you learn to use the computer, and you can both benefit from the shared experience.

Do not eliminate the support you might get from a telephone conversation with a relative or friend hundreds of miles away. Willing friends and neighbors can help by offering to assist with carpools, babysitting, or caring for an older parent. Interested, well-meaning people are not necessarily expecting you to reciprocate in kind, and often are genuinely happy to help and be a part of the endeavor—a true resource.

Health: An Overlooked Resource

One very important resource frequently taken for granted is good health. Despite professional knowledge and experience, nurses can undervalue personal wellness until they have a problem. To maintain physical and mental stamina, students must attend to the basic premises of health promotion and wellness. Disregard for individual health can lead to illness and can negatively influence academic schedules and goals. Regular exercise, good nutrition, and plenty of rest can help you approach responsibilities with a sense of vitality. Cultivate the art of relaxation; it brings a host of physical and mental benefits. Humor can be a healthy coping mechanism that helps put your day in perspective. Laughter often results in a sense of relaxation and defuses stress (Schuster, 2000). With a positive attitude toward personal health, you can achieve a higher level of wellness, feel better, enjoy the college experience, be more productive, and position yourself for academic success (Curry, 2002).

Assembling resources consists of lining up assets and opportunities. It involves drawing on or using the knowledge, service, and access to resources available. Resources can be found as far as the Internet reaches or as near as your personal collection of nursing journals. Interaction and exchange are important in identifying and developing resources. Talking about activities and projects to family, friends, coworkers, and fellow students can increase your "brain power" and extend your network of available assistance. Some resources are readily identified and available, and others may have to be created.

STREAMLINING WORK

The *American Heritage College Dictionary* defines **streamlining** as constructing or designing in a form that offers the least resitance to fluid flow (Pickett, 2002, p. 1366); it connotes concepts such as organization, minimal resistance, efficiency, simplicity, and being unencumbered. These are positive and desirable qualities for work. Try to streamline work in each of the various facets of life—family, social, professional, and educational. Streamlining work in one area of life can positively affect the other areas.

Streamlining involves carefully considering all of your ideas and plans with the coordination of goals, limits, resources, and time management in an action-oriented process geared toward efficiency and saving energy. It requires the organization and fine tuning of how things are usually done. Streamlining means eliminating the unnecessary and making work a pleasant and productive experience. Be careful not to eliminate everything, because functioning with only the absolute essentials can turn work into hard labor. Simplify your life, but do not close down your world.

Educational Streamlining

The educational arena has many requirements and essential activities, yet you can simplify the process and still achieve your objectives. Life and your nursing career provide you with processes integral to streamlining educational activities. Educational streamlining does not focus on the study process per se but rather helps create life circumstances that foster conditions conducive to study. Despite technological advances there is no easy way to acquire and synthesize knowledge. Though individual differences may exist, it requires time and effort. "Knowledge is power, intellect is a gift, but learning is hard work" (Porter-O'Grady & Malloch, 2003).

Accruing Credit

One aspect of streamlining is using resources effectively. This is particularly important in looking at the overall curriculum and various courses involved. The mass of information and number of academic courses necessary may seem overwhelming. You may already possess some of the required knowledge, however, and there is no reason to "reinvent the wheel." Discuss your experience with an advisor and explore the variety of ways, besides taking courses, that you can demonstrate knowledge and receive credits. This can be done during the application and admission process.

Once you have a better understanding of the requirements, you may want to analyze how your experience can earn credits. You may qualify for transfer credits for courses taken at another institution that are comparable in content to those in the curriculum. You may also become eligible for credits by portfolios or challenge exams designed by faculty. These tests are designed to demonstrate knowledge covered in the course.

Course Timing

The time at which a course is offered, especially a required course, is crucial to busy adults. Always check a course's schedule carefully to note whether it has multiple sections, and possibly one at a more convenient time or place. When you have a time conflict for an essential course, talk with your advisor about taking the class at a satellite location, at another school, or via distance education. Distance education programs, which send live video broadcasts to one or more remote classroom locations, or online courses may be viable options. Whenever possible, it is helpful to chain courses together. This minimizes the number of trips to campus and saves transportation time and expense. When there are intervals between classes, it is wise to plan to use the time for a specific task, such as library research, review of notes, or study groups.

Using the Library

Make trips to the campus library as productive as possible. If you did not receive a formal orientation to the library, ask a librarian to describe the policies and features. When using journal articles, e-mail to your computer account or photocopy the material for current and future use at home. Students should make sure the photocopy shows the complete information for citation, including journal volume and edition. For books, note the ISBN number and citation information for quick retrieval in the future. It is helpful to keep a supply of index cards handy to write citations and any pertinent information. Honor due dates. Attach a note with the due date on the front of the book to remind yourself to return it on time and avoid fines.

When you go to the library for one course, check the availability of materials for other courses. Assist other students by being alert for materials relevant to their topics of interest; they can do the same for you. A class list with selected project or paper topics can guide you. Carefully monitor your time in the library. It is easy to spend inordinate amounts of time there because it is usually quiet and serene, with reminders of the passing time.

Portfolio System

Organizing things is just as important as organizing your life. A portfolio system is extremely helpful for easy access to important materials. Devote one portfolio to your academic progress, including such items as letters of acceptance, catalogs, course schedules, an advisement or curriculum plan, and any correspondence with the college. Transcripts, paid receipts, and other relevant materials can be added each semester. Keep a personal copy of any information requested by the college, such as an annual health history and physical forms, immunization records, or documentation of cardiopulmonary resuscitation certification.

A second portfolio should pertain to course work, with pertinent materials for each course, such as a course outline, schedule, reading list, completed assignments, and papers. Copies of relevant course materials can be included for future reference.

Communication

Efficient communication is part of streamlining. Using e-mail and fax communications can save considerable time in transmitting information. Most colleges have a system for student e-mail accounts. Carrying a list of school-related places and people, with their telephone and fax numbers and e-mail addresses, will also enhance communication. The names and numbers of other students, your advisor, the department secretary, and the library are a few frequently used items. Students who do not use business cards in their professional roles may consider having cards with home address and appropriate phone numbers.

Forming a carpool with another student offers several advantages, including the opportunity to discuss class projects and review material. Students who audiotape courses can use travel time for review. As you progress in your educational program, your academic networks will expand, and more people and information will be available for you to use in the process of streamlining.

Professional Streamlining

Even those employed on a part-time basis usually have to assess and reorganize their situations to accommodate school. Adjustments range from exchanging a few hours to taking a leave of absence.

Negotiation with superiors, and sometimes peers, is often a successful approach to resolving the situation. Cost-conscious employers and supervisors can be extremely receptive to innovative plans that maintain quality performance and increase cooperation and morale. If timing of the workday is an issue, flextime may be the answer. Condensing work hours to fewer days may help. Sometimes arriving early or adding an hour on specified days is all that is necessary to allow a student to leave the workplace in time to attend a class. Trading holiday coverage for class time and job-sharing are other options. If you are a manager or supervisor, delegate functions and authority as appropriate. A leave of absence is sometimes the most appropriate method. Most reasonable requests to realign work schedules to gain an education will be considered, and many are granted.

Streamlining Domestic Functions

One of the first tasks of streamlining is to get all those involved in your home life to realize that you cannot continually relegate schoolwork to the end of the night, after everything else is finished, or to an already crammed weekend. Most home tasks can be rearranged, reprioritized, or eliminated to improve your quality of life.

Have a family discussion and encourage new ideas for getting the work done, determining what can be eliminated, or obtaining volunteers. Use incentives and rewards for a job well done. New interests and unrecognized talents may be developed in the streamlining process.

Hiring household help to clean periodically can provide significant assistance at moderate expense. Relatives may be pleased to provide child care for a few hours a week. Arrange with neighbors to exchange child care or carpooling responsibilities.

Thinking in quantities and doing two things at once can help. Buy and prepare food in quantity. One night a week, while you are cooking dinner, it is possible to prepare additional dishes, to be served on another evening. On occasion, ask a family member to do the grocery shopping or to accompany you—to turn the task into a pleasant time to be together. Schedule these activities early in the week, when your ambition and energy are usually high. Plan to eat out once a week, for family enjoyment and less work.

Some basic practices to increase efficiency in domestic responsibilities are as follows:

- Select and lay out clothes the night before each working day.
- Do a morning check to make sure all necessary family items for the day are ready.
- Know the daily schedule and telephone numbers for each family member.
- Plan a route for each day. Chain activities and errands together to avoid driving in circles.
- Handle mail only once—read and relegate.
- Post a list for needed household items, making an automatic grocery list.
- Make a monthly medicine-cabinet check.
- Plan time for routine car maintenance so you can handle daily schedules without delay.

Reorganizing activities can result in better working conditions, greater productivity, more time for the important things and people, and an improved quality of life.

STUDY TIPS

Have a designated area at home that is conducive to studying and concentrating. The room should have functional furniture and should be capable of holding educational equipment and materials. Furniture that is too comfortable may defeat the purpose. Appropriate lighting, room temperature, and noise level should be considered to prevent distractions. A quiet atmosphere is needed for activities involving concentration, although some learners find that background music or sounds are helpful and may even accelerate the pace of activity. Individual differences exist, however, and not every person or all academic activities require total silence or isolation. Whatever your personal preferences, the environment should be designed to signal your brain that it is entering a work zone.

Preparation for Study

Just as you prepare the environment, you must prepare yourself for study. Your body and mind-set have to be open to academic business. Hunger and fatigue are unwelcome distractions and should be addressed before work begins. Any necessary materials should be on hand and within reach to allow an undisturbed flow of work. A positive attitude, a sense of control, and a concrete plan set the stage for a productive session. You will need to acknowledge the transition and allow time to enter into the task. To participate effectively, you must mentally shift gears and assume the appropriate level of concentration. When projects are ongoing, it can be difficult to regain the mental perspective of the previous work session immediately. A quick review of the last section completed helps focus your attention and reduces start-up time. Ending each work session of a continuing project by attaching a note that details specific directions and ideas for the start of the next session may be beneficial.

Ending each work session of a continuing project by attaching a note that details specific directions and ideas for the start of the next session may be beneficial.

Study Process

Although individual study preferences exist and styles emerge, some practices have been successful for many people and can benefit the returning student who has a busy schedule. It is helpful to establish a routine for study. A routine facilitates readiness for the work and helps the student stay on task during the allotted time. Short study sessions interspersed with breaks and alternated with some physical activity are usually more productive than one continuous daylong effort.

Each textbook is a valuable resource. Take advantage of all the information authors provide. Objectives, key words, headings, highlights, and summaries are not window dressing; they provide direction and facilitate understanding. Illustrations clarify concepts. Diagrams, pictures, graphs, listings, and tables expand and enhance the mental images constructed by the written words. A glossary defines terms from the perspective of the subject area. An index assists students in quickly locating relevant information. Marking frequently used pages with a labeled tab or note can be helpful.

Reading the introduction and summary and paying attention to key words and headings before you read a chapter may help you identify the main points and understand the total concept. When questions arise, or you do not understand the material, tab the page, write the question on an index card, and speak with the professor. Most professors routinely interact with their students via e-mail.

Although initial study should be done individually, you may benefit from a study group. To be effective, the group should have an agenda and a set time for each meeting. The gathering gives students an opportunity to compare notes from class, discuss content or questions from readings, and brainstorm about possible test questions. Group study works best when done on a regular, preferably weekly basis.

Besides reading and discussion, you gain a significant amount of information through note taking. It is important to be an active listener and to record pertinent information. Note taking requires listening for and documenting key words and central thoughts and ideas. Verbatim notes are neither efficient nor realistic. Listen and understand first, and then summarize the information presented. Develop a consistent and efficient method of note taking to ease the process and improve the content. Always date your notes and indicate the topic. Use paragraphs and headings to group and identify information. Record any reference your professor makes to pages in the text or names of other works and authors, and be alert to the importance of listings and definitions. Streamline notes to those points that are necessary and meaningful without being too brief or cryptic. Use common abbreviations and symbols, or develop an individual form of shorthand. Drawings and diagrams offer additional perspective on the words. Most important, handwriting must be legible for your notes to be of value.

The Cornell Note Taking Format is a useful tool. The format uses a lengthwise border on the left side of the paper, with notes written on the right side; the left portion is used for questions, comments, and additional information.

Taping lectures reinforces the note-taking process. Tapes allow the student to add to notes already taken

ONLINE CONSULT

To learn the Cornell Note Taking Format, consult the following Web site that offers the steps of the format.
www.ucc.vt.edu/stdysk/cornell.html

and to clarify details. The portable nature of tapes permits convenient repetition of the material in private settings, such as at home or in the car. Some international students may find tapes especially helpful in adapting to the English language and its nuances or to a professor who speaks rapidly. Any student who wishes to tape a lecture should have ample long-playing tapes available and should request permission of the presenter before taping. Some professors do not permit taping, and some students are reluctant to participate in discussion if it is being taped.

Cross-course activities help streamline and add depth to your education. The concept is to use information or processes from one course in another course or academic endeavor. It involves reprocessing information, reframing ideas, and implementing information or methods in new and creative ways. It does not mean submitting the same paper for two courses, but it can involve developing a new perspective on already researched material. For example, if appropriate to course objectives, a topic such as alcoholism could be used for papers in biology, sociology, psychology, and community nursing courses, among others. A different perspective directs the focus in each case. Students could merge aspects of work already produced to develop new perspectives and draw correlations. In the process, they deepen their knowledge, expand the scope of methods, and improve their critical thinking.

Reference or bibliography cards have been a simple, successful, and portable method of storing and transferring information. The process can readily be inplemented by computer. When researching any topic, document the citation in the correct form on an index card or computer, along with notation of any pertinent information, quotes, or statistics. When the project or paper is completed, the list will be complete, and merely rearranging the items will produce the alphabetical order for typing. The information can then be filed according to a variety of categories (by topic, by course, alphabetically, and so forth) to be retrieved for use later. You may also consider using a personal digital assistant to record information.

Advice on how to study could fill volumes, and many good publications on study strategies are available. Effective use of study methods can lead to cognitive energy and success. You must accept the responsibility for determining and implementing the sound study practices most appropriate and realistic for you.

If you honor the commitment to yourself, plan realistic strategies, use time and resources effectively, and maintain a balance in life activities, you can enjoy the challenge of the educational experience and achieve your goals. You are entitled to enjoy, not simply endure, the educational journey.

INTERACTIVE EXERCISES

Go to the Intranet site and complete the interactive exercises provided for this Chapter.

K E Y P O I N T S

■ Personal goals involve commitment, require time and thought to formulate, and should be individualized and feasible. A series of short-term goals can help you accomplish long-term goals.

■ Refining professional identity and role transition involves change that can be an uncomfortable but positive experience with personal and professional rewards.

■ A mentor offers a role model, support, and assistance to avoid pitfalls.

■ Responsibility to yourself can be both a key motivator and a monitor of actions.

■ It is important to plan activities in realistic time frames to achieve goals and to focus on quality rather than be directed primarily by the clock.

■ Recognition of your abilities, limitations, and resources is essential for realistic implementation of personalized strategies and success.

■ Streamline work to direct time and attention to changing priority areas, maintain quality performance, and provide balance in a multiple-role lifestyle.

■ Flexible thinking and change in perspective indicate growth related to the education experience.

Thought and Discussion Questions

1. List the things that you can delegate or eliminate to streamline your life while in school.

2. Start a collection of motivational sayings. Review and add to them each week. For example:
   - Live the life you've imagined.
   - Happiness is not the absence of problems, but the ability to deal with them.
   - It is more important to do your best than to be the best.

3. Review the quotation about change on the first page of the chapter in the context of the rest of the chapter, and be prepared to discuss it in class.

☐ REFERENCES

Astin, A. (2005–2006). Making sense out of degree completion rates. *Journal of College Student Retention, 7*(1–2), 5–17.

Catalano, J. (2003). *Nursing now: Today's issues, tomorrow's trends*. Philadelphia: F. A. Davis.

Covey, S. R., Merrill, A., & Merrill, R. (1994). *First things first* [audiocassette]. New York: Simon & Schuster, Audio Division.

Curry, B. D. (1994). Societal and marketing influences on enrollment into baccalaureate nursing programs. In *Symposium for the marketing of higher education* (pp. 211–216). Chicago: American Marketing Association.

Curry, B. D. (2002). International inroads to wellness. Presentation, Vienna, Austria.

Fawcett, J. (1995). *Analysis and evaluation of conceptual models of nursing* (3rd ed.). Philadelphia: F. A. Davis.

Grzywacz, J., Frone, M. R., Brewer, C. S., & Kovner, C. T. (2006). Quantifying work-family conflict among registered nurses. *Research in Nursing & Health, 29*(5), 414–426.

Holmes, T. H., & Rahe, R. (1967). The social readjustment scale. *Journal of Psychosomatic Research, 2*(4), 213–218.

Jackson, M., Ignatavicius, D. D., & Case, B. (2006). *Critical thinking and clinical judgement*. Sudbury, MA: Jones & Bartlett.

Jeffries, P. R. (2005). A framework for designing, implementing, and evaluating simulations used as teaching strategies in nursing. *Nursing Education Perspectives, 26,* 97–103.

Katz, J. R., Carter, C., Bishop, J., & Kravits, S. L. (2000). *Keys to science success*. Upper Saddle River, NJ: Prentice Hall.

Knowles, M. (1988). *The adult learner: A neglected species*. Houston, TX: Gulf Publishing.

Meltzer, M., & Palau, S. M. (1993). *Reading and study strategies for nursing students*. Philadelphia: W. B. Saunders.

Patton, T., & Goldenberg, D. (1999). Hardiness and anxiety as predictors of academic success in first year, full time, and part time RN students. *Journal of Continuing Education in Nursing, 30,* 158–167.

Pickett, J. P. (Ed.). (2002). *The American heritage college dictionary* (4th ed.). New York: Houghton Mifflin.

Porter-O'Grady, T., & Malloch, K. (2003). Quantum leadership: A textbook of new leadership. Sudbury, Massachusettes: Jones & Bartlett Publishers.

Rubenfeld, M. G., & Scheffer, B. K. (2006). *Critical thinking tactics for nurses*. Sudbury, MA: Jones & Bartlett.

Schuster, P. (2000). *Communication: The key to therapeutic relationships*. Philadelphia: F. A. Davis.

Shane, D. (1980, June). The returning to school syndrome. *Nursing 80,* 86–88.

Strader, M. K., & Decker, P. J. (1995). *Role transition to patient care management*. Norwalk, CT: Appleton & Lange.

☐ BIBLIOGRAPHY

Bunkers, S. S. (2006). The nurse scholar of the 21st century. In W. K. Cody (Ed.), *Philosophical & theoretical perspectives for advanced nursing practice* (pp. 73–84). Sudbury, MA: Jones & Bartlett.

Burkhardt, M., & Nathaniel, A. (1998). *Ethics and issues in contemporary nursing*. Albany, NY: Delmar Publishers.

Covey, S. R. (1995). *Living the 7 habits* [audiocassette]. New York: Simon & Schuster, Audio Division.

Milstead, J., & Furlong, E. (2006). Handbook of nursing leadership: Creative skills for a culture of safety. Sudbury, MA: Jones & Bartlett Publishers.

■ *Rose* **Kearney-Nunnery**

What Is Theory?

> ❝ *Theory and research are not solely the province of the academic, just as practice is not solely the field of the practitioner.* ❞
>
> (Glanz, Rimer, & Lewis, 2002, p. 23)

Chapter Objectives

On completion of this chapter, the reader will be able to:

1. Define key terms in theory development.
2. Discuss Maslow's theory of motivation with the hierarchy of basic needs.
3. Describe the components of developmental theories and their application to individuals across the life span.
4. Describe the components and application of systems theory.
5. Identify the challenges that quantum theory has placed on conventional wisdom.
6. Discuss the impact of theory on practice.

Key Terms

Theory	Construct	Developmental Theories
Model	Variables	General System Theory
Framework	Propositions	Quantum Theory
Conceptual Model or Framework	Theory Description and Evaluation	
Concept	Hierarchy of Needs	

One characteristic of a profession is that it is built on a theoretical base. This base includes theoretical foundations unique to the profession as well as those adapted from other scientific disciplines. Chapter 1 discussed paradigms and the metaparadigm concepts of nursing. Kuhn (1970) described a paradigm as "universally recognized scientific achievements that for a time provide model problems and solutions to a community of practitioners" (p. vii). When the paradigm is no longer useful in explaining phenomena, practice, and research in that particular scientific community, a paradigm shift occurs, and a new structure evolves.

In 1957, Merton used a paradigm to analyze sociological theory. He viewed the paradigm as a "field glass" to illuminate and view concepts and interrelationships and to make assumptions clear on the body of knowledge for analysis and testing. Merton (1957) identified the purposes of a paradigm as providing for the following:

1. Parsimonious arrangement of concepts and propositions showing interrelationships.
2. A logical guide showing derivations and avoiding hidden assumptions and concepts.
3. Culmination in theory development as a building process.
4. Systematic arrangement and cross-tabulation of concepts for analysis.
5. Codification of qualitative research methods (pp. 13–16).

From a cultural perspective, Leininger (2006) defined *worldview* as "the way people tend to look out upon their world or universe to form a picture or value stance about life or the world around them" (p. 15). In the professional culture of nursing, these are the values, attitudes, beliefs, and practices unique to the profession. Thus, a scientific community has the tools to create and test theory for knowledge development and use of this knowledge in practice. The worldview furnishes the philosophical assumptions that are considered "givens" by the theorist or the scientific community. In nursing, this provides us with the process: the metaparadigm concepts to various paradigms, and the development of theory on which to base research, practice, administration, and education.

TERMINOLOGY IN THEORY DEVELOPMENT AND ANALYSIS

Professions such as nursing are based on unique theory. Kerlinger and Lee (2000) defined a **theory** as "a set of interrelated constructs (concepts), definitions, and propositions that present a systematic view of phenomena by specifying relations among variables, with the purpose of explaining and predicting the phenomena" (p. 11). This definition provides us with the components and aims of a theory, which must initially be described and then evaluated for potential use in practice, education, and research in a discipline. Some theorists, however, believe this definition is too narrow and excludes descriptive theories; descriptive theories, which focus on factor naming, are abundant in professional nursing and are often a first step for further research and development where the phenomena is merely being identified or *named*.

Before moving to the components of a theory, we need to address three similar terms frequently associated with theory: model, framework, and conceptual framework or conceptual model. A **model** is a graphic representation of some phenomenon. It may be a mathematical model (A + B = C) or a diagrammatic model, linking words with symbols and lines. A theoretical model provides a visual description of the theory, using limited narrative and displaying components and relationships symbolically. A **framework** is another means of providing a structural view of the concepts and relationships proposed in a theory. Again, use of words and narrative is limited, but the structure of the theory is presented and allows translation, interpretation, and illumination of the narrative or text.

A **conceptual model or framework** is similar to a theory in that it represents some phenomenon of interest and contains concepts and propositions. With a conceptual model or framework, however, the concepts and especially the propositions are broader in scope, less defined, and less specific to the phenomenon of concern than with a theory. As Fawcett (2006) noted, in professional nursing practice, conceptual models provide different ways to view practice and each model provides an alternative guide to the way nurses work with clients (p. 500).

A theory can evolve from a conceptual model or framework as concepts are further defined, specified, tested, and interrelated to represent some aspect of reality. Then, a theory is "one or more relatively concrete and specific concepts that are derived from a conceptual model, the propositions that narrowly describe those concepts, and the propositions that state relatively concrete and specific relations between two or more of the concepts" (Fawcett, 2005, p. 18). Fawcett (2000, 2005) has described the structural hierarchy of contemporary nursing knowledge (Fig. 3–1) with its components, from the most abstract metaparadigm, influenced by different philosophies, to conceptual models that further evolve into theories and specific empirical indicators for testing. Concepts become less abstract, and the population of interest is identified. This increase in specificity is evident in the examples

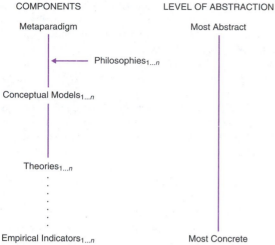

COMPONENTS   LEVEL OF ABSTRACTION

Metaparadigm   Most Abstract

Philosophies$_{1...n}$

Conceptual Models$_{1...n}$

Theories$_{1...n}$

Empirical Indicators$_{1...n}$ Most Concrete

■ **Figure 3.1** The structural hierarchy of contemporary nursing knowledge: Components and levels of abstraction. (From Fawcett, J. [2005]. *Contemporary nursing knowledge: Analysis and evaluation of nursing models and theories* (2nd. ed., p. 4). Philadelphia: F. A. Davis, with permission.)

proposed by Alligood (2006b) who, on the basis of Fawcett's structural hierarchy of nursing knowledge, correlated selected examples in theoretical structures as follows:

- Metaparadigm: Person, environment, health, and nursing
- Philosophies: Nightingale, Watson, Benner
- Conceptual Models: King, Levine, Neuman, Orem, Rogers, Roy
- Grand Theory: Rogers' Theory of Accelerating Change, Roy's Theory of the Person as an Adaptive System, Neuman's Theory of Optimal Client Stability
- Theory: Optimal Client Stability in Specific Settings, Gigliotti's Theory of Women's Multiple Stress Roles, Parse's Theory of Human Becoming, King's Theory of Goal Attainment
- Middle-range Theory: Promoting Optimal Client Stability through Stress Reduction, Medford's Health Promotion for Preterm Infants, Dunn's Theory of Adaptation to Chronic Pain (pp. 44–55)

As more is known about the phenomenon, more can be used in specific, meaningful client applications.

As knowledge about some phenomena increases, a theory is proposed to address phenomena or reality within the discipline. The components of a theory are the constructs (concepts), with their specific definitions, and the propositions that describe or link those constructs (concepts). At the simplest level, a **concept** is a view or idea that we hold about something. It can be something highly concrete, such as a pencil, or

something highly abstract, such as quality. The more concrete the concept, the easier it is understood and consistently used. For instance, we are comfortable envisioning a pencil and can easily describe it to others. This ability to describe something directly in the concrete world shares the "concept." But the concept of quality is more abstract, and ensuring that all individual definitions are the same is difficult, often requiring indirect measures.

We strive to define a concept in operational terms—that is, how we view a specific entity and how it can be measured so that others know exactly what we mean. To meet the criteria of a theory, we need to define the concepts. Consider the concept of a pencil. We think of a pencil as a writing implement. This is the theoretical or conceptual definition of a pencil we read in a dictionary. But what do we truly mean by *pencil*? It is a yellow-painted, wooden-covered graphite instrument that we use to make marks on a paper. Does it have an eraser? Does a mechanical pencil fit into this definition? An operational definition narrows the definition to precisely what we view and how it can be measured for use in practice or research as a measurable, empirical indicator. In addition, concepts are broadened to constructs, such as with quality or identity, which can be multidimensional and difficult, if not impossible, to break down into component parts.

A **construct** is a more complex idea package of some phenomenon that contains many factors but cannot be truly isolated or confined to a more concrete concept. The construct of *identity*, for example, contains many pieces, such as personal perception, role expectations, and status. However, we must still provide an operational definition of a construct by specifying certain elements it contains (as indirect measures), such as self-image, ideal image, group image, role expectations, and status. The same multidimensionality occurs when we assess quality of health care.

In research, we often see the term *variables*, referring to some concept in the theory under study. **Variables** are concepts that can change and contain a set of values that can be measured in a practice or research situation. For example, a client's cholesterol reading is a variable. The concept of blood cholesterol has been operationally defined within certain parameters, and the level of the reading is the value for the variable.

Whether concepts, constructs, or a combination of the two are included in a specific theory, they are the building blocks of the theory. Definitions are provided to help us understand the nature and characteristics of each block in the construction. We then need to relate these building blocks to each other. Describing and stating the relationships between or among the constructs (or concepts) provides the **propositions** of a theory. These are also called the *relational statements,* showing how the concepts are linked in the theory and relate to one another and to the total theoretical structure. They define how the structure is held together. In nursing theory, propositions refer to how the individual is characterized with specific abilities, knowledge, values, and traits and how these interrelate with the characteristics of health, the environment, and nursing.

Research is a means of supporting the concepts and relationships proposed in a theory. It provides supportive evidence and suggests further study and possible gaps or revisions needed in the theoretical structure. We can see this in the next chapters, which cover refinement of nursing and other health models, such as the health-belief model revision. Research can be qualitative and inductive, for generating theory, or more quantitative, for deductively testing hypotheses as theoretical propositions.

As stated previously, Kerlinger and Lee defined the aims or purpose of theory as describing or explaining some phenomena of interest. In nursing, theory is further differentiated into levels that describe, explain, predict, and control. Dickoff and James (1968) developed a classic position paper proposing four levels of nursing theory (Box 3–1). All levels may be present as a practice theory evolves (factor isolating and then relating), is subjected to further research, and is refined, becoming predictive and prescriptive. In application, testing, and refinement, theory is a continuum as long as the content meets the intent of the discipline and metaparadigm.

In addition, theories are classified according to their scope as grand, middle-range, or limited in scope or practice. This is the breadth of coverage of some phenomena. General system theory is an example of a *grand theory*, or one with a broad scope. This theory, discussed later in the chapter, has been used in development, testing, and application in many scientific disciplines.

Merton (1957) was the first theorist to suggest "theories of the middle range: theories intermediate to the minor working hypotheses evolved in abundance during the day-by-day routines of research, and the all

inclusive speculations comprising a master conceptual scheme from which it is hoped to derive a very large number of empirically observed uniformities of . . . behavior" (pp. 5–6). As you will see in the next chapter, *middle-range theories* are narrower in scope, with a limited view of a phenomenon, and contain concepts and propositions that are measurable and can be empirically tested. Some of our traditional nursing theories meet the characteristics of a middle-range theory, as described in Chapter 4. See the "Online Consult" on middle-range nursing theories that follows. Other middle-range theories, some of which you may be familiar with, include developmental theories reviewed later in this chapter. Although these theories address psychosocial, cognitive, and moral development, they apply in interdisciplinary practice areas. More limited nursing practice theories are evolving as hypotheses derived from middle-range theories. These practice theories are tested, clarified, and made specific to certain practice areas or types of health-care client. Chapter 5 shows examples of limited nursing practice models that are being tested and refined into theoretical frameworks, including Pender's health promotion model, the chronic illness trajectory framework, and Campinha-Bacote's model of cultural competence. Even more narrow in scope are *limited practice theories*, which focus on measurable variables and propositions that are based on empirical research and now may be refined further, perhaps to a specific population or group of individuals with a common characteristic.

ONLINE CONSULT

Middle Range Theories at
**http://www.nurses.info/nursing_theory_
midrange_theories.htm**

THEORY DESCRIPTION AND EVALUATION

To understand theories for use and application in practice, we use certain criteria to describe and evaluate them. Theory development is both an inductive and a deductive process. An inductive process is used to generate concepts and make inferences by stating interrelationships (propositions) within a framework to view phenomena. From observations of phenomena, we can name concepts and enumerate proposed relationships. Once the theory is generated, it is applied, in whole or part, for testing as a deductive process. For nursing **theory description and evaluation**, we

Box 3.1 Dickoff and James (1968): Four Levels of Nursing Theory

1. Factor-isolating (naming) theories
2. Factor-relating (situation depicting) theories
3. Situation-relating (predictive or promoting/inhibiting theories)
4. Situation-producing (prescriptive) theories

consider the following three sets of criteria proposed by nursing scholars Chinn and Kramer, Barnum, and Fawcett.

Chinn and Kramer (2004) differentiate between theory description and critical reflection of empiric theory. The theory is described by answering questions in the following areas: purpose, concepts, definitions, relationships, structure, and assumptions. This process provides an understanding of the components and aims of the theory. Once the theory has been described, five issues are addressed in critical reflection:

- Clarity and consistency in presentation
- Simplicity and meaningfulness of structural components and relationships
- Generality or scope of the phenomena addressed
- Accessibility as potential for use with empirically identifiable and applicable concepts
- Significance as leading to the values in practice, education, and research. (Chinn & Kramer, 2004, pp. 118–119)

This differentiation allows us to discriminate between understanding the theoretical structure and evaluating the theory's soundness and usefulness in practice, education, or research. These five areas for evaluation are similarly used by Tomey and Alligood (2006) as clarity, simplicity, generality, empirical precision, and derivable consequences (pp. 9–10).

Barbara Stevens Barnum (1998) proposes two categories of theory: descriptive theory and explanatory theory. *Descriptive theory* is factor-naming and factor-relating theory developed initially to characterize some phenomena. *Explanatory theory* brings us to the situation-relating and situation-producing levels of theory, looking at the "how," the "why," and the interrelationships in the theory (Barnum, 1998). Theory description is delineated as theory interpretation, with questions addressing the following areas:

- Major elements of the theory and their definitions
- Relationships among the elements
- Differentiating between descriptive and explanatory theory
- How the theory addresses, defines, and differentiates nursing
- The focus on the client, nurse, action, or relationship
- Unique language used and defined by the theorist. (Barnum, 1990, 1994, 1998)

For critical analysis, internal criticism and external criticism are differentiated. *Internal criticism* is used to evaluate how the theory components fit together: the clarity, consistency, adequacy, logical development, and, sometimes, level of theory development (Barnum, 1998). *External criticism* deals with real-world issues such as reality convergence, usefulness, significance,

and discrimination from other health-care disciplines (Barnum, 1998). This process allows us to discriminate between understanding the theoretical structure (internal criticism) and evaluating the soundness and usefulness of the theory for application in practice, education, or research (external criticism).

Fawcett (2005) has proposed criteria for theory analysis and evaluation that have undergone several revisions. She further differentiates between analysis and evaluation of conceptual models and nursing theories. Recall that conceptual models are more abstract than theories. As described by Fawcett (2005), a theory is more concrete, specific, and restricted to a more limited range of phenomena than those identified by a conceptual model, with the purpose of middle-range theories to describe, explain, or predict concrete and specific phenomena (p. 24).

Analysis refers to the description of the theory. Fawcett (2005) describes it as "a nonjudgmental, detailed examination of the theory" (p. 442). Theory analysis is followed by theory evaluation, which requires thoughtful interpretation of the theory. Fawcett (2005) identifies a series of questions for analysis and evaluation of nursing theories appropriate to their level of abstraction as compared with conceptual models. In this revision, Fawcett (2005) has proposed the three steps in a framework for the analysis of the nursing theory and six steps for the evaluation of the theory, as follows:

Theory Analysis	Theory Evaluation
Step 1: Scope	Step 1: Significance (importance)
Step 2: Context (basis and origins)	Step 2: Internal Consistency (congruence)
Step 3: Content (concepts and propositions)	Step 3: Parsimony (clear and concise)
	Step 4: Testability
	Step 5: Empirical Adequacy (evidence)
	Step 6: Pragmatic Adequacy (utility)

Application of this framework for theory analysis and evaluation will be evident in Chapter 4, which deals with specific grand and middle-range nursing theories. Each of these sets of criteria involves a careful identification of the components and evaluation components for determination of applicability to nursing practice.

THEORIES FROM OUTSIDE OF NURSING

Nursing and other health-care disciplines have long used a variety of theories to guide practice. Some are discipline-specific, such as the nursing theories reviewed in Chapter 4. Other theoretical structures have been applied from other disciplines. Early nursing theories were described by Barnum (1990) as follows:

> As an applied science, much of nursing's theory is "borrowed" from other disciplines. Every discipline has similar boundary ambiguities, where the inquiry and answers in one field overlap those in another. . . . Nursing's uniqueness in this respect does not lie in boundary overlap but in the number of boundary overlaps with which it must contend. A high number of overlaps occur in the discipline of nursing because it often attempts to deal holistically with a phenomenon (man) that has previously been dealt with in compartmentalized ways by other disciplines. (p. 218)

But, nursing theory has come a long way since that time. As Alligood (2006a) has described the development of nursing theory—from the Curriculum Era in the early 20th century, through the Research and Graduate Education Eras in the middle 20th century, and the Theory Era in the latter part of the 20th century, moving into the 21st century and the Era of Theory Utilization—and "recognizing the importance of a framework for critical thinking and decision making in professional nursing practice" (p. 10). As proposed by Fawcett (2006), nurses must embrace nursing knowledge in the form of explicit nursing conceptual models and theories and that "the use of distinctive *nursing* knowledge in research and practice is the hallmark of professional nursing" (p. 502). Recall the metaparadigm concepts. Borrowed theories may address the human beings, health, and the environment, but what of nursing? With collaborative practice, however, these theories provide a common ground and the opportunity for the application and sharing of middle-range theories. They also enable us to understand human nature, motivation, and development. But as noted by Chinn and Kramer (2004), always consider specific factors that influence a nursing situation.

Several classic theories have been applied in nursing to view the person, family, community, and group. We use Maslow's hierarchy of needs to view the person and basic human needs. Developmental theories have been applied across the human life span as we seek to understand the complexity of human behavior. In looking at the person or group, we have applied systems theory to understand the interaction of person and environment. The following section briefly describes selected theories that are applied in certain areas and have been used in the evolution of nursing models more specific to our metaparadigm concepts.

Maslow's Theory of Human Motivation and Hierarchy of Basic Needs

A theory widely used among disciplines is Maslow's theory of human motivation. In his original 1954 book, *Motivation and Personality*, Maslow described how his work emerged, and the work was published in segments in various journals and books. The book begins by presenting Maslow's philosophy as an approach to science. Human values are prevalent in the philosophy, and his worldview is described as holistic, functional, dynamic, and purposive. In his 1970 revised edition, Maslow reinforced his worldviews and described his theory as holistic-dynamic. He supported his original 16 propositions on motivation, on which his theory was based (see Chapter 10, on motivation in the teaching-learning process). This is a grand theory that views the complexity of human behavior, especially in relation to motivation of behavior. The theory of motivation is based on clinical and experimental data from psychology, psychiatry, education, and philosophy. It does not address specific nursing concerns except as they relate to human behavior with environmental influences.

Maslow's theory includes a hierarchical structure for human needs. This **hierarchy of needs** can be visualized as a pyramid (Fig. 3–2). At the base of the pyramid are the physiologic drives. Higher needs progress upward as safety, love and belonging, esteem, and self-actualization needs. Maslow (1954, 1970) described this as a "hierarchy of prepotency" to explain that the individual concentrates on the physiologic drives. The physiologic drives are considered the most powerful, but as physiologic needs are satisfied, higher needs emerge on which the individual focuses. This is the general structure for the hierarchy.

Individual differences are provided for in this theory. Some individuals have altered placement of needs in the hierarchy. Maslow (1970) described differences among individuals in placement of some of the higher needs, such as a reversal of esteem and love/belonging needs. In addition, individuals may have different levels of need satisfaction. For example, one person might meet the physiologic drives at a 75 percent level, whereas another person's level for satisfaction is 85 percent. Individual differences also apply to the emergence of higher needs. Maslow (1970) regarded this as a gradual process; one person's safety needs may begin to emerge when his or her physiologic needs are being met at 25 percent, whereas another person may not begin to satisfy his or her safety needs until

SELF-
ACTUALIZATION
Meeting one's
full potential

ESTEEM
Feeling competent,
strong self-worth

LOVE and BELONGINGNESS
Feeling worthy of affection and
social support

SAFETY
Feeling free from danger and risk,
secure in one's own environment

PHYSIOLOGIC
Adequate oxygen, food, and water

■ **Figure 3.2** Maslow's hierarchy of human needs.

30 percent of her physiologic needs are met. Levels of satisfaction and emergence of higher needs therefore occur at different points in different people, as do pain thresholds in different people.

Looking again at the theoretical hierarchy, we see at the bottom level of the pyramid the physiologic drives, including the need to maintain homeostasis and the needs of hunger and thirst, sleep and rest, activity and exercise, sexual gratification and sensory pleasure, and maternal responses (Maslow, 1970). Meeting the physiologic hunger drive is very different from meeting one's nutritional requirements or treating anxiety or depression with a chocolate bar. When the individual is truly hungry or thirsty, all energies and thoughts are directed to satisfying that drive for food or water. Consider the physiologic need of an individual with a chemical dependency. The person will focus all efforts on attaining the drug or addictive substance at the required level of satisfaction—while ignoring other needs, including the physiologic need for food or the next level of safety needs. When the physiologic drives and needs are relatively satisfied, higher-level needs emerge.

Safety needs are the next level of the hierarchy. Safety, both physical and emotional, must be achieved. Threats to a person's safety can become all-consuming. Think of an isolated person in an inner-city apartment whose fear for his safety motivates him to place bars on his windows and multiple chains and dead-bolt locks on his door. This person fears for his physical safety from a threat, real or imagined, of bodily harm. This is the main concern, not whether access is impeded in the case of a fire or accident. He places all focus on the quest for freedom from perceived danger.

Perceived safety can also be related to health, as with the fear of the client with chronic obstructive lung disease (COPD) to be near anyone who is coughing or sneezing. This person's safety need is to avoid a respiratory infection that could lead to pneumonia or even diminished oxygenation in an already compromised respiratory system. Even if the other person in the room is experiencing symptoms of a seasonal allergy, the individual with COPD seeks immediate escape from that environment because of the perceived danger of infection. Maslow (1954, 1970) also viewed safety needs more broadly in the need for the familiar and spiritual, religious, or philosophical meaning in life. He describes the use of rituals and ceremonial behaviors in children and individuals with psychological disorders as examples of focusing on safety needs.

Once the person satisfies safety needs, the focus turns to the need for love and belonging. Inclusion and affection are important needs, not the isolated sex act, which is a physiologic drive. Maslow (1970) described the normal person as having a hunger and striving for affectionate relations and a place in a group, as opposed to the maladjusted person (pp. 43–44). Love and affection are manifested in many ways and are individually defined.

Satisfying the need for belonging and love brings us to the next level, esteem needs. Esteem needs involve a sense of dignity, worth, and usefulness in life. Maslow (1970) described two sets of esteem needs: (1) the sense of self-worth, including perceptions of strength, achievement, competence, and confidence; and (2) the esteem of others, including perceptions of deserved respect, status, recognition, importance, and dignity (p. 45). Satisfying the sense of self-worth and respect allows the next, and highest, level of basic needs to emerge.

The need for self-actualization at the top of the pyramid is the desire for self-fulfillment. This is the sense of being able to do all that a person can to answer the "why" of his or her existence. Maslow (1970) defined self-actualization as "the full use and exploitation of talents, capacities, potentialities, etc., such [that] people seem to be fulfilling themselves and . . . developing to the full stature of which they are capable" (p. 150). Originally, Maslow (1954) proposed that self-actualized people include both older people and college students and children. But when he further examined the concept of self-actualization, he separated psychological health from self-actualization, which he limited to older people whose human potentialities have been realized and actualized (Maslow, 1970).

Maslow then developed support for his theory of basic needs and human actions using case studies and other research. Through observation of people, he proposed specific phenomena that are determined by basic gratification of cognitive-affective, cognitive, character traits, interpersonal, and miscellaneous needs. He cited characteristics of people in relation to the hierarchy. For example, the following characteristics of self-actualized people emerged from Maslow's (1970) research and analysis of historical figures, public people, selected college students, and children:

1. More efficient and comfortable perceptions of reality
2. Acceptance of self, others, and nature
3. Spontaneity, simplicity, and naturalness in thoughts and behaviors
4. Problem-centered rather than ego-centered
5. Desire for detachment, solitude, and privacy
6. Autonomy with independence of culture and environment
7. Continued freshness of appreciation
8. Mystic and oceanic feelings with limitless horizons
9. Genuine desire to help people
10. Deeper and more profound interpersonal relationships
11. Democratic character structure
12. Strong ethical sense that discriminates means/ends and good/evil
13. Philosophical and unhostile sense of humor
14. Creativeness
15. Resistance to enculturation with an inner detachment. (pp. 203–228)

Maslow created further hypotheses for testing. He described cases that diverged from his theory, such as the martyr who ignores survival needs for a principle. He called for further research, hypothesizing that satisfying basic needs earlier in life allows the individual to weather deprivation easier in later life (Maslow, 1954, p. 99). Maslow's work continued until his death in 1970. His hierarchy of needs has endured, and its applications have

been extended in health care, education, industry, and marketing to understand people and their motivators. Needs related to individual, environmental, and health concerns are applicable to the nursing discipline. However, this theory is still a grand theory and does not address the specific domain of nursing.

⊙ N L I N E C O N S U L T

Learn more on Maslow and his work at **http://www.maslow.com**

Developmental Theories

A group of theories widely used in health care and education are the **developmental theories**. These middle-range theories address personality (Erikson and Havighurst), cognitive (Piaget), and moral (Kohlberg) development using a life-span perspective. This perspective is based on progression and complexity in motor, personal-social, cognitive, or moral behavior. A brief review of each of the theories demonstrates how the theorist moved from a philosophy or worldview to identify concepts, propositions, and a model or theory based on observations, existing research, or case study presentations. Common to the developmental theories are predictable steps or stages through which the individual progresses during the life cycle. This is a building process. These theories are based largely on research through observation or case studies. Subsequent applications and research have been guided by the use of these theories to explain more specific phenomena or test hypotheses.

Personality Development

Erikson's (1963) eight ages of man represents a theory of psychosocial personality development in which the individual proceeds through critical periods in a step-by-step or epigenetic process (Fig. 3–3). This theory has been and continues to be used widely in health care and psychology. In offering the theory, Erikson presented his philosophy and case studies with Freudian and neo-Freudian applications. Each stage has positive and negative aspects that are defined and described. The basic goal is for the individual to develop a favorable ratio of the positive aspects for a healthy ego. Erikson (1963) further described basic virtues and essential strengths for each of his "ages" or stages of development. These strengths and basic virtues define the positive aspects of ego development required in each stage. Propositions are developed for each of the stages. This theory is supported mainly by case study, with suggestions and encouragement of further hypotheses for research and testing. Erikson's theory has been used

AGES	STRENGTHS & VIRTUES	DEVELOPMENTAL STAGE
8. Ego Integrity vs. Despair	Renunciation & Wisdom	Older Adulthood
7. Generativity vs. Stagnation	Production & Care	Middle Adulthood
6. Intimacy vs. Isolation	Affiliation & Love	Young Adulthood
5. Identity vs. Role Confusion	Devotion & Fidelity	Adolescence
4. Industry vs. Inferiority	Method & Competence	School Age
3. Initiative vs. Guilt	Direction & Purpose	Preschool
2. Autonomy vs. Shame & Doubt	Self-control & Will Power	Toddler
1. Trust vs. Mistrust	Drive & Hope	Infancy

■ **Figure 3.3** Erikson's (1963) eight ages of man.

widely in nursing to foster positive ego development and empowerment in individuals. Although this theory does not specifically address the domain of nursing, common concerns include the human beings, the environment, and psychosocial health.

ONLINE CONSULT

Learn more about child development and Erikson's eight ages at
http://www.childdevelopmentinfo.com/ development/erickson.shtml

Havighurst's developmental tasks and education represent another theory of personality development that includes principles of cognitive and moral development as well. In this perspective, the individual proceeds through six stages, accomplishing critical tasks. Havighurst (1972) described his philosophy, including the origins of the concept, and proposed a method for analyzing individual developmental tasks based on the following five criteria: (1) nature or definition, (2) biologic basis, (3) psychological basis, (4) cultural basis, and (5) educational implications (pp. 17–18). Table 3–1 illustrates the tasks for each of the six age groups.

Although descriptions of the tasks represent some gender bias and cultural limitations, the concept's biologic and psychological bases are applicable to health care. The tasks represent major milestones in biologic, psychological, emotional, and cognitive functioning or development that individuals must negotiate as they progress through life. Human beings, environmental, and health promotion concerns are apparent in the lifespan perspective. Age-specific tasks relate well to activities of daily living during specific life stages and can easily be incorporated in care planning.

Cognitive Development

Piaget's theory of cognitive development focuses on the development of the intellect. Piaget was an example of a self-actualized person. Moving from the publication

of his first monograph on birds at age 10 years, he detailed the development of the intellect in children through observations. His techniques were sometimes criticized by the scientific community. But his theory has since been accepted and used in practice and research by many students and professionals. Piaget's theory looks at the innate and environmental influences on the development of the intellect. This theory has four major periods of cognitive development: sensorimotor, preoperational thought, concrete operations, and formal operations (Table 3–2).

Within his theory, Piaget provided us with the concepts of schema, object permanence, assimilation, and accommodation. *Schemas* are patterns of thought or behavior that evolve into more complexity as more information is obtained through assimilation and accommodation. *Object permanence*, the knowledge that something still exists when it is out of sight, develops when the child is between 9 and 10 months of age. *Assimilation* is the acquisition and incorporation of new information into the individual's existing cognitive and behavioral structures. *Accommodation* is the change in the individual's cognitive and behavioral patterns based on the new information acquired. Piaget's theory has been translated and applied worldwide and across disciplines. His work continued until his death in 1980, and further research and theory are still evolving from his contributions.

Piaget's work concentrated on cognitive development in children, including views on moral development. As such, it is more limited but has provided major insight into working with children. Applications are seen in health teaching, especially in chronic or terminal illness situations. But with these limitations, it can address only a portion of the domain of concern to nursing.

Moral Development

Kohlberg's theory of moral development was an outgrowth of Piaget's work on cognitive development in children. Kohlberg's extensive work on moral development (Kohlberg, 1984; Kohlberg et al., 1987) is based

Table 3.1

Havighurst's Developmental Tasks

Stages	Tasks
I. Infancy and Early childhood	1. Learning to walk 2. Learning to take solid foods 3. Learning to talk 4. Learning to control the elimination of body wastes 5. Learning sex differences and sexual modesty 6. Forming concepts and learning language to describe social and physical reality 7. Getting ready to read 8. Learning to distinguish right and wrong and beginning to develop a conscience
II. Middle childhood	1. Learning physical skills necessary for ordinary games 2. Building wholesome attitudes toward oneself as a growing organism 3. Learning to get along with age-mates 4. Learning an appropriate masculine/feminine social role 5. Developing fundamental skills in reading, writing, and calculating 6. Developing concepts necessary for everyday living 7. Developing conscience, morality, and a scale of values 8. Achieving personal independence 9. Developing attitudes toward social groups and institutions
III. Adolescence	1. Achieving new and more mature relations with age-mates of both sexes 2. Achieving a masculine or feminine social role 3. Accepting one's physique and using the body effectively 4. Achieving emotional independence of parents and other adults 5. Preparing for marriage and family life 6. Preparing for an economic career 7. Acquiring a set of values and an ethical system as a guide to behavior 8. Desiring and achieving socially responsible behavior
IV. Early adulthood	1. Selecting a mate 2. Learning to live with a marriage partner 3. Starting a family 4. Rearing children 5. Managing a home 6. Getting started in an occupation 7. Taking on civic responsibility 8. Finding a congenial social group
V. Middle adulthood	1. Assisting teenage children to become responsible and happy adults 2. Achieving adult social and civic responsibility 3. Reaching and maintaining satisfactory performance in one's occupational career 4. Developing adult leisure-time activities 5. Relating oneself to one's spouse as a person 6. Adjusting and accepting the physiologic changes of middle age 7. Adjusting to aging parents
VI. Later maturity	1. Adjusting to decreasing physical strength and health 2. Adjusting to retirement and reduced income 3. Adjusting to death of a spouse 4. Establishing an explicit association with one's age group 5. Adopting and adapting social roles in a flexible way 6. Establishing satisfactory physical living arrangements

Source: *Developmental Tasks and Education* by Robert J. Havighurst. Copyright © 1948 by the University of Chicago. Copyright © 1950 by Robert J. Havighurst. Copyright © (1952) by David McKay Company, Inc. Copyright © 1972 by David McKay Company. Reprinted by permission of Addison-Wesley Education Publishers, Inc.

Table 3.2

Piaget's Theory of Cognitive Development

Period of Cognitive Development	Age	Stage Description
Sensorimotor Stages		
■ Reflexive	Birth–1 month	Use of primitive reflexes, such as sucking and rooting
■ Primary circular reactions	1–4 months	Repeating an event for the result, such as thumb in mouth
■ Secondary circular reactions	4–10 months	Combining events for a result, such as kicking a mobile over crib
■ Coordination of secondary schema	10–12 months	Creating a behavior for some result, such as standing in crib to reach mobile
■ Tertiary circular reactions	12–18 months	Looking for similar results from varying behaviors, such as shaking crib and jumping to observe movements of mobile
■ Representational thought begins	18–24 months	Symbolic representation in thought, such as hanging objects to create mobile
Preoperational	2–7 years	Making overgeneralizations, such as all cats are named Tiger; egocentric Focuses only on one concrete attribute Magical thought and symbolic play present
Concrete operations	7–11 years	Logical and reversible thought appears; conservation of matter and numbers
Formal operations	After 11 years	Theoretical and hypothetical thinking now possible; higher-order mathematics and reasoning

on research with children given scenarios to describe reactions and make judgments. He initially studied boys 10 to 16 years old from Chicago, later adding research with children of both genders and different backgrounds. Kohlberg's theory consists of six stages grouped into three major levels: preconventional, conventional, and postconventional (Kohlberg, 1984), illustrated in Table 3–3.

Kohlberg's theory confers major insight into moral development. He provided the theoretical structure, the supportive research, and applications in educational practice. The individual progresses through the levels and stages, not as a natural process, but through intellectual stimulation with a central focus on moral justice. This requires thinking about moral problems and issues. Further research and practices have been

based on this theory and are ongoing. Consider the usefulness of this theory when you are working with a child or adolescent whose parent was recently diagnosed with a terminal illness.

As with Piagetian theory, Kohlberg's theory is limited to a specific area of development. The focus is on human beings, such as the child, with ramifications for adult life. Environmental (e.g., social and cultural) factors provide insight for social and psychological health. The limitation to moral development addresses only a portion of the domain of concern to nursing.

Many developmental models are used and applied in nursing. Examine the conceptual models and theories presented in Chapter 4 for their application of developmental concepts. Several nursing theories have a decidedly developmental focus, whether as a main

Table 3.3

Kohlberg's Theory of Moral Development

Level	Stage	Stage Description
Level I: Preconventional morality	1. Heteronomous morality	Egocentrically applies a fixed set of rules from authorities, e.g., parents, to avoid punishment
	2. Individualism, purpose, and exchange	Sees that different individuals have different rules, e.g., parents and teachers, but selection based on individual interests with some fair exchange
Level II: Conventional morality	3. Interpersonal expectations, relationships, and conformity	Motives of other person now emerge when considering right and wrong; use of the Golden Rule in considerations
	4. Social system and conscience	The good of society as a whole now emerges with the individual having certain roles and rules in the system.
Level III: Postconventional morality	5. Social contract and individual rights	Believes in upholding laws and legal contracts, looking at the greatest good for greatest number; sees but cannot deal well with ethical-legal conflicts
	6. Universal ethical principles	Principles of justice and human rights are followed and upheld as a personal and universal ethical system.

Source: Adapted from Kohlberg, L. (1984). *Essays in moral development: Vol. II. The psychology of moral development* (pp. 174–176). San Francisco: Harper & Row, with permission.

component, as in Watson's theory, or with specific concepts included, defined, and built on, as in King's model.

A life-span, developmental, or life-processes focus has major relevance for nursing, because we view human beings in the context of environment and effects on health status. The interrelationships with health and nursing are complex and must be specified for their applicability to the domain of nursing.

Systems Theory

Perhaps the most widely used theory in multiple disciplines is **systems theory**. Systems have been in existence for ages, but in the late 1930s, Bertalanffy introduced systems theory to represent an aspect of reality. Thus, general system theory was incorporated in the paradigms of many scientific communities. This is a grand theory, wide in scope, that has generated numerous theories in many disciplines. Bertalanffy (1968) explained the wide applicability in many scientific communities as the various disciplines

became concerned with "wholeness," not just focusing on isolated parts, but dealing with the interrelationships among them and between the parts and the whole. A system generally contains the following basic components: input, output, boundary, environment, and feedback. Figure 3–4 illustrates a basic view of a simple system.

The initial step in understanding and applying systems theory is to view the grand theory. Bertalanffy (1968) defined a *system* as a complex of interacting elements and proposed that every living organism is essentially an open system. The general system theory applies the following principles to human and organizational systems:

1. *Wholeness:* This indicates that the whole is more than merely the sum of its parts. To understand the whole, one must understand the components and their interactions with each other and the environment.

2. *Hierarchical order:* Some form of hierarchy exists in the system's components, structure, and functions.

Environment

Input ---------> ¦System¦ ----------> Output

Environment

Environment

Feedback

■ **Figure 3.4** General systems model: A simple open system.

3. *Exchange of information and matter (openness):* In an open system, there is an exchange and flow of information and matter with the environment through some boundary that surrounds the system. Inputs come through the boundary from the environment, are transformed through system processes (throughputs), and are sent as outputs through the boundary back into the environment. This exchange of information and matter is goal-oriented, whether to maintain the steady state or to fulfill the functions of the system. An important component of this process is feedback from the environment.

4. *Progressive differentiation:* Differentiation within the system leads to self-organization. Applying the laws of thermodynamics, entropy is a measure of order or organization in the system in the process of seeking equilibrium or some final goal. In an open system, entropy is decreased or negative, allowing for differentiation and self-organization.

5. *Equifinality:* In open systems, the final state can be reached from different initial conditions and in different ways. Initial conditions do not necessarily determine the final state or outcome of the system.

6. *Teleology:* Behavior in the system is directed toward some purpose or goal, as a human characteristic.

Environmental influences are a major consideration in health care. Systems theory provides a useful framework with which to visualize some phenomenon (the system), focusing on the components, structure, and functions as the internal environment (throughputs), and influenced by (inputs and feedback) and influencing (outputs) the environment. It is important to analyze the system carefully for all component parts, structures, and functions. Recall that the basis for general systems theory is that "the whole is greater than the sum of the parts." This brings us to the need for a precise analysis of interrelationships among components and between the parts and the entire system. In addition, an open system has permeable boundaries receiving input and feedback from the environment. Problems occur when environmental factors are unknown, unclear, or ignored. Consider the broad health-service system. Because of

Institute of Medicine reports beginning in 1998, we have become greatly concerned about safety in health care. Systems issues have been a major focus, but moving from a culture of blaming individual practitioners, the challenge became one of improving components in the system, input, feedback, and outputs. In addition, the broader health care environment and societal influences are included and visualized as crossing the system boundaries of an individual hospital setting.

In nursing, systems theory and various applications have been used to explain organizations, nursing and health-care delivery, and groups of people. Several nursing models are based on systems theory. Johnson's behavioral systems conceptual model views the person as a behavioral system and nursing as an external force. It exemplifies how a grand theory (general systems theory) from another scientific community provided a basis for developing the conceptual model of nursing (Johnson's behavioral systems). Specificity to the metaparadigm concepts and interrelationships unique to nursing have provided the basis for the nursing conceptual framework. Further delineation of concepts and propositions leads to more specific nursing theory. Neuman's health-care model, Roy's adaptation model, and King's conceptual framework and theory of goal attainment are examples of nursing conceptual models and theories based on systems models. Other nursing models use various components of general systems theory. Further applications of systems theory are evident in subsequent sections on management in organizations and change.

Theoretical Challenges and a Paradigm Shift

Galbraith (1984) identified conventional wisdom as the structure of ideas that is based on acceptability, and to the people as their reality as they see and articulate it (p. 16). These ideas that people generally consider as "truths" can be obstacles to new theories and the development of new knowledge. Conventional wisdom may be that the current paradigm is on the brink of change. We must be open to new theories with new technology. Knowledge expansion can proceed at a much greater rate, as we have now seen with quantum physics or quantum mechanics.

For years, Newtonian physics provided the conventional wisdom of the three laws of motion: (1) inertia (objects in motion tend to stay in motion, and objects at rest tend to stay at rest unless there is interference from an outside force), (2) net force (the force on an object is mathematically equal to its mass times acceleration), (3) reciprocal actions (for every action there is an equal and opposite reaction).

Based on the work of Galileo and others, Newton's theories from the 17th century prevailed until the 20th century with the addition of Einstein's theory of relativity and the discovery of **quantum theory.** As Laughlin (2005) points out, although applicable to the macroscopic world, Newton's laws are incorrect at the atomic scale (p. 31). How we formerly pictured an atom, as a Newtonian-like solar system, is outdated and incorrect. Researchers and theorists have moved from classical physics to the era of the quantum.

We hear a good deal about the "quantum" nature of our world and universe. But it is all evolving as we develop new insight into the makeup of matter and how particles behave. A quantum is merely an energy bundle at the atomic and subatomic level—neutrons, protons, and electrons. The measurement of the quantum requires high level mathematical computations looking at statistical probabilities of matter and waves. Hence, the discoveries from classic mechanics to quantum mechanics have occurred in areas of physics, chemistry, computers, and biology. This has provided the basis for our certain transformations in health care, such as the introduction of the laser and magnetic resonance imaging (MRI). Biotechnology and advances in physical science will continue with our quest for discovery and knowledge. As noted by Nobel Laureate Robert Laughlin (2005), however, we have experienced a paradigm shift, moving from a reductionist view of science to one of emergence, and, "as in all other human activities, it is necessary in science to take stock now and then and reevaluate what one deeply understands and what one does not" (p. 13).

The language and concepts of quantum theory extend beyond the atom as we look at issues of holism, duality, uncertainty, causality, and probabilities in daily life and practice. Recognition and understanding of the paradigm shift is essential for the health sciences as we seek new knowledge and improvements in patient-care outcomes.

THE IMPACT OF THEORY ON PRACTICE

Alligood (2006a) proposes that "given our history and the challenges of today, utilization and application of nursing's theoretical works are understood to be vital

organizing structures for the critical thinking necessary in professional nursing practice" (p. 3). We use theory every day in our personal and professional lives, from the basic principles of asepsis in hygiene and standard precautions, to understanding the complex communication channels of the organizational system in which we practice.

Theory, practice, and research are interrelated and interdependent. We need theory to guide practice predictably and effectively. We need research to support the significance and usefulness of the theory, because the dynamic nature of our metaparadigm concepts of human beings, environment, health, and nursing makes theories tentative and subject to refinement and revision. Professional practice must provide the questions for study based on problems and phenomena relevant to the discipline. Again, recall that nursing is a profession and a scientific community. We practice using principles provided by our metaparadigm and theoretical bases. This furnishes us with the tools for critical thinking, provision of care, education, administration, research, and interdisciplinary collaboration. We have a paradigm that provides the models for problems and solutions in our knowledge base and practice community in line with Kuhn's (1970) descriptions of a paradigm. Our paradigms and theories are designed to address problems and solutions in practice, or we need to shift to a new structure with different theories and paradigms to explain our concerns for people, environments, health, and nursing.

The theory on which we base practice must be compatible with and must correspond to the phenomena of professional nursing practice. To ensure that the goals of theory and practice are consistent, Alligood (2006b) recommends the following considerations for selecting a framework for practice:

1. Name your values and beliefs held true about nursing.
2. Name your philosophy of beliefs on the metaparadigm concepts.
3. Look at definitions of the metaparadigm concepts in selected models.
4. Select two to three frameworks that are consistent with your beliefs.
5. Look at the assumptions of the models.
6. Apply the models to your practice area—do they work?
7. Compare the models, looking at client focus, nursing action, and outcomes.
8. Read the literature on applications of the selected models to practice.
9. Select the best model appropriate to your practice and implement it. (p. 60)

But recall that conventional wisdom can be an obstacle to the discovery of new knowledge. Practice models are subject to change as new information is discovered and as client needs change. The paradigm concepts must be in a constant state of evaluation to ensure that the model of practice is current and based on nursing science.

In the next chapter, conceptual models and theories unique to nursing are discussed. These models are the guides to practice in our highly complex profession. Implementing models for practice, whether unique to nursing or adapted, is a necessary but arduous and time-consuming task. The process is worth the effort to ensure quality care for recipients, but requires many of the skills addressed in subsequent chapters.

INTERACTIVE EXERCISES

Go to the Intranet site and complete the interactive exercises provided for this Chapter.

K E Y   P O I N T S

■ Kerlinger and Lee (2000) define a theory as "a set of interrelated constructs (concepts), definitions, and propositions that present a systematic view of phenomena by specifying relations among variables, with the purpose of explaining and predicting the phenomena" (p. 11).

■ A model is a graphic representation of some phenomena. A theoretical model provides a visual description of the theory, using limited narrative and displaying components and relationships symbolically. A framework is another means of providing a structural view of the concepts and relationships proposed in a theory.

■ A concept is a view or idea we hold about something, ranging from something highly concrete to something highly abstract. A construct is a more complex idea package of some phenomena. Definitions of concepts and constructs are theoretical or conceptual. An operational definition states precisely what we view as phenomena and how they can be measured as variables in a practice or research situation.

■ Propositions in a theory are the descriptions and relationships among the constructs (or concepts) that propose how the concepts are linked and relate to each other and to the total theoretical structure.

■ Dickoff and James (1968) developed a classic position paper proposing four levels of nursing theory: factor-isolating, factor-relating, situation-relating, and situation-producing theories.

■ Theories are classified as grand, middle-range, or limited (practice) on the basis of their scope or breadth of coverage of phenomena.

■ Theory description is a careful, nonjudgmental analysis of the component parts of a theory—its assumptions, concepts, definitions, propositions, context, and scope.

■ Theory evaluation requires thoughtful interpretation relative to the clarity, significance, consistency, empirical support, and usefulness in explaining a phenomenon of concern.

■ Maslow's theory of human motivation and hierarchy of basic needs proposes a hierarchical structure for human needs.

■ Developmental theories are widely used in nursing and other health-care disciplines and include Erikson's ages of psychosocial development, Havighurst's developmental tasks, Piaget's theory of cognitive development, and Kohlberg's theory of moral development.

■ A system generally contains the following basic component parts: input, output, boundary, environment, and feedback. Bertalanffy's (1968) general system theory is a grand theory applied to many disciplines.

■ Quantum theory, based on quantum physics, uses statistical probabilities for the actions of atomic and subatomic matter and waves and has provided some of the basis for advances in technology.

■ Theory, practice, and research are interrelated and interdependent. When we are selecting a theory on which to base practice, the theory must be compatible and correspond to the phenomena of professional nursing practice.

Thought and Discussion Questions

1. Consider the following statement by Barnum (1990) describing early nursing theories: "A high number of [boundary] overlaps occur in the discipline of nursing because it often attempts to deal holistically with a phenomenon (man) that has previously been dealt with in compartmentalized ways by other disciplines" (p. 218). What did she mean by "holistically"? How do you think other disciplines may deal with the human being in a compartmentalized way?

2. Identify individuals who you think are self-actualized, and explain why.

3. Identify a theory used in your practice setting. Identify the concepts (constructs), how the component concepts are defined, the propositions that link the concepts, and the aims of this theory.

4. Describe how theory is used in your practice setting, and propose how it could be used further.

5. Review the Chapter Thought located on the first page of the chapter, and discuss it in the context of the contents of the chapter.

☐ REFERENCES

Alligood, M. R. (2006a). The nature of knowledge needed for nursing practice. In A. M. Tomey & M. R. Alligood (Eds.), *Nursing theory: Utilization and application* (3rd ed., pp. 1–15). St. Louis: Mosby.

Alligood, M. R. (2006b). Philosophies, models, and theories: Critical thinking structures. In A. M. Tomey & M. R. Alligood (Eds.), *Nursing theory: Utilization and application* (3rd ed., pp. 43–65). St. Louis: Mosby.

Alligood, M. R., & Tomey, A. M. (2006). Introduction to nursing theory: History, terminology, and analysis. In A. M. Tomey & M. R. Alligood (Eds.), *Nursing theorists and their work* (6th ed, pp. 3–13). St. Louis: Mosby/Elsevier.

Barnum, B. J. S. (1990). *Nursing theory: Analysis, application, evaluation* (3rd ed.). Glenview, IL: Scott, Foresman/Little, Brown Higher Education.

Barnum, B. J. S. (1994). *Nursing theory: Analysis, application, evaluation* (4th ed.). Philadelphia: J. B. Lippincott.

Barnum, B. S. (1998). *Nursing theory: Analysis, application, evaluation* (5th ed.). Philadelphia: Lippincott Williams & Wilkins.

Bertalanffy, L. V. (1968). *General system theory: Foundations, development, applications.* New York: George Braziller.

Chinn, P. L., & Kramer, M. K. (2004). *Integrated knowledge development in nursing* (6th ed.). St. Louis: Mosby.

Dickoff, J., & James, P. (1968). A theory of theories: A position paper. *Nursing Research, 17,* 197–203.

Erikson, E. H. (1963). *Childhood and society* (2nd ed.). New York: W. W. Norton.

Fawcett, J. (2000). *Analysis and evaluation of contemporary nursing knowledge: Nursing models and theories.* Philadelphia: F. A. Davis.

Fawcett, J. (2005). *Contemporary nursing knowledge: Analysis and evaluation of nursing models and theories.* (2nd ed.). Philadelphia: F. A. Davis.

Fawcett, J. (2006). Nursing philosophies, models, and theories: A focus on the future. In A. M. Tomey & M. R. Alligood (Eds.), *Nursing theory: Utilization and application* (3rd ed., pp. 499–518). St. Louis: Mosby.

Galbraith, J. K. (1984). *The affluent society.* Boston: Houghton Mifflin.

Glanz, K., Rimer, B. K., & Lewis, F. M. (Eds.). (2002). *Health behavior and health education: Theory, research, and practice* (3rd ed). San Francisco: Jossey-Bass.

Havighurst, R. J. (1972). *Developmental tasks and education* (3rd ed.). New York: David McKay.

Kerlinger, F. N., & Lee, H. B. (2000). *Foundations of behavioral research* (4th ed.). Belmont, CA: Wadsworth Thompson Learning.

Kohlberg, L. (1984). *Essays in moral development: Vol. II. The psychology of moral development.* San Francisco: Harper & Row.

Kohlberg, L., DeVries, R., Fein, G., Hart, D., Mayer, R., Noam, G., Snarey, J., & Wertsch, J. (1987). *Child psychology and childhood education: A cognitive-developmental view.* New York: Longman.

Kuhn, T. S. (1970). *The structure of scientific revolutions* (2nd ed.). Chicago: University of Chicago Press.

Laughlin, R. B. (2005). *A different universe: Reinventing physics from the bottom down.* New York: Basic Books.

Leininger, M. M. (2006). The culture care theory. In M. Leininger & M. R. McFarland (Eds.), *Culture care diversity and universality: A worldwide nursing theory* (2nd ed., pp. 1–41). Boston: Jones and Bartlett.

Maslow, A. H. (1954). *Motivation and personality.* New York: Harper & Brothers.

Maslow, A. H. (1970). *Motivation and personality* (2nd ed.). New York: Harper & Row.

Merton, R. K. (1957). *Social theory and social structure* (Rev. ed.). Glencoe, IL: Free Press.

☐ BIBLIOGRAPHY

Hardy, M. E. (1974). Theories: Components, development, evaluation. *Nursing Research, 23*, 100–107.

Lightman, A. (2000). *Great ideas in physics*. New York: McGraw-Hill.

Power, F. C., Higgins, A., & Kohlberg, L. (1989). *Lawrence Kohlberg's approach to moral education*. New York: Columbia University.

Singer, D. G., & Revenson, T. A. (1998). *A Piaget primer: How a child thinks* (Rev. ed.). Madison, CT: International Universities Press.

Wood, A. F., & Alligood, M. R. (2006). Nursing models: Normal science for nursing practice. In A. M. Tomey & M. R. Alligood (Eds.), *Nursing theory: Utilization and application* (3rd ed., pp. 17–42). St. Louis: Mosby.

☐ ONLINE RESOURCES

Books by A.H. Maslow
http://www.maslow.com

Jean Piaget Society
http://www.piaget.org

Nursing Theories
http://www.nurses.info/nursing_theory.htm

NurseScribe©
http://www.enursescribe.com

Transcultural Nursing Society
http://www.tcns.org

■ Jacqueline **Fawcett**   ■ Barbara **Swoyer**

Evolution and Use of Formal Nursing Knowledge

> **❝** *[T]he need to articulate what nursing is and what nursing can be has never been more critical.* **❞**

(Fawcett, 2005, p. v). Portions of this chapter were adapted from Fawcett, J. (2005). *Contemporary nursing knowledge: Analysis and evaluation of nursing models and theories* (2nd ed.). F. A. Davis; and Fawcett, J. (2005). Appendix N–2: Conceptual models and theories of nursing. In *Taber's cyclopedic medical dictionary* (20th ed., pp. 2588–2618). Philadelphia: F. A. Davis, with permission.

Chapter Objectives

On completion of this chapter, the reader will be able to:

1. Describe the meaning of formal nursing knowledge as the basis for professional nursing practice.
2. Identify the definitions and different functions of conceptual models and theories.
3. Discuss the advantages of using explicit conceptual models of nursing and nursing theories to guide professional nursing practice.
4. Apply a conceptual model of nursing or nursing theory to a particular practice situation.

Key Terms

Formal Nursing Knowledge

Nursing Knowledge

Conceptual Models of Nursing
Johnson's Behavioral System Model
King's Conceptual System
Levine's Conservation Model
Neuman's Systems Model
Orem's Self-Care Framework

Rogers' Science of Unitary Human Beings
Roy's Adaptation Model

Grand Theories of Nursing
Leininger's Theory of Culture Care Diversity and Universality
Newman's Theory of Health as Expanding Consciousness
Parse's Theory of Humanbecoming

Middle-Range Nursing Theories
Orlando's Theory of the Deliberative Nursing Process
Peplau's Theory of Interpersonal Relations
Watson's Theory of Human Caring

This chapter presents a discussion of the evolution of nursing knowledge—as it has been formalized—in conceptual models of nursing and nursing theories, and identifies the impact of that knowledge on professional nursing practice.

FORMAL NURSING KNOWLEDGE

Conceptual models of nursing and nursing theories represent formal nursing knowledge. That knowledge was organized by several nurse scholars who devoted a great deal of time to observing clinical situations, thinking about what is important to nursing in those situations, and then testing their thoughts by conducting nursing research (Fawcett, 1999). Nursing knowledge continues to evolve as nurse researchers and practicing nurses use conceptual models and theories to guide their research and practice and then report the results at conferences and in publications. Consequently, all nurses can contribute to the evolution of nursing knowledge.

Nursing Defined

Nightingale's (1859) book, *Notes on Nursing: What It Is, and What It Is Not*, contains the first ideas that can be considered formal nursing knowledge. More than 100 years later, Henderson (1966) published her definition of nursing, continuing the evolution of formal nursing knowledge. Although the intervening years were filled with many ideas about nursing, most of those ideas unfortunately were not presented as formal conceptual models and theories.

Florence Nightingale's Notes on Nursing

Nightingale's ideas about nursing, first published in 1859, represent the beginning of formal nursing knowledge. Nightingale maintained that every woman is a nurse because every woman, at some time in her life, has charge of the personal health of someone. Nightingale equated knowledge of nursing with knowledge of sanitation. The focus of nursing knowledge was how to keep the body free from disease or in such a condition that it could recover from disease. According to Nightingale, nursing ought to signify the proper use of fresh air, light, warmth, cleanliness, quiet, and the proper selection and administration of diet—all at the least expense of vital power to the patient; that is, she maintained that the purpose of nursing was to put the patient in the best condition for nature to act on him or her. She also asserted that nursing practice encompasses care of both well and sick people, and that nursing actions focus on both patients and their environments. Her 13 "hints" provided the boundaries of nursing practice (Box 4–1).

Box 4.1 Nightingale's 13 Hints

1. *Ventilation and Warming*: The nurse must be concerned first with keeping the air that patients breathe as pure as the external air, without chilling them.
2. *Health of Houses:* Attention to pure air, pure water, efficient drainage, cleanliness, and light will secure the health of houses.
3. *Petty Management:* All the results of good nursing may be negated by not knowing how to manage what you do when you are there and what shall be done when you are not there.
4. *Noise:* Unnecessary noise, or noise that creates an expectation in the mind, is that which hurts patients. Anything that wakes patients suddenly out of their sleep will invariably put them into a state of greater excitement, do them more serious and lasting mischief, than any continuous noise, however loud.
5. *Variety:* The nerves of the sick suffer from seeing the same walls, the same ceiling, the same surroundings during a long confinement to one or two rooms. The majority of cheerful cases are to be found among those patients who are not confined to one room, whatever their suffering, and the majority of depressed cases are seen among those subjected to a long monotony of objects about them.
6. *Taking Food:* The nurse should be conscious of patients' diets and remember how much food each patient has had and ought to have each day.
7. *What Food?:* To watch for the opinions the patient's stomach gives, rather than to read "analyses of foods," is the business of all those who have to decide what the patient should eat.
8. *Bed and Bedding*: The patient should have a clean bed every 12 hours. The bed should be narrow, so that the patient does not feel "out of humanity's reach." The bed should not be so high that the patient cannot easily get in and out of it. The bed should be in the lightest spot in the room, preferably near a window. Pillows should be used to support the back below the breathing apparatus, to allow shoulders room to fall back, and to support the head without throwing it forward.

(box continues on page 52)

Box 4.1 Nightingale's 13 Hints (continued)

9. *Light:* With the sick, second only to their need of fresh air is their need of light. Light, especially direct sunlight, has a purifying effect on the air of a room.
10. *Cleanliness of Rooms and Walls:* The greater part of nursing consists in preserving cleanliness. The inside air can be kept clean only by excessive care to rid rooms and their furnishings of the organic matter and dust with which they become saturated. Without cleanliness, you cannot have all the effects of ventilation; without ventilation, you can have no thorough cleanliness.
11. *Personal Cleanliness:* Nurses should always remember that if they allow patients to remain unwashed or to remain in clothing saturated with perspiration or other excretion, they are interfering injuriously with the natural processes of health just as much as if they were to give their patients a dose of slow poison.
12. *Chattering Hopes and Advices:* There is scarcely a greater worry that invalids have to endure than the incurable hopes of their friends. All friends, visitors, and attendants of the sick should avoid the practice of attempting to cheer the sick by making light of their danger and by exaggerating their probabilities of recovery.
13. *Observation of the Sick:* The most important practical lesson nurses can learn is what to observe, how to observe, which symptoms indicate improvement, which indicate the reverse, which are important, which are not, and which are the evidence of neglect and what kind of neglect.

Source: Nightingale, F. (1859). *Notes on nursing: What it is, and what it is not.* London: Harrison and Sons.
  [Commemorative edition printed 1992, Philadelphia: J. B. Lippincott]

Virginia Henderson's Definition of Nursing

Henderson (1966) contributed to the evolution of nursing knowledge by providing a definition that has been accepted around the world. According to Henderson, the unique function of the nurse is to help individuals, sick or well, to perform those activities contributing to health or its recovery (or to peaceful death) that they would perform unaided if they had the necessary strength, will, or knowledge, and to do so in such a way as to help those individuals gain independence as soon as possible. Henderson maintained that the practice of nursing requires nurses to know and understand patients by putting themselves in the place of the patients. Nurses should not take at face value everything that patients say, but rather should interact with patients to ascertain their true feelings. Basic nursing care involves helping the patient perform certain activities (Box 4–2).

CONCEPTUAL MODELS OF NURSING

The terms *conceptual model, conceptual framework, conceptual system, paradigm,* and *disciplinary matrix* are frequently used interchangeably and have the same definition and functions.

Definition

A conceptual model is defined as a set of relatively abstract and general concepts that address the phenomena of central interest to a discipline, the statements that broadly describe those concepts, and the statements that assert relatively abstract and general relations between two or more of the concepts (Fawcett, 2005).

Each conceptual model presents a particular perspective about the phenomena of interest to a particular discipline, such as nursing. Conceptual models of nursing present diverse perspectives of human

Box 4.2 Virginia Henderson's Activities of Nursing

- Breathe normally.
- Eat and drink adequately.
- Eliminate body wastes.
- Move and maintain desirable postures.
- Sleep and rest.
- Select suitable clothes, and dress and undress.
- Maintain body temperature within normal range by adjusting clothing and modifying the environment.
- Keep the body clean and well groomed and protect the integument.
- Avoid dangers in the environment and avoid injuring others.
- Communicate with others in expressing emotions, needs, fears, or opinions.
- Worship according to one's faith.
- Work in such a way that there is a sense of accomplishment.
- Play or participate in various forms of recreation.
- Learn, discover, or satisfy the curiosity that leads to normal development and health, and use the available health facilities.

beings—including individuals, families and other groups, and communities—who are participants in nursing; the environment of the nursing participant, and the environment in which nursing practice occurs; the health condition of the nursing participant; and the definition and goals of nursing as well as the nursing process or practice methodology used to assess, label, plan, intervene, and evaluate.

Functions

One function of any conceptual model is to provide a distinctive frame of reference, or "a horizon of expectations" (Popper, 1965, p. 47), and "a coherent, internally unified way of thinking about . . . events and processes" (Frank, 1968, p. 45) that tells nurses what to observe and how to interpret what they observe in practice. Each conceptual model, then, presents a unique focus that has a profound influence on nurses' ways of thinking about nursing participants and their environments in matters of health.

Another function of each conceptual model is to identify a particular "philosophical and pragmatic orientation to the service nurses provide patients—a service which only nurses can provide—a service which provides a dimension to total care different from that provided by any other health professional" (Johnson, 1987, p. 195). Conceptual models of nursing provide explicit orientations not only for nurses but also for the general public. They identify the purpose and scope of nursing and provide frameworks for objective records of the effects of nursing assessments and interventions. As Johnson (1987) explained, "Conceptual models specify for nurses and society the mission and boundaries of the profession. They clarify the realm of nursing responsibility and accountability, and they allow the practitioner and/or the profession to document services and outcomes" (pp. 196–197).

Conceptual Models of Nursing

Currently, the works of several nurse scholars are recognized as broad conceptual models that can be used in many different practice situations. Among the best known of those conceptual models are Johnson's (1990) Behavioral System Model, King's (2006) Conceptual System, Levine's (1991) Conservation Model, Neuman's Systems Model (Neuman & Fawcett, 2002), Orem's (2001) Self-Care Framework, Rogers's (1990) Science of Unitary Human Beings, and Roy's Adaptation Model (Roy & Andrews, 1999). An overview of each of these nursing models is presented in the following section, along with the implications of each one for professional nursing practice.

Some nurses use conceptual models that were developed for a particular area of nursing specialty practice. For example, the Synergy Model (Hardin & Kaplow, 2005) was developed by members of the American Association of Critical Care Nurses to guide practice with critically ill patients. Practice guided by the Synergy Model focuses attention on the match between certain characteristics of patients and certain competencies of nurses. According to the model, when nurse competencies are a good match with patient characteristics, the likelihood of attaining optimal patient outcomes is increased.

Dorothy Johnson's Behavioral System Model

Johnson's conceptual model of nursing, the **Behavioral System Model,** focuses on the person as a behavioral system, made up of all the patterned, repetitive, and purposeful ways of behavior that characterize life. Seven subsystems carry out specialized tasks or functions needed to maintain the integrity of the whole behavioral system and to manage its relationship to the environment. The subsystems are:

1. *Attachment or affiliative:* Function is the security needed for survival as well as social inclusion, intimacy, and formation and maintenance of social bonds.
2. *Dependency:* Function is the succoring behavior that calls for a response of nurturance as well as approval, attention or recognition, and physical assistance.
3. *Ingestive:* Function is appetite satisfaction in terms of when, how, what, how much, and under what conditions the individual eats, all of which is governed by social and psychological considerations as well as biologic requirements for food and fluids.
4. *Eliminative:* Function is elimination in terms of when, how, and under what conditions the individual eliminates wastes.
5. *Sexual:* Functions are procreation and gratification, with regard to behaviors dependent on the individual's biologic sex and gender role identity, including but not limited to courting and mating.
6. *Aggressive:* Function is protection and preservation of self and society.
7. *Achievement:* Function is mastery or control of some aspect of self or environment, with regard to intellectual, physical, creative, mechanical, social, and care-taking (of children, partner, home) skills.

The structure of each subsystem involves four elements:

1. *Drive or goal*: The motivation for behavior.
2. *Set*: The individual's predisposition to act in certain ways to fulfill the function of the subsystem.
3. *Choice*: The individual's total behavioral repertoire for fulfilling subsystem functions, which encompasses

the scope of action alternatives from which the person can choose.

4. *Action*: The individual's actual behavior in a situation. Action is the only structural element that can be observed directly; all other elements must be inferred from the individual's actual behavior and from the consequences of that behavior.

The three functional requirements listed below are needed by each subsystem to fulfill its functions:

1. *Protection* from noxious influences with which the system cannot cope
2. *Nurturance* through the input of appropriate supplies from the environment
3. *Stimulation* to enhance growth and prevent stagnation

Implications for Nursing Practice
Nursing practice is directed toward the restoration, maintenance, or attainment of behavioral system balance and dynamic stability at the highest possible level for the individual. Johnson's practice methodology, which is called the **Nursing Diagnostic and Treatment Process,** encompasses the four steps listed in Box 4–3. Each step is discussed in detail below.

Determination of the Existence of a Problem
- The nurse obtains:
  - Past and present family and individual behavioral system histories via interviews, structured and unstructured observations, and objective methodologies
  - Data about the nature of behavioral system functioning in terms of the efficiency and effectiveness with which the client's goals are obtained
  - Information to determine the degree to which the behavior is purposeful, orderly, and predictable
  - Information on the condition of the subsystem structural components to draw inferences about: (1) drive strength, direction, and value; (2) the solidity and specificity of the set; (3) the range of behavior patterns available to the client; and (4) the usual behavior in a given situation
- The client's behavior is compared with the following indices for behavioral system balance and stability,

Box 4.3 Johnson's Behavioral System Model: Diagnostic and Treatment Process

- Determination of the Existence of a Problem
- Diagnostic Classification of Problems
- Management of Nursing Problems
- Evaluation of Behavioral System Balance and Stability

as well as the reorganization and integration of the subsystems:
- The behavior is achieving the consequences sought.
- Effective motor, expressive, or social skills are evident.
- The behavior is purposeful—actions are goal directed, reveal a plan and cease at an identifiable point, and are economical in sequence.
- The behavior is orderly—actions are methodical and systematic, build sequentially toward a goal, and form a recognizable pattern.
- The behavior is predictable—actions are repetitive under particular circumstances.
- The amount of energy expended to achieve desired goals is acceptable.
- The behavior reflects appropriate choices—actions are compatible with survival imperatives and the social situation.
- The client is sufficiently satisfied with the behavior.

Diagnostic Classification of Problems
- Classification occurs in two areas:
  - *Internal subsystem problems*: Functional requirements are not met, inconsistency or disharmony among the structural components of subsystems is evident, and/or the behavior is inappropriate in the ambient culture.
  - *Intersystem problems*: The entire behavioral system is dominated by one or two subsystems, or a conflict exists between two or more subsystems.

Management of Nursing Problems
- The general goals of action are to restore, maintain, or attain the client's behavioral system balance and stability and to help the client achieve an optimum level of balance and functioning when this goal is possible and desired. The nurse determines what nursing is to accomplish on behalf of the behavioral system by determining who makes the judgment regarding the acceptable level of behavioral system balance and stability. Nursing actions may occur in three areas:
  - *Temporary external regulatory or control mechanisms,* by setting limits for behavior by either permissive or inhibitory means, inhibiting ineffective behavioral response, helping the client acquire new responses, and reinforcing appropriate behaviors
  - *Repair of damaged structural components,* by reducing drive strength by changing attitudes, redirecting goal by changing attitudes, altering set by instruction or counseling, and adding choices by teaching new skills
  - *Fulfillment of functional requirements* of subsystems, by protecting the client from overwhelming noxious influences, supplying adequate nurturance,

and providing stimulation to enhance growth and inhibit stagnation
- The nurse negotiates the treatment modality with the client by establishing a contract with the client and helping him or her to understand the meaning of the nursing diagnosis and the proposed treatment.

Evaluation of Behavioral System Balance and Stability
- The nurse compares the client's behavior after treatment with indices of behavioral system balance and stability.

Imogene King's Conceptual System

King's conceptual model of nursing, which she calls the **Conceptual System**, focuses on the continuing ability of individuals to meet their basic needs so that they may function in their socially defined roles. This conceptual model also concentrates on individuals' interactions within three open, dynamic, interacting systems—the personal system, the interpersonal system, and the social system.

Personal Systems
Personal systems are individuals who are regarded as rational, sentient, social beings. Concepts related to the personal system are:

- *Perception*: A process of organizing, interpreting, and transforming information from sense data and memory that gives meaning to one's experience, represents one's image of reality, and influences one's behavior
- *Self*: A composite of thoughts and feelings that constitute a person's awareness of individual existence, of who and what he or she is
- *Growth and development*: Cellular, molecular, and behavioral changes in human beings that are a function of genetic endowment, meaningful and satisfying experiences, and an environment conducive to helping individuals move toward maturity
- *Body image*: A person's perceptions of his or her body
- *Time*: The duration between the occurrence of one event and the occurrence of another event
- *Personal space:* The physical area called territory that exists in all directions as perceived by each individual
- *Learning:* Gaining knowledge

Interpersonal Systems
Interpersonal systems are defined as two, three, or more individuals interacting in a given situation. The concepts associated with this system are:

- *Interaction:* The act of two or more persons in mutual presence; a sequence of verbal and nonverbal behaviors that are goal directed
- *Communication:* The vehicle by which human relations are developed and maintained; it encompasses

intrapersonal, interpersonal, verbal, and nonverbal communications
- *Transaction:* A process of interaction in which human beings communicate with the environment to achieve goals that are valued
- *Role:* A set of behaviors expected of a person occupying a position in a social system
- *Stress:* A dynamic state whereby a human being interacts with the environment to maintain balance for growth, development, and performance, which involves an exchange of energy and information between the person and the environment for regulation and control of stressors
- *Coping:* A way of dealing with stress

Social Systems
Social systems are organized boundary systems of social roles, behaviors, and practices developed to maintain values, and the mechanisms to regulate the practices and rules. The concepts related to social systems are:

- *Organization:* Composed of human beings with prescribed roles and positions who use resources to accomplish personal and organizational goals
- *Authority:* A transactional process characterized by active, reciprocal relations in which members' values, backgrounds, and perceptions play a role in defining, validating, and accepting the authority of individuals within an organization
- *Power:* The process whereby one or more persons influence other persons in a situation
- *Status:* The position of an individual in a group or a group in relation to other groups in an organization
- *Decision-making:* A dynamic and systematic process by which goal-directed choice of perceived alternatives is made and acted on by individuals or groups to answer a question and attain a goal
- *Control:* Being in charge

Implications for Nursing Practice
Nursing practice is directed toward helping individuals maintain their health so they can function in their roles. King's practice methodology, which is the essence of her Theory of Goal Attainment, is called the **Interaction-Transaction Process.** The process encompasses the 10 steps listed in Box 4–4. Each step is discussed in detail below.

Perception
- One aspect of the assessment phase of the interaction-transaction process.
- The nurse and the client meet in some nursing situation and perceive each other.
- Accuracy of perception depends on verifying the nurse's inferences with the client.
- The nurse can use the Goal-Oriented Nursing Record (GONR) to record perceptions.

Box 4.4 King's Conceptual System Practice
Methodology: Interaction-Transaction Process

- Perception
- Judgment
- Action
- Reaction
- Disturbance
- Mutual Goal Setting
- Exploration of Means to Achieve Goals
- Agreement on Means to Achieve Goals
- Transaction
- Attainment of Goals

Judgment
- Another aspect of the assessment phase of the interaction-transaction process.
- The nurse and the client make mental judgments about the other.
- The nurse can use the GONR to record judgments.

Action
- Another aspect of the assessment phase of the interaction-transaction process.
- Action is a sequence of behaviors of interacting persons, including recognition of the situation, activities related to the situation, and motivation to exert some control over the events to achieve goals.
- The nurse and the client take some mental action.
- The nurse can use the GONR to record mental actions.

Reaction
- Another aspect of the assessment phase of the interaction-transaction process.
- The nurse and the client mentally react to each one's perceptions of the other.
- The nurse can use the GONR to record mental reactions.

Disturbance
- The diagnosis phase of the interaction-transaction process.
- The nurse and the client communicate and interact, and the nurse identifies the client's concerns, problems, and disturbances in health.
- The nurse conducts a nursing history to determine the client's activities of daily living, using the Criterion-Referenced Measure of Goal Attainment Tool (CRMGAT); roles; environmental stressors; perceptions; and values, learning needs, and goals. The nurse records the data from the nursing history on the GONR.
- The nurse records the medical history and physical examination data, results of laboratory tests and x-ray examination, and information gathered from

other health professionals and the client's family members on the GONR.
- The nurse records diagnoses on the GONR.

Mutual Goal Setting
- One aspect of the planning phase of the interaction-transaction process.
- The nurse and the client interact purposefully to set mutually agreed on goals.
- The nurse interacts with family members if the client cannot verbally participate in goal setting.
- Mutual goal setting is based on the nurse's assessment of the client's concerns, problems, and disturbances in health; the nurse's and client's perceptions of the interference; and the nurse's sharing of information with the client and his or her family to help the client attain the goals identified.
- Mutual goal setting includes consideration of the ethical aspects of the situation, including:
  - Helping the client and family to sort out the values inherent in the situation and encouraging them to think through their own value system and the consequences of action they decide to take in the situation.
  - Helping the client and family to make decisions that take their value system into consideration by providing information that contributes to their decision, by emphasizing their reality as they have expressed it, and by not making decisions for them.
  - Becoming skillful in identifying options in every nursing situation and exploring those options with the client and family.
  - Identifying those elements in the situation that can be changed and controlled and those that cannot, and concentrating energy and efforts on control and change.
  - Being especially sensitive to the ethical issues that may arise when considering the right to life, the right to die, and the right to information required for informed choice.
- The nurse records the goals on the GONR.

Exploration of Means to Achieve Goals
- Another aspect of the planning phase of the interaction-transaction process.
- The nurse and the client interact purposefully to explore the means to achieve the mutually set goals.

Agreement on Means to Achieve Goals
- Another aspect of the planning phase of the interaction-transaction process.
- The nurse and the client interact purposefully to agree on the means to achieve the mutually set goals.
- The nurse records the nursing orders with regard to the means to achieve goals on the GONR.

Transaction
- The implementation phase of the interaction-transaction process.
- Transaction refers to what is valued in the interaction.
- The nurse and the client carry out the measures agreed upon to achieve the mutually set goals.
- The nurse can use the GONR flow sheet and progress notes to record the implementation of measures used to achieve goals.

Attainment of Goals
- The evaluation phase of the interaction-transaction process.
- The nurse and the client identify the outcome of the interaction-transaction process. The outcome is expressed in terms of the client's state of health, or ability to function in social roles.
- The nurse and the client make a decision with regard to whether the goal was attained and, if necessary, determine why the goal was not attained.
- The nurse can use the CRMGAT to record the outcome and the GONR to record the discharge summary.

Myra Levine's Conservation Model

Levine's conceptual model of nursing, the **Conservation Model**, focuses on conservation of the person's wholeness. Adaptation is the process by which people maintain their wholeness or integrity as they respond to environmental challenges and become congruent with the environment. The three sources of environmental challenges are:

1. *Perceptual environment:* Encompasses that part of the environment to which individuals respond with their sense organs
2. *Operational environment:* Includes those aspects of the environment that are not directly perceived, such as radiation, odorless and colorless pollutants, and microorganisms
3. *Conceptual environment:* The environment of language, ideas, symbols, concepts, and invention

Individuals respond to the environment by means of four integrated processes that constitute the organismic response:

1. Flight-or-flight mechanism
2. Inflammatory-immune response
3. Stress response
4. Perceptual awareness, which includes the basic orienting, haptic, auditory, visual, and taste-smell systems

Implications for Nursing Practice
Nursing practice is directed toward promoting wholeness for all people, well or sick. Patients are partners or participants in nursing care and are temporarily dependent on the nurse. The nurse's goal is to end the dependence as quickly as possible. Levine's practice methodology is **Nursing Process as Conversation** (Box 4–5), which is defined as "keeping together." The three steps of the process are listed in Box 4–5. Each step is discussed in detail below.

Trophicognosis
- Trophicognosis is formulation of a nursing care judgment arrived at by the scientific method. The nurse observes and collects data that will influence nursing practice, using appropriate assessment to establish an objective and scientific rationale for nursing practice. The nurse understands the basis for the prescribed medical regimen, including the medical diagnosis, the medical history, and the laboratory and x-ray examination reports, with specific reference to areas influencing the nursing care plan.
- Assessment skills are directed at four conservation principles:
  - *Conservation of energy* determines the ability to perform necessary activities without producing excessive fatigue. Relevant observations include vital signs, the patient's general condition, the patient's behavior, the patient's tolerance of nursing activities required by his or her condition, and allowable activity for the patient based on his or her energy resources.
  - *Conservation of structural integrity* determines physical functioning. Relevant observations include status of any pathophysiologic processes, status of healing processes, and effects of surgical procedures.
  - *Conservation of personal integrity* determines moral and ethical values and life experiences. Relevant observations include the client's life story, interest in participating in decision making, and identifying sense of self.
  - *Conservation of social integrity* takes the client's family members, friends, and conceptual environment into account. Relevant observations include identification of the client's significant others, participation in workplace and/or school activities, religion, and cultural and ethnic history.
- The basis for implementation of the nursing care plan includes principles of nursing science and adaptation of nursing techniques to the unique cluster of needs

Box 4.5 Levine's Conservation Model Practice Methodology: Nursing Process as Conservation

- Trophicognosis
- Intervention/Action
- Evaluation of Intervention/Action

demonstrated in the individual patient. The nurse identifies the provocative facts—that is, the data that provoke attention on the basis of knowledge of the situation—to provide the basis for a hypothesis, or trophicognosis. Observations are then recorded and transmitted.

Intervention/Action

- Intervention/action is a test of the hypothesis. The nursing care plan is implemented and evaluated within the structure of administrative policy, availability of equipment, and established standards of nursing. The general types of nursing intervention required are therapeutic nursing intervention, which influences adaptation favorably, or toward renewed social well-being, and supportive nursing interventions, which cannot alter the course of the adaptation and can only maintain the status quo or fail to halt a downward course. Nursing interventions are structured according to the four conservation principles:
  - *Conservation of energy* through an adequate deposit of energy resource and regulation of the expenditure of energy
  - *Conservation of structural integrity* through maintenance or restoration of the structure of the body
  - *Conservation of personal integrity* through maintenance or restoration of the patient's sense of identity, self-worth, and acknowledgment of uniqueness
  - *Conservation of social integrity* through acknowledging the patient as a social being

Evaluation of Intervention/Action

- Evaluation of the intervention/action is the nurse's evaluation of the effects of the intervention/action and is used to revise the trophicognosis as necessary.
- An indicator of the success of nursing interventions is the patient's organismic response.

Betty Neuman's Systems Model

Neuman's conceptual model of nursing, the **Neuman Systems Model,** focuses on the wellness of the client system in relation to environmental stress and reactions to stress. The client system, which can be an individual, a family or other group, or a community, is a composite of five interrelated variables:

1. *Physiologic:* Bodily structure and function
2. *Psychological:* Mental processes and relationships
3. *Sociocultural:* Social and cultural functions
4. *Developmental:* Developmental processes of life
5. *Spiritual:* Aspects of spirituality on a continuum from complete unawareness or denial to a consciously developed, high level of spiritual understanding

The client system is depicted as a central core, which is a basic structure of survival factors common to the species, surrounded by three types of metaphorical concentric rings:

1. *Flexible line of defense:* The outermost ring is a protective buffer for the client's normal or stable state that prevents invasion of stressors and keeps the client system free from stressor reactions or symptomatology.
2. *Normal line of defense:* This lies between the flexible line of defense and the lines of resistance and represents the client system's normal or usual wellness state.
3. *Lines of resistance:* The innermost concentric rings are involuntarily activated when a stressor invades the normal line of defense. They attempt to stabilize the client system and foster a return to the normal line of defense. If these rings are effective, the system can reconstitute; if they are ineffective, death may ensue.

Environment represents all internal and external factors or influences surrounding the client system. The *internal environment* is all forces or interactive influences internal to or contained solely within the boundaries of the defined client system; the source of intrapersonal stressors. The *external environment* is all forces or interaction influences external to or existing outside the defined client system; the source of interpersonal and extrapersonal stressors. The *created environment* is subconsciously developed by the client as a symbolic expression of system wholeness, and supersedes and encompasses the internal and external environments; it functions as a subjective safety mechanism that may block the true reality of the environment and the health experience.

Implications for Nursing Practice

Nursing practice is directed toward facilitating optimal wellness through retention, attainment, or maintenance of client system stability. The nurse uses the Neuman Systems Model Assessment and Intervention Tool, the Systems Model Nursing Diagnosis Taxonomy, and any other relevant clinical tools to guide collection of data and facilitate documentation of nursing diagnoses, nursing goals, and nursing outcomes. The three steps of Neuman's practice methodology, which is called the **Nursing Process Format,** are listed in Box 4–6. Each step is discussed in detail here.

Nursing Diagnosis

- The nurse establishes the database, which involves simultaneous consideration of the dynamic interactions of physiologic, psychological, sociocultural, developmental, and spiritual variables. The nurse identifies the client/client system's perceptions and his or her own perceptions, including basic structure factors and energy resources; flexible and

Box 4.6 Neuman's Systems Model Practice Methodology: Nursing Process Format

- Nursing Diagnosis
- Nursing Goals
- Nursing Outcomes

normal lines of defense, lines of resistance, degree of potential or actual reaction, and potential for reconstitution following a reaction; and the internal and external environmental stressors that threaten the stability of the client/client system.

- The nurse compares the client/client system's and the nurse's perceptions by identifying similarities and differences in perceptions. A comprehensive nursing diagnosis is presented that encompasses the client/client system's general condition or circumstances, including identification of actual or potential variances from wellness and available resources.

Nursing Goals

- The nurse prioritizes goals by considering the client/client system's wellness level, the meaning of the experience to the client/client system, system stability needs, and total available resources.
- Outcome goals and interventions are proposed that will facilitate the highest possible level of client/client system stability or wellness, maintain the normal line of defense, and retain the flexible line of defense.
- Desired prescriptive change or outcome goals are developed to correct variances from wellness with the client/client system, taking client/client system needs and resources into account. Specific prevention as intervention modalities are negotiated with the client/client system.

Nursing Outcomes

- The nurse implements nursing interventions through the use of one or more of the three "prevention as intervention" modalities:
  - *Primary prevention*: Nursing actions to retain system stability are implemented through such measures as preventing stressor invasion, providing resources to retain or strengthen existing client/client system strengths, and supporting positive coping and functioning.
  - *Secondary prevention*: Nursing actions to attain system stability are implemented through such measures as protecting the client/client system's basic structure, mobilizing and optimizing the client/client system's internal and external resources to attain stability and energy conservation, and facilitating purposeful manipulation of stressors and reactions to stressors.
  - *Tertiary prevention*: Nursing actions to maintain system stability are implemented through such

measures as attaining and maintaining the highest possible level of client/client system wellness and stability during reconstitution; educating, reeducating, and/or reorienting the client/client system as needed; and supporting the client/client system toward appropriate goals.

- The nurse evaluates the outcome goals by confirming (with the client/client system) their attainment, and reformulating goals as necessary. The nurse and client/client system set intermediate and long-range goals for subsequent nursing action.

Dorothea Orem's Self-Care Framework

Orem's conceptual model of nursing focuses on patients' deliberate actions to meet their own and dependent others' therapeutic self-care demands. The **Self-Care Framework** also focuses on nurses' deliberate actions to implement nursing systems designed to assist individuals and multiperson units who have limitations in their abilities to provide continuing and therapeutic self-care or care of dependent others. The concepts of Orem's conceptual model are:

Self-Care
Self-care is behavior directed by individuals to themselves or their environments to regulate factors that affect their own development and functioning in the interests of life, health, or well-being.

Self-Care Agency
A self-care agency is the complex capability of maturing and mature individuals to determine the presence and characteristics of specific requirements for regulating their own functioning and development, make judgments and decisions about what to do, and perform care measures to meet specific self-care requisites.

Power Components
The person's ability to perform self-care is influenced by 10 power components:

1. Ability to maintain attention and exercise requisite vigilance with respect to self as self-care agent, and internal and external conditions and factors significant for self-care
2. Controlled use of available physical energy that is sufficient for the initiation and continuation of self-care operations
3. Ability to control the position of the body and its parts in the execution of the movements required for the initiation and completion of self-care operations
4. Ability to reason within a self-care frame of reference
5. Motivation (i.e., goal orientations for self-care that are in accord with its characteristics and its meaning for life, health, and well-being)
6. Ability to make decisions about care of self and to operationalize these decisions

7. Ability to acquire technical knowledge about self-care from authoritative sources, to retain it, and to operationalize it
8. A repertoire of cognitive, perceptual, manipulative, communication, and interpersonal skills adapted to the performance of self-care operations
9. Ability to order discrete self-care actions or action systems into relationships with prior and subsequent actions toward the final achievement of regulatory goals of self-care
10. Ability to consistently perform self-care operations, integrating them with relevant aspects of personal, family, and community living

Basic Conditioning Factors
The person's ability to perform self-care also is influenced by 10 internal and external factors called basic conditioning factors:

1. Age
2. Gender
3. Developmental state
4. Health state
5. Sociocultural orientation
6. Health-care system factors, such as medical diagnostic and treatment modalities
7. Family system factors
8. Patterns of living, including regular activities
9. Environmental factors
10. Resource availability and adequacy

Therapeutic Self-Care Demand
The therapeutic self-care demand is the action demand on individuals to meet three types of self-care requisites:

- *Universal self-care requisites*: Actions that need to be performed to maintain life processes, the integrity of human structure and function, and general well-being
- *Developmental self-care requisites*: Actions that need to be performed in relation to human developmental processes, conditions, and events and in relation to events that may adversely affect development
- *Health deviation self-care requisites:* Actions that need to be performed in relation to genetic and constitutional defects, human structural and functional deviations and their effects, and medical diagnostic and treatment measures prescribed or performed by physicians

Self-Care Deficit
The self-care deficit is the relationship of inadequacy between self-care agency and the therapeutic self-care demand.

Nursing Agency
Nursing agency is a complex property or attribute that enables nurses to know and help others to know their therapeutic self-care demands, meet their therapeutic self-care demands, and regulate the exercise or development of their self-care agency.

A nursing system is a series of coordinated deliberate practical actions performed by nurses and patients directed toward meeting the patient's therapeutic self-care demand and protecting and regulating the exercise or development of the patient's self-care agency.

Implications for Nursing Practice
Nursing practice is directed toward helping people meet their own and their dependent others' therapeutic self-care demands. Orem's practice methodology, which is called **Professional-Technologic Operations of Nursing Practice,** involves the seven steps listed in Box 4–7. A detailed discussion of the operations is given below.

Case Management Operations
- The nurse:
  - Uses a case management approach to direct each of the nursing diagnostic, prescriptive, regulatory, and control operations.
  - Maintains an overview of the interrelationships between the social, interpersonal, and professional-technological systems of nursing.
  - Uses the nursing history and other appropriate tools for collection of information, documentation of information, and measurement of the quality of nursing.

Diagnostic Operations
- The nurse:
  - Identifies the unit of service for nursing practice as an individual, an individual member of a multiperson unit, or a multiperson unit.
  - Determines why the individual needs nursing.
  - Collects demographic data about the patient and information about the nature and boundaries of the patient's health-care situation and nursing's jurisdiction within those boundaries.

Box 4.7 Orem's Practice Methodology: Professional-Technologic Operations of Nursing Practice

- Case Management Operations
- Diagnostic Operations
- Prescriptive Operations
- Regulatory Operations: Design of Nursing Systems for Performance of Regulatory Operations
- Regulatory Operations: Planning for Regulatory Operations
- Regulatory Operations: Production of Regulatory Care
- Control Operations

Prescriptive Operations
- In collaboration with the patient or family, the nurse specifies:
  - All care measures needed to meet the entire therapeutic self-care demand.
  - The roles to be played by the nurse(s), patient, and dependent-care agent(s) in meeting the therapeutic self-care demand.
  - The roles to be played by the nurse(s), patient, and dependent-care agent(s) in regulating the patient's exercise or development or self-care agency or dependent-care agency.

Regulatory Operations: Design of Nursing Systems for Performance of Regulatory Operations
- The nurse designs a nursing system, a series of coordinated deliberate practical actions performed by the nurse and the patient. The actions are directed toward meeting the patient's therapeutic self-care demand and protecting and regulating the exercise or development of the patient's self-care agency or dependent-care agency.

The selection of the appropriate nursing system depends on who can or should perform self-care actions.

- The *wholly compensatory nursing system* is selected when the patient cannot or should not perform any self-care actions, and thus the nurse must perform them.
- The *partly compensatory nursing system* is selected when the patient can perform some, but not all, self-care actions.
- The *supportive-educative nursing system* is selected when the patient can and should perform all self-care actions.

Each nursing system is implemented using one or more of the following five *methods of helping:*

- Acting for or doing for the patient
- Providing a developmental environment
- Supporting the patient psychologically
- Guiding the patient
- Teaching the patient

Regulatory Operations: Planning for Regulatory Operations
- The nurse specifies what is needed to produce the nursing system(s) selected for the patient, including:
  - The time during which the nursing system will be produced.
  - The place where the nursing system will be produced.
  - The environmental conditions necessary for the production of the nursing system, as well as the equipment and supplies required.
  - The number and qualifications of nurses and other health-care providers necessary to produce the nursing system and to evaluate its effects.
  - The organization and timing of tasks to be performed.
  - The designation of who (nurse or patient) is to perform the tasks.

Regulatory Operations: Production of Regulatory Care
- Nursing systems are produced by means of the actions of nurses and patients during nurse-patient encounters; the nurse produces and manages the designated nursing system(s) and method(s) of helping for as long as the patient's self-care deficit or dependent-care deficit exists. The nurse:
  - Performs and regulates the self-care or dependent-care tasks for patients or assists patients with their performance of self-care or dependent-care tasks.
  - Coordinates self-care or dependent-care task performance so that a unified system of care is produced and coordinated with other components of health care.
  - Helps patients, their families, and others bring about systems of daily living for patients that support the accomplishment of self-care or dependent-care and are, at the same time, satisfying in relation to patients' interests, talents, and goals.
  - Guides, directs, and supports patients in their exercise of, or in the withholding of the exercise of, their self-care agency or dependent-care agency.
  - Stimulates patients' interests in self-care or dependent-care by raising questions and promoting discussions of care problems and issues when conditions permit.
  - Is available to patients at times when questions are likely to arise.
  - Supports and guides patients in learning activities and provides cues for learning as well as instructional sessions.
  - Supports and guides patients as they experience illness or disability and the effects of medical care measures and as they experience the need to engage in new measures of self-care or change their ways of meeting ongoing self-care requisites.

Control Operations
- The nurse performs control operations concurrently or separately from the production of regulatory care. The nurse makes observations and evaluates the nursing system to determine whether:
  - The nursing system that was designed is actually produced.
  - There is a fit between the current prescription for nursing and the nursing system that is being produced.

- Regulation of the patient's functioning is being achieved through performance of care measures to meet the patient's therapeutic self-care demand.
- Exercise of the patient's self-care agency or dependent-care agency is being properly regulated.
- Developmental change is in process and is adequate
- The patient is adjusting to any decline in powers to engage in self-care or dependent care.

Martha Rogers' Science of Unitary Human Beings

Rogers' conceptual model of nursing, called the **Science of Unitary Human Beings**, focuses on unitary, irreducible human beings and their environments. The four basic concepts are:

1. *Energy fields:* Irreducible, indivisible, pandimensional unitary human beings and environments that are identified by pattern and manifesting characteristics that are specific to the whole and that cannot be predicted from knowledge of the parts. Human and environmental energy fields are integral with each other.
2. *Openness*: A characteristic of human and environmental energy fields; energy fields are continuously and completely open.
3. *Pattern:* The distinguishing characteristic of an energy field. Pattern is perceived as a single wave that gives identity to the field. Each human field pattern is unique and is integral with its own unique environmental field pattern. Pattern is an abstraction that cannot be seen; what is seen or experienced are manifestations of field patterns.
4. *Pandimensionality:* A nonlinear domain without spatial or temporal attributes.

The three principles of homeodynamics, which describe the nature of human and environmental energy fields, are as follows:

1. *Resonancy* asserts that human and environmental fields are identified by wave patterns that manifest continuous change from lower to higher frequencies.

Box 4.8 Rogers' Science of Unitary Human Beings Practice Methodology: The Health Patterning Practice Method

- Pattern Manifestation Knowing and Appreciation—Assessment
- Voluntary Mutual Patterning
- Pattern Manifestation Knowing and Appreciation—Evaluation

2. *Helicy* asserts that human and environmental field patterns are continuous, innovative, and unpredictable, and are characterized by increasing diversity.
3. *Integrality* emphasizes the continuous mutual human field and environmental field process.

Implications for Nursing Practice
Nursing practice is directed toward promoting the health and well-being of all persons, wherever they are. The three steps of Rogers' practice methodology, which is called the **Health Patterning Practice Method,** are listed in Box 4–8. Each step is discussed in detail below.

Pattern Manifestation Knowing and Appreciation—Assessment
- The continuous process of apprehending and identifying manifestations of the human energy field and environmental energy field patterns that relate to current health events.
- The nurse uses one or more research instruments or clinical tools based on the Science of Unitary Human Beings to guide application and documentation of the practice methodology.
- The nurse acts with pandimensional authenticity—that is, with a demeanor of genuineness, trustworthiness, and knowledgeable caring.
- The nurse focuses on the client as a unified whole, a unitary human being.

Voluntary Mutual Patterning
- The continuous process whereby the nurse, with the client, patterns the environmental energy field to promote harmony related to the health events.
- The nurse facilitates the client's actualization of potentials for health and well-being. The nurse has no investment in the client's changing in a particular way.
- The nurse does not attempt to change anyone to conform to arbitrary health ideals. Rather, the nurse enhances the client's efforts to actualize health potentials from the client's point of view.

Pattern Manifestation Knowing and Appreciation—Evaluation
- The nurse evaluates voluntary mutual patterning by means of pattern manifestation knowing.
- Additional pattern information is monitored and collected as it unfolds during voluntary mutual patterning.
- The nurse considers the pattern information within the context of continually emerging health patterning goals affirmed by the client.

Callista Roy's Adaptation Model

Roy's Adaptation Model focuses on the responses of the human adaptive system, which can be an individual or a group, to a constantly changing environment. Adaptation is the central feature of the model.

Problems in adaptation arise when the adaptive system is unable to cope with or respond to constantly changing stimuli from the internal and external environments in a manner that maintains the integrity of the system. Environmental stimuli are categorized as:

- *Focal:* The stimuli most immediately confronting the person.
- *Contextual:* The contributing factors in the situation.
- *Residual:* Other unknown factors that may influence the situation. When the factors making up residual stimuli become known, they are considered focal or contextual stimuli.

Adaptation occurs through innate or acquired coping mechanisms used to respond to changing environmental stimuli:

- *Regulator coping subsystem (for individuals)* receives input from the external environment and from changes in the individual's internal state, and processes the changes through neural-chemical-endocrine channels to produce responses.
- *Cognator coping subsystem (for individuals)* also receives input from external and internal stimuli that involve psychological, social, physical, and physiologic factors, including regulator subsystem outputs. These stimuli then are processed through cognitive/emotive pathways, including perceptual/information processing, learning, judgment, and emotion.
- *Stabilizer subsystem control process (for groups)* involves the established structures, values, and daily activities used by a group to accomplish its primary purpose and contribute to common purposes of society.
- *Innovator subsystem control process (for humans in groups)* involves the structures and processes necessary for change and growth in human social systems.

Responses take place in four modes for individuals and groups:

- *Physiologic/physical mode:*
  - *Physiologic mode (for individuals)* is concerned with basic needs requisite to maintaining the physical and physiologic integrity of the individual human system. It encompasses oxygenation; nutrition; elimination; activity and rest; protection; senses; fluid, electrolyte, and acid-base balance; neurologic function; and endocrine function. The basic underlying need is physiologic integrity.
  - *Physical mode (for groups)* pertains to the manner in which the collective human adaptive system manifests adaptation relative to basic operating resources, including participants, physical facilities, and fiscal resources. The basic underlying need is resource adequacy, or wholeness achieved by adapting to change in physical resource needs.

- *Self-concept/group identity mode:*
  - *Self-concept mode (for individuals)* addresses the composite of beliefs and feelings that a person holds about himself or herself at a given time. The basic underlying need is psychic and spiritual integrity, the need to know who one is so that one can be or exist with a sense of unity, meaning, and purposefulness in the universe. The *physical self* refers to the individual's appraisal of his or her own physical being, including physical attributes, functioning, sexuality, health and illness states, and appearance. It includes the components of body sensation and body image. The *personal self* refers to the individual's appraisal of his or her own characteristics, expectations, values, and worth, including self-consistency, self-ideal, and the moral-ethical-spiritual self.
  - *Group identity mode (for groups)* addresses shared relations, goals, and values, which create a social milieu and culture, a group self-image, and coresponsibility for goal achievement. Identity integrity is the underlying need, which implies the honesty, soundness, and completeness of the group members' identification with the group and involves the process of sharing identity and goals. This mode encompasses interpersonal relationships, group self-image, social milieu, and group culture.
- *Role function mode (for individuals and groups)* focuses on the roles that the individual occupies in society. The basic underlying need is social integrity, the need to know who one is in relation to others so that one can act. For the group, this mode focuses on the action components associated with group infrastructure that are designed to contribute to the accomplishment of the group's mission or the tasks or functions associated with the group. The basic underlying need is role clarity, the need to understand and commit to fulfill expected tasks, so that the group can achieve common goals.
- *Interdependence mode (for individuals and groups)* focuses on the basic underlying need of relational integrity, defined as the feeling of security in nurturing relationships. For the individual, the mode focuses on interactions related to the giving and receiving of love, respect, and value, and encompasses affectional adequacy, developmental adequacy, resource adequacy, significant others, and support systems. For the group, it pertains to the social context in which the group operates, including both private and public contacts both within the group and with those outside the group, and encompasses affectional adequacy, developmental adequacy, resource adequacy, context, infrastructure, and resources.

The four modes are interrelated. Responses in any one mode may have an effect on or act as a stimulus in one or all of the other modes. Responses in each mode are judged as either adaptive or ineffective. A judgment of "adaptive responses" indicates promotion of the goals of the human adaptive system, including survival, growth, reproduction, and mastery. A judgment of "ineffective responses" does not contribute to the goals of the human adaptive system.

Implications for Nursing Practice

Nursing practice is directed toward promoting adaptation in each of the four response modes, thereby contributing to the person's health, quality of life, and dying with dignity. Roy's practice methodology is **Roy's Adaptation Model Nursing Process,** which encompasses the six steps listed in Box 4–9. Each step is discussed in detail below.

Assessment of Behavior

- The nurse systematically gathers data about the behavior of the human adaptive system and judges the current state of adaptation in each adaptive mode.
- The nurse uses one or more of Roy's Adaptation Model-based research instruments or clinical tools to guide application and documentation of the practice methodology.

Assessment of Stimuli

- The nurse recognizes that stimuli must be amenable to independent nurse functions. Consequently, factors such as medical diagnoses and medical treatments are not considered stimuli, because those factors cannot be independently managed by nurses.
- The nurse identifies the internal and external focal and contextual stimuli that are influencing the behaviors of particular interest, in the order of priority established at the end of the Assessment of Behavior component of Roy's Adaptation Model Nursing Process.

Nursing Diagnosis

- The nurse uses a process of judgment to make a statement conveying the adaptation status of the human adaptive system of interest. The nursing diagnosis is a statement that identifies the behaviors of interest together with the most relevant influencing stimuli.

Box 4.9 Roy's Adaptation Model Practice Methodology: The Nursing Process

- Assessment of Behavior
- Assessment of Stimuli
- Nursing Diagnosis
- Goal Setting
- Intervention
- Evaluation

ONLINE CONSULT

North American Nursing Diagnosis Association (NANDA) at
www.nanda.org

- The nurse uses one of the following three different approaches to state the nursing diagnosis:
  - Behaviors are stated within each adaptive mode and with their most relevant influencing stimuli.
  - A summary label for behaviors in each adaptive mode with relevant stimuli is used.
  - A label that summarizes a behavioral pattern across adaptive modes that is affected by the same stimuli is used.
- The nurse may link Roy's Adaptation Model-based nursing diagnosis with a relevant diagnosis from the taxonomy of the North American Nursing Diagnosis Association (NANDA).

Goal Setting

- The nurse articulates a clear statement of the behavioral outcomes in response to nursing provided to the human adaptive system.
- Goals are stated as specific short-term and long-term behavioral outcomes of nursing intervention.
- The goal statement designates the behavior of interest, the way in which the behavior will change, and the time frame for attainment of the goal.
- Goals may be stated for ineffective behaviors that are to be changed to adaptive behaviors and also for adaptive behaviors that should be maintained or enhanced.

Intervention

- The nurse selects and implements nursing approaches that have a high probability of changing stimuli or strengthening adaptive processes.
- Nursing intervention is the management of stimuli. The nurse may alter, increase, decrease, remove, or maintain stimuli.

Evaluation

- The nurse judges the effectiveness of nursing interventions in relation to the behaviors of the human adaptive system.
- The nurse systematically reassesses observable and nonobservable behaviors for each aspect of the four adaptive modes.

NURSING THEORIES

The terms *theory*, *theoretical framework*, *theoretical model*, and *theoretical rationale* frequently are used interchangeably and have the same definition.

Definition

A nursing theory is defined as one or more relatively concrete and specific concepts that are derived from a conceptual model, the statements that describe those concepts, and the statements that assert relatively concrete and specific relations between two or more concepts (Fawcett, 2005). Each theory presents a unique perspective about a particular phenomenon, such as a nursing participant, the environment, health, or a step of the nursing process or practice methodology.

Functions

The function of a nursing theory is to provide considerable specificity in the description, explanation, or prediction of some phenomenon. Theories are more concrete and specific than conceptual models. A *conceptual model* is an abstract and general system of concepts and statements, whereas a *theory* deals with one or more relatively concrete and specific concepts and statements. In addition, conceptual models are general guides that must be specified further by relevant and logically congruent theories before action can occur.

Nursing Grand Theories

Theories vary in scope—that is, they vary in the relative level of concreteness and specificity of their concepts and statements. Theories that are broadest in scope are called grand theories. These theories are made up of rather abstract and general concepts and statements that cannot be generated or tested empirically. Indeed, grand theories are developed through thoughtful and insightful appraisal of existing ideas or creative intellectual leaps beyond existing knowledge. Examples of grand theories of nursing are Leininger's Theory of Culture Care Diversity and Universality (Leininger & McFarland, 2006), Newman's (1994) Theory of Health as Expanding Consciousness, and Parse's (1998) Theory of Humanbecoming. An overview of each grand theory, along with implications for practice, is presented below. The less abstract nature of grand theories compared with conceptual models is illustrated by Parse's (1998) theory, which was derived in part from Rogers' (1970, 1990) conceptual model. Rogers' conceptual model is a frame of reference for all of nursing, whereas Parse's theory limits the domain of interest to the unitary human's experience of becoming.

Madeleine Leininger's Theory of Culture Care Diversity and Universality

Leininger's grand theory focuses on the discovery of human care diversities and universalities and ways to provide culturally congruent care to people. The concepts of the **Theory of Culture Care Diversity and Universality** are described as follows:

- *Care:* Abstract and concrete phenomena related to assisting, supporting, or enabling experiences or behaviors toward or for others with evident or anticipated needs to ameliorate or improve a human condition or lifeway
- *Caring:* The actions and activities directed toward assisting, supporting, or enabling another individual or group with evident or anticipated needs to ameliorate or improve a human condition or lifeway or to face death
- *Culture:* The learned, shared, and transmitted values, beliefs, norms, and lifeways of a particular group that guide thinking, decisions, and actions in patterned ways; encompasses several cultural and social structure dimensions: technologic factors, religious and philosophical factors, kinship and social factors, political and legal factors, economic factors, educational and cultural values, and lifeways
- *Language:* Word usages, symbols, and meanings about care
- *Ethnohistory:* Past facts, events, instances, experiences of individuals, groups, cultures, and institutions that are primarily people-centered (ethno) and that describe, explain, and interpret human lifeways within particular cultural contexts and over short or long periods of time
- *Environmental context:* The totality of an event, situation, or particular experience that gives meaning to human expressions, interpretations, and social interactions in particular physical, ecological, sociopolitical, and/or cultural settings
- *Health:* A state of well-being that is culturally defined, valued, and practiced and that reflects the ability of individuals (or groups) to perform their daily role activities in culturally expressed, beneficial, and patterned lifeways
- *Worldview:* The way people tend to look out on the world or their universe to form a picture of or a value stance about their life or the world around them
- *Cultural care:* The subjectively and objectively transmitted values, beliefs, and patterned lifeways that assist, support, or enable another individual or group to maintain their well-being and health, to improve their human condition and lifeway, and to deal with illness, handicaps, or death; the two dimensions of cultural care are:
  - *Cultural care diversity:* The variabilities and/or differences in meanings, patterns, values, lifeways, or symbols of care within or between collectivities that are related to assistive, supportive, or enabling human care expressions.
  - *Cultural care universality:* The common, similar, or dominant uniform care meanings, patterns,

values, lifeways, or symbols that are manifest among many cultures and reflect assistive, supportive, facilitative, or enabling ways to help people.
- *Care systems:* The values, norms, and structural features of an organization designed for serving people's health needs, concerns, or conditions; the two types of care systems are:
  - *Generic lay care systems:* Traditional or local indigenous health-care or cure practices that have special meanings and uses to heal or assist people, which are generally offered in familiar home or community environmental contexts with their local practitioners.
  - *Professional health-care system:* Professional care or cure services offered by diverse health personnel who have been prepared through formal professional programs of study in special educational institutions.
- *Cultural-congruent nursing care:* Cognitively based assistive, supportive, facilitative, or enabling acts or decisions that are tailor-made to fit with individual, group, or institutional cultural values, beliefs, and lifeways in order to provide or support meaningful, beneficial, and satisfying health-care or well-being services; the three modes of cultural-congruent nursing care are:
  - *Cultural care preservation or maintenance:* Assistive, supportive, facilitative, or enabling professional actions and decisions that help people of a particular culture retain and/or preserve relevant care values so that they can maintain their well-being, recover from illness, or face handicaps and/or death.
  - *Cultural care accommodation or negotiation:* Assistive, supportive, facilitative, or enabling creative professional actions and decisions that help people of a designated culture adapt to, or negotiate with, others for a beneficial or satisfying health outcome with professional care providers.
  - *Cultural care repatterning or restructuring:* Assistive, supportive, facilitative, or enabling professional actions and decisions that help clients reorder, change, or greatly modify their lifeways for a new, different, and beneficial health-care pattern while respecting the clients' cultural values and beliefs and still providing a beneficial or healthier lifeway than before the changes were coestablished with the clients.

Implications for Nursing Practice
Nursing practice is directed toward improving and providing culturally congruent care to people. The components of the practice methodology for the **Theory of Culture Care Diversity and Universality** are shown in Box 4–10. Each component is discussed in detail here.

Goals of Nursing Practice
- To improve and to provide culturally congruent care that is beneficial, will fit with, and will be useful to the client, family, or culture group healthy lifeways.
- To provide culturally congruent nursing care in order to improve or offer a different kind of nursing care service to people of diverse or similar cultures.

Clients
- Clients include:
  - Individuals
  - Families
  - Subcultures
  - Groups
  - Communities
  - Institutions

Culturalogical Assessment
- The nurse maintains a holistic or total view of the client's world by using the Sunrise Enabler to guide assessment of cultural beliefs, values, and lifeways.
- More than one session with the client typically is required to cover all components of the Sunrise Enabler.
- The first session in a hospital or clinic typically is approximately 20 minutes. Subsequent sessions may be longer.
- The nurse knows his or her own culture and subculture with their particular variabilities, strengths, and assets.
- The nurse discovers and remains aware of his or her own cultural beliefs, values, lifeways, biases, attitudes, and prejudices to avoid cultural blindness.
- The nurse clarifies and explains the focus of the assessment to the client, which is the client's internal (emic) world, not the nurse's outsider (etic) world.
- The nurse is aware that the client may belong to a subculture or special group that maintains its own values and beliefs that differ from the values and beliefs of the dominant culture.
- The nurse shows a genuine interest in the client and learns from and maintains respect for the client.
- The nurse asks open-ended questions and maintains the role of an active listener, learner, and reflector.

Box 4.10 Leininger's Theory of Culture Care Diversity and Universality Practice Methodology

- Goals of Nursing Practice
- Clients
- Culturalogical Assessment
- Nursing Judgments, Decisions, and Actions
- Clinical Protocols

The nurse shares professional knowledge only if the client asks about such knowledge.

- The nurse begins the assessment with such questions as the following:
  - "What would you like to share with me today about your experiences or beliefs to help you keep well?"
  - "Are there some special ideas or ways you would like nurses to care for you?"
- The nurse gives attention to client gender differences, communication modes, special language terms, interpersonal relationships, and use of space and foods.

Nursing Judgments, Decisions, and Actions

- Nursing practice requires the coparticipation of nurses and clients working together to identify, plan, implement, and evaluate the appropriate mode(s) of cultural-congruent nursing care.
- Nursing decisions and actions encompass:
  - Assisting
  - Supporting
  - Facilitating
  - Enabling
- Nurse and client select one or more modes of cultural-congruent nursing care:
  - *Cultural Care Preservation or Maintenance,* used when professional decisions and actions are needed to help clients of a designated culture to retain or preserve relevant care values so that they can maintain their well-being, recover from illness, or face handicaps or death.
  - *Cultural Care Accommodation or Negotiation,* used when professional actions and decisions are needed to help clients of a designated culture adapt to, or negotiate with, others for a beneficial or satisfying health outcome.
  - *Cultural Care Repatterning or Restructuring,* used when professional actions and decisions are needed to help clients of a designated culture reorder, change, or greatly modify their lifeways for a new, different, and beneficial health-care pattern, while respecting the clients' cultural values and beliefs and still providing a beneficial or healthier lifeway than before the changes were coestablished with the clients.

Clinical Protocols

- Specific nursing practices or clinical protocols are derived from the findings of research guided by the Theory of Culture Care Diversity and Universality.
- The research findings are used to develop protocols for cultural-congruent care that blends with the particular cultural values, beliefs, and lifeways of the client, and is assessed to be beneficial, satisfying, and meaningful to the client.

Margaret Newman's Theory of Health as Expanding Consciousness

Newman's grand theory, called the **Theory of Health as Expanding Consciousness,** emphasizes the idea that every person in every situation, no matter how disordered and hopeless the situation may seem, is part of the universal process of expanding consciousness. The concepts of the theory are consciousness and pattern.

Consciousness

Consciousness is the informational capacity of human beings; that is, it is the ability of humans to interact with their environments. Consciousness encompasses interconnected cognitive and affective awareness; physiochemical maintenance, including the nervous and endocrine systems; growth processes; the immune system; and the genetic code. Consciousness can be seen in the quantity and quality of the interaction between human beings and their environments. The process of life moves toward higher levels of consciousness. Sometimes this process is smooth, pleasant, and harmonious; other times it is difficult and disharmonious, as in disease.

Pattern

Pattern is information that depicts the whole; it is relatedness. People are identified by their pattern. The evolution of expanding consciousness is seen in the pattern of movement-space-time. Pattern is manifested as exchanging, communicating, relating, valuing, choosing, moving, perceiving, feeling, and knowing. Pattern encompasses three dimensions—movement-space-time, rhythm, and diversity:

- *Movement-space-time:* Movement is an essential property of matter, a means of communicating, the means whereby one perceives reality and becomes aware of self, and the natural condition of life. Space encompasses personal space, inner space, and life space as dimensions of space relevant to the individual, and territoriality, shared space, and distancing as dimensions relevant to the family. Time is the amount of time perceived to be passing (subjective time), and clock time (objective time).
- *Rhythm:* Basic to movement; the rhythm of movement is an integrating experience
- *Diversity:* Seen in the parts

Implications for Nursing Practice

Nursing practice is directed toward facilitating pattern recognition by connecting with the client in an authentic way and assisting him or her to discover new rules for a higher level of organization or consciousness. The components of Newman's research/practice methodology, which is called the **Research as Praxis Protocol,** are listed in Box 4–11. Each component is discussed in detail here.

Box 4.11 Newman's Health as Expanding Consciousness Practice Methodology: Research as Praxis Protocol

- Phenomenon of Interest
- The Interview
- Transcription
- Development of the Narrative: Pattern Recognition
- Diagram: Pattern Recognition
- Follow-up: Pattern Recognition
- Application of the Theory of Health as Expanding Consciousness

Phenomenon of Interest
- The process of expanding consciousness.

The Interview
- The meeting of the nurse and the study participant/client occurs when there is a mutual attraction via congruent patterns, i.e., interpenetration of the two fields.
- The nurse and study participant/client enter into a partnership with the mutual goal of participating in an authentic relationship, trusting that in the process of its unfolding, both will emerge at a higher level of consciousness.
- The nurse explains the study.
- The study participant/client agrees to continue in the study and agrees to recording the interview on tape.
- The nurse begins the initial interview with a simple, open-ended statement, such as "Tell me about the most meaningful persons and events in your life." This question may be modified to fit the focus of the study.
- The nurse continues the interview in a nondirectional manner, although more direct questions may be used occasionally. Examples of additional questions are: "Tell me what it has been like living with [a particular medical diagnosis, clinical condition, or life circumstance]." "What is meaningful to you?" "What do you think about what we have been talking about?"
- The nurse may prompt the study participant/client to bring to mind something from childhood that stands out in memory, if he or she needs help in thinking of something considered important.
- The nurse acts as an active listener and clarifies and reflects as necessary.
- The nurse is fully present in the moment, is sensitive to intuitive hunches about what to say or ask, and waits for insight into the meaning of the pattern.
- The nurse is free to disclose aspects of himself or herself that are deemed appropriate.
- The initial interview lasts 45 to 60 minutes.

Transcription
- The nurse listens carefully to and transcribes the tape of the interview soon after the interview is completed.
- The nurse is sensitive to the relevance of the data and may omit comments made by the study participant/client that do not directly relate to his or her life pattern, with an appropriate note to the place on the tape where such comments occurred, in case those comments seem important later.

Development of the Narrative: Pattern Recognition
- The nurse selects the statements deemed most important to the study participant/client and arranges the key segments of the data in chronological order to highlight the most significant events and persons.
- The data remain the same except in the order of presentation. Natural breaks where a pattern shift occurs are noted and form the basis of the sequential patterns. Recognition of the pattern of the whole, made up of segments of the study participant/client's relationships over time, will emerge for the nurse.

Diagram: Pattern Recognition
- The nurse then transmutes the narrative into a simple diagram of the sequential pattern configurations.

Follow-up: Pattern Recognition
- The nurse conducts a second interview with the study participant/client to share the diagram or other visual portrayal of the pattern.
- The nurse does not interpret the diagram. Rather, it is used simply to illustrate the study participant/client's story in graphic form, which tends to accentuate the contrasts and repetitions in relationships over time.
- The mutual viewing of the graphic form is an opportunity for the study participant/client to confirm and clarify or revise the story being portrayed.
- The mutual viewing also is an opportunity for the nurse to clarify any aspect of the story about which he or she has any doubt.
- The nature of the pattern of person-environment interaction will begin to emerge in terms of energy flow, e.g., blocked, diffuse, disorganized, repetitive, or whatever descriptors and metaphors come to mind to describe the pattern.
- The study participant/client may express signs that pattern recognition is occurring (or already has occurred in the interval following the first interview) as the nurse and study participant/client reflect together on the study participant/client's life pattern.

- If no signs of pattern recognition occur, the nurse and study participant/client may want to proceed with additional reflections in subsequent interviews until no further insight is reached.
- Sometimes, no signs of pattern recognition emerge, and if so, that characterizes the pattern for that person. It is not to be forced.

Application of the Theory of Health as Expanding Consciousness

- The nurse undertakes more intense analysis of the data in light of the Theory of Health as Expanding Consciousness after the interviews are completed.
- The nurse evaluates the nature of the sequential patterns of interaction in terms of quality and complexity, and interprets the patterns according to the study participant/client's position on Young's spectrum of consciousness.
- The sequential patterns represent presentational construing or relationships.
- Any similarities of pattern among a group of study participants/clients having a similar experience may be designated by themes and stated in propositional form.

Rosemarie Parse's Theory of Humanbecoming

Parse's grand theory, called the **Theory of Humanbecoming** focuses on human experiences of participation with the universe in the cocreation of health. The concepts of the theory are:

- *Humanbecoming:* A unitary construct referring to the human being's living health.
- *Meaning:* The linguistic and imagined content of something and the interpretation that one gives to something.
- *Rhythmicity:* The cadent, paradoxical patterning of the human-universe mutual process.
- *Transcendence:* Reaching beyond with possibles— the hopes and dreams envisioned in multidimensional experiences and powering the originating of Transforming.
- *Imaging:* Reflective-prereflective coming to know the explicit-tacit all-at-once.
- *Valuing:* Confirming-not confirming cherished beliefs in light of a personal worldview.
- *Languaging:* Signifying valued images through speaking-being silent and moving-being still.
- *Revealing-concealing:* Disclosing-not disclosing all-at-once.
- *Enabling-limiting:* Living the opportunities-restrictions present in all choosings all-at-once.
- *Connecting-separating:* Being with and apart from others, ideas, objects, and situations all-at-once.

- *Powering:* The pushing-resisting process of affirming-not affirming being in light of nonbeing.
- *Originating:* Inventing new ways of conforming-nonconforming in the certainty-uncertainty of living.
- *Transforming:* Shifting the view of the familiar-unfamiliar, the changing of change in coconstituting anew in a deliberate way.

The three major principles of the theory of humanbecoming are as follows:

1. *Structuring meaning multidimensionally* is cocreating reality through the languaging of valuing and imaging. It means that humans construct what is real for them from choices made at many realms of the universe.
2. *Cocreating rhythmical patterns of relating* is living the paradoxical unity of revealing-concealing and enabling-limiting while connecting-separating. It means that humans live in rhythm with the universe coconstituting patterns of relating.
3. *Cotranscending with the possibles* is powering unique ways of originating in the process of transforming. It means that humans forge unique paths with shifting perspectives as a different light is cast on the familiar.

Implications for Nursing Practice

Nursing practice is directed toward respecting the quality of life as perceived by the person and the family. Parse's **Practice Methodology** is summarized in Box 4–12. Each aspect of the practice methodology is discussed in detail below.

PART 1

Theory of Humanbecoming Principle	Practice Methodology Dimension	Practice Methodology Process (Empirical Activity)
1: Structuring meaning mutidimensionally	*Illuminating meaning:* Explicating what was, is, and will be	*Explicating:* Making clear what is appearing now through languaging
2: Cocreating rhythmical patterns	*Synchronizing rhythms:* Dwelling with the pitch, yaw, and roll of the human-universe process	*Dwelling with:* Immersing with the flow of connecting-separating
3: Mobilizing transcendence	*Mobilizing transcendence:* Moving beyond the meaning moment with what is not yet	*Moving beyond:* Propelling with envisioned possibles of transforming

Box 4.12 Parse's Theory of Humanbecoming
Practice Methodology

- Explicating
- Dwelling with
- Moving beyond
- Contexts for nursing
- Goal of the discipline of nursing
- Goal of the humanbecoming nurse
- True presence
- Ways of changing health patterns in true presence

PART 2
Contexts for Nursing

- Nurse-person situations
- Nurse-group situations
- Participants: Children, adults
- Locations: Homes, shelters, health-care centers, parish halls, all departments of hospitals and clinics, rehabilitation centers, offices, other milieus where nurses are with people

Goal of the Discipline of Nursing
- Quality of life from the person's, family's, and community's perspective.

Goal of the Humanbecoming Nurse
- To be truly present with people as they enhance the quality of their lives.

True Presence
- A special way of "being with" in which the nurse is attentive to moment-to-moment changes in meaning as she or he bears witness to the person's or group's own living of value priorities
  - *Coming-to-be-present:* An all-at-once gentling down and lifting up. True presence begins in the coming-to-be-present moments of preparation and attention; an all-at-once gentling down and lifting up. True presence begins in the coming-to-be-present moments of preparation and attention. Preparation involves an emptying to be available to bear witness to the other or others, and being flexible, not fixed but gracefully present from one's center, as well as dwelling with the universe at the moment, considering the attentive presence about to be. Attention involves focusing on the moment at hand for immersion.
  - *Face-to-face discussions:* Nurse and person engage in dialogue, and the nurse tries to understand the person's perspective by initiating discussions. Conversation may be through discussion in generalor through interpretations of stories, films, drawings, photographs, music, metaphors, poetry, rhythmical movements, and other expressions. The nurse really listens to the person,

without interrupting. The nurse may seek clarification of the person's comments.
  - *Silent immersion:* A process of the quiet that does not refrain from sending and receiving messages; a chosen way of becoming in the human-universe process lived in the rhythm of speaking-being silent, moving-being still as valued images incarnate meaning; true presence without words
  - *Lingering presence:* Recalling a moment through a lingering presence that arises after an immediate engagement; a reflective-prereflective "abiding with" attended to through glimpses of the other person, idea, object, or situation

Ways of Changing Health Patterns in True Presence
- *Creative imagining:* Picturing, by seeing, hearing, and feeling, what a situation might be like if lived in a different way.
- *Affirming personal becoming:* Uncovering preferred personal health patterns by critically thinking about how or who one is.
- *Glimpsing the paradoxical:* Changing one's view of a situation by recognizing incongruities in that situation.

Middle-Range Theories

Middle-range theories are narrower in scope than grand theories, encompassing a smaller number of concepts and a limited aspect of the real world. Middle-range theories are, therefore, made up of concepts that are empirically measurable and statements that are empirically testable. Examples of middle-range nursing theories are Orlando's (1961) Theory of the Deliberative Nursing Process, Peplau's (1952, 1992) Theory of Interpersonal Relations, and Watson's (2006) Theory of Human Caring. An overview of each of these middle-range theories is given below, along with implications for practice.

Many other middle-range nursing theories and middle-range theories from other disciplines are used by nurses (Peterson & Bredow, 2004; Smith & Liehr, 2003; Ziegler, 2005). Some of those theories can be linked with nursing conceptual models and others may not be able to be so linked. For example, the theory of planned behavior, which is a middle-range theory developed by social psychologists, has been linked with Neuman's Systems Model and Orem's Self-Care Framework (Villarruel, Bishop, Simpson, Jemmott, & Fawcett, 2001).

The specificity of middle-range theory concepts and statements is illustrated by Orlando's (1961) theory. This theory predicts that using a particular communication technique is effective in identifying the patient's immediate need for help. The technique requires the nurse, using a personal pronoun, to share with the patient his or her perceptions, thoughts, or feelings about the patient's behavior and to ask the patient whether those perceptions, thoughts, or feelings are correct. An example is, "I think you do not want to exercise today. Am I correct?"

Ida Jean Orlando's Theory of the Deliberative Nursing Process

Orlando's middle-range predictive nursing theory, called the **Deliberative Nursing Process**, focuses on an interpersonal process between people. It helps identify the nature of the patient's distress and his or her immediate needs for help. The concepts of the theory are:

Patient's Behavior
The patient's behavior is behavior observed by the nurse in an immediate nursing-patient situation. The two dimensions are:

1. *Need for help:* A requirement of the patient that, if supplied, relieves or diminishes immediate distress or improves immediate sense of adequacy or well-being.
2. *Improvement:* An increase in the patient's mental and physical health, well-being, and sense of adequacy.

The need for help and improvement can be expressed in both nonverbal and verbal forms. Visual manifestations of nonverbal behavior include such motor activities as eating, walking, twitching, and trembling as well as such physiologic forms as urinating, defecating, temperature and blood pressure readings, respiratory rate, and skin color. Vocal forms of nonverbal behavior—nonverbal behavior that is heard—include crying, moaning, laughing, coughing, sneezing, sighing, yelling, screaming, groaning, and singing. Verbal behavior refers to what a patient says, including complaints, requests, questions, refusals, demands, and comments or statements.

Nurse's Reaction
The nurse's reaction is the nonobservable response to the patient's behavior. The three dimensions are:

1. *Perception:* Physical stimulation of any one of the five senses by the patient's behavior.
2. *Thought:* An idea that occurs in the nurse's mind.
3. *Feeling:* A state of mind inclining the person toward or against a perception, thought, or action. It occurs in response to the nurse's perceptions and thoughts.

Nurse's Activity
Nurse's activity is the observable actions taken by the nurse, including instructions, suggestions, directions, explanations, information, requests, and questions directed toward the patient; making decisions for the patient; handling the patient's body; administering medications or treatments; and changing the patient's

immediate environment. The two dimensions of nurse's activity are:

1. *Automatic nursing process:* Actions decided on by the nurse for reasons other than the patient's immediate need.
2. *Deliberative nursing process (process discipline):* A specific set of nurse behaviors or actions directed toward the patient's behavior that ascertain or meet the patient's immediate needs for help.

Implications for Nursing Practice
Nursing practice is directed toward identifying and meeting the patient's immediate needs for help through use of **Orlando's Practice Methodology.** The components of the practice methodology are listed in Box 4–13. Each component is discussed in detail below.

Observations
Encompass any and all information pertaining to a patient that the nurse acquires while on duty; form the raw material with which the nurse makes and implements plans for the patient's care.

- *Direct observations*— nurse's reaction to patient's behavior: Consists of any perception, thought, or feeling the nurse has from her own experience of the patient's behavior at any or several moments in time.
- *Indirect observations*—other information about the patient's behavior: Consists of any information that is derived from a source other than the patient. This information pertains to, but is not directly derived from, the patient.

Actions
Carried out with or for the patient

- *Nurse's activity—deliberative nursing process:* This is the process used to share and validate the nurse's direct and indirect observations.
- *Clinical protocols:* These contain the specific requirements for the deliberative nursing process.
- *Direct help:* The nurse meets the patient's need directly when the patient is unable to meet his or her own need and when the activity is confined to the nurse-patient contact.
- *Indirect help:* The nurse meets the patient's need indirectly when the activity extends to arranging the services of a person, agency, or resource that the patient cannot contact by himself or herself.

Box 4.13 Orlando's Practice Methodology

- Observations
- Actions
- Reporting
- Recording

Reporting

The nurse receives reports about the patient's behavior from other nurses and from other health professionals and reports observations.

Recording

The nurse records the nursing process, including:

- The nurse's perception of or about the patient.
- The nurse's thought and/or feeling about the perception.
- What the nurse said and/or did to, with, or for the patient.

Hildegard Peplau's Theory of Interpersonal Relations

Peplau's middle-range descriptive nursing theory, called the **Theory of Interpersonal Relations,** focuses on the phases of the interpersonal process that occur when an ill person and a nurse come together to resolve a health difficulty. The one concept of the Theory of Interpersonal Relations is the *nurse-patient relationship,* which is an interpersonal process made up of four components—two persons, the professional expertise of the nurse, and the client's problem or need for which expert nursing services are sought—and which has three discernible phases:

1. *Orientation phase:* The phase in which the nurse first identifies herself or himself by name and professional status and states the purpose, nature, and time available for the patient. This is the phase during which the nurse conveys professional interest and receptivity to the patient, begins to know the patient as a person, obtains essential information about the patient's health condition, and sets the tone for further interactions.
2. *Working phase:* The phase in which the major work occurs. The two subphases are:
   - *Identification:* The subphase during which the patient learns how to make use of the nurse-patient relationship.
   - *Exploitation:* The subphase during which the patient makes full use of available professional services (Peplau, 1952).
3. *Termination phase:* The phase in which the work accomplished is summarized and closure occurs.

Implications for Nursing Practice

Nursing practice is directed toward promoting favorable changes in patients, which is accomplished through the nurse-patient relationship. Within that relationship, the nurse's major function is to study the interpersonal relations between the patient/client and others. The components of **Peplau's Clinical**

Methodology, which can be used for both nursing practice and research, are listed in Box 4–14. Each component is discussed in detail below.

Observation

Identification, clarification, and verification of impressions about the interactive drama, of the pushes and pulls in the relationship between nurse and patient, as they occur.

- *Nurse's behavior:* Observation of the nurse's words, voice tones, body language, and other gestural messages.
- *Patient's behavior:* Observation of the patient's words, voice tones, body language, and other gestural messages.
- *Interpersonal phenomena:* Observation of what goes on between the patient and the nurse.
- *Reframing empathic linkages:* Occurs when the nurse's and/or the patient's ability to feel in self the emotions experienced by the other person in the same situation is converted to verbal communications by the nurse asking, "What are you feeling right now?"

Communication

Aims are the selection of symbols or concepts that convey both the reference, or meaning in the mind of the individual, and referent, the object or actions symbolized in the concept; and the wish to struggle toward the development of common understanding for words between two or more people.

- *Interpersonal techniques:* Verbal interventions used by nurses during nurse-patient relationships, aimed at accomplishing problem resolution and competence development in patients.
- *Principle of clarity:* Comments and questions to force the patient to think, to respond, and to use those capacities that will produce the necessary data.
- *Principle of continuity:* Occurs when language is used as a tool for the promotion of coherence or connections of ideas expressed, and leads to discrimination of relationships or connections among ideas and the feelings, events, or themes conveyed in those ideas. Continuity is promoted when the nurse is able to pick up threads of conversation that the patient offers in the course of a conversation and

---

Box 4.14 Peplau's Clinical Methodology

- Observation
- Communication
- Recording
- Data Analysis

over a longer period, such as a week, and when she aids the patient to focus and to expand those threads.

Recording
The written record of the communication between nurse and patient, or the data collected through participant observation and reframing of empathic linkages. The aim is to capture the exact wording of the interaction between the nurse and the patient.

Data Analysis
Focuses on testing the nurse's hypotheses, which are formulated from first impressions or hunches about the patient.

- *Phases of the nurse-patient relationship:* Identify the phase of nurse-patient relationship in which communication occurred: orientation phase; working phase, identification subphase, exploitation subphase; termination phase.
- *Roles:* Identify the roles taken by the nurse and the patient in each phase of the nurse-patient relationship.
- *Relations:* Identify the connections, linkages, ties, and bonds that go on or went on between a patient and others, including family, friends, staff, and the nurse.
- *Pattern integrations:* Identify the patterns of the interpersonal relation between two or more people that together link or bind them and that enable the people to transform energy into patterns of action that bring satisfaction or security in the face of a recurring problem.

Jean Watson's Theory of Human Caring

Watson's middle-range explanatory nursing theory, called the **Theory of Human Caring**, focuses on the human component of caring and the moment-to-moment encounters between the one who is caring and the one who is being cared for, especially the caring activities performed by nurses as they interact with others. The concepts of the Theory of Human Caring are:

Transpersonal Caring Relationship
Human-to-human connectedness, whereby each person is touched by the human center of the other. This is a special kind of relationship involving a high regard for the whole person and his or her being-in-the-world. The concept of transpersonal caring relationship encompasses three dimensions:

- *Self:* Transpersonal-mind-body-spirit oneness, an embodied self, and an embodied spirit.
- *Phenomenal field:* The totality of human experience, one's being-in-the-world.
- *Intersubjectivity:* "Transpersonal" refers to an intersubjective human-to-human relationship in which

the person of the nurse affects and is affected by the person of the other, both of whom are fully present in the moment and feel a union with the other.

Caring Occasion/Caring Moment
The coming together of nurse and other(s), which involves action and choice both by the nurse and the other. The moment of coming together in a caring occasion presents them with the opportunity to decide how to be in the relationship—what to do with the moment.

Caring (Healing) Consciousness
A holographic dynamic that is manifest within a field of consciousness and that exists through time and space and is dominant over physical illness.

Clinical Caritas Processes
Those aspects of nursing that actually potentiate therapeutic healing processes for both the one caring and the one being cared for. The 10 clinical caritas processes used by nurses when caring for people are:

1. Practice of loving kindness and equanimity within the context of caring consciousness.
2. Being authentically present and enabling and sustaining the deep belief system and subjective life world of self and one-being-cared-for.
3. Cultivation of one's own spiritual practices and transpersonal self, going beyond ego self, opening to others with sensitivity and compassion.
4. Developing and sustaining a helping-trusting, authentic caring relationship.
5. Being present to, and supportive of, the expression of positive and negative feelings as a connection with deeper spirit of self and the one-being-cared-for.
6. Creative use of self and all ways of knowing as part of the caring process; to engage in artistry of caring-healing practices.
7. Engaging in genuine teaching-learning experience that attends to unity of being and meaning, attempting to stay within others' frames of reference.
8. Creating healing environments at all levels (physical as well as nonphysical, subtle environment of energy and consciousness, whereby wholeness, beauty, comfort, dignity, and peace are potentiated).
9. Assisting with basic needs, with an intentional caring consciousness, administering "human care essentials," which potentiate alignment of mind-body-spirit, wholeness, and unity of being in all aspects of care, tending to both embodied spirit and evolving spiritual emergence.
10. Opening and attending to spiritual-mysterious, and existential dimensions of one's own life-death; soul care for self and the one-being-cared-for.

>5

Implications for Nursing Practice

Nursing practice is directed toward helping persons gain a higher degree of harmony within the mind, body, andsoul. This in turn generates self-knowledge, self-reverence, self-healing, and self-care processes while increasing diversity, which is pursued through use of the 10 clinical caritas processes. The components of **Watson's Practice Methodology** are listed in Box 4–15. Each component is discussed in detail below.

Requirements for a Transpersonal Caring Relationship

- The nurse considers the person to be valid and whole, regardless of illness or disease.
- The nurse makes a moral commitment and directs intentionality and consciousness to the protection, enhancement, and potentiation of human dignity, wholeness, and healing, such that a person creates or co-creates his or her own meaning for existence, healing, wholeness, and caring.
- The nurse orients intent, will, and consciousness toward affirming the subjective/intersubjective significance of the person; a search to sustain mind-body-spirit unity and I-Thou versus I-It relationships.
- The nurse has the ability to realize, accurately detect, and connect with the inner condition (spirit) of another. The nurse recognizes that actions, words, behaviors, cognition, body language, feelings, intuition, thought, senses, and the energy field gestalt all contribute to the interconnection.
- The nurse has the ability to assess and realize another's condition of being-in-the-world and to feel a union with the other. This ability is translated via movements, gestures, facial expressions, procedures, information, touch, sound, verbal expressions, and other scientific, aesthetic, and human means of communication into nursing-art acts wherein the nurse responds to, attends to, or reflects the condition of the other. Drawn from the ontological caring-consciousness stance and basic competencies of the nurse, this ability expands and translates into advanced caring-healing modalities, nursing arts, advanced nursing therapeutics, and healing arts.
- The nurse understands that the caring-healing modalities potentiate harmony, wholeness, and comfort and produce inner healing by releasing some of the disharmony and blocked energy that interfere with the natural healing processes.
- Transpersonal caring-healing modalities include:
  - Intentional conscious use of auditory modalities, such as music; sounds of nature, wind, sea, chimes, and chants; and familiar sounds.
  - Intentional conscious use of visual modalities, such as light, color, form, texture, and works of art.
  - Intentional conscious use of olfactory modalities, such as aromatherapy, breathwork, breathing fresh air, and inhalation-exhalation.
  - Intentional conscious use of the tactile modality, including such body touch therapies as acupressure, body therapy, caring touch, foot reflexology, shiatsu, and therapeutic massage.
  - Intentional conscious use of gustatory modalities, with a focus on particular foods in one's diet.
  - Intentional conscious use of mental-cognitive modalities, with a focus on the importance of the mind and the imagination through story.
  - Intentional conscious use of kinesthetic modalities, such as basic skin care, deep massage and deep cellular tissue work (e.g., Rolfing), movement, dance, yoga, Tai Chi, applied kinesiology, chiropractic, Feldendrais work, Jin shin jyutsu, polarity work, Reiki, and Trager work.
  - Intentional conscious use of "caring consciousness" as modality, with a focus on physical presence, psychological presence, and therapeutic presence.
- The nurse understands that his or her own life history and previous experiences, including opportunities, studies, consciousness of having lived through or experienced human feelings and various human conditions, or of having imagined others' feelings in various circumstances, are valuable contributors to the transpersonal caring relationship.

Authentic Presencing

The nurse:

- Is authentically present as self and other in a reflective mutuality of being and becoming.
- Centers consciousness and intentionality on caring, healing, and wholeness, rather than on disease, problems, illness, complications, and technocures.
- Attempts to:
  - Stay within the other's frame of reference
  - Join in a mutual search for meaning and wholeness of being
  - Potentiate comfort measures, pain control, a sense of well-being, or spiritual transcendence of suffering.

Box 4.15 Watson's Practice Methodology

- Requirements for a Transpersonal Caring Relationship
- Authentic Presencing

ADVANTAGES OF USING FORMAL NURSING KNOWLEDGE

Recognition of nursing as a profession confers a certain status on nurses. The status conferred by being a member of a profession, rather than having an occupation or a trade, carries with it the responsibility to use formal nursing knowledge. Anderson (1995) explained that, as members of a profession, nurses "must ensure that we have a solid scholarly and scientific foundation upon which to base our practice" (p. 247). Conceptual models of nursing and nursing theories are that foundation; they provide explicit frames of reference for professional nursing practice by delineating the scope of nursing practice. Furthermore, conceptual models of nursing and nursing theories (1) specify innovative goals for nursing practice, (2) introduce ideas that are designed to improve practice (Lindsay, 1990), and (3) enhance the quality of people's lives by facilitating the identification of relevant information, reducing the fragmentation of health care, and improving the coordination of all aspects of health care (Chalmers, as cited in Chalmers, Kershaw, Melia, & Kendrich, 1990).

More specifically, the use of formal nursing knowledge to guide nursing practice "represents nursing's unique contribution to the health-care system" (Parse, 1995, p. 128). It is the hallmark of professional nursing practice. As Chalmers pointed out, "Nursing models [and theories] have provided what many would argue is a much needed alternative knowledge base from which nurses can practice in an informed way. An alternative, that is, to the medical model which for so many years has dominated many aspects of health care" (Chalmers et al., 1990, p. 34).

Formal nursing knowledge also provides an alternative to the institutional model of practice, in which "the most salient values [are] efficiency, standardized care, rules, and regulations" (Rogers, 1989, p. 113). The institutional model, moreover, typically upholds, reinforces, and supports the medical model (Grossman & Hooton, 1993). Thus, the use of conceptual models of nursing and nursing theories moves the practice of nursing away from that driven by a medical or institutional model and, therefore, fosters autonomy from medicine and a coherent purpose of practice (Bélanger, 1991; Bridges, 1991; Ingram, 1991; Parse, 1995).

The major practical advantage of using a conceptual model of nursing is the identification of a comprehensive nursing process format or practice methodology that encompasses particular parameters for assessment, labels for problems, a strategy for planning nursing interventions, a typology of nursing interventions, and criteria for evaluation of the outcomes of nursing practice. More specifically, whereas the generic nursing process tells the nurse only to assess, label, plan, intervene, and evaluate, the nursing process associated with a particular conceptual model tells the nurse what to assess, what labels are possible, how to plan, what interventions are appropriate, and what outcomes to evaluate.

The major practical advantage a nursing theory provides is greater specificity in one or more phases of the nursing process. For example, Orlando's (1961) Theory of the Deliberative Nursing Process tells the nurse exactly how to identify the patient's immediate need for help. Orlando's theory can be used very effectively in combination with Roy's Adaptation Model (Roy & Andrews, 1999) and other conceptual models of nursing.

It should be obvious by now that formal nursing knowledge identifies the distinctive nursing territory within the vast arena of multidisciplinary health care (Feeg, 1989). Each conceptual model of nursing and nursing theory provides a holistic orientation for nursing practice and reinforces the view that nursing practice ultimately is "for our patients' sake" (Dabbs, 1994, p. 220). In addition, the use of formal nursing knowledge "help[s] nurses better communicate what they do" (Neff, 1991, p. 534) and why they do it. The importance of communicating what nursing is and what nurses do was underscored by Feeg (1989), who identified three reasons for implementing conceptual model-based or theory-based nursing practice that are as relevant today as they were in the 1980s. The three reasons are:

1. In this time of information saturation and rapid change, we know it is not valuable to focus on every detail and, therefore, we need [conceptual models and theories] to help guide our judgments in new situations.
2. In this time of technologic overdrive, we need a holistic orientation to remind us of our caring perspective.
3. In this time of professional territoriality, it has become even more important to understand our identity in nursing and operationalize our practice from a [formal nursing] knowledge base. (p. 450)

The number of nurses throughout the world who recognize the advantages of using formal nursing knowledge is rapidly increasing. Indeed, although some clinicians continue to hold the "unfortunate view [that nursing models and theories] are the inventions and predictions only of scholars and academics [that have] little significance for their own practice environments," many other clinicians recognize the beneficial effects of formal nursing knowledge on practice (Hayne, 1992, p. 105). Moreover, Cash's (1990) claim that "there is no central core that can distinguish nursing theoretically from a number of other occupational activities"

(p. 255) is readily offset by many claims to the contrary. In particular, Cash's claim clearly fails to take into account the contributions made by formal nursing knowledge to the development of practices that enable all nurses to talk nursing (Chalmers et al., 1990), to think nursing (Nightingale, 1993; Perry, 1985), and to engage in thinking nursing (Allison & Renpenning, 1999), rather than just doing tasks and carrying out physicians' orders (Le Storti et al., 1999).

Nurses are able to think nursing and talk nursing because the conceptual models and theories that constitute formal nursing knowledge provide a distinctive nursing language. The lack of a nursing language in the past, and in the present when conceptual models of nursing and nursing theories are not used, "has been a handicap in nurses' communications about nursing to the public as well as to persons with whom they work in the health field" (Orem, 1997, p. 29). Thus, the content of each conceptual model of nursing and nursing theory, which is stated in a distinctive vocabulary, should not be considered jargon. Rather, the terminology used by the author of each conceptual model or theory should be recognized as the result of considerable thought about how to convey the meaning of that particular perspective to others (Biley, 1990). "The attention to language," Watson (1997) maintained, "is especially critical to an evolving [profession], in that during this postmodern era, one's survival depends on having language; writers in this area remind us 'if you do not have your own language you don't exist'" (p. 50). Elaborating, Akinsanya (1989) explained, "Every science has its own peculiar terms, concepts, and principles which are essential for the development of its knowledge base. In nursing, as in other sciences, an understanding of these is a prerequisite to a critical examination of their contribution to the development of knowledge and its application to practice" (p. ii). Indeed, the differences in the vocabularies of the various conceptual models and theories are the same as the differences in the vocabularies of diverse medical specialties, such as obstetrics, gynecology, cardiology, neurology, psychiatry, and geriatrics.

Thinking nursing within the context of formal nursing knowledge helps nurses to "clarify their thinking on their role, especially at a time when the roles of many health professionals are becoming blurred" (Nightingale, 1993, p. 2). Moreover, thinking nursing within the context of formal nursing knowledge may shape the way in which specialized nursing practice is viewed. Indeed, nurses may elect to specialize in the use of a particular conceptual model of nursing or nursing theory, or they may elect to specialize in a particular concept of a particular conceptual model of nursing or nursing theory. A nurse could, for example, specialize in one behavioral subsystem of Johnson's Behavioral System Model (Rogers, 1973).

Risks and Rewards of Using Formal Nursing Knowledge

Johnson (1990) noted that although individual clinicians and nursing departments take risks when the decision is made to implement conceptual model- or theory-based nursing practice, the rewards far outweigh the risks. She stated:

> To openly use a nursing model [or theory] is risk-taking behavior for the individual nurse. For a nursing department to adopt one of these models [or theories] for unit or institution use is risk-taking behavior of an even higher order. The reward for such risk-taking for the individual practitioner lies in the great satisfaction gained from being able to specify explicit concrete nursing goals in the care of patients and from documenting the actual achievement of the desired outcomes. The reward for the nursing department is having a rational, cohesive, and comprehensive basis for the development of standards of nursing practice, for the evaluation of practitioners, and for the documentation of the contribution of nursing to patient welfare. (Johnson, 1990, p. 32)

Accumulating anecdotal and empirical evidence indicates that additional rewards of using formal nursing knowledge to guide nursing practice include reduced staff nurse turnover, more rapid movement from novice to expert nurse, greater patient and family satisfaction with nursing, increased nurse job satisfaction, and considerable cost savings (Fawcett, 2005). Furthermore, as the use of formal nursing knowledge grows, both nurses and participants in nursing are empowered. Indeed, "[nursing] knowledge is power" (Orr, 1991, p. 218), and it can be used to empower individuals, families, and communities to fully participate in decisions about their health care (Lister, 1991; Malin & Teasdale, 1991). The challenge, then, is to help each nurse select an explicit nursing model or theory to guide his or her nursing practice.

SELECTING A CONCEPTUAL MODEL OR NURSING THEORY FOR PROFESSIONAL NURSING PRACTICE

Although formal nursing knowledge is made up of many conceptual models and theories, using more than one model or theory at the same time will create much confusion. Therefore, each nurse should select just one as a guide for professional practice. The following six steps can help you select an appropriate conceptual model of nursing or nursing theory:

1. Identify your own beliefs and values related to the phenomena of interest to all nurses. State your

beliefs about the participants in nursing, the relevant environment, health, and the goals of professional nursing practice.

2. Identify the patient population with which you would like to work. The population may be based on a specific medical diagnosis, such as cancer or renal failure; an age group, such as children and adolescents or the elderly; a type of illness, such as an acute crisis or chronic illness; or a particular symptom, such as chest pain or an elevated temperature.

3. Systematically analyze and evaluate the content of several conceptual models of nursing and nursing theories. Review the summaries of the conceptual models and theories presented in the chapter as well as the primary source material for each conceptual model and theory. This review will provide a firm foundation for your selection of the conceptual model or theory.

4. Compare your own beliefs and values with the philosophical claims undergirding the selected conceptual model.

5. Identify the conceptual models and nursing theories that are appropriate guides for nursing with the patient population in which you are interested.

6. Choose the conceptual model or theory that most closely matches your beliefs and values and the patient population with which you want to work. Then use the model or theory to guide your practice with several nursing participants so that you can determine its utility. If you find that the conceptual model or theory you have chosen is not useful, select another model or theory and test its utility.

USING CONCEPTUAL MODELS TO GUIDE PROFESSIONAL NURSING PRACTICE

The use of an explicit conceptual model of nursing to guide professional nursing practice is exemplified in the following case study.

Research findings indicate that nurses feel vulnerable and experience a great deal of stress when they attempt to achieve professional aspirations within a rapidly changing, medically dominated, bureaucratic health-care delivery system (Graham, 1994). As a structure for

CASE STUDY | Orem's Self-Care Framework

Gerry Smith is a 64-year-old, well-nourished man with long-standing non-insulin dependent diabetes mellitus (NIDDM). He underwent emergency open-heart bypass graft surgery 7 weeks ago and remains hospitalized with a serious leg wound. Mr. Smith had an uneventful cardiac recovery after his surgery, but the graft site on his left leg became infected and failed to heal properly. Two weeks after the open-heart surgery, Mr. Smith underwent emergency arterial bypass surgery to improve circulation to his left lower limb.

He currently is a patient on the rehabilitation unit for management of the leg wound. Sterile dressing changes are required three times daily. Mr. Smith transfers with moderate assistance, and ambulates using a walker and minimal to moderate assistance, depending on his pain and fatigue level. He requires moderate assistance for dressing, toileting hygiene, and bathing, and minimal assistance for meal set-up. Mr. Smith has urinary and bowel control with occasional urgency of bowel secondary to diarrhea caused by multiple antibiotics. Mr. Smith has the support of his wife of 42 years and four grown sons.

Mrs. Smith is currently learning skin-care dressing techniques. She will be the primary caregiver when Mr. Smith is discharged in approximately 2 weeks. Mr. Smith has been experiencing periods of moodiness and depression since his operations. He admits that the long hospitalization has left him feeling overwhelmed at times, but he is hopeful for the future. He expresses gratitude that his leg was saved. More than anything else, Mr. Smith wants to regain enough ability to enjoy a hunting trip.

Initial assessment of Mr. Smith's self-care agency—that is, his ability to perform self-care—reveals that he currently is unable to meet what Orem calls his therapeutic self-care demand. Therapeutic self-care demand is defined as "the known self-care requisites [that are] particular for individuals in relation to their conditions and circumstances" (Orem, 1995, pp. 65, 123). Three types of self-care requisites make up the therapeutic self-care demand: universal, developmental, and health deviation. Comparing the therapeutic self-care demand with Mr. Smith's current self-care agency reveals several self-care deficits.

(case study continues on page 78)

CASE STUDY Orem's Self-Care Framework (continued)

Mr. and Mrs. Smith, along with his nurse, agree that the goal is to enhance Mr. Smith's self-care agency and Mrs. Smith's dependent-care agency through the use of all three types of nursing systems. The wholly compensatory nursing system is needed to provide both blood glucose monitoring and sterile dressing changes three times daily. The partly compensatory nursing system is needed to assist Mr. Smith with dressing, toilet transfers, bathing, and ambulation. The supportive-educative nursing system is needed to teach Mr. and Mrs. Smith about his personal care and to provide psychological support to facilitate coping with a chronic illness. Consequently, the nursing staff will initially provide wound care to Mr. Smith's leg, but will teach Mrs. Smith how to perform sterile dressing care when Mr. Smith goes home. In summary, the nursing staff will give Mr. and Mrs. Smith the necessary guidance and teaching to allow them to meet his therapeutic self-care demand once he is discharged from the hospital. ■

critical thinking within a distinctively nursing context, formal nursing knowledge provides the intellectual skills and points to the practical skills that nurses need to survive at a time when cost containment through reduction of professional nursing staff is the modus operandi of managed care and the administrators of health-care delivery systems, including hospitals, home health-care agencies, and health-maintenance organizations.

As a novice user of a conceptual model of nursing or nursing theory, you should not become discouraged if your initial experiences with the model or theory seem forced or awkward. Adopting an explicit nursing model or theory does require using a new vocabulary and a new way of thinking about nursing situations. Repeatedly using the conceptual model or theory should, however, lead to more systematic and organized applications. Broncatello's (1980) words, written more than 20 years ago, continue to provide the encouragement needed to start using a conceptual model of nursing or nursing theory to guide professional nursing practice.

The nurse's consistent use of any model [or theory] for the interpretation of observable [patient] data is most definitely not an easy task. Much like the development of any habitual behavior, it initially requires thought, discipline, and the gradual evolvement of a mind-set of what is important to observe within the guidelines of the model [or theory]. As is true of most habits, however, it makes decision making less complicated. (p. 23)

Using formal nursing knowledge allows the nursing profession to be clear about its mission in the constantly changing health-care arena. Now, perhaps more than ever before, it is crucial that nurses explicate what they know and why they do what they do. In other words, it is crucial that all nurses communicate distinctive nursing knowledge and explain how that knowledge governs the actions performed on behalf of or in conjunction with people who require nursing. Thus, it is incumbent on all nurses to use formal nursing knowledge. Only if they do so can nurses continue to claim a place on the multidisciplinary health-care team.

KEY POINTS

■ Conceptual models of nursing present diverse perspectives of the participant in nursing, who can be an individual, a family, or a community; the environment of the nursing participant and the environment in which professional nursing practice occurs; the participant's health state; and the definition and goals of nursing as well as nursing actions or interventions.

■ The most practical function of a conceptual model is its delineation of goals for nursing practice and a nursing process format or practice methodology that encompasses parameters for assessment, labels for problems, a strategy for planning nursing interventions, a typology of nursing interventions, and criteria for evaluation of the outcomes of nursing practice. A conceptual model of nursing provides a structure for documentation of all aspects of the nursing process, from patient assessment to evaluation of outcomes. A conceptual model also helps identify standards of nursing practice and criteria for quality assurance reviews.

(Key points continue on page 79)

K E Y   P O I N T S   (continued)

■ The function of a nursing theory is to provide considerable specificity in the description, explanation, or prediction of some phenomenon. Theories are more concrete and specific than conceptual models. A conceptual model is an abstract and general system of concepts and statements, whereas a theory deals with one or more relatively concrete and specific concepts and statements. In addition, conceptual models are general guides that must be specified further by relevant and logically congruent theories before action can occur.

■ Conceptual models of nursing and nursing theories move the professional practice of nursing away from that which is driven by a medical or institutional model and, therefore, foster autonomy from medicine and a coherent purpose for professional nursing practice.

■ Six steps are used to select a conceptual model or nursing theory to guide professional nursing practice: (1) state your philosophy of nursing, in the form of beliefs and values about the nursing participant, the environment, health, and nursing goals; (2) identify the particular patient population with which you wish to practice; (3) thoroughly analyze and evaluate several conceptual models of nursing and nursing theories; (4) compare the philosophical claims on which each conceptual model and nursing theory is based with your own philosophy of nursing; (5) determine which conceptual models or nursing theories are appropriate for use with the patient population you are interested in; and (6) select the conceptual model or nursing theory that most closely matches your philosophy of nursing and the patient population of interest.

Thought and Discussion Activities

1. List two ways in which a conceptual model differs from a grand theory or a middle-range theory.

2. Many people select nursing as a career because they enjoy "taking care of" other people. Orem's conceptual model of nursing focuses on individuals with limited abilities to provide continuing self-care or care of dependent others. Describe the difference between "taking care of people" as a general term and professional nursing practice directed toward helping people meet their own and their dependent others' therapeutic self-care demands.

3. Describe the focus of Orem's Self-Care Framework in relation to chronically ill patients and their families as they struggle to adjust to changes in the patients' ability to meet self-care demands.
   - Do you let your own beliefs interfere with how you interact with these patients? Explain your answer.
   - Is your practice standard for all patients? Explain your answer.

4. Explain how conceptual models of nursing provide a framework for objective measurement of the effects of your nursing assessments and interventions.

☐ REFERENCES

Akinsanya, J. A. (1989). Introduction. *Recent Advances in Nursing, 24,* i–ii.

Allison, S. E., & Renpenning, K. (1999). *Nursing administration in the 21st century.* Thousand Oaks, CA: Sage.

Anderson, C. A. (1995). Scholarship: How important is it? *Nursing Outlook, 43,* 247–248.

Bélanger, P. (1991). Nursing models—A major step towards professional autonomy. *AARN Newsletter, 48*(8), 13.

Biley, F. (1990). Wordly wise. *Nursing (London), 4*(24), 37.

Bridges, J. (1991). Working with doctors: Distinct from medicine. *Nursing Times, 87*(27), 42–43.

Broncatello, K. F. (1980). Auger in action: Application of the model. *Advances in Nursing Science, 2*(2), 13–23.

Cash, K. (1990). Nursing models and the idea of nursing. *International Journal of Nursing Studies, 27,* 249–256.

Chalmers, H., Kershaw, B., Melia, K., & Kendrich, M. (1990). Nursing models: Enhancing or inhibiting practice? *Nursing Standard, 5*(11), 34–40.

Dabbs, A. D. V. (1994). Theory-based nursing practice: For our patients' sake. *Clinical Nurse Specialist, 8,* 214, 220.

Fawcett, J. (1999). *The relationship of theory and research* (3rd ed.). Philadelphia: F. A. Davis.

Fawcett, J. (2005). *Contemporary nursing knowledge: Analysis and evaluation of nursing models and theories* (2nd ed.). Philadelphia: F. A. Davis.

Feeg, V. (1989). From the editor: Is theory application merely an intellectual exercise? *Pediatric Nursing, 15*, 450.

Frank, L. K. (1968). Science as a communication process. *Main Currents in Modern Thought, 25*, 45–50.

Graham, I. (1994). How do registered nurses think and experience nursing: A phenomenological investigation. *Journal of Clinical Nursing, 3*, 235–242.

Grossman, M., & Hooton, M. (1993). The significance of the relationship between a discipline and its practice. *Journal of Advanced Nursing, 18*, 866–872.

Hardin, S. R., & Kaplow, R. (2005). *Synergy for clinical excellence: The AACN synergy model for patient care.* Boston: Jones and Bartlett.

Hayne, Y. (1992). The current status and future significance of nursing as a discipline. *Journal of Advanced Nursing, 17*, 104–107.

Henderson, V. (1966). *The nature of nursing. A definition and its implications for practice, research, and education.* New York: Macmillan.

Ingram, R. (1991). Why does nursing need theory? *Journal of Advanced Nursing, 16*, 350–353.

Johnson, D. E. (1987). Evaluating conceptual models for use in critical care nursing practice [Guest editorial]. *Dimensions of Critical Care Nursing, 6,* 195–197.

Johnson, D. E. (1990). The behavioral system model for nursing. In M. E. Parker (Ed.), *Nursing theories in practice* (pp. 23–32). New York: National League for Nursing.

King, I. M. (2006). Part One: Imogene M. King's theory of goal attainment. In M. E. Parker, *Nursing theories and nursing practice* (2nd ed., pp. 235–243). Philadelphia: F. A. Davis.

Leininger, M. M., & McFarland, M. R. (2006). *Culture care diversity and universality: A worldwide nursing theory* (2nd ed.). Boston: Jones and Bartlett.

Le Storti, L. J., Cullen, P. A., Hanzlik, E. M., Michiels, J. M., Piano, L. A., Ryan, P. L., & Johnson, W. (1999). Creative thinking in nursing education: Preparing for tomorrow's challenges. *Nursing Outlook, 47*, 62–66.

Levine, M. E. (1991). The conservation principles: A model for health. In K. M. Schaefer & J. B. Pond (Eds.), *Levine's conservation model: A framework for nursing practice* (pp. 1–11). Philadelphia: F. A. Davis.

Lindsay, B. (1990). The gap between theory and practice. *Nursing Standard, 5*(4), 34–35.

Lister, P. (1991). Approaching models of nursing from a postmodernist perspective. *Journal of Advanced Nursing, 16*, 206–212.

Malin, N., & Teasdale, K. (1991). Caring versus empowerment: Considerations for nursing practice. *Journal of Advanced Nursing, 16*, 657–662.

Neff, M. (1991). President's message: The future of our profession from the eyes of today. *American Nephrology Nurses Association Journal, 18*, 534.

Neuman, B., & Fawcett, J. (2002). *The Neuman systems model* (4th ed.). Upper Saddle River, NJ: Prentice Hall.

Newman, M. A. (1994). *Health as expanding consciousness* (2nd ed.). New York: National League for Nursing Press.

Nightingale, F. (1859). *Notes on nursing: What it is, and what it is not.* London: Harrison and Sons. [Commemorative edition printed 1992, Philadelphia: J. B. Lippincott]

Nightingale, K. (1993). Editorial. *British Journal of Theatre Nursing, 3*(5), 2.

Orem, D. E. (1997). Views of human beings specific to nursing. *Nursing Science Quarterly, 10*, 26–31.

Orem, D. E. (2001). *Nursing: Concepts of practice* (6th ed.). St. Louis: Mosby.

Orlando, I. J. (1961). *The dynamic nurse-patient relationship: Function, process and principles.* New York: G. P. Putnam's Sons. [Reprinted 1990, New York: National League for Nursing]

Orr, J. (1991). Knowledge is power. *Health Visitor, 64*, 218.

Parse, R. R. (1998). *The humanbecoming school of thought: A perspective for nurses and other health professionals.* Thousand Oaks, CA: Sage.

Parse, R. R. (1995). Commentary. Parse's theory of humanbecoming: An alternative guide to nursing practice for pediatric oncology nurses. *Journal of Pediatric Oncology Nursing, 12,* 128.

Peplau, H. E. (1952). *Interpersonal relations in nursing.* New York: G. P. Putnam's Sons. [Reprinted 1991, New York: Springer]

Peplau, H. E. (1992). Interpersonal relations: A theoretical framework for application in nursing practice. *Nursing Science Quarterly, 5*, 13–18.

Perry, J. (1985). Has the discipline of nursing developed to the stage where nurses do 'think nursing'? *Journal of Advanced Nursing, 10*, 31–37.

Peterson, S. J., & Bredow, T. S. (2004). *Middle-range theories: Application to nursing research.* Philadelphia: Lippincott Williams and Wilkins for an overview of the theory.

Popper, K. R. (1965). *Conjectures and refutations: The growth of scientific knowledge.* New York: Harper and Row.

Rogers, C. G. (1973). Conceptual models as guides to clinical nursing specialization. *Journal of Nursing Education, 12*(4), 2–6.

Rogers, M. E. (1990). Nursing: Science of unitary, irreducible, human beings: Update 1990. In E. A. M. Barrett (Ed.), *Visions of Rogers' science-based nursing* (pp. 5–11). New York: National League for Nursing.

Rogers, M. E. (1989). Creating a climate for the implementation of a nursing conceptual framework. *Journal of Continuing Education in Nursing, 20*, 112–116.

Rogers, M. E. (1970). *An introduction to the theoretical basis of nursing.* Philadelphia: F. A. Davis.

Roy, C., & Andrews, H. A. (1999). *The Roy adaptation model* (2nd ed.). Stamford, CT: Appleton and Lange.

Smith, M. J., & Liehr, P. R. (Eds.). (2003). *Middle range theory for nursing.* New York: Springer for an overview of the theory.

Villarruel, A. M., Bishop, T. L., Simpson, E. M., Jemmott, L. S., & Fawcett, J. (2001). Borrowed theories, shared theories, and the advancement of nursing knowledge. *Nursing Science Quarterly, 14,* 158–163.

Watson, J. (1997). The theory of human caring: Retrospective and prospective. *Nursing Science Quarterly, 10,* 49–52.

Watson, J. (2006). Part One: Jean Watson's theory of human caring. In M. E. Parker, *Nursing theories and nursing practice* (2nd ed., pp. 295–302). Philadelphia: F. A. Davis.

Ziegler, S. M. (Ed.). (2005). *Theory-directed nursing practice* (2nd ed.). New York: Springer.

☐ BIBLIOGRAPHY

Alligood, M. R., & Marriner-Tomey, A. (2006). *Nursing theory: Utilization and application* (3rd ed.). St. Louis: Mosby Elsevier.

Parker, M. E. (Ed.). (1993). *Patterns of nursing theories in practice*. New York: National League for Nursing Press.

Parker, M. E. (2006). *Nursing theories and nursing practice* (2nd ed.). Philadelphia: F. A. Davis.

Parker, M. E. (Ed.). (1990). *Nursing theories in practice*. New York: National League for Nursing.

■ *Rose* **Kearney-Nunnery**

Models for Health and Illness

5

> ❝ *I can enter your world, as one who invites your growth or as a strangler of your possibilities, a prophet of stasis.* ❞
>
> Sidney M. Jourard

Chapter Objectives

On completion of this chapter, the reader will be able to:

1. Differentiate among the various health and illness models for applicability to professional nursing practice.
2. Discuss the advantages and disadvantages of the various models.
3. Apply a health belief or health promotion model to a given nursing care situation.
4. Analyze differences in health beliefs held by members of various cultural groups and the application of models for cultural competence.

Key Terms

Health
Health Promotion
Health Protection
Preventive Services
Primary Prevention

Secondary Prevention
Tertiary Prevention
High-Level Wellness
Health Belief Model
Health Promotion Model

Chronic Illness Trajectory Framework
Functional Health Patterns
Cultural Competence
Models for Culture Care

ealth is a condition we seek, promote, and hope to maintain. Health is more than the absence of illness, or infirmity. A multidimensional construct of health is determined by the individual's worldview and philosophical assumptions. Consider the four metaparadigm concepts of nursing and that health is specified in the nursing theory that guides our practice. Health as a part of the metaparadigm is interrelated with concepts of human beings, environment, and nursing. Considering your particular view of the world and your concept of health, we can now approach ways of promoting health using a sample of different models. The selection of a model is, again, determined by one's worldview and theoretical guide.

In Chapter 4, health is illustrated within individual theoretical structures. For example, compare the definitions of health provided by King, Roy, and Leininger. King (1981) defines health as "dynamic life experiences of a human being, which implies continuous adjustment to stressors in the internal and external environment through optimum use of one's resources to achieve maximum potential for daily living" (p. 5). Here we have the focus on human beings. Roy (2006) defines health as a state and process of being and becoming integrated and whole with a focus on the mutuality between human beings and the environmental (p. 4). The central focus is adaptation. Leininger (2002b) defines health as "a state of well-being or restorative state that is culturally constituted, defined, valued, and practiced by individuals or groups that enables them to function in their daily lives" (p. 84). Care, rather than health, is considered the central concept. It refers to the secondary concepts of nursing—health, curing, and well-being, especially culture care (Leininger and McFarland, 2006, p. 3).

In other nursing theories and models, the concept of health may not be well defined but is interpreted, as in Rogers' theory, as a "value term defined by the culture or individual" (Gunther, 2002, p. 229). Or, in Parse's (1981) theory, health is a process of becoming (p. 159). Still, health or well-being is represented in each framework on which practice is based. Before delving into the theories of health and illness—in the context of health promotion and illness prevention—and cultural perceptions of health, it is first important to understand the different levels and types of health promotion and illness prevention activities.

LEVELS OF PREVENTION

When considering health promotion activities, we frequently refer to illness and disability prevention. In 1990, national health promotion and disease prevention activities were developed under the auspices of the U.S. Department of Health and Human Services (USDHHS) and later published as Healthy People 2000 (1992). Interestingly, the publication distinguished between health promotion and health protection strategies, with an individual versus a community focus, as follows:

> **Health promotion** strategies are those related to individual lifestyle—personal choices made in a social context—that can have a powerful influence over one's health prospects. These include physical activity and fitness, nutrition, tobacco, alcohol and other drugs, family planning, mental health and mental disorders, and violent and abusive behavior. . . . **Health protection** strategies are those related to environmental or regulatory measures that confer protection on large population groups. These strategies address issues such as unintentional injuries, occupational safety and health, environmental health, food and drug safety, and oral health. **Preventive services** include counseling, screening, immunization, or chemoprophylactic interventions for individuals in clinical settings. (USDHHS, 1992, pp. 6–7)

These preventive activities and services address the three levels of prevention: primary, secondary, and tertiary. Health promotion activities are both protective and preventive, but they require consumers actively involved in all levels of prevention. And this focus on health promotion and health protection strategies became an important component of Healthy People 2010 (2000) with the national goals to increase the quality and years of healthy life and to eliminate health disparities. See Chapter 16 for more information.

Primary Prevention

Primary prevention refers to healthy actions taken to avoid illness or disease. Examples are healthy nutrition, smoking cessation, exercise programs, parenting classes, community awareness programs, and mental health programs and activities. Primary prevention refers to the individual lifestyle health promotion strategies recommended in Healthy People 2010. These are becoming more popular and prevalent as people take responsibility for their own health. Health columns have appeared more frequently in publications. We have also seen a growing number of health food and holistic health stores, "healthy" fast food options, Web sites, and educational programs for the general public. But consumers can still have difficulty acquiring sufficient information on a selected topic before they become frustrated.

Secondary Prevention

Secondary prevention involves screening for early detection and treatment of health problems. With secondary prevention, the individual is seeking health care not for a specific problem but, rather, for early detection of a potential problem to mobilize resources and reduce its intensity or severity if the problem is identified. Secondary prevention usually involves use of some procedure or measurement tool in addition to the health history and physical assessment. Examples of secondary prevention are screening procedures used by health-care consumers or health-care professionals for physiologic, developmental, or environmental problems. Physiologic procedures include screening for hypertension or specific forms of cancer. Mental health screening procedures range from simple tests for orientation to more elaborate instruments such as mental status questionnaires for aging clients. In young children, examples of secondary prevention activities are use of growth charts to assess growth along established percentiles and developmental screening tests to detect problems in the areas of personal-social skills, motor activities, and language. Note the difference between using parenting classes as primary prevention for developmental stimulation and screening for developmental problems as secondary prevention. Environmental screening procedures include testing air and water quality and home safety assessments. If a problem is detected, a referral is made for a differential diagnosis and institution of early treatment.

Tertiary Prevention

Tertiary prevention occurs during the rehabilitative phase of an illness to prevent complications or further disability. The individual has already entered the health-care system and is recovering from or learning to cope with a health deficit. Tertiary prevention builds on this care to prevent further deficits. Examples of tertiary prevention are counseling and teaching after recovery from a cardiovascular event, an accident or injury, an abusive situation, or any other physical, psychosocial, mental, or environmental disruption from usual health and functioning. Support from self-help groups is a large component of tertiary prevention. An example of tertiary prevention is family counseling after identification of a child in an abusive situation.

Professional nursing practice involves not only health promotion but also all three levels of preventive activities. Because the health of individuals, families, communities, and groups is a major concern in nursing, professional skill and expertise in the area of prevention activities are presumed in practice, education, research, and administrative functions.

THEORIES OF HEALTH AND ILLNESS

Aside from the nursing conceptual or theoretical frameworks, different models are available to guide assessment of health factors and promote and preserve health. Interestingly, Benner and Wrubel (1989) described five theories of health as (1) an ideal, (2) the ability to fulfill social roles, (3) a commodity, (4) a human potential, and (5) a sense of coherence. Health is more than an ideal. We strive for the person, family, community, or group to reach a positive state of well-being. Defining health as the ability to perform one's role is limiting and fails to meet our holistic concern for human beings. As Benner and Wrubel (1989) observe, "this view focuses on doing rather than being and ignores the person's sense of fulfillment and well-being" (p. 151). Health as a commodity implies that it can be bought, sold, traded, and withheld. This view fails to meet the intent of a caring professional practice discipline. Health as a commodity is described as a "medicalized view," promising instant cures without personal involvement (Benner & Wrubel, 1989, pp. 151–153).

Health defined as a human potential is consistent with the beliefs of many in nursing and other health-care disciplines and is the basis of the first three health models presented here. Health as a human potential includes physical, mental, and spiritual health. Benner and Wrubel (1989) describe the limitation of this model by saying that although all people have the potential for health, they are continually pursuing increasing levels of health but not attaining health as a state or condition (pp. 156–157). This definition depends on whether health is viewed as a defined goal or a dynamic state that we continue to strive toward. Dunn's high-level wellness model, the health belief model, and Pender's health promotion model are consistent with health viewed as human potential.

The fifth view of health takes a phenomenologic approach. *Phenomenology* is the lived experience of the individual, from his or her unique perspective. This view focuses on one's lived experience rather than on an opinion derived from another person's observations of the experience. Benner and Wrubel's (1989) approach to health as a mind-body-spirit integration in a state of becoming is an example of health as a sense of coherence. A focus on the person's belonging to a sociocultural group makes this integration unique. Benner and Wrubel define the term *well-being* as a better indication of health with challenges and involvement in the following definition: "Well-being is defined as congruence between one's possibilities and one's actual practices and lived meanings and is based on caring and feeling cared for" (Benner & Wrubel, 1989, p. 160).

In this view, a model must be based on a qualitative approach to address individuals' well-being, because it depends on the lived experience of those persons in their context. As Benner and Wrubel (1989) state.

"health as well-being comes when one engages in sound self-care, cares, and feels cared for—when one trusts the self, the body, and others. Breakdown occurs when that trust is broken. Well-being can be restored" (p. 165).

The chronic illness trajectory framework is consistent with the view of health as coherence.

Model of High-Level Wellness

Dunn developed his model of high-level wellness starting with the 1947 definition of health from the World Health Organization that emphasized physical, mental, and social well-being. He stressed that well-being includes the positive, dynamic, and unique integration of mind, body, and spirit of the individual within his or her environment, including work, family, community, and society. Dunn (1973) defined high-level wellness for an individual as "an integrated method of functioning which is oriented toward maximizing the potential of which the individual is capable. It requires that the individual maintain a continuum of balance and purposeful direction within the environment where he is functioning" (pp. 4–5).

Dunn regarded high-level wellness as an ongoing challenge to the highest level possible, the individual's maximum potential. Meeting basic needs and striving for higher needs were components of his view of individual health and well-being. Dunn (1973) viewed high-level wellness as "an open-ended and ever-expanding tomorrow with its challenge to live at full potential" (p. 223). He also considered high-level wellness, with similar components, for the family, community, environment, and society.

Dunn's beliefs about high-level wellness evolved into a health grid (Fig. 5–1) that demonstrates a person or group at some point along a health continuum or horizontal axis, from death at the left side to peak wellness at the right. The person or group was further influenced by the environment (the vertical axis), from a very favorable environment at the top to a very unfavorable environment at the bottom. This grid illustrates the person or group in context, within one of the four

quadrants ranging from poor health to protected poor health, high-level wellness, and emergent high-level wellness. The high-level wellness model provides an explanation of the person-environment relationship in health but gives no direction as to movement among quadrants, and it also compartmentalizes wellness.

The model could be used effectively to address health disparities for the client who is currently in an unfavorable environment (poorly accepted services related to language) to a favorable environment where we strive to promote more culturally relevant, understandable, and acceptable services and health care.

Health Belief Model

The health belief model is a valuable tool for looking at both health promotion and actions directed at maintaining or restoring health. Originally, the model was based on the following hypothesis:

Persons will not seek preventative care or health screening unless they possess minimal levels of relevant health motivation and knowledge, view themselves as potentially vulnerable and the condition as threatening, are convinced of the efficacy of intervention, and see few difficulties in undertaking the recommended action. (Becker, Haefner, Kasl, Kirscht, Maiman, & Rosenstock, 1977, p. 29)

The health belief model was designed as an organizing framework to advance health promotion activities by targeting interventions on certain individual variables. The three major concepts in the model were individual perceptions, modifying factors, and likelihood of action. Individual perceptions involve how the person considers the risk of susceptibility or the severity of the illness— in other words, how likely he or she believes it is that the disease or condition could happen to him or her. Modifying factors are a set of demographic, sociopsychological cues to action from family, friends, professionals, or the media relative to the perceived threat of the disease. Sociopsychological variables include personality, interpersonal influences, and socioeconomic status. The modifying factors, along with individual perceptions, lead to the likelihood of action in the direction of health. The concept of motivation is central to this model (Becker et al., 1977, p. 31).

An extensive review of research on variables in the health belief model led to a subsequent revision. The model was expanded from a diagram of health belief concepts and their relationships to a full explanation of and prediction about health-related behaviors (Fig. 5–2). The three major concepts were (1) readiness to undertake recommended compliance behavior, (2) modifying and enabling factors, and (3) compliant behaviors. On

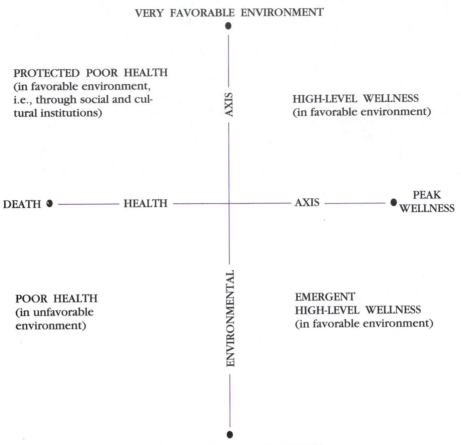

VERY FAVORABLE ENVIRONMENT

PROTECTED POOR HEALTH
(in favorable environment,
i.e., through social and cultural institutions)

HIGH-LEVEL WELLNESS
(in favorable environment)

AXIS

DEATH ●——————HEALTH——————AXIS——————● PEAK WELLNESS

POOR HEALTH
(in unfavorable
environment)

EMERGENT
HIGH-LEVEL WELLNESS
(in favorable environment)

ENVIRONMENTAL

VERY UNFAVORABLE ENVIRONMENT

■ **Figure 5.1** Dunn's high-level wellness. (From U.S. Department of Health, Education, and Welfare. Public Health Service, National Office of Vital Statistics.)

the basis of research, readiness to undertake recommended compliance behavior broadened individual perceptions from perception of susceptibility and severity to perceptions of motivations, values for threat reduction, and subjective risk/benefit considerations that the compliant behaviors would be safe and effective. Modifying factors were expanded to more inclusive modifying and enabling factors on the basis of research findings. A reciprocal relationship between readiness and modifying/enabling factors also became more apparent in the revised model. The outcome in the revised model was the likelihood of compliant behaviors with preventive recommendations or prescribed regimens.

The original version of the health belief model focused on health promotion or preventive behaviors. Since its inception, the model has been widely used in research and practice. In addition to use in understanding utilization of health-care services and health promotion behaviors, the model has guided research in client compliance to health care. An extensive body of research

on patient compliance for the revised model demonstrated applicability in a wide range of health-care situations. Insights for use of the model in practice and education were offered. Concerning client education, Becker and associates (1977) recommended that health-care providers understand the following principles:

1. Behavior is motivated.
2. Certain beliefs seem central to a client's decision to act.
3. Not all persons possess these beliefs and motives to equal degrees.
4. Intellectual information, although necessary, is often not sufficient to stimulate needed beliefs.
5. Health providers need to view the importance of client education and accept substantial responsibility in this activity. (p. 42)

These principles are consistent with the discipline of professional nursing practice and are routinely incorporated into plans for care and health teaching. Consideration of the belief systems of the individual,

READINESS TO
UNDERTAKE RECOMMENDED
COMPLIANCE BEHAVIOR

MODIFYING AND
ENABLING FACTORS

COMPLIANT
BEHAVIORS

Motivations
Concern about (salience of) health
matters in general
Willingness to seek and accept
medical direction
Intention to comply
Positive health activities

Demographic (very young or
old)

Structural (cost, duration,
complexity, side effects, accessibility of regimen, need for
new patterns of behavior)

Attitudes (satisfaction with
visit, physician, other staff,
clinic procedures, and facilities)

*Value of Illness Threat
Reaction*
Subjective estimates of:
 Susceptibility or unsusceptibility
 (incl. belief in diagnosis)
 Vulnerability to illness in general
 Extent of possible bodily harm*
 Extent of possible interference with
 social roles*
Presence of (or past experience
with) symptoms

Interaction (length, depth,
continuity, mutuality of expectation; quality and type of
doctor-patient relationship;
physician agreement with patient; feedback to patient)

Enabling (prior experience
with action, illness, or regimen;
source of advice and referral
(incl. social pressure)

Likelihood of:
Compliance with preventa-
tive health recommendations
and prescribed treatment:
e.g., screening, immunizations, prophylactic exams,
drugs, diet, exercise, personal
and work habits, follow-up
tests, referrals and follow-up
appointments, entering
or continuing a treatment
program

*Probability That
Compliant Behavior Will Reduce
the Threat*
Subjective estimates of:
 The proposed regimen's safety
 The proposed regimen's efficacy to
 prevent, delay, or cure (incl. "faith
 in doctors and medical care" and
 "chance of recovery")

■ **Figure 5.2** Health belief model for explaining and predicting individual health-related behaviors. (From Becker, M. H., Haefner, D. P., Kasl, S. V., Kirscht, J. P., Maiman, L. A., & Rosenstock, I. M. [1977]. Selected psychosocial models and correlates of individual health-related behaviors. *Medical Care, 15*[5], 30. Reproduced with permission, Philadelphia: Lippincott-Raven Publishers.)

family, or group is essential in assessing a client and choosing interventions. The extent of detail and inclusion of this information is the challenge to the nurse, whose health-teaching role is an integral component of professional practice.

As a part of the health history, readiness, as motivations in health behaviors, is easily included in the interview. The client's "subjective estimates" of the potential to reduce the threat and care options are less commonly included in the assessment, depending on the professional's impressions of time restraints and knowledge of the client, or even on cultural or interpersonal

differences between the professional and the client. In a nursing health assessment, we frequently acquire demographic information and some structural information that provides insight into modifying and enabling factors. The challenge is to acquire the additional structural information, such as cost and accessibility, and to seek information from the client about quality, satisfaction, and social pressures for additional knowledge of attitudinal, interaction, and enabling factors. This information can be used to increase compliant behaviors.

Nevertheless, the model has limitations. First, the language is directed to physician-patient relationships, quite possibly a product of the roles and functions of other health-care providers in 1977. More recently, the health belief model has been used in further research consistent with views of nursing. Ongoing research and applications of health behavior have been demonstrated at the level of the individual, dyad, group, organization, and community (Glantz, Rimer, & Lewis, 2002). Second, as Pender (1987, 1996; Pender, Murdaugh, & Parsons, 2002, 2006) indicates, the health belief model is directed at preventive services or health protection behaviors in the context of a provider-consumer relationship rather than individual health promotion behaviors. To be empowered consumers in today's health-care system, individuals must take personal responsibility for their own health long before they seek care from a health professional. This concept is now beginning to be addressed in the health belief model, especially in application related to health education.

Health Promotion Model

Pender's health promotion model, an outgrowth of the health belief model, is based on research and information on health and health-protecting behaviors. It is primarily a nursing model and has been revised with evolving knowledge. In the health promotion model, health promotion is motivated by the desire to increase the level of wellness and actualization of an individual or an aggregate group (Pender, 1996, p. 7). Pender describes the health promotion model as a "competence- or approach-oriented model with applicability across the life span for motivating overall healthy lifestyles (Pender et al., 2006, p. 48). She points out that "unlike the health belief model, the health promotion model does not include 'fear' or 'threat' as a source of motivation for the health behavior" (Pender et al., 2006, p. 48).

Structurally, the model had been designed as a schematic representation similar to the original health belief model. After extensive research, however, the model was revised, and significant variables were reorganized (Fig. 5–3). The knowledge obtained through research led to the later addition of three new variables in the health promotion model: activity-related affect, commitment to a plan of action, and immediate competing demands and preferences.

The revised health promotion model contains two principal components that interact for participation in health-promoting behaviors: (1) individual characteristics and experiences, and (2) behavior-specific cognitions and affect. Individual characteristics and experiences are similar to the individual perceptions in the health belief model, in that they involve looking at health through past experiences (prior related behavior) and personal factors.

Pender points out that "research indicates that often the best predictor of behavior is the frequency of the same or a similar behavior in the past" (Pender et al., 2006, p. 51–52). Personal factors include biologic variables (age, gender, body mass, etc.), psychological variables (such as self-esteem, self-motivation, perceived health status), and sociocultural variables (race, ethnicity, aculteration, education, socioeconomic status) (Pender et al., 2006, p. 52).

On the basis of research evidence, these biologic, psychological, and sociocultural personal factors were included in the model as further predictors of individual health perceptions and behaviors. For example, consider the health-seeking behaviors demonstrated by clients of different socioeconomic groups, family backgrounds, and experiences in the health-care system. A later section of this chapter addresses specific cultural differences in health beliefs that also influence health-seeking behaviors.

The behavior-specific cognitions and affect are similar to the health belief model's modifying or enabling factors but relate more to the nomenclature of nursing. As Pender has indicated, this category of variables is of "major motivational significance" and provides the critical "core," because they are subject to modification based on nursing interventions (Pender et al., 2006, p. 52). These behavior-specific cognitions and affects include perceived benefits, perceived barriers, perceived self-efficacy, activity-related affect (subjective feelings), interpersonal influences, and situational influences. Interpersonal and situational influences are identified as having both direct and indirect effects on health promotion behaviors. Consider the older adult walking through a shopping mall and noticing a free hypertension screening clinic. Indirect situational influences to obtain a screening test may include the perceived camaraderie of people in the clinic compared with a tedious wait for an office appointment. The direct influence is the availability of the screening during this older adult's routine exercise program at the mall.

The variables of perceived benefits, perceived barriers, self-efficacy, interpersonal influences, and situational influences have been supported in research studies as predictors of health promotion behaviors (Pender, 1996; Pender et al., 2002, 2006). Activity-related affect, a variable added in the revised health promotion model, addresses the individual's subjective feelings related to the health promotion behavior. Because of the recent inclusion of this variable in the model, limited support is available for it as a predictor of health promotion behaviors (Pender, 2006).

Behavioral outcome, the third component of the model, includes actions toward the healthy behavior. These actions lead to the attainment of a positive health outcome. Two variables (immediate competing

INDIVIDUAL
CHARACTERISTICS
AND EXPERIENCES

BEHAVIOR-SPECIFIC
COGNITIONS
AND AFFECT

BEHAVIORAL
OUTCOME

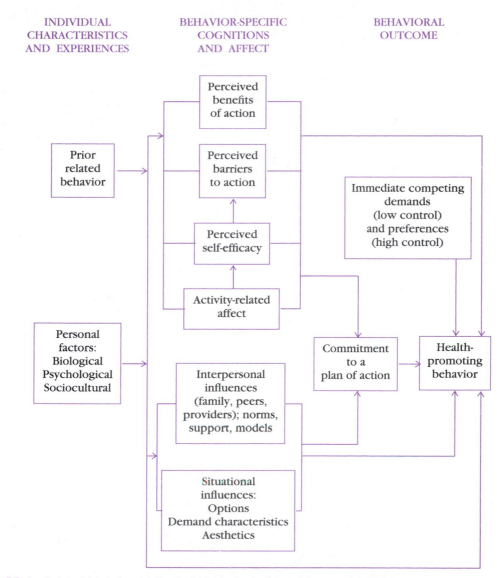

■ **Figure 5.3** Pender's health belief model. (Pender, N. J., Murdaugh, C. L., and Parsons, M. A. [2006]. *Health promotion in nursing practice* [5th ed.] Upper Saddle River, NJ: Pearson Prentice Hall. Reprinted with permission.)

demands and preferences; and commitment to a plan of action) were added to the revised health promotion model to explain further the behavioral outcome of the health-promoting behavior. Pender describes the commitment to the plan of action with two distinct cognitive processes: "(a) commitment to carry out a specific action at a given time and place and with specified persons or alone, irrespective of competing preferences; and (2) identification of definitive strategies for eliciting, carrying out, and reinforcing the behavior" (Pender et al., 2006, p. 56).

The health-promoting behavior can be affected by the immediate competing demands and preferences the

individual perceives. These are viewed as alternate behaviors. Competing demands are behaviors over which the person has little control because of environmental factors, like family commitments. Competing preferences are behaviors with powerful reinforcing properties—such as a sudden urge for a particular food—over which the person has a high level of control (Pender et al., 2006, pp. 56–57). This component is greatly influenced by nursing interventions related to values clarification, encouragement, and reinforcement of healthy behaviors.

In the earlier version of the health promotion model, Pender (1987) described the model as a flexible organizing framework, subject to revision after further testing. This was followed by the identification of theoretical basis from both the Expectancy-Value Theory and the Social Cognitive Theory with the specification of first seven assumptions (Pender, 1996), then 15 theoretical propositions (Pender, et. al., 2002). Research has been ongoing for testing of the model. With the empirical support of variables, the revised model has greater potential to predict and intervene for health promotion activities. Health promotion settings are the social environment in which we live, work, and play, such as family, school, workplace, health-care agencies, and the community at large. Ongoing research studies have focused on a variety of client populations to target health promotion activities.

Comparison of the Two Models

Table 5–1 compares the health belief model and the health promotion model. Both models propose that the health professional must understand how the person perceives the world and that the person makes personal decisions through identified readiness or individual characteristics and experiences. The modifying factors

or behavior-specific cognitions and affect are the social, situational, and environmental influences related to the person's conception of healthy behavior. Both models include demographic variables, because research supports the importance of differences. For example, the choice between surgery and irradiation is very different for a 28-year-old patient and an 88-year-old patient, in terms not only of physiologic differences but also of past experiences. Attention to these differences turns the focus of health-care consumers to their specific outcomes and increases chances of success in the health promotion activity.

Chronic Illness Model

Although the health belief model has been used in research and practice settings with clients who have chronic illnesses, Corbin and Strauss's chronic illness model is specific to chronicity. Despite its focus on chronic illness, it is still a health promotion model. As Corbin and Strauss (1992a) have stated:

> The focus of care in chronicity is not on cure but first of all on the prevention of chronic conditions,

Table 5.1

Comparing the Health Belief Model and the Health Promotion Model

Model	Individual Characteristics	Mediating Factors	Outcomes
Health Belief Model (Becker et al., 1977)	Readiness for Recommended Behavior: Motivations, including general health concerns, willingness and compliance behaviors, positive health attitudes Value of illness threat reduction, including subjective estimates and past experiences Probability that compliant behavior will reduce threat (subjectively)	Modifying/Enabling Factors: ■ Demographic ■ Structural ■ Attitudes ■ Interaction ■ Enabling	Compliant Behaviors: Likelihood of compliance with preventive health recommendations and prescribed regimens
Pender's Health Promotion Model (1996)	Individual Characteristics and Experiences: Prior related behavior Personal factors ■ Biologic ■ Psychological ■ Sociocultural	Behavior-Specific Cognitions and Affect: ■ Perceived benefits ■ Perceived barriers ■ Perceived self-efficacy ■ Activity-related affect ■ Interpersonal influences ■ Situational influences	Behavioral Outcomes: ■ Commitment to a plan of action ■ Immediate competing demands and preferences ■ Health promoting behaviors

then on finding ways to help the ill manage and live with their illness should these occur. Interventions are aimed at fostering the prevention of, living with, and shaping the course of chronic illnesses, especially those requiring technologically complex management, while promoting and maintaining quality of life. (p. 20)

The **chronic illness trajectory framework** (Corbin & Strauss, 1992a), shown in Table 5–2, is a substantive theory that applies to individuals with a broad range of chronic conditions. Benner and Wrubel's (1989) concept of health as coherence applies to this model. Corbin and Strauss (1992a) describe the development of the framework as based on 30 years of qualitative, grounded theory research. The original framework was developed with the following concepts: key problems, basic strategies, organizational or family arrangements, and consequences (Strauss & Glaser, 1975; Strauss, Corbin, Fagerhaugh, Glaser, Maines, Suczek, et. al., 1984). It evolved into a nursing theory through its use and research base, but the developers maintain that potentially it applies to all health-care disciplines. The framework or model is based on the following assumptions:

1. The course of chronic conditions varies and changes over time.
2. The course of a chronic condition can be shaped and managed.

3. The technology involved is complex and can potentially create side effects.
4. The illness and technology pose potential consequences for the individual's physical well-being, biographical fulfillment (identity over time), and performance of daily activities.
5. Biographical needs and performance of daily activities can affect illness management choices and the course of the illness.
6. The course of illness is not inevitably downward.
7. Chronic illnesses do not necessarily end in death. (Corbin & Strauss, 1992a, p. 10; 1992b, p. 97)

Corbin and Strauss (1992a) described the framework as a conceptual model organized under the central concept of trajectory. This central concept was proposed to indicate the management of the evolving course of the chronic condition, as "shaped" by the person, family members, and health-care providers. From this central organizing or umbrella concept flow the other major theoretical concepts.

These concepts are described as leading to the structure of the nursing process, with the following steps:

1. Locating the client and family, and setting goals
2. Assessing conditions influencing management
3. Defining the intervention focus, the target of intervention

Table 5.2

The Chronic Illness Trajectory Framework (Corbin & Strauss, 1992a)

Trajectory phasing	Eight phases: pretrajectory, trajectory onset, crisis, acute, stable, unstable, downward, dying; subphasing within each phase for fluctuations as improvements, plateauing, reversals, or deterioration occurs during course of illness
Trajectory projection	Vision of the illness course
Trajectory scheme	Shaping the course, controlling symptoms, and handling disability
Conditions influencing management	Technology used, resources, past experience, motivation, setting of care, lifestyle/beliefs, interactions/relationships, type of chronic condition and physiologic involvement, symptoms, political and economic climate affecting legislation
Trajectory management	Management of symptoms, side effects, crises, and complications through the trajectory scheme
Biographical and everyday living impact	Identity adjustments and management of limitations
Reciprocal impact	Consequences with management and problems related to illness, biography, and everyday activities

4. Intervention

5. Evaluating the effectiveness of intervention.

This model focuses on the person to illustrate the management of an evolving course of a chronic condition the individual experiences that is influenced by that individual, the family, and health-care providers. It takes us a step further than the health belief model because this model is more grounded in the individual's unique, personal history and patterns of life. Individuals with various chronic illnesses have been studied in many countries around the world using grounded theory and Corbin and Strauss' Chronic Illness Trajectory Framework. Their framework has also been used in National Institute of Nursing Research (NINR) funded research focused on the chronic illness experience and placement decisions for relatives with dementia (Winslow, 2002). The use of grounded theory as an inductive approach to understanding the individual's experience with chronic illness and all the associate contextual factors is predominant in these research studies. For example, the chronic illness experience is distinctively different for an elderly, frail Anglo-American woman living in an urban high-rise apartment than for the African-American elder with a physical disability living in a rural farm area. The difference involves more than the issue of compliance; it focuses on quality. This model is extremely relevant to nursing care as we experience the rising numbers of chronic illnesses managed in contemporary practice and the growing population of aging adults who are living longer while dealing with a chronic illness. In addition, the importance of cultural relevance, the beliefs and values of individuals, families, communities, and groups, and environmental factors, are major considerations in health care.

All of these models require a thoughtful and thorough nursing assessment. Valid data are needed for their application. As part of the nursing assessment, the application of Gordon's (2006) functional health patterns could assist in this application (Box 5–1). Nursing assessment of each of these areas provides valuable data for application of a health or illness model to address health and illness focused on human potential or a sense of coherence.

CULTURAL INFLUENCE ON HEALTH PERCEPTIONS AND PROMOTION

Healthy People 2000 and Healthy People 2010 targeted selected groups of at-risk populations requiring special health promotion strategies. These reports illustrated significant health problems in some minority groups,

but more importantly, they emphasized individuals within subgroups. As originally reported in Healthy People 2000, individual differences—beyond racial group, socioeconomic status, and educational level—affect health status and access to health care. These reports pointed out that "our health-care programs are characterized by unacceptable disparities linked to membership in certain racial and ethnic groups" (USDHHS, 1992, p. 31). To address this issue, the Commonwealth Foundation conducted a field study, reporting that "minorities have difficulty getting appropriate, timely, high-quality care because of language barriers and that they may have different perspectives on health, medical care, and expectations about diagnosis and treatment" (Betancourt, Green, & Carrillo, 2002, p. 3). Further research into managed care, education, and government illustrated "a clear link between cultural competence, improving quality, and eliminating racial and ethnic disparities in health care" (Betancourt, Green, Carrillo, & Park, 2005, p. 1). The issue then goes beyond access to the need for the provision of acceptable health care to address the existing disparities.

These reports highlight the need for a concerted effort to understand and embrace diversity in our daily personal and professional lives. But much is implied within the construct of "diversity." When people speak of ethnicity and race, they generally refer to a group, tribe, or nation of people united by some common characteristics, whether biologic, environmental, or social. In the United States, we tend to classify people into five ethnic groups: African-Americans, Asian-Americans and Pacific Islanders, Hispanic-Americans, Native Americans, and white Americans. But this tendency does little to help us understand the health

Box 5.1 Functional Health Patterns

Gordon (2006) has identified 11 functional health patterns for inclusion in the nursing assessment and diagnosis process:

- Health perception and health management
- Nutrition and metabolic
- Elimination
- Activity and exercise
- Sleep and rest
- Cognitive and perceptual
- Self-perception and self-concept
- Role and relationship
- Sexuality and reproductive
- Coping and stress tolerance
- Values and beliefs

ONLINE CONSULT

Agency for Healthcare Research & Quality at
www.ahrq.gov

The Commonwealth Fund at
www.cmwf.org

Healthy People at
www.healthypeople.gov

U.S. Department of Health and Human Services at
www.hhs.gov

beliefs, practices, needs, or diversity represented within each of these population classifications. It may, in fact, encourage us to impose stereotypical judgments on persons within these groups.

This point leads us to the concept of culture as a way of life and the increasing focus on **cultural competence**. Betancourt and associates (2002) describe three components of cultural competence—organizational, systemic, and clinical—with clinical cultural competence as "health professionals' awareness of cultural issues and health beliefs while providing methods to elicit, negotiate, and manage the information once it is obtained" (Betancourt et al., 2002, p. 17).

Our cultural inheritance has a powerful influence on our health beliefs, both conscious and unconscious. We bring into our personal and professional lives the influences from our ancestors, family, peers, and colleagues. We are affected by history, genetics, social customs, religion, language, politics, law, economics, education, and many other factors. We mutually influence and are influenced by others because of these endowments. When we talk about cultural diversity, we mean more than an inherited background. "Culture" implies social, familial, religious, national, and professional characteristics that affect the way we think and act; it is a combination of all these things.

Research demonstrating individual differences and perceptions provided valuable data for the revision of the health belief model. Educational, ethnic, and social class differences were identified for careful assessment of client beliefs and perceptions (Becker et al., 1977). These data are significant whether one is dealing with individual clients or families with a specific health-care deficit or a larger population group with informational needs for health promotion activities.

But it is important to consider the characteristics of both the client and the health professional. The values for cultural diversity and culturally sensitive care are clearly illustrated in position statements of our nursing organizations. As Andrews (2003) indicates, however, "health professionals must have positive experiences

with members of other cultures and learn to value genuinely the contributions all cultures make to our multicultural society" (p. 9).

One's health beliefs are the result of cultural inheritance, education, reasoned opinions, and, often, unfounded impressions. The proportion of each of these factors is individually determined. Babcock and Miller (1994) describe three paradigms for cultural influence on health care: (1) magico-religious, (2) scientific or biomedical, and (3) holistic. The three different views show us how individuals differ in their beliefs in the supernatural, the scientific community, or the holistic mind-body-spirit interrelationship. It is worth noting that the traditional health-care system operates from the scientific worldview, which diverges from that of many cultures and their subgroups.

The *magico-religious paradigm* of health and healing focuses on the supernatural. It can include ancient rites and rituals, reliance on prayer and the will of a supreme being, pilgrimages, spiritual healing, and the like. The *scientific or biomedical paradigm* is the dominant one for the health-care system, with reliance on allopathic medicine and biomedical treatments for illness and disease. As noted by Spector (2000), the allopathic philosophy is predicated on a dualistic view of body and mind and adherence to scientific and technological norms of the system for acute care, chronic care, rehabilitation, psychiatric/mental health, and community/public health—and is a culture onto itself (pp. 110–111). The *holistic paradigm* sees health as a balance of the physical, mental, and spiritual whole and includes both alternative and complementary therapies (e.g., aroma or massage therapy) and ethnocultural practices (e.g., herbals or voodoo) (Spector, 2000). The holistic aim is for a sense of harmony and treatment is to correct an imbalance. Significant differences can exist in health beliefs and roles between the client with a health-care need and the health-care provider, considered the "expert."

In our health-care system, we generally view the roles of health-care providers and those of consumers in traditional ways. We consider the disease or illness, including all the pathophysiology and treatment modalities. We are aware of health-care and health-promotion services in both the hospital and community setting. We usually present them through our words and behaviors as norms to which clients must adhere. Otherwise, they are termed "bad patients," "noncompliant," or even "problem cases." For example, the health-care community carefully conducts, evaluates, and uses research to identify biologic, chemical, structural, and physical factors to treat, manage, or cure a disease. Faced with clients whose belief system includes the "hot/cold" theory of disease causation and treatment—which holds that imbalance of the four body humors of yellow and black bile, phlegm, and blood resulting in a "hot" infectious condition must be treated with appropriate foods or herbs—we may ignore or patronize the client. Many scientific minds reject this theory, creating conflict and failure to provide health care. As Benner and Wrubel (1989) observe, "changes in lifestyles and health habits work best when they are integrated into the person's own cultural patterns and traditions [for] it is hard to sustain new patterns if they go against the grain of one's normal social patterns" (p. 155).

Models of Cultural Care and Competence in Practice

The movement for culturally competent care is an imperative and the focus of the following selected models.

Culture Care Diversity and Universality

Madeleine Leininger proposed a transcultural nursing theory with the central focus on care, especially the concept of *culture care*. Leininger's (1970) early definition of *culture* referred to a way of "life belonging" to a designated group, through accumulated traditions, customs, and the ways the group solves problems that are learned and transmitted systematically, largely through socialization practices that are reinforced through social and cultural institutions (pp. 48–49). Within her culture care theory, Leininger (2002b) defined culture as "patterned lifeways, values, beliefs, norms, symbols, and practices of individuals, groups, or institutions that are learned, shared, and usually transmitted intergenerationally over time" (p. 83). Taking this one step further as a health belief, Leininger (2002b) defined *cultural care* as "the synthesized and culturally constituted assistive, supportive, and facilitative caring acts toward self or others focused on evident or anticipated needs for the client's health or well-being or to face disabilities, death or other human conditions" (p. 83). To this end, she states that "the purpose of the theory of Culture Care was to discover, document, know and explain the interdependence of care and culture phenomena with differences and similarities between and among cultures" (Leininger and McFarland, 2006, p. 4).

On the basis of in-depth qualitative research, Leininger has identified dominant cultural values and culture care meanings and action modes for many different American subculture groups, showing differences with the Anglo-American health-care value structure. She defines *subcultures* as "small or large groups living in a dominant culture that retain certain values and beliefs that are different from the dominant culture" (Leininger, 2002a, p. 122). The Anglo-American cultural values include individualism,

independence and freedom, competition and achievement, materialism, technology, instant time and actions, youth and beauty, equal rights (gender), leisure time, scientific facts and numbers, and a sense of generosity in time of crisis; action modes include stress alleviation, personalized acts, self-reliance, and health instruction. These characteristics are consistent with the prevailing culture of the practitioners and organizations that make up the health-care system. In her book, *Culture, Care, Diversity, and Universality: A Theory of Nursing,* Leininger lists information on a sample of some American subgroups (Leininger, 1991a, p. 355). She has identified further special groups as subgroups, such as the homeless, drug users, homosexuals, the deaf, those infected with acquired immunodeficiency syndrome and human immunodeficiency virus (HIV-AIDS), and nurses. Valencia-Go (2006) supports the identification of these subgroups as *emerging populations* in health care to include ethnic minorities, the homeless, and those afflicted with HIV-AIDS (p. 24).

Difficulties arise when significant values are unknown, in conflict, or poorly understood. The client's cultural values can be quite different from those of the health-care provider. As Leininger (1991a) details in her book, of the 15 sample subgroups presented, 10 share none of the dominant characteristics of health-care systems and Anglo-American clients, and few characteristics are shared by the remaining subgroups. In addition, consider the importance of religious or dominant spiritual influence in all but three of the cultural subgroups she described. Knowledge of the dominant values can assist in providing health promotion or health maintenance information, activities, and programs. An example can be seen with the increasing importance of the use of the faith communities in health promotion activities. Leininger (1994) stresses that nurses as primary, secondary, and tertiary care providers, through their close and continuous contact with culturally diverse clients, must move from unicultural personal and professional knowledge to provide meaningful culturally based nursing care (p. 255). Time, openness, and a growing understanding are critical components of a clinician's development of higher levels of cultural competence.

The Giger and Davidhizar Transcultural Assessment Model

Another nursing model directed at the importance of culture and care focuses on the assessment process. Giger and Davidhizar have identified a variety of cultural behavior patterns relevant to health assessment that have an influence on the delivery of care. They define culture as "a patterned behavioral response that develops over time as a result of imprinting the mind through social and religious structures and intellectual and artistic manifestations" (Giger and Davidhizar, 2006, p. 3). Their assessment model has been used in a variety of research and clinical practice settings and includes the concepts listed in Box 5–2. Cultures of origin, subcultures, and acculturalization are important considerations in this assessment model.

Notice that in this assessment model, the focus is on the cuturally unique individual. The initial area for assessment is on individual characteristics, including the individual's definition of culture. The next assessment areas include specifics on communication patterns and use of space, in which we see cultural differences but which also have a profound influence on interactions and acceptability of information sharing. Social organization is designed to obtain information on current health status as well as family, work, social, political and religious affiliations, practices, and preferences. Assessment of time consideration also looks at cultural patterns, practices, and preferences. Environmental control focuses on the individual's perception of locus of control (internal versus external as with the magico-religious paradigm), values and supernatural influences, and their description of their environment and their concept of health. The area of biologic variations includes a complete physical examination with particular attention to cultural variations, physical, metabolic, genetic, and sociocultural. The final area of this assessment model focuses on clinical judgment of the individual and the assessment data for incorporation into the plan of care. Although identified in their assessment model as nursing assessment, applications have been extended to other health-care areas. As reported by Giger and Davidhizar (2006), application of the model in diverse settings is producing a means for clinical understanding and application of culturally competent care (p. 13).

Personal Health Traditions of a Unique Cultural Being

Using the same concepts of communication, space, time, biologic variations, and social orientation, Spector (2000) views a person as a unique cultural

Box 5.2 Patterns for Assessment in the Giger & Davidhizar (2006) Transcultural Assessment Model

- Culturally unique individual factors
- Communication
- Space
- Social orientation
- Time
- Environmental control
- Biologic variations
- Nursing assessment

being, as having personal health traditions and by how he is affected by cultural phenomena. Her model is an oval with the outer band containing the five concepts of communication, space, time, biologic variations, and social orientation, and with the middle band containing the concepts of culture, religion, and ethnicity. At the center of the model is the person as a unique being with personal health traditions. Culture, heritage, and health traditions are important foci for this view of culture and the development of cultural awareness. She provides a heritage assessment tool to understand a person's traditional health and illness beliefs and practices, and to determine appropriate community care resources (Spector, 2000, p. 295).

The Process of Cultural Competence in the Delivery of a Health-Care Services Model

Campinha-Bacote (2003) has proposed a model specifically to address becoming culturally competent. She describes cultural competence as "the process in which the health-care professional continuously strives to achieve the ability and the availability to effectively work within the cultural context of a client (individual, family, or community)" (Campinha-Bacote, 2006, p. 1). The five constructs of cultural competence are identified as:

- Cultural awareness as a self-examination process
- Cultural knowledge and learning about other cultures
- Cultural skill in the assessment process
- Cultural encounter or interactions with culturally diverse others
- Cultural desire or motivation. (Campinha-Bacote, 2006, pp. 1–2)

The model is illustrated as a volcano; as cultural desire erupts, it leads to becoming culturally competent. Time, openness, and a growing level of understanding are required of the clinician to develop the cultural skills. This ongoing process of becoming culturally competent is similar to Maslow's Hierarchy of Needs and the quest for self-actualization at the top of the hierarchy. Cultural competence is the pursuit of a goal. Campinha-Bacote broadened the focus of her model to health-care practitioners and services rather than restricting her model to the practice of nursing.

The Purnell Model for Cultural Competence

Purnell (2005) describes cultural competence as a conscious process, one that is not necessarily linear in nature, and one with many definitions and terminology (p. 7). The Purnell model was originally designed as an organizing framework, as a wheel with four rims representing the society, community, family, and the person, and spokes as 12 wedges representing cultural constructs, to the unknown dark core at the center as illustrated in Figure 5–4. Seven primary concepts (e.g., age and gender) and 13 secondary concepts (e.g., marital status) of culture are identified with cultural competence as a nonlinear process as the road below the wheel. The development of cultural competence is implicit as noted in one of 21 assumptions upon which the model is based, "when individuals of dissimilar cultural orientations meet in a work or therapeutic environment, the likelihood for developing a mutually satisfying relationship is improved if both parties in the relationship attempt to learn about each other's culture" (p. 12).

As Purnell (2005) states, unlike Leininger, his model is in line with the four metaparadigm concepts of nursing in that they provide a wholistic perspective; however, the model is not restricted to nursing and is applicable across many disciplines (p. 12). Information provided in the model is designed to understand holistically human beings with health issues within the various broad constructs.

What each of the models seems to have in common is a directive to seek actively to understand the uniqueness of human beings in their context, as cultural competence. And in doing this, care for individuals, families, and groups will result in more positive outcomes. They also point to the fact, however, that individuals within a selected culture are very different. As we seek to understand different cultures and heritages, we must still focus on human beings. Consider the results of a research study to validate an instrument used with hospitalized clients on advance directives. The researchers found that the instrument was valid, in both the English and Spanish versions. But differences were also found in the preferences, in that the Hispanic adult participants had less knowledge of advance directives and a higher preference for life-support interventions. Froman and Owen (2003) were able to support the validity of the instrument but did recommend further study to address the "great diversity among Hispanic regions and culture" (p. 36). Consider the following variables for culturally competent care:

- Time with clients to become accepted and gain an understanding of their belief system
- Differences in belief systems among generations and geographic origin
- Past experiences and current situation
- Religious influences
- Familial influences
- Understanding of advance directives
- Acceptance of the health-care services, systems, and practitioners
- Linguistic issues

Other individual values may not be initially apparent or may grow more dominant. Complementary and alternative medicine (CAM) and health-care practices, such as acupuncture, imagery, and herbal medicines, are being tried as people become dissatisfied with the biomedical view and move to holistic care. These practices may differ from a client's inherited cultural background but may be adopted or become more dominant. In addition, they may be used along with (complementary) or instead of (alternative) conventional medicine, and their use may or may not be reported by the client to the health-care provider. Spector (2000) reports the rapidly growing use of homeopathic health-care choices as alternative or complementary (e.g., aromatherapy, biofeedback, hypnotherapy, massage) and ethnocultural or traditional (e.g., herbals and holistic healing practices and rituals). And the research and body of knowledge on many of these practices is growing. This increase in use and acceptance of CAM also points to the need for a comprehensive cultural assessment with the client and may require of the clinician great openness, sensitivity, and time.

THE NURSE'S ROLE

Nurses have a primary responsibility in health promotion, health maintenance, and prevention activities; in fact, such activities represent the essence of professional nursing practice. The focus of nursing is on the health of the individual, family, community, and societal group. Health promotion roles are guided within the theoretical framework on which nursing practice is based, including how you, as the professional, view the client, the concept of health, the environment, and the

ONLINE CONSULT

The Center for Cross-Cultural Health at
www.crosshealth.com

Initiative to Eliminate Racial & Ethnic Disparities in Health at
http://www.cdc.gov/omh/AboutUs/disparities.htm

Office of Minority Health at
http://www.omhrc.gov

National Center for CAM at
http://nccam.nih.gov

Transcultural C.A.R.E. Associates at
http://www.transculturalcare.net

The Purnell Model for Cultural Competence

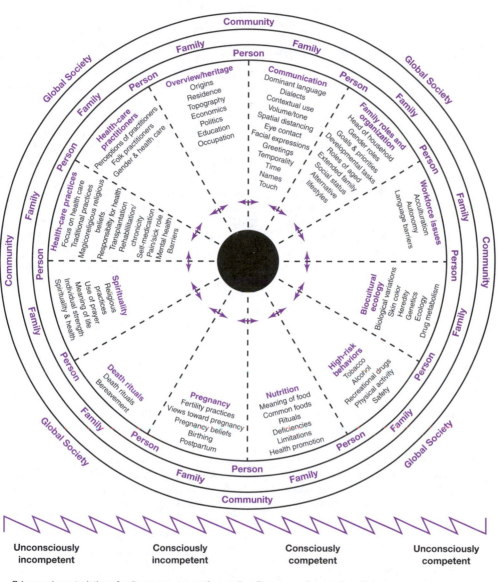

Primary characteristics of culture: age, generation, nationality, race, color, gender, religion

Secondary characteristics of culture: educational status, socioeconomic status, occupation, military status, political beliefs, urban versus rural residence, enclave identity, marital status, parental status, physical characteristics, sexual orientation, gender issues, and reason for migration (sojourner, immigrant, undocumented status)

Unconsciously incompetent: not being aware that one is lacking knowledge about another culture
Consciously incompetent: being aware that one is lacking knowledge about another culture
Consciously competent: learning about the client's culture, verifying generalizations about the client's culture, and providing culturally specific interventions
Unconsciously competent: automatically providing culturally congruent care to clients of diverse cultures

■ **Figure 5.4** The Purnell Model for Cultural Competence. (Purnell, L. D, & Paulanka, B. J. (2003). Transcultural health care: A culturally competent approach (2nd ed.). Philadelphia: F. A. Davis.)

practice of nursing as well as your accord with a model's definitions and relationships. This is the purpose of the middle-range theories discussed in Chapter 3, from which you can move to a practice model that is applicable to your specific function or practice setting. Before you decide on the best framework to guide your own professional practice, consider the following two examples.

Example 1

Suppose your practice is guided by King's Theory of Goal Attainment. In this theory, nursing is defined as "a process of human interactions between nurse and client whereby each perceives the other and the situation, and through communications, they set goals, explore the means to achieve them, agree to the means, [and] their actions indicate movement toward goal achievement" (King, 1987, p. 113). Health promotion, health maintenance, and prevention activities are all implied in this definition of *health* as adjustment to stressors in the system environments and use of resources. Health is viewed as a potential and the goal of the process.

Specific assessment and intervention activities must address the theory's theoretical concepts and propositions. Selected health and illness models can be used to guide practice. Personal perceptions of the client are important components of the Health Belief Model, Pender's Health Promotion Model, and the Chronic Illness Trajectory Framework. If your practice setting is a clinic with a large population that needs health promotion strategies addressing individual lifestyles and the preventive services identified in Healthy People 2010, you may find the health belief model or Pender's Health Promotion Model quite useful with your clients. These same models can address health maintenance as secondary and tertiary prevention. On the other hand, if your practice setting is a hospice or you work primarily with patients with cancer and their families, you may find the chronic illness trajectory framework more useful for guiding your practice and use of the nursing process.

Example 2

If your practice is guided by Leininger's (1991b, 2002b) Culture Care Diversity and Universality model, three modes of cultural care guide your nursing judgment, decisions, and actions: preservation and maintenance, accommodation and negotiation, and repatterning or restructuring. In Leininger's concept of culturally congruent nursing care, these modes all focus on health promotion, health maintenance, and prevention activities within the context of the client's cultural belief system. She defines *culturally congruent nursing care* as the specific use of "culturally based care, knowledge, acts and decisions in sensitive and knowledgeable ways to appropriately and meaningfully fit the cultural values, beliefs, and lifeways of clients for their health and well-being, or to prevent illness, disabilities, or death" (Leininger and McFarland, 2006, p. 15). The practice models and assessment tools you select must be culturally sensitive and must include individual focus on each of the assessment factors in the Sunrise Enabler, which is used by Leininger (1991b, 2002b) and Leininger and McFarland, 2006) to depict the dimensions of her theory visually.

Selecting a health model involves a deliberate and reflective process that takes into account your views, the theory that guides your professional practice, and the unique characteristics of the people and environment in which you work. You may practice under several similar models, depending on a changeable environment or client group interactions.

INTERACTIVE EXERCISES

Go to the Intranet site and complete the interactive exercises provided for this Chapter.

KEY POINTS

■ Health promotion and health protection strategies relate to individual lifestyle and environmental influences on health status and health prospects. Preventive activities and services address three areas of prevention. Primary prevention consists of healthy actions taken to avoid illness or disease. Secondary prevention involves screening for early detection and treatment of health problems. Tertiary prevention during the rehabilitative phase of an illness prevents complications and further disability.

■ Health is more than the absence of illness, disease, or infirmity. A concept of health is determined by one's worldview and philosophical assumptions.

■ Benner and Wrubel (1989) have described five theories of health as (1) an ideal, (2) the ability to fulfill social roles, (3) a commodity, (4) a human potential, and (5) a sense of coherence.

(Key points continue on page 99)

K E Y   P O I N T S   (continued)

■ Dunn's high-level wellness emphasizes well-being, including the positive, dynamic, and unique integration of mind, body, and spirit of the individual functioning within her environment and the individual's maximum potential.

■ The health belief model was designed as an organizing framework to advance health promotion activities by targeting interventions to certain individual variables. Three major concepts explain and predict health-related behaviors: (1) readiness to undertake recommended compliance behavior, (2) modifying and enabling factors, and (3) compliant behaviors.

■ Pender's health promotion model is a schematic representation with three components for health-promoting behaviors. Individual characteristics and experiences include prior related behavior and personal factors (biologic, psychological, and sociocultural factors). Behavior-specific cognitions and affect include perceived benefits, perceived barriers, perceived self-efficacy, activity-related affect interpersonal influences, and situational influences. The behavioral outcome is attainment of a positive health outcome through commitment to the plan of action and competing demands and preferences.

■ The chronic illness trajectory framework (Corbin and Strauss, 1992a) is a conceptual model organized under the main concept of trajectory for managing an evolving course of a chronic condition.

■ Gordon's (2006) 11 functional health patterns can be used as a valuable tool in the nursing assessment and diagnosis process and in the application of models to address health and illness focused on human potential or a sense of coherence.

■ Culture involves a combination of social, familial, religious, national, and professional characteristics that affect the way we think, act, and interact with others. Differences among groups and subgroups produce diversity that can lead from uniculturalism to appreciation of a multicultural environment and health-care behaviors.

■ Leininger and McFarland (2006) define culturally congruent nursing care as "culturally based care, knowledge, acts and decisions in sensitive and knowledgeable ways to appropriately and meaningfully fit the cultural values, beliefs, and lifeways of clients for their health and well-being, or to prevent illness, disabilities, or death" (Leininger and McFarland, 2006, p. 15).

■ The Giger and Davidhizar Transcultural Assessment Model, directed at the importance of culture and care, focuses on the assessment process and patterns of culturally unique individual factors, communication, space, social orientation, time, environmental control, biologic variations, and nursing assessment.

■ Using the same concepts of communication, space, time, biologic variations, and social orientation, Spector (2000) views a person as a unique cultural being with personal health traditions and how he is affected by cultural phenomena.

■ Campinha-Bacote (2003) has proposed the process of Cultural Competence in the Delivery of Healthcare Services Model to accompany the central concepts of cultural awareness, knowledge, skill, encounters, and desire.

■ The Purnell Model for Cultural Competence (2005) was originally designed as an organizing framework, as a wheel with four rims representing the society, community, family, and the person, and spokes as 12 wedges representing cultural constructs, to the unknown dark core at the center.

■ Complementary and alternative medicine (CAM) and health-care practices are being tried as people become dissatisfied with the biomedical view and move to holistic care.

■ Nursing focuses on the health of the individual, family, community, and societal group. Health promotion roles are guided by the theoretical framework on which practice is based.

Thought and Discussion Questions

1. Select a definition provided for health from the nursing theories presented in Chapter 4. Discuss which of the five models of health they fit into, and suggest health promotion models for each.

2. Use Pender's health promotion model to plan a health promotion campaign for one of the following situations:
   - Immunization program in an urban apartment complex with a high density of families with young children
   - Home safety program at a senior citizens' center
   - Wellness program for employees in a manufacturing company

3. Recall a client with a chronic illness for whom you have provided nursing care in the past. Retrospectively apply the chronic illness trajectory framework to the client's experiences that you were able to observe.

4. Think of an example from your experience in which culture affected perception of health, illness, or treatment. How did you or could you alter your approach to the client?

5. Review the Chapter Thought located on the first page of the chapter, and discuss it in the context of this chapter.

☐ REFERENCES

Andrews, M. M. (2003). Theoretical foundations of transcultural nursing. In M. M. Andrews & J. S. Boyle, *Transcultural concepts in nursing care* (4th ed.). Philadelphia: Lippincott Williams & Wilkins.

Babcock, D. E., & Miller, M. A. (1994). *Client education: Theory and practice.* St. Louis: Mosby.

Becker, M. H., Haefner, D. P., Kasl, S. V., Kirscht, J. P., Maiman, L. A., & Rosenstock, I. M. (1977). Selected psychosocial models and correlates of individual health-related behaviors. *Medical Care, 15*(Supplement 5), 27–46.

Benner, P., & Wrubel, J. (1989). *The primacy of caring: Stress and coping in health and illness.* Menlo Park, CA: Addison-Wesley.

Betancourt, J. R., Green, A. R., & Carrillo, J. E. (2002, October). *Cultural competence in health care: Emerging frameworks and practical approaches* (Field Report, Publication No. 576). New York: The Commonwealth Fund.

Betancourt, J. R., Green, A. R., Carrillo, J. E., & Park, E.R. (2005, March/April). Cultural competence and health care disparities: Key perspectives and trends. (The Commonwealth Fund Publication #821). *Health Affairs, 24*(2), 499–505. Retrieved June 23, 2006, from *http://content.healthaffairs.org/content/vol24/issue2/*

Campinha-Bacote, J. (2003, January 31). Many faces: Addressing diversity in health care. *Online Journal of Issues in Nursing, 8*(1), Manuscript 2. Retrieved September 26, 2007 from *http://nursingworld.org/MainMenuCategories/ANAMarketplace/ANAPeriodicals/OJIN/TableofContents/Volume82003/Num1Jan31_2003/AddressingDiversityinHealthCare.aspx*

Campinha-Bacote, J. (2006). The process of cultural competence in the delivery of healthcare services: A culturally conscious model of care. Retrieved June 22, 2006, from *http://www.transculturalcare.net/*

Corbin, J. M., & Strauss, A. (1992a). A nursing model for chronic illness management based upon the trajectory framework. In P. Woog (Ed.), *The chronic illness trajectory framework: The Corbin and Strauss nursing model* (pp. 9–28). New York: Springer.

Corbin, J. M., & Strauss, A. (1992b). Commentary. In P. Woog (Ed.), *The chronic illness trajectory framework: The Corbin and Strauss nursing model* (pp. 97–102). New York: Springer.

Dunn, H. L. (1973). *High level wellness.* Arlington, VA: Beatty.

Froman, R. D., & Owen, S. V. (2003). Validation of the Spanish Life Support Preference Questionnaire (LSPQ). *Journal of Nursing Scholarship, 35*(1), pp. 33–36.

Giger, J.N., & Davidhizar, R.E. (2006). *Transcultural nursing: Assessment and intervention* (4th ed.). St. Louis: Mosby.

Glanz, K., Rimer, B. K., Lewis, F. M. (Eds.) (2002). *Health behavior and health education: Theory, research, and practice* (3rd ed). San Francisco: Jossey-Bass.

Gordon, M. (2006). *Nursing diagnosis: Process and application* (11th ed.). St. Louis: Elsevier Science.

Gunther, M. E. (2002). Martha E. Rogers: Unitary human beings. In A. M. Tomey & M. R. Alligood (Eds.), *Nursing theorists and their work* (5th ed., pp. 226–249). St. Louis: Mosby.

Jourard, S. M. (1971). *The transparent self.* New York: Litton Educational.

King, I. M. (1987). King's theory of goal attainment. In R. R. Parse (Ed.), *Nursing science: Major paradigms, theories, and critiques* (pp. 107–113). Philadelphia: W. B. Saunders.

King, I. M. (1981). *A theory for nursing: Systems, concepts, process.* New York: John Wiley & Sons.

Leininger, M. (2002a). Culture care assessments for congruent competency practices. In M. Leininger & M. R. McFarland,

Transcultural nursing: Concepts, theories, research, and practice (3rd ed., pp. 117–143). New York: McGraw-Hill.

Leininger, M. (2002b). The theory of culture care and ethnonursing research method. In M. Leininger & M. R. McFarland, *Transcultural nursing: Concepts, theories, research, and practice* (3rd ed., pp. 71–98). New York: McGraw-Hill.

Leininger, M. M. (1994). Transcultural nursing education: A worldwide imperative. *Nursing and Health Care, 15,* 254–257.

Leininger, M. M. (1991a). Selected culture care findings of diverse cultures using culture care theory and ethnomethods. In M. M. Leininger (Ed.), *Culture care diversity and universality: A theory of nursing* (Pub. No. 15–2402, pp. 345–371). New York: National League for Nursing.

Leininger, M. M. (1991b). The theory of culture care diversity and universality. In M. M. Leininger (Ed.), *Culture care diversity and universality: A theory of nursing* (Pub. No. 15–2402, pp. 5–68). New York: National League for Nursing.

Leininger, M. (1970). *Nursing and anthropology: Two worlds to blend.* New York: John Wiley & Sons.

Leininger, M. M., & McFarland, M. R. (2006). *Culture care diversity and universality: A worldwide nursing theory* (2nd ed.). Boston: Jones and Bartlett.

Parse, R. R. (1981). *Man-living-health: A theory of nursing.* New York: John Wiley & Sons.

Pender, N. J. (1996). *Health promotion in nursing practice* (3rd ed.). Stamford, CT: Appleton & Lange.

Pender, N. J. (1987). *Health promotion in nursing practice* (2nd ed.). Norwalk, CT: Appleton & Lange.

Pender, N. J., Murdaugh, C. L., and Parsons, M. A. (2006). *Health promotion in nursing practice* (5th ed.). Upper Saddle River, NJ: Pearson Prentice Hall.

Pender, N. J., Murdaugh, C. L., and Parsons, M. A. (2002). *Health promotion in nursing practice* (4th ed.). Upper Saddle River, NJ: Pearson Prentice Hall.

Purnell, L. (2005). The Purnell model for cultural competence. *Journal of Multicultural Nursing & Health, 11*(2), 7–15.

Purnell, L. D, & Paulanka, B. J. (2003). Transcultural health care: A culturally competent approach (2nd ed.). Philadelphia: F. A. Davis.

Roy, C. (2007). The Roy adaptation model. Retrieved September 26, 2007 from http://www.bc.edu/schools/son/faculty/theorist/Roy_Adaptation_Model.html

Spector, R. E. (2000). *Cultural diversity in health & illness* (5th ed.). Upper Saddle River, NJ: Prentice Hall Health.

Strauss, A. L., Corbin, J., Fagerhaugh, S., Glaser, B. G., Maines, D., Suczek, B., & Wiener, C. L. (1984). *Chronic illness and the quality of life* (2nd ed.). St. Louis: C. V. Mosby.

Strauss, A. L., & Glaser, B. G. (1975). *Chronic illness and the quality of life.* St. Louis: C. V. Mosby.

U.S. Department of Health & Human Services. (2000). *Healthy people 2010: Understanding and improving health.* Retrieved June 22, 2006, from *http://www.healthypeople.gov/Document/tableofcontents.htm#under*

U.S. Department of Health & Human Services, Public Health Service, (USDHHS, PHS). *Healthy people 2010* (Conference Edition, in Two Volumes). Washington, DC: U.S. Government Printing Office. Retrieved June 22, 2006, from *http://www.healthypeople.gov/Document/tableofcontents.htm#volume1*

U.S. Department of Health & Human Services, Public Health Service. (1992). *Healthy people 2000: Summary report.* Boston: Jones & Bartlett.

Valencia-Go, G. (2006). Emerging populations and health. In C. L. Edlman & C. L. Mandle (Eds.), *Health promotion throughout the lifespan* (6th ed., pp. 23–49). St. Louis: Mosby.

☐ BIBLIOGRAPHY

Baldwin, D. M. (2003). Disparities in health care: Focusing efforts to eliminate unequal burdens (Continuing Education). Retrieved June 22, 2006, from *http://www.nursingworld.org/mods/mod560/cebrdnfull.htm*

Burton, C.R. (2000). Rethinking stroke rehabilitation: The Corbin and Strauss chronic illness trajectory framework. *Journal of Advanced Nursing, 32*, 595–602.

Campinha-Bacote, J. (2003). *The process of cultural competence in the delivery of healthcare services: A culturally competent model of care* (4th ed.). Cincinnati, OH: Transcultural C.A.R.E. Associates.

Endelman, C. L., & Mandle, C. L. (2006). *Health promotion throughout the lifespan* (6th ed.). St. Louis: Mosby.

Clark, C. C. (2000). *Integrating complementary health procedures into practice*. New York: Springer.

Halcomb, E., & Davidson, P. (2005). Using the illness trajectory framework to describe recovery from traumatic injury. *Contemporary Nurse: A Journal for the Australian Nursing Profession, 19*(1–2), 232–241.

Munro, B. H. (2003). Caring for the Hispanic populations: The state of the science. *Journal of Transcultural Nursing, 14*, 174–176.

Snyder, M., & Lindquist, R. (2002). *Complementary/alternative therapies in nursing* (4th ed.). New York: Springer.

Tate, D. M. (2003). Cultural awareness: Bridging the gap between caregivers and Hispanic patients. *Journal of Continuing Education in Nursing, 34*, 213–217.

Winslow, B. J. W. (2002). Placement decisions for relatives with dementia (NINR Grant #1R15NR005306-01A2). Retrieved June 23, 2006, from *http://crisp.cit.nih.gov/crisp/CRISP_LIB.getdoc?textkey=6504667&p_grant_num=1R15NR005306-01A2*

☐ ONLINE RESOURCES

Agency for Healthcare Research and Quality
www.ahrq.gov

The Center for Cross-Cultural Health
http://www.crosshealth.com

The Commonwealth Fund
www.cmwf.org

Healthy People
www.healthypeople.gov

Initiative to Eliminate Racial & Ethnic Disparities in Health
http://www.cdc.gov/omh/AboutUs/disparities.htm

National Center for Complementary and Alternative Medicine
http://nccam.nih.gov

National Center for Cultural Competence
http://www.georgetown.edu/research/gucdc/nccc

Office of Minority Health
http://www.omhrc.gov

Transcultural C.A.R.E. Associates
http://www.transculturalcare.net

U.S. Department. of Health & Human Services
http://www.hhs.gov

■ *Rose* **Kearney-Nunnery**

Evidence-Based Practice

>❝*We may search for information,*
> *but once gained how does*
> *it become wisdom?*❞
>
> Author

On completion of this chapter, the reader will be able to:

1. Explain the importance of evidence-based practice for the profession of nursing.
2. Define basic terminology used in research for application of findings in practice.
3. Describe legal and ethical considerations applicable to research with human subjects.
4. Describe different ways to participate in nursing research.
5. Analyze barriers to evidence-based practice.
6. Prepare a basic critique of a published research study.
7. Plan for the inclusion of a higher level of evidence-based care in her practice setting.

Key Terms

Evidence-Based Practice	Minimal Risk	Research Design
Research	Empirical Research	Operational Definition
Ethical Codes	Qualitative Research	Variables
Basic Human Rights	Knowledge Transformation	Sampling
Beneficence	Critique	Data Collection Procedures
Full Disclosure	Research Problem	Instruments
Self-Determination	Literature Review	Descriptive Statistics
Privacy and Confidentiality	Hypotheses	Inferential Statistics

Theory guides practice, but current knowledge and practice must be based on evidence of efficacy rather than intuition, tradition, or past practice. Out of a national concern for safety initiatives in 1999 and a focus on systems issues in 2001, the national call came for changes in the education and competencies of health professionals in all disciplines in 2003. The result was the identification of the five core competencies for health professionals identified in Chapter 1. The importance of employing evidence-based practice (EBP) was described as follows:

> The committee feels that it is critical for interdisciplinary health teams and each of the disciplines to be able to tap this evidence base effectively at the point of patient care, determining whether an intervention, such as a preventive service, diagnostic test, or therapy, can be expected to produce better outcomes than alternatives—including the alternative of doing nothing. (Greiner & Knebel, 2003, p. 56)

Sigma Theta Tau (2005), the International Honor Society of Nursing, defines the use of **evidence-based practice** as "an integration of the best evidence available, nursing expertise, and the values and preferences of the individuals, families, and communities who are selected" (p. 2). This does not sound unique to our view of nursing and quality health care. The problem is that we are not consistently *using* the best evidence available to guide care to clients. And the next questions become: Do we have the best evidence available? Where is the information? And, are we applying appropriate knowledge in clinical situations?

As proposed by Hegyvary (2006), evidence-based practice must be more than a "buzzword" and focus on understanding and alleviating the problems that impede health. An actual paradigm shift has occurred, with the call for evidence-based practice. As will be discussed in subsequent chapters, Magnet Status also supports the use of evidence-based practice for enhanced outcomes for both clients and nurses (American Nurses Credentialing Center [ANCC], 2006, p. 5).

Theory guides practice, but current knowledge and practice must be based on evidence of efficacy rather than intuition, tradition, or past practice.

Research supports our knowledge base and answers questions of clinical concern. It provides sound information on which to base practice, as evidence-based nursing practice. Porter-O'Grady (2006) describes evidence-based practice as requiring " a degree of flexibility and fluidity based on firm scientific and clinical evidence validating appropriate and sustainable clinical practice (p. 3). Evidence can come from a number of sources, but we need both seekers and users of the information in practice to develop knowledge. Clinicians in the practice setting have the questions. These questions must be refined and studied so that nurse researchers can find solutions to health-care practice problems. And we need further validation from the consumer as to the appropriateness of the intervention. This is truly evidence-based practice.

THE EVOLUTION OF NURSING RESEARCH

Research has been defined as a "systematic, controlled, empirical, amoral, public, and critical investigation of natural phenomena guided by theory and hypotheses about the presumed relations among such phenomena" (Kerlinger & Lee, 2000, p. 14). Given this definition, research is still viewed by some as an academic exercise. But it is much more in nursing. The purposes of research are to describe, explain, predict, and control phenomena and to provide information for future use in practice or for expansion of the knowledge base.

Nursing research began with Florence Nightingale and her identification of environmental influences on health and illness. In her classic *Notes on Nursing: What It Is, and What It Is Not* (1859), Nightingale identified factors that influence health and wellness, supporting them with observational accounts, statistics, and deductive reasoning. Following her landmark efforts, non-nurse researchers performed limited research on nurses and nursing education. Then in the mid-20th century, graduate nursing programs began to proliferate, as did nurses' involvement in research studies, often on nurses and delivery of nursing services. The introduction of the journal *Nursing Research* in 1952 provided a specific channel for disseminating research findings to other nurses.

During the second half of the 20th century, the number of graduate and baccalaureate nursing programs grew. Content on research became prevalent in baccalaureate nursing curricula during the 1970s and early 1980s. Graduate student enrollments increased with the growth in doctoral programs in the 1980s. Research findings were used to develop and refine conceptual and theoretical models. More nurses were now doing research, and the American Nurses Association (ANA) Cabinet on Nursing Research identified research expectations by level of education in 1981. The primary focus of research changed during this time from educational programs and methods to the focus of nursing: people as patients, clients, and members of society. Support has grown for research as we see the needs to investigate the domain of nursing, test theories and interventions, and demonstrate efficacy and efficiency of nursing actions and client outcomes.

Nursing research is supported further in the position statement of the American Association of Colleges of Nursing (AACN, 2006). This organization has identified research expectations and competencies of graduates from baccalaureate through postdoctoral programs, moving from evaluation and utilization of research to generating new knowledge with advanced preparation (AACN, 2006, p. 5). This concept has implications for the baccalaureate-prepared nurse in the identification of research problems, the support of ongoing research, the use of applicable findings in practice, and the expansion of the knowledge base following preparation at the graduate level.

Development of Nursing Research Organizations

The establishment of the National Center for Nursing Research (NCNR) as part of the National Institutes of Health (NIH) in April 1986, under the Health Research Extension Act of 1985 (PL99–158), demonstrated the importance of research for and by the profession. In 1993, the National Institute of Nursing Research (NINR) was established, a change from the former divisional and center status, with fiscal year appropriations from Congress growing, thus further demonstrating the importance of generating knowledge in nursing. An important component of the mission of the NINR is to "promote and improve the health of individuals, families, communities, and populations [through] . . . clinical and basic research and research training on health and illness across the lifespan . . . " (NINR, 2007, p. 2). Extramural research programs for the NINR concern health promotion and disease prevention, acute and chronic illness, and nursing systems.

Research proposals are highly competitive at NINR, as with other areas of NIH. Research proposals are reviewed by a panel of experts and scored according to the consistency with the mission of NINR and the merit of the research project. During the initial phase of NINR initiatives, research priorities were specified for investigations. In 2004, the NINR issued research opportunities to focus on chronic illnesses or conditions, behavioral changes and interventions, and responding to compelling public health concerns. Important information is evolving with results presented to Congress and other audiences. Reports on these projects are available and are making a difference, as are the continued federal appropriations that are committed to the NINR. Areas of science continue to be identified as focus areas.

A vital issue is the need for reliable and valid research on questions of clinical concern for decision-making and change. In nursing, research must be directed at interventions over which nursing has control so that the knowledge developed can lead to needed

ONLINE CONSULT

American Nurses Foundation at
http://www.anfonline.org/anf/nrggrant.htm

Federal Opportunities for Research Funding at
www.grants.gov

National Institute of Nursing Research at
http://ninr.nih.gov

National League for Nursing at
http://www.nln.org

Sigma Theta Tau International at
http://www.nursingsociety.org/research

change. This is the essence of evidence-based professional nursing practice.

For some time, Sigma Theta Tau has recognized the importance of generating and using research. The purposes of this honor society include encouraging scholarly and creative work. This purpose is applicable to both the conduct and utilization of research. Scholarship involves discovery, integration, application, and teaching. Utilizing and communicating research in nursing practice projects and conferences have been foci of Sigma Theta Tau International. The organization also supports research investigations that generate nursing knowledge through competitive extramural grants for researchers, as does the American Nurses Foundation. Now there is a resurgence of the need for research on nursing education outcomes with support available from the National League for Nursing. Nurses have a major responsibility to identify research problems, support ongoing research, and use applicable findings in practice, along with continuing to learn in this area of scholarly nursing practice.

LEGAL AND ETHICAL CONSIDERATIONS IN RESEARCH

An essential responsibility in professional nursing practice is protecting the rights of research subjects.

Background

The rights of people in research have been of great concern to ethicists, legislators, and professionals, leading to ethical codes and guidelines for the protection of research subjects. History has provided much of the impetus for our professional codes and federal regulations. During World War II, experiments noted for the unethical treatment of subjects included the Nazi medical experiments and the Japanese concentration camp experiments on human subjects. As a result, international **ethical codes** evolved. In 1949, the Nuremberg Code set standards for involving human subjects in research, with guidelines for consent, protections, risks and benefits, and qualifications of researchers. For example, true informed and voluntary consent became an essential requirement. The Declaration of Helsinki (1990), made in 1964 and revised in 1975 and 1989, provided guidelines on therapeutic and nontherapeutic research, along with the requirements for disclosing the risks and potential benefits of the research and obtaining written consent for participation from research subjects.

Safety, Health, and Welfare

In the United States, the Tuskegee syphilis study, the Jewish Chronic Disease Hospital study, and the Willowbrook hepatitis study are further examples of unethical treatment of research subjects (Box 6–1). In the quest for knowledge, researchers failed to consider the basic human rights of their subjects, especially the right of informed consent and considerations for vulnerable populations. Federal regulations evolved from the original guidelines of the former Department of Health, Education, and Welfare, culminating in the National Research Act in 1974. This law specified the composition and authority of institutional review boards (IRBs). IRBs were now mandated as oversight bodies to ensure protection of research subjects, especially for research projects seeking federal funding.

The Belmont Report was the outcome of a National Commission for the Protection of Human Subjects of Biomedical and Behavioral Research assembled by the National Research Act. This commission was charged with identifying principles and developing guidelines. The report specified boundaries between practice and research. Basic ethical principles were reinforced, highlighting respect for persons and defining the principles of beneficence (doing no harm, with maximum benefits and minimal risks) and justice (fairness relative to one's share, need, effort, contribution, and merit). Specific applications that resulted from the Belmont Report (1979) were: (1) guidelines on informed consent, including provision of information and ensuring comprehension and voluntariness; (2) assessment of risks and benefits; and (3) selection of subjects. The Belmont Report provided the basis for federal laws.

All activities involving humans as subjects must provide for the safety, health, and welfare of every individual. Subjects do not abdicate rights with their participation in a research study. Four **basic human rights** must be ensured for research subjects. These principles speak to ethical considerations and human rights:

1. **Beneficence** (Do no harm.)
2. **Full Disclosure**
3. **Self-determination**
4. **Privacy and confidentiality**

The "do no harm" concept includes careful consideration of the risk-benefit ratio with any research project. One must keep in mind that **minimal risk** requires that "the probability and magnitude of harm or discomfort anticipated in the research are not greater in and of themselves than those ordinarily encountered in daily life or during the performance of routine physical or psychological examinations or tests" (Protection of Human Subjects, 45 CFR 46, §42.102 [i]). Full disclosure of information and self-determination by potential subjects are necessary conditions for informed consent. In addition, subjects' rights to privacy and confidentiality must be ensured throughout the process. As protections for these four rights, the guidelines must be considered by researchers and their respective IRBs (Box 6–2).

The issue of privacy of personal health information (PHI) was the focus of the Health Insurance Portability and Accountability Act (HIPAA) of 1996. PHI is "individually identifiable health information transmitted by electronic media, maintained in electronic media, or transmitted or maintained in any other form or medium" (USDHHS, 2004, p. 6). The Act's Privacy Rule establishes:

[M]inimum federal standards for protecting the privacy of individually identifiable health information.

Box 6.1 Examples of Unethical Use of Vulnerable Populations in Research

1932–1972   Tuskegee, Alabama

Longitudinal clinical study by the Public Health Service of untreated syphilis in sharecroppers, mostly African Americans, who did not receive full disclosure, did not give informed consent, and received deceptive and ineffective treatments.

1963   Brooklyn, New York

In a short-term study, debilitated patients at the Jewish Chronic Disease Hospital, who did not have cancer, were injected with live cancer cells to study their response. This study also had partial federal funding with subjects who were indigent and did not receive full disclosure or informed consent.

1963–1966   Staten Island, New York

At Willowbrook State School, a school for the mentally retarded, healthy children were intentionally injected with the hepatitis virus to study the disease and treatment process. Parents did not receive full disclosure, and needless to say, subjects were harmed.

Box 6.2 General Principles/Ethical Guidelines for Research on Human Subjects

- Risks to the subjects are minimized.
- Risks are reasonable in relation to anticipated benefits to subjects.
- Selection of subjects is equitable.
- Informed consent is sought from each prospective subject or the legally authorized representative.
- Informed consent is appropriately documented.
- The research plan makes adequate provision for monitoring the data collected to ensure the safety of subjects.
- Adequate provisions exist to protect the privacy of subjects and maintain the confidentiality of data.
- Special protections are in place for populations that are vulnerable, e.g., children, prisoners, pregnant women, mentally disabled persons, or economically or educationally disadvantaged persons, because these subjects are vulnerable to coercion or undue influence.

Source: Title 45 Code of Federal Regulations Part 46 (45 CFR 46), §46.111

ONLINE CONSULT

Federal Guidelines for the Protection of Human Subjects including the Belmont Report, the Declaration of Helsinki, and the Nuremberg Code at
http://ohsr.od.nih.gov/guidelines/

The Ethical and Legal Implications of Programs to Redress Injured Subjects, Volume 1, a report by the U. S. President's Commission for the Study of Ethical Problems in Medicine and Biomedical and Behavioral Research, Washington, DC, June 1982, at
http://www.gwu.edu/~nsarchiv/radiation/dir/ mstreet/commeet/meet16/brief16/tab_b/ br16b1a.txt

The Rule confers certain rights on individuals, including rights to access and amend their health information and to obtain a record of when and why their PHI has been shared with others for certain purposes. (USDHHS, 2004, p. 6)

For researchers, informed consent is a necessary process. HIPAA's privacy provisions require further language in the consent process, with required elements for access to and use of PHI. A privacy authorization may be incorporated into the consent form or maintained as a separate document. De-identifying PHI before revealing it to others requires the removal of 18 specific data identifiers that could link the individual to their PHI. The privacy rules do allow, however, for the use of selected categories of PHI, as a *Limited Data Set* that may be used or disclosed, for purposes of research, public health, or health-care operations, without obtaining either an individual's authorization or a waiver for its use and disclosure, with the removal of 16 data identifiers and a data use agreement (USDHHS, 2004, p. 19).

As with other areas of nursing practice, legal and ethical considerations are deliberated with any research activity. These issues occur in the planning, implementation, analysis, and reporting stages for a research endeavor. In the proposal or planning stage of any research study, the researcher must consider the rights of the subjects and the ethical nature of the study. When a researcher defines the problem and purpose of the research, the significance of the problem for the body of knowledge and the ethical issues associated with the proposed investigation are vital considerations.

The Institutional Review Board

Once the basic research plan is developed, an IRB must review and approve the start of the study. Strict federal guidelines for review by an IRB must be adhered to, especially in agencies seeking funding for research. Human subjects' rights of full disclosure, self-determination (informed consent), privacy and confidentiality, and safety (not to be harmed) must be ensured. The research proposal, with statements of the problem and purpose or significance, literature support, theory and definitions, specific research questions or hypotheses, design, sampling plans, and data collection and analysis methods must be approved by the IRB for use with human subjects. The researcher submits a proposal to an IRB for approval to proceed to the next steps of subject selection and data collection. During this stage of implementing the research project, the investigator must adhere to the procedures specified for data collection and analysis. The IRB performs evaluations throughout the project to ensure that subjects are not placed at risk and that the integrity and confidentiality of the data are maintained during collection, analysis, and dissemination of the findings.

ONLINE CONSULT

Office of Civil Rights—HIPAA at
http://www.hhs.gov/ocr/hipaa/

ANA Guidelines

In addition to basic ethical principles, federal, state, local, and institutional regulations, in 1985 the ANA specified human rights guidelines for nurses in research. Ten years later, and with the consideration of societal and professional practice changes that had occurred, new guidelines based on nine principles were published (Silva, 1995, p. 2). As shown in Box 6–3, these principles address beneficence, full disclosure, self-determination, privacy and confidentiality, and the skills of the researcher.

Each of the nine principles charges the investigator with specific responsibilities. Explanatory commentary and specific research guidelines are presented for each of the nine principles. For example, with the protection of subjects against harm, it discusses specifically several vulnerable groups, such as pregnant women, children, persons with human immunodeficiency virus (HIV) or acquired immunodeficiency syndrome (AIDS), and the elderly. All of the principles require that professionals in a practice setting be aware of any ongoing research and its associated risks to both subjects and participants. And nurses have both the right and the responsibility to participate in research. Participation of nurses should be evident; for example, they should function as members of research teams and IRBs. Nurses also can actively participate by giving support and assistance to others involved in research for the advancement of knowledge and enhancement of professional practice. The process of

ONLINE CONSULT

Agency for Healthcare Research and Quality at
http://www.ahrq.gov/

National Institutes of Health at
http://www.nih.gov/

U.S. Department of Health & Human Services at
http://www.hhs.gov

Office for Human Research Protections (OHRP) at
http://www.hhs.gov/ohrp/

research with human subjects must be diligent and must benefit subjects and participants through the acquisition and use of new knowledge.

Consult the government and your institutional Web sites for information on protections for human subjects in research.

PROCESSES OF NURSING RESEARCH

The actual research process is generally thought of as the scientific method. This can be misleading, however, when one considers the different types of research. To understand the basics of nursing research, first think about the scientific method as a systematic process for answering a question or testing a hypothesis. One

---

Box 6.3 Ethical Principles in the Conduct, Dissemination, and Implementation of Nursing Research

The Investigator:

1. Respects autonomous research participant's capacity to consent to participate in research and to determine the degree and duration of that participation without negative consequences.
2. Prevents harm, minimizes harm, and/or promotes good to all research participants, including vulnerable groups and others affected by the research.
3. Respects the personhood of research participants, their families, and significant others, valuing their diversity.
4. Ensures that the benefits and burdens of research are equitably distributed in the selection of research participants.
5. Protects the privacy of research participants to the maximum degree possible.
6. Ensures the ethical integrity of the research process by the use of appropriate checks and balances throughout the conduct, dissemination, and implementation of the research.
7. Reports suspected, alleged, or known incidents of scientific misconduct in research to appropriate institutional officials for investigation.
8. Maintains competency in the subject matter and methodologies of research as well as in other professional and societal issues that affect nursing research and the public good.
9. If involved in animal research, maximizes the benefits of the research with the least possible harm or suffering to the animals.

Reprinted with permission from Mari Silva, *Ethical Guidelines in the Conduct, Dissemination, and Implementation of Nursing Research,* ©1995 Nursesbooks.org, Silver Spring, MD.

problem emerges: this is done more easily in a controlled laboratory setting, with variables such as chemicals, than in a natural setting in which the variables involve people, well or ill, who need nursing interventions. With this in mind, it is easier to begin with empirical research using quantitative methods.

The Empirical Method

First, consider the steps of research. **Empirical research** is based on the strict rules of the scientific method and on the philosophical perspective of positivism. With this perspective, the focus is on an observable, measurable, and predictable world. It is guided by a controlled set of steps that one goes through to observe something or test a hypothesis. It is a deductive and linear method with the following steps:

1. Identification of the problem
2. Statement of the purpose
3. Review of the literature
4. Description of the theoretical framework
5. Definition of terms
6. Statement of the hypothesis(es)
7. Selection of the research design, population, and sample
8. IRB approval
9. Collection of data
10. Analysis and interpretation of data
11. Presentation of findings and recommendations

Using this empirical approach, the researcher may return to a prior step in the planning stage, for example, to refine the problem after the review of the literature, but will still go through all successive steps in a systematic and controlled manner to maintain the integrity of the process. Once the plans for the study are finalized, strict research protocols are adhered to with quantitative methods to reduce threats to the validity of the study. Although some of the steps may be combined, nurse researchers using quantitative methods engage in the same process to describe, explain, predict, and control phenomena of concern to nursing. The following is a review of the research process.

In the initial step of *problem identification*, the researchers specify what they are interested in studying. This is the "what" that will be done as the study progresses. For example, a specific nursing intervention is compared with a traditional nursing intervention for a selected group of clients. Next, researchers specify the reason they are interested in this problem, or the *purpose of the research*. At this time, the significance of the problem for the body of knowledge and ethical issues associated with the proposed investigation are considerations. This is "why" the researchers want to investigate the new intervention, for example, to effectively improve the health awareness or healthy behaviors of the client group.

The researchers next search the *literature* to discover what is known on the topics: the interventions, the client group, cultural factors, useful theoretical bases (e.g., self-care), and what problems have been studied in the area. This provides context and the current information known on the topic. This is a time-intensive process that requires absorbing a great deal of information for the planning stage of the project. Researchers perform literature searches, followed by careful critique and assimilation of the information. Next, researchers specify the philosophical orientation that will guide the research, the *theoretical framework*. For example, the study may be guided by one of the middle-range or practice theories discussed in Chapter 4. The *defining terms and variables* specific to the study emerge from the theoretical framework, as do specific research questions that will be addressed or the *hypotheses* (predictions) the study will test.

So far we have the basic idea for the investigation, but the researchers must select a design or plan for the study that is appropriate for the problem in light of the theoretical framework. For example, when studying the efficacy of an intervention with two groups of clients, the researcher may use an experimental control group design. However, true experiments require manipulation of the independent variable, control of other variables, and random assignment to study group. Often we see quasi-experimental designs in nursing, as perhaps use of a nonequivalent control group, due to the nature of the intervention.

Once the appropriate *design* has been selected, the researchers must *define the population*—those individuals or groups to whom the findings will be applicable or generalizable. Researchers know that not all the people to whom the research applies can be studied, so they must study a select group of the population: the *sample*. The researchers' decision about the type and the size of the sample is based on the research design, the theoretical framework, research purpose, and research problem. It all relates back in a linear manner, but the goals in sampling are to limit bias and statistical error and for the sample to be representative of the population.

The researchers now have the basic plan for their investigations, but no one has been studied yet. The rights of human subjects must be considered and protected. At this point the researcher submits a proposal to an IRB for approval or exemption to proceed to the next step of data collection. Once IRB approval has been secured, the researcher is ready to begin *collecting data*.

Plans for data collection and analysis have already been made in the research proposal and are strictly adhered to. Researchers must follow the proposed design when data are collected; for example, they cannot decide to replace interviews that were planned with a questionnaire. Data must be collected in an orderly and systematic manner and must be recorded before analysis and decision-making begin.

Measurement issues are of prime concern. The type of data collected and the measurement instruments are, again, determined before the study is started, on the basis of the research problem, literature review, theoretical basis, research questions or hypotheses, research design, and sampling method. Issues of reliability (consistency of measurement) and validity (measuring the variable of interest properly) are considered by the researcher from prior methodological studies, use in similar research, or a pilot study as a small-scale version or a formal trial to resolve any methodological issues. Measurements may be self-reported, in writing, by the subjects in the sample (tests, questionnaires, diaries, etc.) or may require taping or note-taking by researchers in personal or telephone interviews.

Measurements can also be observations of behavior (ability to perform a skill, such as a dressing change), responses by subjects on a scale (such as a Likert scale or a scale for pain perception from 0 to 10), physiologic measures (such as blood pressure, electrocardiogram, electroencephalogram, or oxygen saturation), review of records, or a number of other types of methods. Research protocols are strictly adhered to: the identical and detailed process is used with each research subject. Scripts are used to read instructions to subjects to ensure that each subject has been given the same information for the data collection process.

Once all subjects have been investigated and all data collected, the researcher moves into the *analysis stage*. The analysis provides information to answer the research questions or support or refute the hypotheses. The analysis stage seems to be the most threatening to the research novice. Keep in mind that the research depends on a good analysis of the data so that reliable, valid information is made available on the topic. The most important decisions for this stage were made before the study was started, with the selection of the correct statistical tests. In addition, computers or statisticians can easily perform calculations. Try to see this stage as one of discovery and understanding how the data provide answers to the research questions or hypotheses. The findings are reported objectively for each research question or hypothesis.

The results of the descriptive statistics (such as frequencies, means, standard deviations, correlations) are reported to characterize the sample. Appropriate inferential statistics are used to generalize to the population (such as t-test, analysis of variance, correlations, and multivariate analysis), according to the type of measurement scale, the sample size, and the assumption of a normal distribution. From the point of reporting the statistics, the researcher then *interprets the meaning* and implications relative to the stated research questions or hypotheses. Recommendations for use of the findings and further research are then presented in the research report.

Disseminating the findings to others is the final responsibility of the researcher as part of the particular study. The findings can be disseminated locally, regionally, nationally, and globally through presentations or publications. It is vital that the information be shared with others. If the findings are important and point to a need for change, practicing nurses must have the opportunity and responsibility to implement the information as appropriate to their practice settings. Further research is also needed. If the findings were not significant or were indifferent, then further research is needed, perhaps further specification of the problem, better measurement instruments, or a different environment or sample. If the research findings were negative, the new intervention was less effective than current ones. Still more research may be needed if there were problems with reliability and validity. If a safety issue emerged during the research, a subject would have been withdrawn from the study or the study halted. Still, it is necessary for others to know all situations to make use of good information or avoid problem areas.

Qualitative Research

The research process using qualitative research methods is somewhat different. These methods are inductive and theory-generating research. **Qualitative research** is used to generate theory to explore, describe, and illuminate phenomena. The basis of qualitative research focuses on the meaning and interpretation of experiences to understand some phenomena. Types of research classified as qualitative include ethnography, field studies, grounded theory, historical research, analytic induction, and phenomenology.

Major data collection methods are naturalistic observation (hence the term field studies) and on-site interviewing. Some researchers describe the data that emerge from this research as "information rich," because the researcher begins a study with a need to understand from the perspective of people in the environment. The researcher is not limiting the data collection to a few variables. Rather, he or she is trying to have the people in their environment describe the phenomena; the researcher then classifies concepts, identifies themes, and generates theory. This is why some also see qualitative research as a "humanistic" form of research that discovers people and their unique experiences.

In qualitative research, the linear steps of the process are not the procedure. The researcher must still complete the initial process of developing the project, with *identification of a "problem"* of a little-understood area or phenomena, and the *statement of purpose as an inquiry* for "discovery" of the phenomena. The *review of the literature* looks at what is known, which is often tangential, because little may be known before the research "uncovers" the phenomena. The *theory* will evolve from this research, rather than be driven by it, as are the *terminology* and *future study hypotheses* that use quantitative methods for theory testing. The process of IRB approval is still required prior to data collection, for the protection of human subjects.

Qualitative methods have different inquiry forms and processes. *Data collection* and *analysis* are driven by the particular qualitative method, as with an ethnography to describe the phenomena from the perspective of the subjects. Reliability and validity issues can be difficult with this form of research, and investigators frequently use triangulation of data to provide valid

results. *Triangulation* involves the use of multiple data sources, complementary investigations, or theoretical perspectives to improve the data's validity. Dissemination of the findings through presentations and publication is the final step in the process, along with identification of future areas for inquiry.

Choice of Research Method

Whether quantitative or qualitative research methods are selected depends on the phenomena of interest and the purpose of the research. For example, the researcher may select or use qualitative methods to investigate health beliefs of a particular cultural group, but would use quantitative methods to test a new intervention designed to enhance the functional independence of older adults with a limitation in mobility. Comparisons of qualitative research to the empirical research process are illustrated in Table 6–1. Regardless of the methods selected to address the need for information on the problem, the research must respect the individual or group in the quest for knowledge.

Table 6.1

Empirical and Qualitative Research Methods

	Empirical Research	**Qualitative Research**
Identification of the problem	Narrowly specify what is to be studied.	Identify little understood area or phenomena.
Statement of the purpose	Specify reason the problem is of interest; significance.	Specify the inquiry for discovery of the phenomena.
Review of literature	Discover what is already known about the problem.	Using tangential subjects, demonstrate why little is known on the phenomena.
Theoretical framework	Select and apply a theory or model.	Theory will evolve from the research.
Definitions and terminology	Define terms and variables to be studied, consistent with the theoretical model.	Terminology will emerge from the findings.
Questions and hypothesis(es)	Specify questions or hypotheses to be tested, consistent with the theoretical model.	Develop broad questions to be asked that will lead to others during the research as discovery.
Selection of the research design, population, and sample	Select specific design and study instruments. Specify population of interest. Identify group and number of research subjects (sample).	Select a qualitative method and a group to seek their descriptions of their human experience, and propose methods to access the group.

(Table continues on page 112)

Table 6.1

Empirical and Qualitative Research Methods (continued)

	Empirical Research	Qualitative Research
Approval of Internal Review Board	Submit and obtain approval of research proposal.	Submit and obtain approval of research proposal.
Collection of Data	Strictly adhere to research protocol, controls, and steps specified with the study's measurement instruments; for example, the experimental group of subjects has one intervention while the control group received the usual treatment or intervention. Systematically record data,	Gain entry to the group, propose broad questions, receive information, and seek meaning. Further questions emerge as the study progresses and are pursued in search of meaning and understanding. For example, use grounded theory to see the data falling into differing categories.
Data analysis and interpretation	Apply the statistical tests on the specific study variables specified in the research proposal and drawing conclusions from these tests.	Create meaning and themes from information in transcripts and documents that evolve into different areas and emerge into a theoretical framework.
Presentation of findings	Report the statistics on the questions or hypotheses as findings. Draw conclusions based on the findings and proposing applications and further investigation.	Propose a theoretical framework to pursue further investigation of the categories of meaning discovered, thus adding to our theoretical bases described in Chapter 4.

THE ROAD TO EVIDENCE-BASED PRACTICE

We have a responsibility to base nursing practice on current knowledge. This responsibility highlights an accountability issue for the profession and focuses the direction of nursing research on issues for improved patient outcomes and effective care in a time when resources are stretched beyond limits. We have evolved from the landmark work for research-based nursing practice that began in the 1970s. The federally funded WICHE (Western Interstate Commission for Higher Education) Project between 1971 and 1975 focused on both the conduct of research projects and the utilization of research findings, to support collaborative research endeavors followed by a focus on using research findings in practice (Lindeman & Krueger, 1977). The second federally funded CURN (Conduct and Utilization of Research in Nursing) Project, between 1975 and 1981, focused on use in the hospital setting of the knowledge from research already available. Finding the information and the applicability to the practice setting were the skills of concern. This led to the development of guidelines and specific protocols for research-based nursing

interventions and educational media to help nurses base their practice and interventions with clients on research evidence. Since the 1970s, there has been a growing number of professional journals dedicated to publishing research findings. Specialty journals include special columns or research features. Professional conferences, both general and specialty, now provide more research presentations as special and concurrent offerings. A focus on research has also emerged in certification examinations.

Then in 1981, the ANA Cabinet for Nursing Research developed guidelines for involvement in research based on level of nursing education, as mentioned earlier in the chapter. Subsequently, both the ANA (1997) and the AACN (2006) have delineated expectations for nurses' involvement in research according to level of educational preparation. In these guidelines, the graduate with doctoral or postdoctoral preparation is seen as providing leadership on investigations, applying theory, and developing methods to generate knowledge for the discipline. With an expertise in specialty practice, the master-prepared nurse is the facilitator for using research findings and conducting investigations. Associate degree and baccalaureate nursing graduates are research consumers.

Baccalaureate graduates are also responsible for identifying researchable problems and findings from prior research on which to base practice.

Nevertheless, there have been problems with disseminating findings and applying them in practice. National practice guidelines have been available since the 1990s, but studies have shown they have not been incorporated consistently in practice. Evidence-based practice is fundamental to contemporary nursing, providing a firm foundation for nursing interventions and quality improvement in health care. It has been identified as one of the core competencies for health professionals in all disciplines.

To address this core competency, the Academic Center for Evidence-based Practice (ACE) led the way with a project to establish a national consensus on essential competences for EBP for use in education and practice (Stevens, 2005, p. 1). Competencies by educational level (undergraduate, 20; masters, 32; and doctoral, 31) have been identified based on their ACE Star Model of knowledge transformation with five stages (Fig. 6–1). **Knowledge transformation** is defined as "the conversion of research findings from primary research results, through a series of stages and forms, to impact on health outcomes by way of EB care" (Stevens, 2005, p. 25). As new knowledge is transformed through the five stages— discovery, evidence summary, translation, integration, and evaluation—the outcome is quality improvement of care (Stevens, 2005, pp. 25–27). Discovery is primary research whereas the evidence summary is the available body of knowledge. Stevens (2005) describes the process with evidence summary as the synthesis of the primary research and the body of knowledge leading to translation into practice guidelines and then integrated in practice and evaluation of outcomes (pp. 26–27).

When systematic reviews of research are available, more is known on the body of knowledge and the evidence is stronger for clinical application, based on the unique needs of the client population. Proficiency

ONLINE CONSULT

ACE: Learn about EBP at
http://www.acestar.uthscsa.edu/about.htm

in critiquing or evaluating research or the evidence summaries is central to the ability to translate and integrate the evidence in professional practice.

SKILLS FOR A THOUGHTFUL CRITIQUE

Consider both the objective process of critiquing a research study and the subjective process of evaluating its application to practice. An objective analysis looks at the content as available to the reader. This analysis is required to have the information for making a judgment as to whether the information is applicable to your practice area and setting.

Objective Evaluation

A **research critique** is an objective analysis of a published research report. The reader must critically consider all components of the report—problem, purpose, supporting literature, theoretical framework, definitions, study questions or hypotheses, design, population and sample, data collection methods and procedures, analysis, and interpretation of findings (Box 6–4). The ultimate goal of a research critique is to evaluate applicability of appropriate scientific findings to one's own professional practice and knowledge base.

Thoughtful critique is based on critical thinking skills used to address the steps of the research process. When publishing research reports, researchers must provide the essential information gained from the study within the given space. This can create a challenge for the reader attempting to glean the vital information for a critique. A published research report is frequently organized into the following sections: abstract, introduction, review of literature, theoretical framework, methods, results, discussion, and references.

Preliminary information provides valuable information for the reader. First, the title of the study should clearly reflect the problem area and capture the reader's interest. Information provided about the researcher includes his background and qualifications in the practice area and for conducting the research study. The abstract briefly reviews the problem, purpose, methodology, findings, and conclusions, summarizing the content and also capturing the reader's attention.

Next comes the introduction to the research report. The opening paragraphs outline the background of the

ACE Star Model of Knowledge Transformation

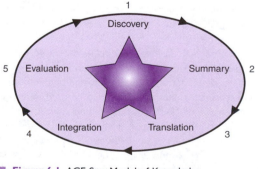

■ **Figure 6.1** ACE Star Model of Knowledge Transformation.

Box 6.4 Areas to Address in a Thoughtful Critique*

Areas to address while doing a thoughtful critique of a research study as a component of evidence-based practice include:

- Title and abstract
- Introduction, problem, and purpose
- Literature review
- Theoretical framework
- Research questions or hypotheses
- Methods: design, ethics, sampling, data collection
- Results and analysis
- Discussion and recommendations

And now, are the findings applicable to use in your practice?

*Further information on the areas to address in a research critique are located on the Intranet site.

problem, including its purpose and significance to nursing and the care of clients. The **research problem** is the central question that the research has been designed to answer. It is the "what" that is being done in the study to describe, explain, predict, or control some phenomenon of concern to nursing. The research problem contains the major variables and the population of concern to the researcher. The author may also identify specific research aims in this introductory section.

Next, a **review of literature** pertinent to the research problem is provided. The literature review is a report and comparison of all pertinent prior investigations on the topic, variables of interest, theoretical models, and methods used. Unlike the library research done for a paper, a research literature review concentrates on primary references. A *primary* literature source is the actual report of an investigation or development of an instrument or theory written by the researcher or theorist. Using the primary source eliminates the chance of error in interpretation that could occur through analyses by others or loss of the context of the original work.

The literature review should provide a critical appraisal and synthesis of what is already known on the topic. Thus, the literature review supports the study and how the investigation proposes to contribute to the existing body of nursing knowledge. A review of literature may be conducted electronically with the availability of online databases, resources, and articles. Caution is recommended on the use of research reports found in chat rooms, on personal Web pages, or other sources that have not been subjected to a thoughtful peer review process before being accepted for publication.

The theoretical framework may be described in a separate section or may be included with the literature review. As was discussed in Chapters 3 and 4, a theoretical framework or model is the way the researcher views the concepts and their interrelationships; it may be described in words or displayed symbolically. This underlying view drives the research in describing, explaining, predicting, or controlling the phenomena, as in the case of empirical research studies.

At this point, the researcher may present specific questions to address in the study or hypotheses to be tested. Specific research questions must flow from, and relate back to, the main research problem or purpose. **Hypotheses** are predictions about the variables that the investigation is testing with a subject group. Hypotheses may be null (statistical), predicting no relationship; conversely, the researcher may state research (alternative) hypotheses that do predict a difference and, in some cases, the direction of the difference (increase, decrease, greater, less). Both null and research hypotheses can be either simple (stating a prediction between two variables) or complex (stating a difference between more than two variables). Hypothesis testing uses inferential statistics, inferring from the sample to make generalizations about the population. Both research questions and hypotheses must be consistent with the framework that provides the theoretical guidance for the investigation. The variables to be investigated should be readily apparent in either the stated research questions or hypotheses.

The next major section in a published research report describes the methodology or methods. This section contains information on the research design, research subjects (including ethical considerations and sampling), and data collection and procedures used. The **research design** is the overall blueprint for the study. The design specifies the setting for the study, the subjects (sample group), the experimental or nonexperimental treatment or grouping methods, the data collection methods, and procedures or protocol. The research design is selected to address the variables of concern to answer the research questions or test the hypotheses. Study designs may be experimental or nonexperimental. Qualitative research studies are also useful in aiding the understanding of a phenomenon that is relevant to your practice area.

Experimental designs are classified as true experiments, quasi-experiments, and pre-experiments, with varying degrees of control, manipulation, and randomization. Nonexperimental study designs may be used to answer the research questions with less human subject involvement or intervention; such designs are ex post facto, correlational, survey, case study, needs assessment, secondary analysis, and evaluation studies. Additional designs you may see in the literature are methodological (studies on research tools or instruments) and meta-analysis, which uses many previous studies to determine the overall effect. The design must "fit" the research problem, purpose, and theoretical framework. You may refer to a nursing research text for more information on these various designs.

The researcher provides definitions for all major variables included in the study. Both theoretical and operational definitions may be provided in the introduction or the review of the literature. Theoretical, or in some cases conceptual, definitions are the general description of a term, that is, the term as defined in a specific theoretical framework or the dictionary. Researchers must provide operational definitions of the major variables of interest, especially when quantitative research methods are used. An **operational definition** is the description specific to the use of the variable in the study. It is precisely what the researchers are looking at and how they are measuring it. For example, consider the term *stethoscope*. Every nurse knows it is an acoustical instrument used to measure heart rate apically or blood pressure peripherally. But the type of stethoscope must be specified in the operational definition, for example, bell-diaphragm combination, electronic, or pediatric. The specification ensures controls in quantitative methods, describing exactly what the researcher used and enabling others to reproduce the study results given a similar set of circumstances or apply to a specific practice setting.

Generally, the researcher provides operational definitions of the study variables in the section on methodology. **Variables** are concepts and constructs defined and manipulated, controlled, or measured in a research study. Independent variables are variables manipulated by the researcher, such as the cause, treatment, or difference between the groups (for example, the type of dressing used). Dependent variables are the outcome variables that the researcher is measuring and analyzing. The researcher wishes to see whether or not the change in the independent variable (type of dressing) caused a difference in the dependent variable (healing time or bacterial colony count). Uncontrolled or confounding variables (such as nutritional status) must also be considered because they can have extraneous and unwanted effects on the dependent variable (healing time). The researcher often attempts to control the extraneous effects by selecting a population or study procedures that meet specific criteria, to reduce the chance of occurrence of the unwanted influences. In the methods section, special attention is given to the descriptions of the subjects. Ultimately, this allows the readers to determine the applicability of results to practice with their specific client group. Ethical considerations specific to the sample should also be described.

Sampling is the use of a subset (sample) of the population as a feasible group to study, ultimately generalizing the findings to the population. The population is the total group to which the researcher wishes the results of the research to be generalized. For example, not all cardiac patients in a rehabilitation program can be interviewed in person. Yet the researcher would like the study results to be applicable to all patients similar to the subjects interviewed in the study, so that the information will add to the body of nursing knowledge. Samples may be selected by probability (based on statistical chance of selection) or they may be nonprobability samples. Types of probability samples are random, systematic, stratified, and cluster. Nonprobability samples include convenience, purposive, snowball, quota, and expert samples. Each type of sample has advantages and disadvantages that must be considered. At this point, look for the sample size. Smaller sample sizes are associated with qualitative methods. On the other hand, minimum sample sizes are necessary with some statistical procedures in quantitative methods and analysis.

Specific research methods are described as **data collection procedures**. *Data* are the measures or responses obtained from the subjects in the study. Analyzed data become information. Research methods may be quantitative or qualitative. Quantitative methods focus on numerical data that can be obtained from subjects using any one or a combination of measurement instruments. Qualitative methods focus on information gathered from individuals and groups, often in their natural environment, to explore their unique qualities in depth and generate theory on a little-known topic or construct. The different research methods can use similar or different instruments to obtain or measure data.

Instruments are the measurement tools for collecting data. They include paper-and-pencil instruments (such as questionnaires, diaries, or scales), biophysiologic instruments (such as a stethoscope, sphygmomanometer, pulse oximeter, electrocardiograph, or electroencephalograph), interview guides, videotapes and audiotapes, and others, depending on the specific investigation and variables. Important considerations for use of any instrument, including an observer as data collector, are the reliability and validity of the measurement. Researchers report the reliability and validity tests before they discuss the findings of their study.

Instrument reliability describes whether the instrument provides consistent measurement. The reliable instrument measures the variable consistently over time. The need for instrument reliability is apparent in examples of a calibrated scale that dependably provides a reading of the client's weight or the test that consistently estimates the client's stress level. The types of instrument reliability that are reported in studies are test-retest (stability of the measure over time), internal consistency or alpha (statistical measure on items or parts of a test), equivalent forms of tests, and interrater (equivalence among data collectors).

Instrument validity considers whether the instrument measures what it is intended to measure, such as body surface area and not weight. Types of instrument validity include content, construct, and criterion-related. A panel of experts may assess the content validity of an instrument, ensuring that it adequately addresses the variable or area of interest. Construct validity is described with prior research on the instrument and may be reported as findings from a factor analysis or other statistical test. Criterion-related validity is important when the variable cannot be measured directly, such as family and visitor contacts, cards and gifts, and discussions (as another criterion) to discover social support for a study on the psychosocial stress of the hospitalized client.

Once the data collection methods have been described, the researcher describes methods used to analyze the data and reports the results in the findings or results section. Methods for analysis of the data are based on the specified research methods and the type of data involved. For numerical data, statistics are used in the analysis of quantitative research methods. **Descriptive statistics** are used to summarize and describe data through graphic displays of the information (percentages and frequency counts), measures of central tendency (means, medians, modes), and measures of dispersion (ranges, variances, and standard deviations). **Inferential statistics** are used to test hypotheses, make predictions, and infer from the sample (statistic) to the population (parameter). Depending on the variables, data, and sample size and distribution, inferential statistics used include nonparametric tests (chi square, Spearman rho, median test) and parametric tests (t test, analysis of variance [ANOVA], Pearson r correlation coefficient®). The results are reported for each research question or hypothesis in an objective manner.

Finally, the researcher presents his or her interpretation of the results in a discussion section. Conclusions should be consistent with the theoretical framework used to guide the study. The discussion also includes the researcher's identification of limitations and recommendations for using the findings in practice, teaching, administration, and further research.

Guidelines to assist with a thoughtful critique of a research study have been posted on the Intranet site.

Subjective Evaluation: Incorporating Evidence-Based Practice

At this point, the reader must determine the applicability of the results to the individual practice area. A research critique is an objective assessment of the information presented in the report against some criterion, such as the critique questions. The subjective evaluation for use of the findings in one's own practice area is made after the objective critique of the value of the study's process and results. If the critique is positive, you must decide whether the results are applicable in your practice area. If so, it is a professional responsibility to implement information found to be beneficial to clients, rather than to continue to practice on the basis of tradition instead of fact and efficacy—your competence in evidence-based practice.

Reading professional journals and keeping abreast of current knowledge are essential in contemporary nursing practice. Acquiring critique skills is integral for good clinical decisions. Access to quality journals and the depth of reading must also be considered. Look carefully at the professional journals to which you subscribe and the journals that are available at your work site or online. Do they contain research reports? If so, are you reading research studies as well as the narrative and practice articles? Consider different levels of reading, from skimming the information to a careful analysis of the content or a comparison with other literature to synthesize the information known on the topic. At what level are you reading? Critiquing a research article is at the level of analytic reading rather than merely looking for articles of interest to your practice area. Make time, on a consistent basis, to look for and evaluate research in the professional literature.

As an additional aid to the implementation of evidence-based practice, alternate sources beyond traditional research articles are available to assist the clinician. Pape (2003) identifies cognitive clustering for integration of findings on a specific research topic through sources such as published meta-analyses, systematic reviews, practice guidelines, online reviews, and Internet searches. As noted by Stevens (2005), systematic reviews have been greatly advanced and produce new knowledge. They combine findings from all studies, identify bias and limit chance effects, and increase reliability and replication of the results (Stevens, 2005, p. 26).

As mentioned previously, national clinical guidelines have been available since the 1990s but are not consistently accessed or used. The National Guideline Clearinghouse provides archives of current practice guidelines that have been reviewed, revised, or deleted

ⓄNLINE ⒸONSULT

Agency for Healthcare Research and Quality at **http://www.ahrq.gov/**

The Cochrane Collaboration at **http://www.cochrane.org/**

National Guideline Clearinghouse at **http://www.guideline.gov/**

within the past five years, organized by health conditions and national organizations. The AHRQ also provides useful information for clinicians on current research and quality measures for application in evidence-based practice. The Cochrane Collaboration also provides internationally and interdisciplinary leading evidence-based practice information.

Once you have obtained the information from the professional literature or resources, the issue is implementation and sharing. Are you sharing the information with colleagues? This can be done informally among your colleagues or formally presented at a unit conference or during an interdisciplinary grand rounds session. Having access to "user-friendly" databases or a library is essential for acquiring information on a clinical issue. Investigate what is available in your environment. Attending "brown bag lunches" and participating in a journal club focused on research studies are ways of making this activity more enjoyable and rewarding.

Obtaining new information is the intended aim of attending a clinical conference, whether or not you need continuing education units for relicensure or recertification. Quality of programs and significance of the topics to your practice area must be considered for evidence-based practice. Selecting EBP concurrent sessions is a good way to hear current research information. Attendance at grand rounds in an institution committed to research is also a valuable experience. Research questions specific to nursing or interdisciplinary collaboration may become available. Your work setting may have a nursing or interdisciplinary research committee. Participating on a research committee can be a challenging and rewarding experience. Nurses can collaborate on different stages of the research process. In addition, the practice problems specific to your setting can emerge, be developed, and be investigated when professionals start the discussion and raise the issues. It can be quite a stimulating and fun experience.

ELIMINATING BARRIERS TO EVIDENCE-BASED NURSING PRACTICE

Barriers to evidence-based nursing practice should be diminished or removed. Such barriers are a real and perceived lack of educational preparation, administrative support, resources, and time. In this time of diminishing resources, the use of the most reliable and accurate information is crucial. Trial-and-error strategies as the basis for a client intervention waste valuable resources and are unconscionable if there is contrary evidence. We need an increasing sense of professional commitment to practice based on evidence of effective outcomes for our clients.

Negative attitudes toward research or researchers must be replaced with greater collaboration among clinicians, researchers, administrators, and educators. Barnsteiner and Prevost (2002) have proposed the following strategies for facilitating evidence-based practice:

- Change viewpoints about research
- Increase knowledge about the EBP process
- Harness new knowledge
- Consider potential consequences
- Institute system changes
- Collaborate locally and globally

Clinicians have firsthand awareness of problem areas but must be assisted in accessing the current knowledge base, looking at problems in the domain of nursing that address the need for improved client outcomes, having the professional commitment to go the extra mile and take time to get involved with research activities, basing their nursing interventions on the current evidence of efficacy, and receiving some form of recognition for their efforts.

The support and encouragement of the chief nurse administrator or executive are a must to ensure that the organizational climate, resources, and philosophy of practice are present in the practice setting. Moving to evidence-based practice will not be an easy transition without a dynamic person spearheading the process. Clinicians must keep an open mind and make a professional commitment to identify problems and search the current knowledge base for information. Researchers must collaborate with clinicians to address nursing questions and avoid speaking or talking in "researchese," thus providing clear practice implications in publications and presentations. Educators must also assist in the development of critique and EBP skills.

Commitment must be made to the ongoing nature of building knowledge and basing practice on evidence of efficacy. Our knowledge base has been evolving since the time of Nightingale and before. It will constantly evolve because of the nature of the information and our focus on people in a dynamic environment. The profession needs more extensive research that is generalizable to and supportive of nursing as a major player in health-care issues. We need more replications to add reliability and validity to instruments and information. Constant updating and modification of any protocol is needed as more information becomes available. Gaining critique skills and learning the language of EBP are components of this process.

INTERACTIVE EXERCISES

Go to the Intranet site and complete the interactive exercises provided for this Chapter.

EVIDENCED-BASED PRACTICE: CONSIDER THIS . . .

*C*oopey, Nix, and Clancy (2006) from the Agency for Healthcare Research and Quality have described the process for translating research into EBP. They have identified the following five steps in a cyclic evidence process:

1. Body of individual evidence (multiple individual studies)
2. Systematic review to synthesize the body of evidence
3. Translating evidence into action and tools, such as guidelines
4. Implementation in practice
5. Evaluation of effectiveness for quality improvement. (Coopey, Nix, & Clancy, 2006, p. 196).

   Suppose you have selected an AHRQ EBP guideline with the systematic review of the literature and suggested tools for implementation that are appropriate for your setting.

   Question: How will you use this information and include an evaluation process to promote quality improvement?

Source: Coopey, M., Nix, M., & Clancy, C. (2006). Translating research into evidence-based nursing practice and evaluating effectiveness. *Journal of Nursing Care Quality, 21*(3), 195–202.

KEY POINTS

■ Evidence-based practice, core competency for health professionals, is defined as the use of clinical expertise and interventions that are based on evidence of efficacy for client outcomes and the preferences of the clients served.

■ Research is a process for generating scientific knowledge and utilizing the knowledge on which to base practice. Using evidence of efficacy for practice is a vital professional attribute and a responsibility.

■ Nursing research began with Florence Nightingale and has become vital to both professionals and consumers in investigating the domain of nursing, testing theories and interventions, and demonstrating the efficacy and efficiency of nursing actions.

■ Ethical considerations in research must include the four basic human rights:
   ■ Do no harm (beneficence)
   ■ Full disclosure
   ■ Self-determination
   ■ Privacy and confidentiality

■ A professional nurse should be an active consumer of nursing research, promoting use of current and valid scientific knowledge and identifying the questions to be addressed in further research. Professional accountability demands that one read the literature, attend educational sessions, use critique skills, participate in investigations, and promote evidence-based interventions.

■ Empirical research is based on the strict rules of the scientific method, with the following steps:
   ■ Identification of the problem
   ■ Statement of the purpose
   ■ Review of the literature
   ■ Description of theoretical framework
   ■ Definition of terms
   ■ Statement of hypothesis(es)
   ■ Selection of the research design, population, and sample
   ■ Approval by the IRB

(Key points continue on page 119)

K E Y   P O I N T S   (continued)

- ■ Collection of data
- ■ Analysis and interpretation of data
- ■ Presentation of findings and recommendations

■ Knowledge transformation is defined as "the conversion of research findings from primary research results, through a series of stages and forms, to impact on health outcomes by way of EB care" (Stevens, 2005, p. 25).

■ A critique is an objective analysis of a research report. The reader must critically consider all components of the report.

■ A research problem is the main issue or central question that the researcher addresses in the investigation. Specific research questions or hypotheses flow from the main research problem.

■ The literature review is a report and comparison of all pertinent prior investigations on the topic, variables of interest, theoretical models, and methods used.

■ Variables are concepts and constructs defined and manipulated, controlled, or measured in a research study. Independent variables are manipulated by the researcher.

■ Hypotheses are predictions about the variables that the researcher is testing with a subject group.

■ The research design is the overall blueprint and methods for the study.

■ Research methods may be quantitative or qualitative. Quantitative methods focus on numerical data that can be obtained from subjects through any one or a combination of measurement instruments. Qualitative methods focus on information gathered from individuals and groups, often in their natural environment, to explore in depth their unique qualities and generate theory on a little-known topic or construct.

■ Sampling is the use of a subset (sample) of the population as a feasible group to study and ultimately generalize findings to the population.

■ Instruments are the measurement tools for collecting data. Important considerations for use of any instrument are the reliability and validity of the measurement.

■ Statistics are used in analyzing quantitative research methods. Descriptive statistics are used to summarize and describe data. Inferential statistics are used to test hypotheses, make predictions, and infer from the sample to the population.

Thought and Discussion Questions

1. Describe activities present in your practice setting that demonstrate the use of evidence-based practice.

2. Develop a plan to encourage or promote evidence-based practice in your nursing practice environment. Select a clinical protocol or problem. Use the following six phases of the research utilization process to organize your plan: (1) identification of clinical problems and access to research bases; (2) evaluation of the knowledge and the potential for application in the organization, along with policy and cost determinants; (3) planning for implementation and evaluation of the innovation; (4) clinical trial and evaluation; (5) decisions to adopt, modify, or reject innovations on the basis of evaluation; and (6) if the innovations are adopted, planning for their extension to other units (Horsley, Crane, & Bingle, 1978). Describe who will be involved in the process and how the new practice or protocol will be implemented. Finally, identify evaluation criteria.

3. Identify practice issues that can be developed into a nursing research problem for investigation.

(Thought and Discussion Questions continue on page 120)

Thought and Discussion Questions (continued)

4. Find the requirements for the IRB at your college or institution. Be prepared to participate in a discussion on the requirements for the preparation of a research proposal for consideration by the IRB.

5. Look further at PHI and current privacy issues. Be prepared to participate in a discussion as scheduled by your instructor.

6. Review the Chapter Thought located on the first page of the chapter and discuss it in the context of the contents of the chapter.

REFERENCES

American Association of Colleges of Nursing (AACN). (2006). Position statement on nursing research. Retrieved June 3, 2006, from *http://www.aacn.nche.edu/ publications/positions/NsgRes.htm*

American Association of Critical-Care Nurses. (AACN). (2004). Practice alert: Family presence during CPR and invasive procedures. Retrieved October 8, 2006, from *http://www.aacn.org/AACN/practiceAlert.nsf/Files/FP/ $file/Family Presence During CPR 11–2004.pdf*

American Nurses Association. (1997). Position statement: Education for participation in nursing research. Retrieved June 1, 2006, from *http://nursingworld.org/ readroom/position/research/rseducat.htm*

American Nurses Association Commission on Nursing Research. (1981). *Guidelines for the investigative function of nurses.* Kansas City, MO: American Nurses Association.

American Nurses Credentialing Center (ANCC). (2006). Introduction to the magnet credentialing program for student of nursing. Retrieved June 3, 2006, from *http://www.nursingworld.org/ancc/magnet/forms/ StudentManual.pdf*

Barnsteiner, J., & Prevost, S. (2002). How to implement evidence-based practice: Some tried and true pointers. *Reflections on Nursing Leadership, 28*(2), 18–21.

Coopey, M., Nix, M., & Clancy, C. (2006). Translating research into evidence-based nursing practice and evaluating effectiveness. *Journal of Nursing Care Quality, 21*(3), 195–202.

Greiner, A. C., & Knebel, E. (Eds.). (2003). *Health professions education: A bridge to quality.* Washington, DC: Institute of Medicine.

Hegyvary, S. T. (2006). Editorial: A call for papers on evidence-based problems. *Journal of Nursing Scholarship, 38,* 1–2.

Horsley, J. A., Crane, J., & Bingle, J. D. (1978). Research utilization as an organizational process. *Journal of Nursing Administration, 8*(7), 4–6.

Kerlinger, F. N., & Lee, H. B. (2000). *Foundations of behavioral research* (4th ed.). Belmont, CA: Wadsworth Thompson Learning.

Lindeman, C. A., & Krueger, J. C. (1977). Increasing the quality, quantity, and use of nursing research. *Nursing Outlook, 25,* 450–454.

National Institute of Nursing Research. (2007). National Institute of Nursing Research mission statement. Retrieved September 26, 2007, *from http://www.ninr.nih.gov/ AboutNINR/NINRMissionandstrategicPlan*

Nightingale, F. (1859). *Notes on nursing: What it is, and what it is not.* London: Harrison and Sons. [Commemorative edition printed 1992, Philadelphia: J. B. Lippincott]

Pape, T. M. (2003). Evidence-based nursing practice: To infinity and beyond. *Journal of Continuing Education in Nursing, 34,* 154–161, 189–190.

Porter-O'Grady, T. (2006). A new age for practice: Creating the framework for evidence. In K. Mallock & T. Porter-O'Grady (Eds.), *Introduction to evidence-based practice* (pp. 1–29). Boston: Jones and Bartlett.

Protection of Human Subjects, 45 CFR 46 (2005). Title 45 Code of Federal Regulations Part 46 (45 CFR 46), §46.101. Retrieved June 1, 2006, from *http://www.hhs .gov/ohrp/humansubjects/guidance/45cfr46.htm*

Sigma Theta Tau. (2005). Evidence-based nursing position statement. Retrieved June 3, 2006, from *http://www .nursingsociety.org/research/main.html#ebp*

Silva, M. (1995). *Ethical guidelines in the conduct, dissemination, and implementation of nursing research.* Washington, DC: American Nurses Association.

Stevens, K. R. (2005). *Essential competencies for evidence-based practice in nursing.* San Antonio, TX: Academic Center for Evidence-Based Practice, UTHSCSA.

United States Department of Health & Human Services (USDHHS). (2004). *Protecting personal health information in research: Understanding the HIPAA privacy rule* (NIH Pub. No. 03–5388). Retrieved June 4, 2006, from *http://privacyruleandresearch.nih.gov/pr_02.asp*

BIBLIOGRAPHY

Academic Center for Evidence-Based Practice, UTHSCSA. Retrieved June 28, 2006, from *http://www.acestar. uthscsa.edu/About.htm*

American Nurses Association. (1985). *Human rights guidelines for nurses in clinical and other research* (Pub. No. D-46 3M 9/87R). Kansas City, MO: American Nurses Association.

Belmont Report: Ethical principles and guidelines for the protection of human subjects of research, 79 Fed. Reg. 12065 (1979).

Burns, N., & Grove, S. (2004). *The practice of nursing research: Practice, critique, and utilization* (5th ed.). Philadelphia: Saunders.

Crane, J. (1985). Research utilization: Theoretical perspectives. *Western Journal of Nursing Research, 7,* 261–268.

Declaration of Helsinki. (1990). Recommendations guiding physicians in biomedical research involving human subjects. *Bulletin of Pan American Health Organization, 24*(4), 606–609.

DiCenso, A., Guyatt, G., & Cilska, D. (2005). *Evidence-based nursing: A guide to clinical practice*. St. Louis, MO: Mosby.

Lobiondo-Wood, G., & Haber, J. (2006). *Nursing research: Methods and critical appraisal for evidence-based practice* (6th ed.). St. Louis, MO: Mosby.

McCann, T.V., & Clark, E. (2003). Grounded theory in nursing research: Part 3 application. *Researcher, 11* (3), 29–39.

Schreiber, R. S., & Stern, P. N. (2001). *Using grounded theory in nursing*. New York: Springer.

Streubert Speziale, H. J., & Carpenter, D. R. (2006). *Qualitative research in nursing: Advancing the humanistic imperative* (4th ed.). Philadelphia: Lippincott Williams & Wilkins.

Thomas, S. P., & Pollio, H. R. (2002). *Listening to patients: A phenomenological approach to nursing research and practice*. New York: Springer.

Thompson, C., Cullum, N., McCaughan, D., Sheldon, T., & Raynor, P. (2004). Nurses, information use, and clinical decision making–the real world potential for evidence-based decisions in nursing. *Evidence Based Nursing: EBN Online*. Retrieved June 3, 2006, from *http://ebn.bmjjournals.com/cgi/content/full/7/3/68*

U.S. President's Commission for the Study of Ethical Problems in Medicine and Behavioral Research. (1982). *Compensating for research injuries: The ethical and legal implications of programs to redress injured subjects* (Vol. 1). Retrieved June 3, 2006, from *http://www.gwu.edu/~nsarchiv/radiation/dir/mstreet/commeet/meet16/brief16/tab_b/br16b1a.txt*

☐ ONLINE RESOURCES

Academic Center for Evidence-Based Practice (ACE)
http://www.acestar.uthscsa.edu

Agency for Healthcare Research and Quality
http://www.ahrq.gov/

American Nurses Foundation
http://www.anfonline.org/nrggrant.htm

The Cochrane Collaboration
http://www.cochrane.org/

Federal Guidelines for the Protection of Human Subjects
http://ohsr.od.nih.gov/guidelines/.html

Federal Opportunities for Research Funding
http://www.grants.gov

National Institute of Nursing Research
http://ninr.nih.gov

National Institutes of Health
http://www.nih.gov/

National League for Nursing
http://www.nln.org

Office for Human Research Protections (OHRP)
http://www.hhs.gov/ohrp/

Office of Civil Rights
http://www.hhs.gov/ocr/hipaa/

Sigma Theta Tau International
http://www.nursingsociety.org/research

U.S. Department of Health & Human Services
http://www.hhs.gov

■ *Jacqueline* **Owers Favret**

Effective Communication

> " *Silence at the proper season is wisdom, and better than any speech.* "

Plutarch (46–120 A.D.) Greek Essayist and Biographer

Chapter Objectives

On completion of this chapter, the reader will be able to:

1. Describe and understand the various communication models.
2. Explain the various forms of communication, such as verbal and nonverbal communication.
3. Evaluate the use of therapeutic communication in the health-care setting.
4. Differentiate between ways the nurse receives information from the client.
5. Discuss the various types of barriers to communication.
6. Identify past life experiences that influence communication skills.
7. Evaluate your current communication skills with clients and colleagues and propose refinements as a part of advancing your career in nursing.

Key Terms

Communication	Relationships	Facial Expressions
Communication Models	Transactions	Physical Appearance
Source	Contexts	Therapeutic Communication
Encoder	Metacommunication	Active Listening
Message	Verbal Communication	Questions
Channel	Nonverbal Communication	Silence
Receiver	Proxemics	Barriers to Communication
Decoder	Cultural Variations	Collaboration
Noise	Kinesics	Workplace Collaboration

Communication is a comprehensive and complex process. The word *communication* is similar to words like love, health, and freedom; intuitively, each of us thinks that we know what it means, but really people base their definitions on their own life experiences, cultures, and surroundings. For the nurse, communication is an essential element, not only in the relationship with the client but also in working effectively with the interdisciplinary health team. The process of interactions between humans can be verbal or nonverbal, written or unwritten, planned or spontaneous. It is therefore essential for communication to be defined within the context of nursing. **Communication** consists of "all the cognitive, affective, and behavioral responses used to convey a message to another person" (Watson, 1979, p. 33). Within this context there is no such thing as "no communication" between individuals. All behavior, whether verbal or nonverbal, has both meaning and a message value.

Effective communication within the client-nurse relationship is not necessarily a natural process; it is a learned skill. Clear and appropriate communication is essential for providing effective nursing care and presents a unique challenge to nurses today. Society is composed of many different cultures using many different languages. "Nearly 32 million people in the United States speak a language other than English at home" (Andrews & Boyle, 1999, p. 37). For example, in the aftermath of the September 2001 terrorist attack in New York, one of the biggest challenges faced by the Red Cross workers was communicating with individuals who spoke so many different languages. When a nurse is giving care to a client, the nurse's message must be understandable to the client and the nurse should be adept at understanding whatever the communication is from the client. Nurses must be aware not only of what they are saying in their words but also of what their body language is saying to their clients and other members of the health interdisciplinary team.

The 21st century poses an additional challenge to nurses in communicating via technology. Nurses also use many different types of communication in their care of clients—in person, the written word, telephone, facsimile (fax), and electronic mail. Finding effective ways to overcome communication barriers, discussed later in this chapter, gives nurses the opportunity to bridge culture gaps within their community and provide care to a larger number of individuals. The chapter will cover various techniques of communication and offer tools to assist you in your professional relationships with others.

COMMUNICATION MODELS

The chapter first presents an overview of basic **communication models** to help the reader understand the complex process of communication in the health-care setting.

Basic Components

Whether or not sources of communication are effective depends on a combination of factors (Berlo, 1960). All types of communication require the following components:

- **Source:** The individual who decides what message is to be sent
- **Encoder:** The person who interprets the message
- **Message:** The content of meaning
- **Channel:** The medium or way chosen to convey the message
- **Receiver:** The one who receives the message
- **Decoder:** The one who interprets the message sent

In intrapersonal communication, the source and the encoder are the same person. The message is then communicated either by verbal or nonverbal language. The message may be sent to any or all of a person's five senses. The receiver is also the decoder. According to Berlo (1960), in effective communication, the receiver is the most important component in the communication process. If the source does not reach the receiver with the intended message, the source might just as well have talked to himself or herself.

In written communication, the reader receiver is most important. In spoken communication, the listener receiver is most important. When the source chooses a "code" for his message, he must choose one that is familiar to his receiver. An example of poor communication in the health-care setting is when a nurse gives information to a client using as a code only the jargon or terms known within the profession. The client can receive the information but does not have the knowledge to decode the message.

Human communication is a two-person process in which both individuals influence and are influenced by each other.

Shannon-Weaver Model

Claude Shannon, a mathematician, and Warren Weaver, an electrical engineer, developed one of the early contemporary communications models in 1947. Both men were employed by Bell Telephone Laboratory and were referring to electronic communication, not interpersonal human communication (Berlo, 1960). Yet behavioral scientists have found the linear Shannon-Weaver Model (Fig. 7–1) very useful in describing human communication. They defined communication in a "very broad sense to include all of the procedures by which one mind may affect another" (Shannon & Weaver, 1949, p. 95). In this model, the *information source* selects a desired *message* out of a set of possible messages. The *transmitter* changes this

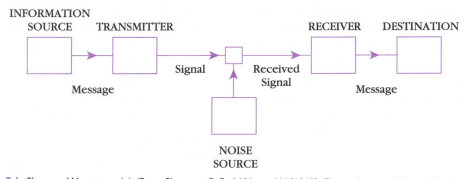

■ **Figure 7.1** Shannon-Weaver model. (From Shannon, C. E., & Weaver, W. [1949]. *The mathematical theory of communication.* [p. 720]. Champaign, IL: University of Illinois Press. Copyright 1949 by the Board of Trustees of the University of Illinois. Used with permission of the University of Illinois Press.)

message into the *signal* that is then transmitted to the *receiver.* The transmitter is the encoder of the message; the receiver is the decoder (Shannon & Weaver, 1949). Noise is a distinctive entity of this model. In the process of transmission of the message, certain things are added to the signal that were not intended by the information source. **Noise** refers to any disturbances, such as actual static, environmental noises, or the psychological or perceptual distortion of the receiver. In a nurse-client interaction, noise could represent an environment that is not conducive to receiving the message, such as a room that is too cold or a loud television playing in the background. This model does demonstrate a communication path but fails to show any type of reciprocal interaction on the part of the receiver.

Source-Message-Channel-Receiver Model

David Berlo (1960), a professor at Michigan State University, developed the source-message-channel-receiver (SMCR) model of the communication process (Fig. 7–2). This paradigm emphasizes the importance of a thorough understanding of human behavior as a prerequisite to communication analysis. The SMCR model represents a communication process that occurs as a *source* formulates *messages* based on the source's communication skills, attitudes, knowledge, and sociocultural system. These messages, which have unique elements, structure, content, treatment, and codes, are then transmitted along channels. *Channels* are the various senses, such as seeing, hearing, touching,

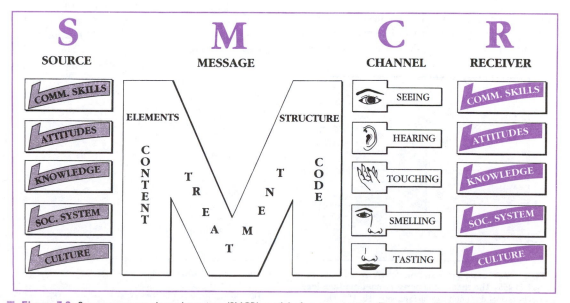

■ **Figure 7.2** Source-message-channel-receiver (SMCR) model of communication. (From Berlo, D. K. [1960]. The process of communication: An introduction to the theory and practice [p. 7]. New York: Holt, Rhinehart & Winston, with permission.)

smelling, and tasting. The *receiver* interprets messages on the basis of his or her own communication skills, attitudes, knowledge, and sociocultural system.

The strength of the SMCR model is that it demonstrates the complex process of communication and shows that communication is not a static event. It incorporates the sociocultural context of both sender and receiver as a critical component in the communications process. The model comes up short, however, by omitting the feedback component of communication (Northouse & Northouse, 1992).

Leary Model

According to Timothy Leary (1955), interpersonal communication is the aspect of personality psychology that is concerned with the social effect that one human being has on another. Leary developed a model that is truly a transactional and multidimensional model, stressing the relationship aspect of interpersonal communication. It demonstrates that human communication is a two-person process in which the two individuals influence and are influenced by each other (Leary, 1955).

As a psychotherapist, Leary noted that patients influenced the way he behaved toward them. He concluded that individuals actually "train" others to respond to them in ways that are pleasing for the individuals' own preferred interpersonal behaviors. From this perspective, according to the Leary model, every communication message can be viewed as occurring along two dimensions: dominance/submission and hate/love (Fig. 7–3). Leary (1955) stated that two rules govern how these dimensions function in human interaction:

- *Rule 1:* Dominant or submissive behavior usually stimulates the *opposite* behavior in others. For example, if we prefer to be dominant, we condition

others to behave submissively; conversely, if we like to be submissive, we condition others to behave in a way that is dominant towards us.
- *Rule 2:* Loving or hateful behavior usually stimulates the *same* behavior from others. Being kind to another individual usually encourages kindness from others, but if we display aggressive behavior, the other person will usually react in a hostile manner.

Leary says that these rules operate reflexively; our own responses toward one another are involuntary and immediate.

The Leary model of communication can be directly applied to the health-care arena. In the past, clients were generally passive about their health care and needs, and often assumed a submissive role, allowing the health-care professionals to assume the dominant role. Amidst current trends of consumerism and the availability of information about health care, however, clients are tending to take a more active role in their health care. When consumers become more assertive, the health-care providers have to relinquish some of their own control and authority. The strength of Leary's model is the transactional way in which he describes these power and affiliation issues in our everyday interactions with others. It is important to be aware of what each person brings to interactions with others.

Health Communication Model

The models previously described provided the foundation for Northouse and Northouse (1992) to construct the health communication model (HCM) (Fig.7–4), which specifically applies to transactions between participants in health care about health-related issues. The HCM's primary focus is on the health communication that occurs within the various kinds of relationships in health-care settings. This model also takes a broader systems view of communication and emphasizes the way in which a series of factors can affect the interactions in the health-care setting. Three major factors illustrate the health communication process: relationships, transactions, and contexts.

Relationships

From a systems perspective, the HCM illustrates four major types of **relationships** that exist in the health-care setting:

- Professional/professional
- Professional/client
- Professional/significant other
- Client/significant other

When an individual is involved in health communication, he or she is involved in one of these types of

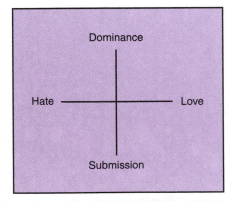

■ **Figure 7.3** Leary's reflexive model. (Adapted from Leary, T. [1955]. The theory and measurement methodology of interpersonal communication. *Psychiatry,* 18, 152. The William Alanson White Psychiatric Foundation, Inc.)

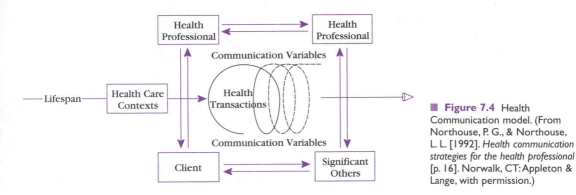

■ **Figure 7.4** Health Communication model. (From Northouse, P. G., & Northouse, L. L. [1992]. *Health communication strategies for the health professional* [p. 16]. Norwalk, CT: Appleton & Lange, with permission.)

relationships. In this model, the term *health professional* is any individual who has the education, training, and experience to provide health services to others. *Health professionals* include a wide range of individuals such as nurses, health administrators, social workers, physicians, and occupational and physical therapists (Northouse & Northouse, 1992). Each of these professionals brings unique characteristics and beliefs to health-care settings that affect the way they interact with the client and with the other members of the interdisciplinary health-care team.

Clients are the people who are the focus of the health-care services being provided. The term also encompasses the characteristics, values, and beliefs that these individuals bring to the health-care setting. Just as the personal characteristics of the nurse and other professionals influence their interactions, the characteristics of clients influence their interactions with others. Within the social network of the client, the client's *significant others* include family members and friends who have been found to be essential in supporting clients as they maneuver through the health-care system. Significant others are all of the people who are significant in clients' lives but are not health professionals.

The client's self-esteem, emotional stability, and sense of identity will define how the client relates to the health-care professionals as well as those significant individuals in his or her life.

Northouse and Northouse (1992) realized that too often, health professionals overlook the important role played by family members and other significant individuals in enhancing the health of the person. Their model includes this aspect because as clients live longer with chronic health problems, significant others assume an even more central role as patient advocates and are more involved in the direct care of the client. This concept is also true when the nurse is visiting the client in the home. The dynamics within the family and

the support of the significant others around the client can help the client realize the full potential of a healthy lifestyle.

Transactions

Transactions, the second major element in the HCM, are the health-related interactions between the nurse or other health professional, the client, and the client's significant others. These transactions about health can include both verbal and nonverbal communication behaviors, which are equally important and are most effective when they are compatible with each other. Northouse and Northouse (1992) represent these health transactions with a circle from which an unending spiral emerges, signifying that communication is not static but is an interactive process that occurs at various points in a person's life. This continuous feedback allows the message to be changed in accordance with the situation.

Contexts

Contexts, the third major element in the model, is defined as the settings where the health communication takes place and includes the properties of these settings. At one level, context can refer to the health-care setting, such as a hospital room or the client's home. For example, if the professional is communicating with the client in an ambulatory clinic, there may be many distractions and infringements of privacy. Each particular health-care setting affects the dynamics of the transactions that take place. At another level, however, health-care contexts can refer to the number of participants within the particular health-care setting. Communication can take place in a one-to-one situation or in small groups. The number of participants present influences the overall interactions in the setting.

The health communication model is based on the assumption that communication is ongoing, dynamic, and always changing. It is transactional, in that each participant affects the other participants, and it has both a content and relationship dimension that are inextricably bound together in the interactions. It is a model that incorporates the thoughts, feelings, attitudes, and current roles of the participants and demonstrates that all of these things can affect the accuracy of the communication.

FORMS OF COMMUNICATION

In order to share information, people express messages in a complex composite of both verbal (spoken or written) and nonverbal behaviors. Individuals express themselves through language, gestures, voice inflection, facial expressions, and use of space. Within the nurse-client relationship, information exchanged between two individuals must be interpreted not only by the nurse but also by the client. The health-care provider should be aware of styles of communication and should have observational skills that enhance the encounter.

Metacommunication

Metacommunication is a broad term used to "describe all of the factors that influence how the message is perceived" (Arnold & Boggs, 2007, p. 186) and has long been recognized as being of enormous value in the nurse-client therapeutic relationship. Metacommunication includes all things taken into account when the receiver is interpreting a message, such as the role of the communicator, the nonverbal messages sent, and the context in which the communication is taking place. These messages may be hidden within verbal messages or conveyed by nonverbal expressions or gestures. An example is the "play fighting" observed in children and animals. Bateson noted that for an organism to "play" at fighting, it must be able to both appear that it is fighting and simultaneously appear not to be fighting but merely simulating the act of fighting (Mitchell, 1991).

In the nurse-client relationship, metacommunication conveys messages about how to interpret both verbal and nonverbal communication clues. For example, a nurse can convey a message of caring by saying to the client, "That's important. Let's talk about it." If the nurse sits in a chair and uses nonverbal cues such as maintaining eye contact, smiling, having a relaxed posture, and listening intently, the verbal and nonverbal messages are congruent. If the same verbal message is delivered while the nurse fidgets and looks at a watch, the nurse may provide a nonverbal message that he or she does not have time or is not willing to listen. Metacommunication is the message conveyed when both verbal and nonverbal communication are perceived together.

Nurses must make sure that their verbal and nonverbal messages to clients are consistent and congruent in order to be sure that the clients interpret the messages clearly. Suppose you walk into a room and ask a client whether he is in pain and he answers no, but you observe that he is thrashing in bed, clutching his incision, and has deep grimaces on his face. How would you interpret this behavior? A nurse who is skilled in communication would realize that the verbal answer and the nonverbal cues are inconsistent and would clarify the situation. If the nurse points out the incongruent form of communication that he or she observed, the client may admit that he is in pain (Arnold & Boggs, 2007).

Metacommunication is the message conveyed when both verbal and nonverbal communication are perceived together.

Verbal Communication

Verbal communication takes place when people use words to share experiences with others. Without the use of spoken language, individuals are severely limited in means of sharing with others what they are feeling. The choice of words that a person uses is based on language, educational background, age, race, and socioeconomic background, as well as by the situation in which the communication takes place.

According to the individual's background and experience, interpretation of the words may also vary. One cannot assume that words have the same meaning to everyone who hears them. "Language is useful only to the extent that it actually reflects the experience it is designed to portray" (Arnold & Boggs, 2003, p.218). If a person speaks a different native language, consider the difficulty that person will have expressing his or her thoughts in English. This could also apply to a small child or a person who is afflicted with Alzheimer's disease.

Keep in mind that the intended meaning of the message may be represented in the emphasis placed on a particular word. The pitch and tone of a word can suggest mood and can either support or contradict the content of the verbal message. When a client is explaining something to the nurse, the nurse must consider that certain phrases and words may have entirely different meanings for the client and the nurse.

Potter and Perry (1999) state that the six most important aspects of verbal communication are (1) vocabulary, (2) denotative and connotative meanings, (3) intonation, (4) pacing, (5) clarity and brevity, and (6) timing and relevance.

Vocabulary

Vocabulary consists of the words or phrases that a person chooses and uses to communicate a message. Communication is unsuccessful if the receiver cannot translate or understand the sender's words and phrases. Nurses work with individuals of various ages, developmental stages, cultures, and educational backgrounds as well as individuals who have physical problems that distort their communication skills.

Nurses must be very aware of their use of nursing or medical jargon. Consider the nurse who is instructing a client before an operation. If the nurse says, "You are to be NPO after midnight and you are to void prior to the pre-op injection," what will the client be able to decipher from this instruction? At the same time, the nurse must not "talk down" or patronize the client. The nurse must respect the client and understand the best way to provide the information in a manner that can be understood readily.

Meaning

A single word may have several different meanings. The denotative meaning is the meaning that is shared by individuals who use a common language. The word *football* may be understood by all individuals who speak English but denotes a different meaning to individuals of different countries. The word *code* denotes a cardiac arrest to members of the health-care profession but has different meaning outside the health community. The connotative meaning is the interpretation or the way one's feelings, thoughts, experiences, or ideas about the word influence the meaning of the word. When a family is told that their loved one is in a "serious condition," they may interpret that phrase to mean that their loved one is near death. To the nurse, however, the term may merely describe the nature of the illness. Nurses should be extremely cautious to use words and phrases that will not be misinterpreted, especially when explaining a client's condition.

When a nurse is giving instructions to a client, the nurse must use terms and phrases that the client understands. The best way to ensure that the client has understood the instructions is have the client repeat the instructions to the nurse. At that time, any questions can be answered and the nurse can be assured that the client has the correct information.

Intonation

Intonation is the cadence and tone of the spoken word. The intonation of words in a message can readily change the meaning. Take the phrase "He is." If spoken one way it can be a sentence, but with a different tone it can be a question. Emphasizing the "he" or the "is" also changes the meaning of the phrase. The tone of voice can also dramatically affect the message's meaning, and emotions directly influence the tone of voice. Emotions such as anger, enthusiasm, and concern may be gleaned from the tone of voice that one uses. Nurses must be aware of this fact to avoid sending an unintended message. The nurse must also realize that the client's intonation may reflect the client's emotional state, even if the client's words do not.

Pacing

Pacing is the speed and rate of the spoken word. Communication is more successful when words are spoken at an appropriate speed or pace. Talking too rapidly or too slowly may express an inadvertent message. When the nurse is communicating important information to a client, the nurse must speak slowly and clearly and must pause at appropriate points to give emphasis. This approach allows the client time to absorb the message and to understand it more clearly. Pacing is better if the nurse thinks the message out before delivering it.

The nurse should also be aware of the pace of the client's spoken word. The speech may be slow and slurred if the client has some type of neurologic problem or is under the influence of drugs or alcohol. The client who is scared and nervous may speak very rapidly. Cultural variables may also influence the pace of the words; people from the southern part of the United States sometimes speak in a slow manner, and someone from the Northeast may speak very quickly. It is important for the nurse to be aware of these differences and be able to interpret the meanings of a person's pace of speaking.

Clarity, Timing, and Relevance

The nurse should use words and phrases that express an idea simply and directly. Using examples tends to make a message clearer. Timing and relevance are likewise critical in communication. The client must be ready to hear what the nurse has to say. If a patient is distracted by pain, the nurse must realize that it is not the right time to give detailed instructions. Often the best time to communicate is when the client has expressed interest in a particular topic. Choosing this timing tends to make the client more attentive.

Nurses should also demonstrate *credibility*, which is defined as a sense of trustworthiness, sincerity, reliability, and integrity. The nurse must be dependable and believable. If the client asks the nurse a question that the nurse does not know the answer to, it is much better for the nurse to answer, "I do not know the answer to that but I will find out for you" than to give erroneous information. When a nurse establishes credibility in a nurse-client relationship, the communication is more reliable and can have more substantial meaning for both the client and the nurse.

Nonverbal Communication

Nonverbal communication is communication without words; it includes messages that are created through body motions, facial expressions, use of space and sounds, and the use of touch. Birdwhistell (1970) studied the area of body movement and suggested that 65 to 70 percent of the social meaning of an interaction is transmitted by nonverbal communication. Although nonverbal communication does not include language, it can be either vocal or nonvocal. For example, if a client is moaning in pain, he is giving a nonverbal cue that the nurse should ask more questions about his condition.

Nonverbal communication can be intentional or unintentional. If a nurse is giving important information to a client, the nurse should intentionally have a serious facial expression. A client who is giving the nurse information in an apparently relaxed and gleeful manner but whose face shows expressions of fear and uncertainty demonstrates unintentional nonverbal communication. A prime example of nonverbal communication is Holly Hunter's 1993 role in the movie "The Piano." For the entire length of the movie, she does not speak one word of language, yet her nonverbal communication in the role is so effective that it earned her an Oscar for the best actress performance.

Monitoring subtle nonverbal communication clues accounts for the vast majority of communication between individuals.

Most Americans are only dimly aware of their use of nonverbal language, although they use it every day. We are constantly communicating our real feelings in nonverbal ways (Hall, 1959). Arnold and Boggs (2003) categorize four areas in which nonverbal behaviors are used: (1) proxemics, (2) cultural variations, (3) kinesics, which include body language and facial expression, and (4) appearance.

Proxemics

Proxemics refers to how individuals use and interpret space in the communication process. Some areas of proxemics address questions of territoriality, personal space, and distance relevant to the health-care setting. Each culture has expectations for appropriate distance, depending on the context of communication. Personal space, or one's own territory, is important because it gives one a sense of identity, security, and control. A person may feel threatened or simply irritated when his or her personal space is invaded.

When people enter the health-care setting, they are required to give up their privacy and personal space. They are required to give personal and intimate information to strangers and may undergo procedures that

further compromise their sense of privacy and personal space. Although nurses and other health professionals may not be able to eliminate these problems of personal space, the health-care professional should respect the client's territory, belongings, and right to privacy. The client should be given as much control over the situation as possible. For example, the client should be allowed to decide whether the door to the room is left open or closed and where personal items are placed. The client's body should be exposed as little as possible to minimize the discomfort involved with procedures that invade his or her privacy.

Cultural Variations

Cultural variations are learned subconsciously through the observations of behavior of significant individuals in the client's culture. Communication patterns vary in different cultures, even for such conventional social behaviors as smiling, a handshake, and direct eye contact. For many Hispanic clients, smiling and shaking hands are considered an integral part of sincere interaction and trust, whereas a Russian-American client might perceive this behavior to be inappropriate (Andrews & Bolye, 1999).

Sometimes a nonverbal *gesture*—a body movement usually with the hand—is totally acceptable in one culture and truly offensive in another one. For example, the nurse may mean to signal to a Brazilian client that things went well by making an "OK" circle with the thumb and index finger; in Brazil, however, this movement is considered an obscene gesture (Arnold & Boggs, 2003).

Cultural taboos can inhibit nonverbal behaviors. Different cultures have different rules about *eye contact*—looking directly into another person's eyes. In many Western cultures, making direct eye contact is interpreted as being interested and attentive. The use of eye contact is one of the most culturally variable nonverbal behaviors, however. Although most nurses have been taught to look directly at the client when speaking, individuals from other cultures may attribute other culturally based meanings to this behavior. Asian, Native American, Arab, and Appalachian clients may consider eye contact impolite or antagonistic, and they may divert their own eyes when talking to a nurse or physician. In some cultures, showing respect to the nurse dictates that the client should cast the eyes downward. Hispanic clients may expect eye contact from the nurse but will not necessarily reciprocate it (Andrews & Boyle, 1999).

In some cultures, *touching*—coming into physical contact with another person—is one of the most powerful means of nonverbal communication, but the nurse must give careful consideration to issues surrounding touch. Touch can take a variety of forms and can convey a range of meanings, but it is a powerful tool in health care when it communicates caring and respect. Touch can ease a client's sense of isolation and can make procedures seem less invasive. Care must be taken, however, to understand individual cultural customs about touching, which can vary dramatically. For example, the cultures of Muslim and Orthodox Jewish men dictate that they do not touch women outside their families. Such men may be very uncomfortable even shaking the hand of a female health-care provider (Arnold & Boggs, 2003).

Unfortunately, there is no precise formula to determine when or when not to touch a client, and no universal meaning can be given to a touch. In order for clients to perceive touch positively in a therapeutic relationship, Northouse and Northouse (1992) suggest that nurses use the following guidelines:

- *Use a form of touch that is appropriate to the particular situation:* There are many types of touch that can be used in various ways. The nurse should use touch that is fitting to the situation. For example, if a woman has just been told distressing information (e.g., that her child is diagnosed with leukemia), she may respond positively to the nurse's hand being placed on her arm. However, this type of touch may not be therapeutic or well received by a male adolescent who has just been told that he has diabetes and who is in the process of venting anger. It is better to let him get the anger out than to try to console him.
- *Do not use a touch gesture that imposes more intimacy on a client than he or she desires:* To some people, certain gestures may imply a level of intimacy or degree of closeness. When the touch suggests a degree of closeness that is not equally shared or agreed upon by both parties, distress may occur. The client may be offended if his personal space is violated.
- *Observe the client's response to the touch:* Assessment of a touch is especially important in the initial meeting with clients, when the nurse does not know how the client will respond. The nurse should observe the client's nonverbal behaviors. For example, if the client pulls away or displays a tense facial expression, he or she may be having a negative reaction or response to the touch. On the other hand, if a client appears relaxed and more comforted after the touch, it is likely that he or she is receiving the touch positively.

In health-care situations in which both the nurse and the client are comfortable with touch, and the use of touch is assessed for therapeutic effect, touch can be a very valuable mode of human communication.

Kinesics

Kinesics, commonly referred to as body language, is an important component of nonverbal communication (Arnold & Boggs, 2003). **Kinesics** is also defined as involving the conscious or subconscious body positioning and actions of the individual giving the message. Some dimensions of kinesics are posturing and gait, gestures, and facial expressions. Body stance can convey a message about the nurse or the client. If the client is in a slumped, head-down position, the nurse may assess that the client may have low self-esteem, whereas an erect posture and decisive movements may suggest confidence and self-control. Rapid, diffuse, or agitated body movements may indicate anxiety.

Facial expressions, the various movements in the face, provide emotional undertone and feeling whether or not they are accompanied by verbal communication. Throughout life, individuals respond to the expressive qualities of another face, often without realizing it. Mehrabian (1971), in studying the impact of words, vocalization, and facial expressions, noted that the power of the facial expression supporting the verbal content far outweighs the impact of the actual words.

Facial expression is important in conveying a message; it either reinforces or changes the verbal message that the listener hears. When the verbal message is inconsistent or different from the individual's facial expression, the nonverbal expressions assume more prominence and meaning and are generally perceived as more trustworthy and meaningful than the spoken word (Mehrabian, 1971).

The face is the most expressive part of the body, adding obvious and subtle cues to the real focus of the message. Common facial expressions are surprise, sadness, anger, happiness and joy, disgust and contempt, and fear (Arnold & Boggs, 2003). A client's facial expression should be part of the nursing assessment. For example, if a client frowns after receiving information, he or she may be experiencing confusion or anger. The nurse can intervene by saying, "I see that you are frowning. Is something wrong?" The question would encourage the client to clarify his or her response.

In the health-care profession, it is very important for the nurse's facial expression to be congruent with the verbal message given to the client. When a nurse walks into a client's hospital room, the client will "search" the nurse's face for clues before the nurse can even speak. For example, if the client asks the nurse, "Do I have cancer?" the slightest change in the nurse's facial features can reveal the nurse's answer. Although it is difficult to control all facial expressions, the nurse should try to avoid showing overt shock, revulsion, dismay, and other distressing reactions in the client's presence. If the nurse comes into a client's room with an expression of anger, stress, or disgust, the client and his family may perceive the nurse to be uncaring.

Appearance

The nurse's **physical appearance,** including dress, grooming, posture, gestures, and ease of movements, makes an important impact on the client and conveys the nurse's attitudes about himself or herself and others. Studies have shown that spoken words account for only seven percent of the message.

The business world has been aware of the "dress for success" rule and has noted the role clothes play in projecting the image of the serious professional. Nursing is no different; the client reacts to the way a nurse is dressed. In the past, nurses wore white uniforms and caps in designs that represented their various schools of nursing. In today's health-care environment there is no standard uniform for the professional nurse—a fact that does tend to confuse the layperson. What nurses wear is usually determined by the area of the hospital in which they work or the role they have in the community. Mangum, Garrison, Lind, Thackeray, and Wyatt (1991) surveyed clients, nurses, and administrators to determine whether or not different styles of nursing uniforms are associated with the professional image of nursing. In their summary, they noted that the nurse is judged primarily by what is worn and presented at the bedside. The nurse should make a conscious effort to dress in a professional way.

THERAPEUTIC COMMUNICATION

Therapeutic communication, a term coined by Ruesch (1961), is defined as a purposeful form of communication between the health professional and the client that allows them to reach health-related goals through participation in a focused relationship. "Therapeutic communication differs from ordinary communication in that the intention of one or more of the participants is clearly directed at bringing about a change in the system and manner of communication" (Ruesch, 1961, p. 460). This type of communication differs from a social communication, because there is a specific purpose or planned direction to the communication. The nurse uses therapeutic communication to promote a psychological setting that allows positive change, growth, and healing for the client. As the professional caregiver, the nurse comes to know the client as an individual who has unique health needs, responses, and patterns of living. With this knowledge, the nurse uses a goal-directed approach when communicating with the client.

Therapeutic communication can take place in a variety of clinical settings, ranging from the acute care system to nursing homes. As health-care delivery moves to a community focus, therapeutic communication can take place in nontraditional health-care settings such as the client's home, schools, and ambulatory care settings. Therapeutic conversations in health-care settings are designed to help clients maintain healthy habits, learn about their illness, and learn ways of coping. The communication is goal-oriented and client-centered, has rules and boundaries, and uses individualized strategies (Arnold & Boggs, 2003).

Therapeutic Communication Techniques

A number of techniques are used in therapeutic communication (Box 7–1). Nurses should familiarize themselves with and make it a habit to use these techniques both in and outside of therapeutic situations.

Active Listening

Effective therapeutic communication between the nurse and client begins with **active listening** (Bush, 2001). Listening actively means that the listener is communicating interest and attention to the client. The goal of active listening is to comprehend and understand fully what the other person is trying to communicate.

Two important techniques used by the nurse in active listening are restatement and reflection (Craven & Hirnle, 1996). *Restatement* takes place when the nurse listens carefully to the client and then restates some or all of the content back to the client to ensure that the nurse has the correct understanding of what the client has said. When the content is restated, the client has the opportunity to hear what he or she has said and therefore gains an understanding of how the nurse has perceived what he or she has communicated.

The nurse listens to the client for both content and emotions expressed through nonverbal facial expression, body posture, and emotional status.

Reflection is the process of identifying the main emotional themes in the conversation and directing them back to the client (Box 7–2). The nurse listens for the underlying feeling that the client is conveying and then shares this with the client in a nonjudgmental, open manner. This process allows the client to explore his or her own ideas and gives the client a clearer understanding of the feelings being experienced.

Box 7.1 Therapeutic Communication Techniques

- Active listening
- Restatement
- Reflection
- Focusing
- Encouraging elaboration
- Looking at alternatives
- Use of silence
- Appropriate questions

Box 7.2 Reflection and Restatement

Client: I don't want to eat anything today. I can't even begin to think about food.

Nurse: You don't want to eat and you can't think about food. *(Restatement)*

Client: All I can think about is what the doctor will tell me about the biopsy. *(Client is wringing her hands and almost crying)*

Nurse: The news about the biopsy result is worrying you and makes you unable to eat. *(Reflection)*

Client: Yes, I'm very nervous that it will mean that I have to have more surgery. I'm really frightened.

Questions

Questions are an important part of all phases of therapeutic communication because they allow the nurse to obtain information from the client. The nurse needs to ask pertinent questions but not to the point that the client feels that he or she is being interrogated.

Arnold & Boggs (2003) suggest that questions can be divided into three categories: open-ended, close-ended, and circular. *Open-ended questions* are phrases stated in such a way that the client is able to elaborate beyond a simple yes or no answer. This gives the client a way to "tell a story." Think of such a question as an essay question on a test. It gives the client a chance to express thoughts about a problem or health need. Open-ended questions usually begin with words like "how," "what," "when," and "can you tell me about." Examples of open-ended questions are, "What brought you to the hospital?" and "Can you tell me about your being diagnosed with diabetes?" These questions are general, rather than specific, and are open to the client's interpretation.

Closed-ended questions require specific answers and limit a client's response. These types of questions are best used in emergency situations, and it may take more of them to get the desired response. In this situation, the nurse wants to obtain information quickly and the client's emotional reactions are secondary. Examples of closed-ended questions are "When did the pain start?" and "How long has it been since you saw the doctor?"

Circular questions focus on the impact of the illness or injury and how it will affect the family and significant others. Circular questions differ from open-ended questions because the nurse is intentionally asking specific questions to elicit responses from the client or a family member. The nurse uses circular questions as a type of family interviewing strategy. The nurse can use the information that the family or others provide as a basis for additional questions about the client or other family members. For example, the nurse asks family members about the care of a terminally ill client (the mother) in their home. From the family's response, the nurse may receive multidimensional information about the family that could not be learned by asking specific questions. This approach provides a basis for open discussion of the client and the family's circumstances.

Other Therapeutic Communication Techniques

Other techniques the nurse may use in therapeutic communication are focusing, encouraging elaboration, and looking at alternatives. Focusing means asking goal-directed questions that help keep the client focused on the subject at hand. The nurse is also conveying that she is helping the client discuss the main areas of concern. The nurse can also encourage elaboration. This technique allows the client to describe the concerns or problems under discussion in a more detailed manner. The nurse can look attentively at the client and use short responses like "I see" and "Go on" to allow the client to continue to explore feelings. Looking at alternatives allows the nurse to help the client increase the client's perceived choices. This technique should not be used until the client has a clear understanding of the current situation. Sometimes the client has to deal with emotions such as anger and denial before alternatives come into play.

Probably one of the most difficult techniques the nurse must learn is the use of **silence,** that period when no words are being spoken between the nurse and the client. For Americans in particular, it takes experience to become comfortable with pauses in the conversation. Most people have a natural tendency to try to fill up the empty spaces with words. By contrast, many Native Americans consider silence essential to understanding and respecting what the nurse has said. In traditional Chinese and Japanese cultures, silence may mean that the speaker wants the listener to consider the importance of the content before continuing. British and Arab people may use silence as a sign of respect for the individual's privacy; whereas French, Spanish, and Russian individuals may consider silence a sign of agreement. Among some African Americans, silence is used to respond to what is perceived as an inappropriate statement (Andrews & Boyle, 1999).

In therapeutic relations, silent moments give the nurse and the client time to observe each other, digest what messages have been communicated, and think of things to say. Silence can be used deliberately and thoughtfully and can be a powerful listening tool. On the other hand, long silences may be very uncomfortable. By pausing briefly before continuing a conversation with a client, the nurse gives the client a chance to reflect and come up with questions of her own.

Barriers to Communication

In the therapeutic communication setting, the nurse must be aware of certain responses that may lower the client's self-esteem and limit full disclosure of client information. Among the responses that tend to block or present barriers to communication are the following (Box 7–3):

- *False reassurance* is the use of clichés or comforting phrases in order to attempt to reassure the client. These types of responses invalidate the client's feelings or fears. Expressions such as "Everything will be okay" and "Don't worry" send a message to the client that the nurse is not interested in the client's true feelings.
- *Giving advice* is telling the client what to do or making a decision for the client. The nurse should avoid offering personal opinions to the client. Avoid phrases such as "should do" or "ought to do." These types of responses tend to center the interaction on the nurse's needs and perspective rather than on the client's. If a client asks a nurse for specific advice, the nurse can use a reflective statement and explore the various choices the client has in that situation.
- *Probing* is asking questions out of curiosity rather than for information needed to assist the client. Many of these questions begin with the word "Why?" These types of questions from the nurse tend to put the client in a defensive mode and also violate the client's privacy.
- *Stereotyping* is the process of attributing characteristics to a group of people as though all people in that group possess those features. Stereotyping groups clients in a category and does not value or recognize their individuality. Stereotypes lead the nurse to false conclusions about the client, and if they are based on strong emotions, stereotypes can be identified as prejudices. It is important that the nurse convey acceptance of the client as a unique individual.
- *Social comment* is the use of polite, superficial comments that do not focus on what the client is feeling or trying to express to the nurse. The nurse can use social comments at the beginning of an interaction to make a connection with the patient. However, the nurse should focus on a therapeutic interaction with

the client when talking about issues or concerns that affect the client's health. Socialization is inappropriate when a more serious approach to the client's situation is suitable.

- *Changing the subject* when the client is trying to communicate about another topic is rude and shows lack of sensitivity. Changing the subject tends to block communication; the client may withhold information about important issues and fail to express his feelings openly. If the nurse does have to change the subject, the reason for this change should be given to the client.
- The nurse should not use *nursing or medical jargon*—terminology that is used among nurses and other health professionals—when addressing the client. These unfamiliar words can cause confusion and anxiety for clients. They also may be frightening to some clients. Nurses should try to use common terms with which the client is familiar. And if nurses need to use jargon, they should make sure that they carefully explain what the terms mean.

A valuable tool to evaluate communication patterns is a process recording where verbal and nonverbal behavior interactions are analyzed (Table 7–1).

COMMUNICATION WITH COLLEAGUES

Nurses must communicate effectively with a diverse group of professionals and unlicensed personnel in caring for clients. When members of the health-care team communicate ineffectively with one another, delivery of health care to the client suffers.

The nurse must use effective communication skills with all colleagues, regardless of their position, and must regard each individual with an attitude of respect. "Using clear, simple messages and clarifying the intent of others constitutes a positive goal in all personal and professional communication"(Chitty, 1997, p. 391). Just as a client must have trust in the health professional administering care, trust and respect must exist between colleagues for effective communication.

Collaboration, the collegial working relationship with other health-care providers, is intrinsic to nursing. Henneman, Lee, and Cohen (1995) state that collaboration implies working in cooperation with other personnel and viewing them as a team. The relationship between individuals who are collaborating is nonhierarchical. The power is shared and is based on the knowledge and expertise that each individual brings to the setting, not on role or title (Henneman et al., 1995). In this team approach, each person recognizes the boundaries of

Box 7.3 Communication Barriers

- False reassurance
- Giving advice
- Probing
- Stereotyping
- Social comment
- Changing the subject
- Use of jargon

Table 7.1

Sample Process Recording for Evaluation of Communication

Select a 10–15 minute section of verbal therapeutic interaction that meets all of the evaluation criteria. Goals for the interaction should be specific, realistic, and therapeutic for the patient. The goal is short term and is related only to this particular interaction.

Body of Recording:
Client and Student Response Column:
- Record as accurately as possible what was said *verbally*.
- Record the feeling that accompanied the verbal message.
- Record the nonverbal message that was sent.
- Record periods of silence when they occurred.

   Analysis Column
   - CT: Identify the interviewing/communication technique used by the student.
   - R: What is the rationale for using this technique?
   - V: State the student's perception of the messages sent *verbally* by the student/client. Include silence.
   - NV: State the student's perception of messages sent *nonverbally* by the student/client.

Client Response	Verbal/ Nonverbal	Student Response	Verbal/ Nonverbal	Analysis (CT; R; V; NV)
		"How are you this morning, Ms. G?"	Happy voice; nurse is smiling	Nurse is trying to ascertain client's condition
"Okay."	Client is slumped in the bed and is looking toward wall. Answered very reluctantly	"You're only okay?"	Nurse can see that there is something on the client's mind; student is concerned.	Reflective question. Get client to open up.
"My doctor was in a few minutes ago."	Looks at the nurse with worried and grimaced face	"What did he have to say to you?"	Nurse showing concern; perhaps info from doctor was upsetting	Direct question; student needs info

each discipline and values the contribution that every person makes.

Because nurses are the managers of client care in acute care settings and are with the client for 24 hours, they obtain a lot of information that must be communicated to other health-care providers. Nurses must make a concerted effort to have a collaborative relationship with the team members, not just work in cooperation with others (Silva & Ludwick, 2002). Collaboration allows the nurse to identify the contributions of the other disciplines and permits the integration of this information into the health-care plan for the client. It also helps enhance problem-solving skills by utilizing insights from other disciplines and health-care workers who deal with the client. Collaboration with other members of the health-care team is essential for the nursing profession to provide excellent health care to all clients.

Workplace Collaboration

In 1972, the American Medical Association and the American Nurses Association formed the National Joint Practice Commission (NJPC). The purpose of the NJPC was to describe, research, and define the value of collaborative practice for physicians and nurses. It also described collaborative practices and guidelines for the establishment of these practices. NJPC concluded that joint practice directly affects the quality of care, provides satisfaction to the patient and the provider, and decreases time of stay in the acute care facility (Buttaro, 2003).

As nurses, we know that health care is in persistent change and this brings us to visit the important concept of professional collaboration in the context of today's workplace. **Workplace collaboration** can be reflected on every level of health care and is demanded for cost effectiveness, quality improvement, and the demand of efficiency. Improving patient care and creating gratifying work roles are added benefits. What does one have to do to be part of the collaborative effort?

Webster's New World College Dictionary (2001) has two definitions of the word collaboration: "1) to work together, esp. in some literary, artistic, or scientific undertaking; and 2) to cooperate with an enemy invader" (p. 286). Sometimes, when there is a need for nurses and physicians to communicate, it can seem like an "invader" is around and collaboration can become very difficult. One must realize that collaboration is a complex process that requires individuals to be willing to share information about the client from their own area of expertise. Each discipline that cares for the client has its own knowledge, skill, and clinical experiences.

"Collaboration is significantly more complex than simply working in close proximity to one another. It implies a bond, a joining together, a union, and a degree of caring about one another and the relationship. A collaborative relationship is not merely the sum of its parts, but it is a synergistic alliance that maximizes the contributions of each participant resulting in action that is greater than the sum of individual works." (Evans, 1994, p. 23)

Some *characteristics of collaboration* include clarity of communication, accountability, and mutual respect. In our daily work we realize how important it is for each of us to communicate in a clear fashion. We need to think about the information that needs to be shared and use a technique that other individuals will be able to hear and accept. Each person must also be accountable for her actions and accept the results of her decision or action. Respect for each other's knowledge, skill, background, and clinical decision is the backbone of a positive collaborative arrangement. It is also important to find the common ground between disciplines because there may be differing patterns of communication (Grover, 2005). Individuals caring for the client bring unique contributions from the various disciplines.

ⓞ N L I N E ⓒ O N S U L T

Communication Resources at
http://carbon.cudenver.edu/~mryder/itc/comm_theory.html

The American Communication Journal at
http://www.acjournal.org/

Nonverbal Communication at
http://stephan.dahl.at/nonverbal/

The challenge is to make the most of each encounter and interaction so that the best knowledge and ability of each team member is recognized and valued. In the interest of the care of the client, no profession stands alone and the use of good collaborative skills is essential (Lindeke & Sieckert, 2006). Mutual respect is of utmost importance among all members of the health-care team, and must be of value to each individual.

There are many *barriers to collaboration* in the workplace. The first barriers to come to mind are gender issues and hierarchy issues. Some old school physicians may still think that the nurse (traditionally a position dominated by women) should be subservient and have no contribution on a professional level. Nurses should continue to demonstrate that the nursing profession is unique and that nurses bring a different perspective to the client's care. Organize factual data when presenting information to other team members. Also take the time and effort to learn from the other's perspective and encourage new team members to share their experiences. In collaboration there is no implied supervision; it is a two-way exchange of information. One must value the other person's suggestions and the fact that the individuals are coming from two different perspectives.

A health-care system that is hierarchal in nature does not encourage collaborative practice; therefore, the individuals must have the specific intention of working together. The dominance of the medical profession leads to a lack of understanding and appreciation of the value of nursing and other professions (Stapleton, 1998). The attitudes and skills associated with collaborative relationships can be learned if all parties are willing to participate.

When there is true *collaboration in the workplace*, the responsibility for the client is shared; the professionalism of all is strengthened when each member of the group has participated and has obtained success. The unique perspective that each profession brings to a situation tends to result in creative and practical solutions, and in turn, the client's well-being is of utmost importance. In order to practice effective communication in the workplace setting, each individual must be willing to participate equally. Basic therapeutic technique of communication is essential; we must be aware of the variables of gender, hierarchy, and collegiality and have basic mutual respect for each member of the health team.

INTERACTIVE EXERCISES

Go to the Intranet site and complete the interactive exercises provided for this Chapter.

EVIDENCED-BASED PRACTICE: CONSIDER THIS . . .

M anojlovich (2005) reports original research investigating relationships among factors in the practice environment that contribute to job satisfaction. Although the importance of nurse-physician communication has been supported in prior research, this study reported that over 60% of the variance in nurses' job satisfaction was explained by a combination of practice environment factors and nurse-physician communication (Manojlovich, 2005, p. 372).

Question: How will you use this information as a nurse or nurse-manager?

Source: Manojlovich, M. (2005). Linking the practice environment to nurses' job satisfaction through nurse-physician communication. *Journal of Nursing Scholarship, 37,* 367–373.

KEY POINTS

■ Effective communication within the client-nurse relationship is a learned skill and is essential for providing effective nursing care.

■ Communication models illustrate the complex process of communication with the basic components: source/encoder, the message, the medium, and the receiver/decoder.

■ The health communications model uses a broad systems view of communication and emphasizes the way in which a series of factors (relationships, transactions, and contexts) can affect interactions in the health-care setting.

■ When people share information, they express messages in a complex composite of both verbal (spoken or written) and nonverbal behaviors. Individuals express themselves through language, gestures, voice inflection, facial expressions, and use of space.

■ Metacommunication is a broad term used to "describe all of the factors that influence how the message is perceived" (Arnold & Boggs, 2003, p. 217).

■ Oral communication is the use of words by people to think about ideas, to share experiences with others, and to validate the perceptions of the world.

■ Potter and Perry (1999) state that the six most important aspects of verbal communication are (1) vocabulary, (2) denotative and connotative meaning, (3) intonation, (4) pacing, (5) clarity and brevity, and (6) timing and relevance.

■ Nonverbal communication is communication without words and includes messages that are created through body motions, facial expressions, use of space and sounds, and use of touch. Arnold and Boggs (2007) categorize areas in which nonverbal behaviors are used: touch, proxemics, nonverbal body clues, facial expression, and clothing.

■ In order for clients to perceive touch in a positive therapeutic relationship, Northouse and Northouse (1992) suggest that nurses use the following guidelines: use touch that is appropriate to the particular situation, do not use a touch that imposes more intimacy on a client than he or she desires, and observe the client's response to the touch.

■ Therapeutic communication is a purposeful form of communication that serves as a point of contact between the health professional and the client and allows them to reach health-related goals through participation in a focused relationship. Techniques include active listening, restatement, reflection, focusing, encouraging elaboration, looking at alternatives, use of silence, and use of appropriate questions.

(Key Points continue on page 138)

K E Y   P O I N T S   (continued)

■ Barriers to communication are certain responses that may lower the client's self-esteem, limit full disclosure of client information, and block communication. These barriers include false reassurance, giving advice, probing, stereotyping, social comment, changing the subject, and use of jargon.

■ Collaboration in the workplace depends on working in cooperation with other members of the health-care team. The power is shared and is based on the knowledge and expertise that each member brings to the setting; mutual respect is of utmost importance for successful communication.

Thought and Discussion Questions

1. Contrast the various communication models for use in the hospital versus the home setting.

2. Explain how nonverbal communication may be more "powerful" than spoken words.

3. Describe a collaborative relationship that you have experienced in your work setting.

4. Prepare a Process Recording of a five-minute intervention with a client. Use the format shown in Table 7–1.

5. Read Coeling and Cukr's January, 2000, article, "Communication Styles that Promote Perceptions of Collaboration, Quality, and Nurse Satisfaction" in the *Journal of Nursing Care Quality* (14[2], 63–74). Form a study group and discuss the various aspects of this evidence-based practice study. How does this affect your workplace issues? What new techniques could you introduce in your workplace?

6. Review the Chapter Thought on the first page of the chapter and discuss it in the context of the contents of the chapter.

☐ REFERENCES

Andrews, M., & Boyle, J. (1999). *Transcultural concepts in nursing care* (3rd ed.) Philadelphia: Lippincott.

Arnold, E., & Boggs, K. (2003). *Interpersonal relationships: Professional communication skills for nurses* (4th ed.) Philadelphia: W. B. Saunders.

Arnold, E., & Boggs, K. (2007). *Interpersonal relationships: Professional communication skills for nurses* (5th ed.) Philadelphia: Saunders/Elsevier.

Berlo, D. K. (1960). *The process of communication: An introduction to theory and practice.* New York: Holt, Rinehart & Winston.

Birdwhistell, R. L. (1970). *Kinesics and context.* Philadelphia: University of Pennsylvania Press.

Bush, K. (2001). Do you really listen to patients? *RN 2001, 64* (3), 35–37.

Buttaro, T. (2003) *Primary care: A collaborative practice* (2nd ed.) St. Louis, MO: Mosby.

Chitty, K. K. (1997). *Professional nursing concepts and challenges* (2nd ed.). Philadelphia: W. B. Saunders.

Coeling, H., & Cukr, P. (January, 2000). Communication styles that promote perceptions of collaboration, quality, and nurse satisfaction. *Journal of Nursing Care Quality 14*(2), 63–74.

Craven, R., & Hirnle, C. (1996). *Fundamentals of nursing: Human health and function* (2nd ed.). Philadelphia: Lippincott-Raven.

Evans, J. (1994) The role of the nurse manager in creating an environment for collaborative practice. *Holistic Nursing Practice, 8,* 22–31.

Grover, S. (2005) Shaping effective communication skills and therapeutic relationships at work. *American Association of Occupational Health Nurses Journal, 53* (4), 177–187.

Hall, E. T. (1959). *The silent language.* Garden City, NY: Doubleday & Company.

Henneman, E. A., Lee, J. L., & Cohen, J. I. Collaboration: A concept analysis. *Journal of Advanced Nursing, 21,* 103–109, 1995.

Leary, T. (1955). The theory and measurement methodology of interpersonal communication. *Psychiatry, 18,* 147–161.

Lindeke, L., & Sieckert, A. (2006). Nurse-physician workplace collaboration. *Online Journal of Issues in Nursing.* Retrieved August 11, 2006, from *http://www.nursingworld.org/ojin/topic26/tpc26_4.htm*

Mangum, S., Garrison, C., Lind, A., Thackeray, R., & Wyatt, M. (1991). Perceptions of nurses' uniforms. *Image: The Journal of Nursing Scholarship, 23*(2), 127–130.

Mehrabian, A. (1971). *Silent messages.* Belmont, CA: Wadsworth Publishing.

Mitchell, R. W. (1991). Bateson's concept of metacommunication in play. *New Ideas in Psychology, 9*(1), 73–87.

Northouse, P. G., & Northouse, L. L. (1992). *Health communication strategies for health professionals* (2nd ed.). Norwalk, CT: Appleton & Lange.

Potter, A., & Perry, G. (1999). *Basic nursing: A critical thinking approach* (4th ed.). St. Louis, MO: Mosby.

Ruesch, J. (1961). *Therapeutic communication.* New York: W. W. Norton.

Shannon, C. E., & Weaver, W. (1949). *The mathematical theory of communication.* Urbana, IL: University of Illinois Press.

Silva, M., and Ludwick, R. (August 30, 2002). Ethics Column: Ethical grounding for entry into practice: Respect, collaboration, and accountability. *Online Journal of Issues in Nursing.* Retrieved August 11, 2006, from *http://www.nursingworld.org/ojin/ethicol/ethics_9.htm*

Stapleton, S. (1998) Team-building: Making collaborative practice work. *Journal of Nurse-Midwifery, 43*(1), 12–18.

Watson, J., (1979). *Nursing: The philosophy and science of caring.* Boston: Little, Brown.

Webster's New World College Dictionary (4th ed.) Cleveland, OH: IDG Books Worldwide.

☐ BIBLIOGRAPHY

Benson, A., & Latter, S. (1998). Implementing health promoting nursing: The integration of interpersonal skills and health promotion. *Journal of Advanced Nursing, 27,* 100–107.

Brown, G. (1995). Understanding barriers to basing nursing practice upon research: A communication model approach. *Journal of Advanced Nursing, 21,* 154–157.

Ceccio, J., & Ceccio, C. (1982). *Effective communication in nursing: Theory and practice.* Canada: John Wiley & Sons.

Craven, R., & Hirnle, C. (1996). *Fundamentals of nursing: Human health and function* (2nd ed.). Philadelphia: Lippincott-Raven.

Crowther, D. (1991). Metacommunication a missed opportunity? *Journal of Advanced Nursing, 20,* 703–706.

Davidhizar, R., & Giger, J. (1994). When your patient is silent. *Journal of Advanced Nursing, 20,* 703–706.

Edwards, B., & Brilhart, J. (1981). *Communication in nursing practice.* St. Louis, MO: C. V. Mosby.

Leininger, M., & McFarland, M. (2002). *Transcultural nursing: Concepts, theories, research and practice* (3rd ed.). New York: McGraw-Hill.

Lindberg, J., Hunter, M., & Kruszewski, A. (1983). *Introduction to person-centered nursing.* Philadelphia: J. B. Lippincott.

Long, L. (1992). *Understanding/responding: A communication manual for nurses.* Boston: Jones and Bartlett.

Mehrabian, A. (1981) *Silent messages: Implicit communication of emotions and attitudes* (2nd ed.). Belmont, CA: Wadsworth Publishing.

Mulaik, J., Megenity, J., Cannon, R.B., Chance, K. S., Cannella, K. S., Garland, L. M., et al. (1991). Patients' perceptions of nurses' use of touch. *Western Journal of Nursing Research, 13*(3), 306–323.

Peplau, H. (1952). *Interpersonal relations in nursing.* New York: G. P. Putnam's Sons.

Peplau, H. (1960). Talking with patients. *American Journal of Nursing, 60,* 964–966.

Salle, A. (1999). Effective communication. In B. Cherry & S. Jacob (Eds.), *Contemporary nursing issues, trends, & management* (pp. 378–402). St. Louis, MO: Mosby.

Sieh, A., & Brentin, L. (1997). *The nurse communicates.* Philadelphia: W. B. Saunders.

Steel, J. E. (1986). *Issues in collaborative practice.* Orlando, FL: Grune & Stratton, Inc.

☐ ONLINE RESOURCES

Communication Resources
http://carbon.cudenver.edu/~mryder/itc/comm_theory.html

The American Communication Journal
http://www.acjournal.org/

Nonverbal Communication
http://stephan.dahl.at/nonverbal/

Working with Groups

> **❝** *We communicate in many ways, especially when working with others toward a common goal.* **❞**
>
> Author

Chapter Objectives

On completion of this chapter, the reader will be able to:

1. Explain the techniques for effective communication in group settings.
2. Evaluate personal communication patterns used with clients and colleagues in a group.
3. Describe different types of groups, including their characteristics and roles of group members.
4. Differentiate between effective and ineffective groups and the characteristics of an effective group leader.
5. Evaluate communication patterns in a group for effective functioning in meeting the group's common goals.

Key Terms

Group
Group Process
Group Structure
Group Composition
Group Roles
Group Focus
Professional Groups
Work Groups
Educational Groups
Therapeutic Groups

Effective Groups
Goal Attainment
Member Participation
Cohesiveness
Decision-making
Communication Patterns
Attendance
Creativity
Power

Ineffective Groups
Stages of Group
  Development
Functional Task Roles
Functional Group-Building
  Roles
Nonfunctional Group Roles
Organizational Group
Virtual Meetings

Communication—verbal, nonverbal, and written—is integral to working with individuals and groups. DeWine, Gibson, and Smith (2000) identify four contexts or environments in which communication takes place: interpersonal, group, organizational, and mass communication. Nurses must be skilled in each of these areas, from the interpersonal situation with a client or colleague, to small client or colleague groups, to larger organizational settings and, finally, to mass communications with the public.

The concepts of effective group process are important components in professional nursing practice and require understanding of the types of groups, their composition and functions, and the roles played by the members. As nurses, we need to develop skills to use as both leaders and members of various work and professional groups, as well as to apply group process to intervene therapeutically with clients. Examining the group's characteristics and evaluating the group's effectiveness provide the knowledge and skills needed to accomplish these goals. Note that understanding groups is an initial step in addressing the core competency of working in interdisciplinary health-profession teams.

GROUPS

A **group** consists of three or more individuals with some commonality, such as shared goals or interests. Living in society, we are members of many groups—family, work, professional, and social. Each type of group has a specific goal and membership. As nurses, we are involved as participants in work groups and interact with groups of clients in their health-care activities. We may also participate in therapy or support groups. We use the principles of group process in all of these activities and in assisting our clients. Some of these groups are structured loosely, with minimal rules, whereas others have clearly defined roles and limits. It is essential for the nurse to understand group processes to communicate and function effectively in the group as both an individual and a professional.

Group Process

Group process is the dynamic interplay of interactions within groups of humans. Interplay includes what is said and done in groups, as well as how members interact with one another and the group leader. A group is actually a social system. Recall from Chapter 3 that systems theory is concerned with holism as opposed to the isolated parts. The basic components of a system are the input, output, boundary, environment, and feedback. A group, as a social system, is composed of people with their unique characteristics and communication styles but focused on the group goals as the output from the system. And as Berlo (1960) pointed out in his classic work on communication, "a knowledge of the composition and workings of a social system is useful in making predictions about how members of that system will behave in a given communication situation" (p. 135). This is particularly applicable to professional practice with the nurses' focus on the importance of working with groups in a variety of practice settings—client, family, self-help, self-awareness, peer, and task groups.

Group Characteristics

Groups can be classified according to structure, composition, roles, and focus. A particular group often fits more than one classification, especially in terms of its roles. For example, the initial purpose of developing a cancer support group might have been to provide the members with a sense of sharing and support. But this type of group often fills many other functions, such as education regarding medications, traditional and nontraditional treatment programs, and health-care providers; information sharing about benefits, wills, and finances; and strategy sharing on coping with symptoms and managing daily life.

Group Structure

Groups may be differentiated by **group structure**, such as whether a group is formal or informal. Formal groups are highly structured, with functions specified in job descriptions, contracts, policies, and procedures. Formal groups associated with nursing are the entire nursing staff and the professional standards committee. Each of these groups has particular requirements for membership and specific rules, procedures, and standards of practice. A professional group can also be viewed as a formal group, with requirements for membership, rules that govern meetings, and specific member expectations. An advantage of structured groups is their clear understanding of roles and expectations. This same benefit may become a disadvantage, if the group is not open to changing to meet the needs of the members. The leaders of more structured groups tend to have greater power. By contrast, informal groups are more loosely structured, at times disbanding or reconvening according to the needs of the membership. Examples of informal groups are special interest groups and support groups. Informal groups benefit from some degree of flexibility in roles, expectations, and leadership.

Composition of Groups

Groups can also be differentiated by the unique composition of the membership. **Group composition** may be homogeneous or heterogeneous, depending on the characteristics of the members. Members of homogeneous groups are similar in some aspect, such as all adolescent male clients or female nurses employed in the intensive care units. A benefit of working with a homogeneous group is the sense of shared connection that the members typically feel from the beginning. This sense may be expressed as "He has the same problem" or "She thinks the same way I do." Heterogeneous groups consist of a mix of individuals, such as clients with various diagnoses or ages, or a work group of both nurses and physicians working with patients in a cardiac intensive care unit. This type of group has a wider range of diversity and therefore usually a greater variety of opinions, beliefs, and needs. Facilitating a sense of connection among members is a key challenge for the heterogeneous group. With a heterogeneous group, however, group members have the advantage of learning from many different perspectives.

Roles for Members of the Group

A third way to classify groups is in terms of the leader and participant **group roles**. Some groups are led by a professional who is responsible for instituting the rules, establishing the structure, and determining the membership. There are clear expectations for the leader and the participants. An example is an outpatient recovery group, in which a cardiac rehabilitation counselor leads the group, initiates themes for discussion, and often sets criteria for member participation. Other groups have informal leadership as well as rules for members. Peer support groups are an example of this type. Traditionally, the leadership may be shared by members, who are usually working on a common issue. Members are free to attend or not, depending on their own needs and schedules. At times, the group may become engulfed in struggles for leadership, which can compromise the group's effectiveness.

Group Focus

Groups may also be classified according to their focus or approach. The **group focus** can be work-related, educational, therapeutic, or professional. Professional nursing groups were described in Chapter 1, along with their unique missions and membership requirements. These professional groups are generally formal and are directed at professional issues and at the objectives stated in their mission statements. Work groups are task oriented, focused on a particular work-related activity, as with a nursing department budget committee and the task of allocating resources.

Many of us are members of a variety of work groups. Nurses on a particular unit constitute one group, whereas the nursing department as a whole is another functioning work group. Committees that meet monthly are probably commonly viewed as work groups. They may be convened ad hoc (as needed), or they may be more or less a permanent standing group, such as the nursing standards committee, the safety committee, or the quality assurance committee. The membership changes over time, and the structure varies in level of formality. If the group is focusing on one specific issue or task, members may be expected to fulfill assigned roles. At other times there may be a more informal, shifting assignment of roles, as occurs in monthly staff meetings on a care unit. Attendance varies, depending on schedule, client load, and the issues involved.

Educational groups have a teaching focus, whether members are teaching clients about medications, treatments, parenting skills, or a variety of health promotion activities, or educating their colleagues in areas of expertise. This type of group may actually convene only for an individual session, if held in a clinic or institutional setting, or it may have a series of sessions. An example is a stress reduction class for clients diagnosed with hypertension, which is scheduled on a weekly basis in a clinic or outpatient department. Membership and attendance vary depending on educational needs and appointment schedules. Although the group leader is a professional, the structure is typically less formal and directed at the learning needs of the audience. Teaching and learning principles, discussed in Chapter 10, are important considerations, along with the group process.

Therapeutic groups vary in nature, depending on the specific treatment or client needs. This group is led by a professional and is a formally structured group that typically specifies when members can join and when they can leave the group. Examples of these groups are cognitive therapy groups for depressed clients, behavioral therapy groups for anger management, and therapeutic activity groups, such as a music therapy group for clients who have suffered cerebral vascular events. The group leader has special training in the different therapeutic approaches used. Advanced Practice Nurses (APRNs) can lead groups in specific therapies as defined in practice standards and as recognized by their state practice act.

Effective Groups

Effective groups have an identified purpose or need for the group and a commitment to the process. Once the decision is made to form a new group, several issues are involved in setting up or structuring the group. Arnold (2007) terms this the pregroup phase, in which the following activities occur:

- Alignment of purpose and membership
- Determination of appropriate group size
- Creation of the appropriate environment

The first consideration is the purpose for forming the group. This purpose must be clearly stated for specification of the membership. Once the intended membership is determined, members can be recruited and goals set for the group. The size of the membership must be appropriate to addressing the group goals effectively. A professional group must be larger to effect change than a work group. A work or therapeutic group becomes less effective when it grows too large, becoming more heterogeneous and unable to focus on the task or treatment aims. For some groups, the leader also spends time interviewing potential members before the initial meeting. This step serves as an orientation to the group as well as a way to determine whether the individual will "fit in."

The room arrangement is another important factor for creating the appropriate environment. When the room is being set up, the goals of the group and interactions needed among members should be considered. A large conference table and chairs may be needed for a work group, whereas placing chairs in a circle to allow individuals to make eye contact without the barrier of a table is imperative in many therapeutic groups. Neither of these arrangements may be feasible or essential in an educational group.

Other factors to consider in creating an effective group include:

- The best meeting place and time for meetings
- Fees, dues, or cost factors
- Frequency and length of meetings
- Documentation needed for third-party payers or sponsoring organizations

An effective group will also determine whether there will be a single leader or coleaders. Those in favor of two-leader groups cite the enhanced ability to examine dynamics, provide feedback, and manage absences of the leader. Those against this style look at the possibility of problems arising between these two individuals in terms of power, equality, and accountability, with the potential for splitting of the group, creating factions, and ineffectiveness. The goal is to form a strong, viable group. Before initiating a group, a nurse should consider all of these concerns.

Evaluating Effectiveness of Groups

Effective groups are those that work toward the stated goals and whose members derive a sense of belonging and acceptance. How these outcomes can be accomplished requires a closer look at behaviors, strategies, and goals. In addition, organizations and third-party payers may determine their own criteria of effectiveness. General factors to consider in determining effectiveness of any group are identified in Box 8–1.

Box 8.1 Factors to Consider in Evaluating Effectiveness of Groups

- Goal attainment
- Member participation
- Cohesiveness
- Decision-making
- Communication patterns
- Attendance
- Creativity
- Power

Goal attainment is the initial and most important criterion in determining the effectiveness of any group. It is an evaluation of whether the intended task or goal was accomplished, especially in a work group. In a professional association, goal attainment is focused on the activities related to the organization's mission and strategic initiatives. In a therapeutic group, goal attainment relates to the focus of the group, such as gaining insight, awareness, or skills.

Member participation is another important criterion for assessing the effectiveness of a group. Consider whether all members are included in the discussions and what roles they are playing as group members. On the other hand, think about a situation in which an autocratic leader limits the members' ability to participate in the group discussions. In an effective group, there is evidence of belonging, camaraderie, and acceptance. But participation does not imply that all members should be in agreement on all issues. "Group think" is the phenomenon by which all members are in constant agreement, which can limit creativity and lead to stagnation.

Cohesiveness among the group members indicates that they are working together toward the group's common purpose or goal. If all members are not focused on the purpose, the original goal for which the group was formed will be difficult to attain, and conflict may arise. To achieve cohesiveness, the group members must be refocused on the original intent for the group, with the leader and members supporting one another in their actions and demonstrating agreement on the common goal.

In an effective group, **decision-making** must occur at the group level, with all members being involved in decisions rather than unilateral actions being taken by the leader or a disruptive member. A democratic leader and involved, cohesive members directed toward the common goal usually signify effective group functioning as they actively work toward that goal.

The **communication patterns** among the members provide valuable information on whether there is a common focus, respect, and decision-making. Evaluate how the group's decisions are made. The group leader should facilitate effective communication patterns, thus allowing all members to be heard and involved in the group process. In an effective group, members are actively involved in a mutual communication process.

Attendance is regular and active in an effective group. Members are punctual and involved, energetically focused on the task or purpose of the group. When a group meeting is arranged in advance, members in an effective group honor their commitments to the meeting rather than making excuses for not attending or demonstrating routine tardiness.

A high level of **creativity** among the members is another sign of an effective group. The group members are spontaneously generating novel ideas for solutions on the common problem. Brainstorming sessions are focused on the goals, and communication is encouraged, with all ideas and contributions from members considered.

Typically, the leadership style in more effective groups is described as democratic, and the interactions among the members are interdependent and collaborative. **Power** is distributed, on the basis of the common purpose and abilities of the members to achieve their goal in an effective group. Power struggles disrupt group process, with members focusing inwardly rather than working collaboratively on the group's goals.

Ineffective groups have low levels of productivity. These groups contain much unrest and stagnation, and members feel that they do not belong or that it is not safe for them to share their thoughts, ideas, and feelings. The group members demonstrate an uncaring attitude toward one another, have little spontaneous involvement, or are reluctant participants. The members do not appear to trust one another, seem unwilling to take risks and, in work groups, rarely volunteer for or willingly accept assignments. The attendance may be uneven, with a high rate of dropout and tardiness. The leadership style in less effective groups is often described as autocratic or laissez-faire, and the group interactions as independent and competitive.

THE BASICS OF GROUP PROCESSES

Skills in group process are tailored to the developmental stage of the group, and require effective leadership and participation by the members.

The Stages of Group Development

Understanding the expected stages of group development and how to facilitate groups during these stages is essential to nursing practice, when the nurse is a group

member or a leader. As with the developmental stages of individuals, groups go through predictable stages. In his classic work, Tuckman (1965) identified five **stages of group development**: forming, storming, norming, performing, and mourning or termination. Yalom and Leszcz (2005) further describe the storming stage as one of conflict that arises in the group. Arnold (2007) has further clarified the stage of termination as one of adjournment that is more applicable to the professional or work group. An effective group leader must be aware of these stages and must motivate members and modify approaches accordingly.

We can use the traditional stages of the nurse-client relationship (initial, working, and termination), with the addition of the conflict and norming stages before the working phase, to understand the process of group development better. The stages of group development, along with expected goals and examples of appropriate nursing approaches, are illustrated in Table 8–1. Now, consider the five stages of group development: initial or forming, conflict or storming, norming, working or performing, and termination or adjourning.

Forming

In the initial or forming stage, the group is being formed. The members are becoming acquainted with one another, the group, and the purpose and outcomes. Arnold (2007) identifies the major group tasks during this forming stage as establishing the group contract, developing trust, and identification. The leader focuses on orienting the members and determining the structure in terms of time, duration, and frequency of meetings, as well as the goals for the group. Cohesiveness of the group is enhanced by clearly stated goals and group norms. Work groups require an introduction, identification of goals and expectations, and orientation to the structure. Client groups also require this introduction and orientation information, but issues of confidentiality and personal disclosure are important considerations in the forming stage. Another factor to consider is whether members can join or leave at different times or whether all members must begin and terminate together.

Storming and Norming

The next phase is the conflict or storming stage. This is the time when members become more comfortable with the group but may be ambivalent about the need for the group and its intended goals. This ambivalence can be demonstrated by "testing" the authority of the leader through questioning, skipping sessions, or coming late. These issues must be dealt with openly and clearly so that the group can settle into its work. This becomes the time of norming, with the identification of standards and expectations of behavior. Some level of

Table 8.1

Group Stages, Expected Goals, and Nursing Techniques

Stage	Expected Goals	Nursing Techniques
Initial/forming	Sense of trust	Making introductions Structuring group Defining parameters and goals Encouraging the sense of group
Conflict/storming	Sense of commitment	Encouraging verbalizations Allowing interactions and role development Handling confrontations and setting limits
Norming	Sense of purpose	Setting limits, rules, and expectations Encouraging group cohesion
Working/performing	Sense of hope	Facilitating discussion Identifying themes and progress Refocusing as needed Identifying processes
Termination/adjourning	Sense of accomplishment	Summarizing and evaluating goals Facilitating transfer of knowledge and skills Supporting closure

discomfort or conflict is often expressed overtly or covertly, until the group becomes functional. All groups need this time to set norms such as roles, rules, and structure.

Performing

The working or performance stage involves exactly that—performance of the work of the group. In this stage, the leader becomes less involved in running the group. The members themselves decide what to discuss and how to address the goals and, to some degree, manage the group themselves. Cohesiveness and creativity should be apparent and encouraged. The leader's role is to refocus and clarify as needed, handle problems and conflicts if they arise, and identify the process as it develops. In this process, members may avoid issues or tasks and engage in disruptive reactions and behaviors. By bringing problems and conflict out in the open, the participants can examine these issues and make changes. Some groups have established dates for each stage; others depend on the tasks and type of group.

Adjourning

Termination or adjourning is the formal ending of the group. How long this stage lasts depends on the purpose of the group and its duration. As in the orientation stage, the group leader assumes an active role at this stage. The goals are to assist the members in expressing what has been accomplished and preparing for closure. This can be an emotional stage, with some members striving for continual closeness in some therapeutic groups or the continued camaraderie that is not experienced in the work setting. On the other hand, some work-group members are relieved at having accomplished the intended goals.

The Role of the Group Leader

Role theory is applicable to groups in terms of both leader and member roles. Recall that a group is a social system. As such, the leader and the members will assume selected roles based on expectations, gender, and learning. Roles are organized behavioral patterns and expectations for a given position and accompany a specific situation or circumstance (Bailey & Yost, 2004, p. 1). In the case of the group, the roles of the leader and members reflect the group's identified structure, composition, focus, and associated expected roles. The role of the leader can set the expectations for the group as the social system.

Leadership is an essential consideration for the viability of many groups. One consideration is whether the leader has been selected externally or determined internally through group consensus. This appointment status may affect both the leader and member behaviors within the group. Other factors that may influence the particular leadership style adopted by an individual are the person's personality and skills, the purpose of the group, and the characteristics of the group and the participants or members.

Traditional group leadership styles have been described as democratic, autocratic, or laissez-faire. Group leaders often use a combination of styles or modify their style, depending on the group membership or the topic being discussed. With a democratic leadership style, the leader shares the authority and decision-making tasks with members. A democratic leader seeks greater participation by and feedback from group members. One of the benefits of this style is that it typically produces a greater sense of satisfaction among members. On the other hand, the need to have consensus or agreement may impede the progress of the group by monopolizing the discussion.

An autocratic leadership style is one in which the leader makes all pertinent decisions, informs members of the rules, and structures the sessions. This style can facilitate the group effectiveness and goal achievement because the expectations have been clearly delineated and actions controlled. At the same time, it may limit group interaction and lead some members to feel that they are disenfranchised and that their opinions are not valued.

The laissez-faire leadership style is unstructured, allowing members a great deal of freedom and the ability to come and go at will. This style might also involve a change of leader from session to session, which can be effective with a highly functional, goal-directed population but will not work well with poorly focused or unmotivated groups.

Regardless of the leadership style, characteristics of an effective group leader include the ability to understand the dynamics of the group, listen attentively, focus on the goals, and facilitate the progress of the group. Again, effective communication and interpersonal skills are vital attributes of an effective leader. Interestingly, McKay, Davis, and Fanning (1995) have proposed that every meeting have two purposes, (1) the group goal, and (2) maintenance of the group morale. The maintenance of group morale is a major role of the group leader.

Leadership Tasks and Skills

Consider the leadership tasks and skills necessary to manage a group successfully by analyzing the group's purpose, structure, member participation, communication, and goal attainment. One of the first tasks for the group leader is to establish a structure that will promote an effective working relationship. The leader is also responsible for securing a meeting place, deciding the length and frequency of meetings, and determining the goals for the group. These goals must be clearly communicated to the members so that they can assume their roles. At times, goal determination may be delayed to allow members to participate in goal development. The leader must also physically set up the room. As discussed earlier, the arrangement of the physical environment is crucial in some groups.

Another critical task for the group leader at this point is to orient the members to the group and its expectations and to allot sufficient time for the group to form before initiating work. The leader can accomplish this by ensuring that the interactions among the members during the initial period of forming remain on a superficial level while the members become acquainted. The stages of forming, storming, and norming may be much briefer in a work group, but the leader must ensure that there is some time for the members to settle in. This may be accomplished in one meeting, but some allowance for introductions and getting to know one another is important, regardless of the group's focus.

Leadership skills are essential to facilitate the group in its deliberation and discussion for decision-making. Ensuring participation by all members, avoiding premature closure on the topic, and recognizing the recurring themes are important activities for an effective group leader. The leader can set the tone for the level of communication, whether superficial or personal, as well as set limits on appropriate and unacceptable communication styles. The leader uses techniques such as restatement, reflection, clarification, collaboration, and problem-solving while always attempting to promote open communication among the members. Another useful technique for the leader is role modeling for the group members on how to provide constructive feedback. In this way, the group leader is actually teaching the members effective communication skills.

Attaining group cohesiveness is another skill of the successful group leader. Coming together as a group and focusing on the common goal or purpose are reinforced by the effective group leader. This cooperative and cohesive group esprit de corps can occur and endure when the group leader provides the positive, supportive, and encouraging lead or model for the group. Conflict can arise in any type of group and must be managed. The best resolution entails a "win-win" situation with a solution satisfying to both sides. Conflict is a challenge for the group leader to direct the members in creative problem-solving for both effective and satisfying group process. Nurses commonly face conflict situations in work-group settings and need to keep in mind the four functional problems that Turniansky and Hare (1998) have identified—meaning, resources, integration, and goal attainment—as well as the four "must" activities to address these problems with groups in organizations:

- An overall meaning of the activity that sets both a direction and boundaries for the group
- Resources adequate for the task
- Integration in the form of role differentiation and level of morale for the group members to work together
- Enough coordination of the resources and the integration functions to provide for goal attainment. (Turniansky & Hare, 1998, p. 111)

The Conflict Resolution Network (CRN) also identifies 12 skills useful in a conflict situation (Box 8–2). The CRN (2003) is an international organization whose purpose is to research, develop, teach, and implement the theory and practice of conflict resolution through a national and international network. Other techniques to use when dealing with difficult people are discussed later in this chapter.

Leaders should avoid using the following ineffective communication techniques: giving advice, giving approval, blaming, and scapegoating. Giving advice and blaming are considered nontherapeutic. Group leaders must be vigilant not to scapegoat a member or allow other group members to do so, especially a disruptive member. The leader needs to recognize these dynamics and intervene appropriately, creating a safe, open, and productive environment for the group. Giving approval is, perhaps surprisingly, not helpful. Giving approval can interfere with the group process and goal accomplishment by focusing on one individual. Rather than express approval for an individual's efforts or successes, the leader can reflect back the accomplishment to the person

Box 8.2 The Conflict Resolution Network's 12 Useful Skills

The Conflict Resolution Network recommends the following 12 skills for dealing with conflict situations:

- The win-win approach
- Creative response
- Empathy
- Appropriate assertiveness
- Cooperative power
- Managing emotions
- Willingness to resolve
- Mapping the conflict
- Developing options
- Negotiation
- Mediation
- Broadening perspectives

ONLINE CONSULT

Visit the CRN at
http://www.crnhq.org/twelveskills.html

or other members, allowing them to express their feelings. The leader can use the group format as a means of teaching effective communication skills, such as how to listen, give and receive feedback, and express feelings or opinions.

Goal accomplishment has already been identified as a benchmark of success for groups. Giving assignments, such as recording the group's discussion or trying out a particular suggestion from the group, is one helpful measure. The use of assignments communicates the belief that members are capable and that change involves work on the part of group members. In a work group, members are given specific areas to work on or research, with the expectation that the group will reconvene to put these pieces together. Ultimately, the leader is responsible for ensuring that activities in the group remain focused on the common goals that were set for the group.

CASE STUDY

Identify possible conflict situations in your next work or group session. Which techniques would you use for effective resolution?

Another leadership activity is facilitating closure. To provide for group closure, the leader must summarize progress at the end of each session as well as at the official termination of the group. If the members enter and leave the group at various individual points, the leader may actually summarize at the start of each session to orient newer and continuing members to current status, goals, and tasks. This approach is also highly effective in educational groups as it serves to reorient learners to prior content. Regardless of the focus of the group, periodic summaries and closure can be essential for the successful functioning of both the group and its members.

Group members need an opportunity to acknowledge their accomplishments.

Roles of Group Members

Group members demonstrate a variety of roles during particular meetings. These roles may be either functional or nonfunctional for the group process. They may remain similar or constant over the life of the group, or individuals may alter their role from meeting to meeting. It is vital for nurses to recognize the roles assumed in groups and to interact purposefully when necessary. Consider the last unit meeting you attended. Who led the group? Did anyone stall or disrupt the

Table 8.2
Functional Task Roles

Initiator/contributor	Makes suggestions and proposes new ideas, methods, or problem-solving approaches
Information giver	Offers pertinent information from personal knowledge appropriate to the group topic or task
Information seeker	Requests information or suggestions from other members appropriate to the group topic or task
Opinion giver/seeker	Offers or requests views, judgments, or feelings about the topic or suggestions under consideration by the group. Provides the opportunity for values clarification by the group members
Disagreer	Identifies errors in statements made or proposes a different viewpoint
Coordinator	Suggests relationships between the different suggestions or comments made by the group members
Elaborator	Elaborates or expands on suggestions already made
Energizer	Stimulates the group into action toward the goals either by introducing certain issues or topics or by behavior
Summarizer	Summarizes suggestions, actions, and accomplishments that have occurred in the group
Procedural technician	Provides the technical tasks needed for the group functions, such as arrangement of the group, including media, equipment, and work supplies
Recorder	Takes notes to record the progress, suggestions, and decisions of the group

Adapted from Tappen, R. M. (2001). *Nursing leadership and management: Concepts and practice* (4th ed.). Philadelphia: F. A. Davis. Reprinted with permission.

discussion? Were the topics discussed major issues for the unit or "pet peeves" of one individual? Did all members participate in the discussion? How could you, if you had been the group leader, have changed this meeting?

Functional Group Roles

Functional group roles facilitate the group process and determine the ultimate effectiveness of the group, especially in accomplishing a task or attaining a goal. In any type of group, members may play both functional and nonfunctional roles for various periods. For the effectiveness of the group process, the goal is for members to demonstrate predominantly functional group roles. For nursing work groups, Tappen (2001, p. 125) differentiates between **functional task roles** (Table 8–2), which contribute to completion of the task, and **functional group-building roles** (Table 8–3), which support development and meet relational needs.

Observe these roles in any work-group setting, such as a committee or unit meeting. Many functional task and group-building roles are demonstrated by the group leader. The leader may start out as the information giver and standard setter during the forming

stage, but then function as an information seeker, gatekeeper, and encourager as the group process evolves in the working stage. The leader may also demonstrate the functional roles of coordinator, energizer, summarizer, and consensus taker to facilitate group process and attainment of the group goals. Other group members will also serve in these functional roles as they become more active and progress toward the achievement of the group's goals. Observe who acts as the procedural technician, helping the leader organize the group and supplying needed equipment and materials. Examine who appears to be the more passive follower in the group, who cracks jokes as the tension reliever, and who records the actions and progress of the group.

Although these roles have been discussed mainly for the work setting, they also apply to professional, educational, and therapeutic group settings. In a professional group, observe the leadership roles shared by the officers, procedural technician roles performed by the aides or room monitors, and the standard setter role taken by the parliamentarian. In an educational group, consider the specific content and the size of the audience. Observe the roles taken by the teacher or facilitator, the people who are seated close to the teacher, the people in the back of the room, and the

Table 8.3
Functional Group-Building Roles

Encourager	Accepts and praises contributions of the group and other group members
Standard setter	Reinforces the standards or processes for effective group functioning
Gatekeeper	Ensures that all members have contributed to the discussion and that the group is not being monopolized by the views of more verbal members
Consensus taker	Seeks the weight of group sentiments or consensus on the issues
Diagnoser	Identifies barriers or blocks to group progress that are occurring
Expresser	Restates or identifies and expresses the feelings of the group
Tension reliever	Uses humor and mediation when group tensions rise and interfere with the group process and accomplishment of tasks
Follower	Consents to whatever is proposed by others in the group. Demonstrates no active participation without great encouragement

Adapted from Tappen, R. M. (2001). *Nursing leadership and management: Concepts and practice* (4th ed.). Philadelphia: F. A. Davis. Reprinted with permission.

people who are asking most of the questions or cracking jokes. In a therapeutic group, observe the particular role of the leader and how he or she facilitates sharing of the members' feelings and beliefs. Observe the members who verbalize supportive comments versus those who disagree or give further information about similar feelings.

Nonfunctional Group Roles

At times, group members demonstrate nonfunctional roles when they interrupt the group process. An example is the individual who provides negative comments on whatever other group members propose. **Nonfunctional group roles** generally are disruptive to group-building, task accomplishment, and progress toward goal attainment. A group can actually be mobilized to act in response to the unacceptable actions of one member, however, such as speaking up to the individual who repeatedly comes late and then insists on being updated on what already occurred. Tappen (2001) has identified the following nonfunctional roles: dominator, monopolizer, blocker, aggressor, recognition seeker, zipper-mouth, and playboy. Smith (2001) lists similar disruptive roles in a meeting as latecomers/early leavers, silent/shy persons, whisperers/side conversationalists, and talk-a-lots, including loudmouths, know-it-alls, and hostiles.

- The *dominator* or *know-it-all* controls conversations, determines what will be discussed, and may control or intimidate other members. The dominator is often focused on his own needs. An example of the dominator in a work group is a unit coordinator at a quality assurance meeting who suggests that the group focus on the number of requests for schedule changes. An example in a therapeutic group is a client who opens the group by describing her plans with her family for the upcoming holidays rather than addressing the group leader's question on the assigned activity from last week.
- The *monopolizer*, or *loudmouth*, seeks attention and demands that the group focus on him. He may repeatedly interrupt others and perceive his issues and problems as the most important. A work-group example is the nurse who goes on and on about how he always has to work overtime. In a therapeutic group, an example is a client who repeatedly interrupts and insists the group listen to his problem.
- The *blocker* interrupts the discussion, often focusing on another topic or personal concerns. The blocker can do this overtly or through side conversations, which can be highly disruptive to the group.
- The *aggressor* or *hostile* attacks during the discussion, making comments that may or may not be relevant to it. Often this individual is focused inwardly

on personal needs and demands to be heard, regardless of relevance to the discussion. This member criticizes other group members because they do not have the same insights or experiences as the aggressor. This individual is readily identified in professional, work, educational, and therapeutic groups by his hostile comments. Signs of discomfort or counterattacks may be apparent among other group members.

- The *recognition seeker* consistently attempts to draw the group's attention to his personal beliefs, values, and concerns. This individual has a need to stand out among the group members and be heard, respected, and perhaps admired. This member sometimes sounds like the leader but is usually working on personal issues. In a work-group example, this is the nurse who declares, "It's not all shifts that are short-staffed. Mine is the one that's always short-staffed with temps, but I am able to orient them successfully after all."
- The *zipper-mouth* is a nonparticipant (Tappen, 2001, p. 126). In either a work or a therapeutic group, this is the silent individual who sits quietly, feeling unlucky to be in the group. This is not the *shy person*, who is tracking the meeting content and perhaps needs more time in the group to develop trust, reflection, and opportunity.
- The *playboy* makes irrelevant remarks and does not take the group seriously (Tappen, 2001, p. 126). Unfortunately, we have all experienced these jokers in a group setting and can easily recognize the disruption they make in the group process. These individuals may also be consistently late without notice or may frequently leave early.

Dealing with Difficult People

The group setting is no different from routine interpersonal interactions. You will inevitably encounter people who are difficult to work with. Whether a leader or a group member, you will inevitably encounter thorny personalities in the group setting. One of the most effective means of dealing with a difficult member is when the leader, as well as the members, address behavior destructive to the group process. Lundin and Lundin (1995) propose that there is no "one-size-fits-all" answer to dealing with the many categories of difficult people (Box 8–3). Awareness of your own reactions, identification of the real problem, preparation, experimentation, and problem-solving are the steps toward resolution (p. 87). And in the group setting, this can make all the difference between stagnation or dissolution, and meeting group goals.

As with interpersonal communication skills, there are effective ways to deal with difficult and disruptive group members. Consider the suggestions in Box 8–4. The skillful and effective group leader or member can

Box 8.3 Categories of Difficult People

• Mean and angry	• Whiner
• Cynic	• Politician
• Pessimist	• Manipulator
• Unresponsive	• Procrastinator
• Suspicious	• Staller
• Negativist	• Exploder
• Know-it-all	• Sniper
• Indecisive	• Sarcastic
• Complainer	• Thin-skinned
• Sneak	• Shy and quiet

From Lundin, W., & Lundin, K. (1995). *Working with difficult people.* New York: American Management Association.

Box 8.4 Communication Techniques in a Group When Dealing with Difficult Members

- Make observations and acknowledge contributions.
- Use the communication techniques of reflection and restatement.
- Refocus the discussion if it is getting off track.
- Set limits and adhere to the ground rules agreed upon by the group.
- Focus on potential solutions raised.
- Provide constructive feedback, not corrective feedback, which should be done privately.
- Promote balanced participation from members.
- Assign functional group roles to members displaying nonfunctional behaviors.
- Plan ahead and anticipate for the next group session.

use a variety of these techniques, depending on the group structure, composition, roles, focus, and situational factors. In addition, Streibel (2003) suggests the inclusion of a "timeout" rule set at the first group meeting with periodic reminders of this rule at subsequent meetings, so "that any member of the group who feels at any time that the situation is getting out of control can call for a timeout" (p. 154). Having this rule empowers any member of the group to intervene in a conflict situation. Effective communication techniques and interpersonal skills are critical to success in group process, whether a small working group or a larger organizational setting.

ORGANIZATIONAL GROUPS

Communication issues among the larger **organizational group** and less tangible groups are also worth exploring.

Interorganizational versus Intraorganizational Groups

Interorganizational groups are those that occur between systems or organizations. Communication is a vital activity to reach out to these other groups or systems. The interorganizational groups may consist of the hospital and the community mental health center, the home health agency, or the various subgroups of a health department. Outpatient hospital groups and inpatient unit groups also fit this category. These groups are often highly structured, with functions specified in job descriptions, policies, and procedures.

Nurses are involved with and provide leadership for effective functioning between or among systems in interorganizational groups. Communication and interpersonal skills are valuable attributes of professional nurses in this process. Along with these skills, a full awareness of each system or organization and its interrelationships is needed. This awareness involves an understanding of each organization's goals and values, hierarchial structure, leadership and management, interpersonal and communication systems, resources and technology, boundaries, and external environments, as illustrated in Chapter 12. In addition, consider the environment in which the different organizations or systems exist. Nursing involvement in interorganizational groups is growing as the complexity of health care and professional practice expand among different systems.

Collaboration among organizational groups is vital for the client and for effective use of resources.

Intraorganizational groups are those that exist within a single, overall system or organization. The nursing, housekeeping, and physical therapy departments are intraorganizational groups within a hospital system. These groups are somewhat similar in terms of their structure, with specified roles, policies, and procedures. It is imperative for nurses to learn how to interact and negotiate effectively with these intraorganizational groups. An example is how to obtain needed supplies and services from the housekeeping department. Accomplishing this task often depends on the ability of members of each department to collaborate with the others. Activity for clients is a major consideration and incentive to work effectively together. For example, the client is the focus for physical therapy and nursing departments. A physical therapist has certain scheduling needs based on individual client progress. The nurse manager has different needs in scheduling staff for treatments, which may be predetermined by client census, staffing, and care needs. Collaboration in this process is vital for the client and effective use of resources.

Communication in Organizational Groups

In addition to the verbal and nonverbal interpersonal communication techniques, additional methods of communication are routinely used in large groups and organizations. The information we compile and the method we use to transmit it vary. Considering the purpose of communication in an organization is indispensable. Whether we are involved in health teaching or the transmission of physiologic findings, the method and receiver of the information are important. Clear, concise, and timely transmission of information is necessary for an effective process. The time frame and ongoing evaluation are also factors in the initial communication phase as well as in the feedback phase of the process.

Specifically, information can be sent or received by telephone, facsimile (fax), electronic mail, or instant messaging, depending on sender's and receiver's access to and skill with the available technology. A classic problem in some organizational settings is fear of technology. Another problem is overuse. Consider the use of e-mail in organizations. The intent is to deliver information efficiently and rapidly to other individuals or groups of individuals in the sender's network while reducing paper and administrative costs. But some people avoid this form of mail, whereas others regularly check for messages, and still others *Reply to All* or copy (or blind copy) multiple recipients creating great volumes of unnecessary messages. If the information is not sent correctly or received appropriately, the message is not communicated and the process is ineffective.

Personal skills in verbal and written communication must be developed continually and refined through specific techniques or technologies. For example, keep in mind that e-mail can be forwarded easily to others, thus communicating with a larger group. The original sender's message will be evaluated by others on the appropriateness of content, format, and presentation (including grammar and appearance). Evaluating the appropriate channels or pertinent audiences and preparing the information in the correct format are vital for effective communication in the organizational setting.

In essence, organizational communication can be thought of as being similar to the rights of administering medications. In organizational communications, these rights are:

1. Information or content
2. Communication channel
3. Format, including use of correct grammar, terms, and language
4. Level of understanding
5. Technology

It is a professional responsibility to transmit a correct, credible, properly delivered message. The appropriate communication channel must be selected, using the appropriate chain of command to convey the message. The correct format is essential for decision-making. One must decide whether to use an interdepartmental memorandum or a formal letter. The nature of the message dictates the format or type of communication. Correct grammar, terminology, and language are essential to present a professional image. Knowing the level of understanding of your intended audience is vital so that they can process the information. This means using the appropriate reading level and vocabulary. And finally, selecting the appropriate technology is important. Without the appropriate technology, recipients may not even receive your message and evaluation of the process should be ongoing.

Virtual Group Meetings

Groups are traditionally viewed as necessitating face-to-face meetings. This situation has changed. Technology now allows groups to meet electronically, whether in real time or asynchronously. Electronic communications have provided the means for **virtual meetings**, by which people connect with others not in the same physical environment. Virtual meetings can be used by work, educational, therapeutic, or professional groups. The group is still focused with a common goal, and members interact with some leadership to organize and maintain the group. Ideas can be exchanged, experiences and information shared, and a common concern discussed. Many nursing groups now have Web sites and provide opportunities for students and professionals in groups to "discuss" core issues. Clients can interact with other clients and professionals via e-mail, chat rooms, and scheduled Internet meetings.

Virtual groups meet the same characteristics as face-to-face groups, in terms of group structure (formal or informal), composition (membership), roles (leader as facilitator and participants), and focus (work-related, educational, therapeutic, or professional). The virtual group experiences the same five stages of group development—initial, conflict, norming, working, and termination. The same set of evaluation criteria can be used to assess effectiveness of the virtual group. The role of the leader is more intense as a facilitator in the group process. The leader must employ a variety of the group-building roles, time and distance being major considerations.

Like those of distance learning, the advantages of virtual meetings are savings in time and travel and, perhaps, the opportunity for involvement in which the travel distance would have been prohibitive. Because these groups do not meet face-to-face, preparation time and follow-up are more intensive to allow all group members to have equivalent information and participation opportunities.

Disadvantages of virtual meetings include the need for all members to have access to similar technologies and the individual's comfort level with their application. Analyzing the functional and nonfunctional roles of the members as virtual participants can be a bit challenging without the face-to-face assessment of interactions. The functional role of a participant can be identified in the text or content communicated, for example as information giver/seeker or elaborator. The nonfunctional members—dominator, monopolizer, blocker, aggressor, and recognition seeker—may appear to have a smaller impact (after all, members can delete their messages), but the leader must still address the underlying issues.

Any group—whether virtual or traditional, organizational, work, professional, educational, or therapeutic—demands the use of skills in observation, interpersonal communication, and group process that are essential characteristics of the involved professional nurse. These skills are tailored to the developmental stage of the group and the unique characteristics of its individual members. Professional nurses function as both members and leaders of such groups, and constant attention to these skills allows them to be integral components of effective groups in the profession and throughout the health-care delivery system.

INTERACTIVE EXERCISES

Go to the Intranet site and complete the interactive exercises provided for this Chapter.

EVIDENCED-BASED PRACTICE: CONSIDER THIS . . .

*T*he American Association of Critical-Care Nurses (AACN) issued a practice alert on severe sepsis. In addition to listing expected practices and the supporting evidence, they provide the following recommendations:

1. Educate all nursing staff on the risk factors and clinical signs
2. Create an interdisciplinary team to develop protocols or guidelines for the initial identification and management of the client presenting with signs of sepsis
3. Consider the development of a rapid response team. (AACN, 2006, p. 2)

Question: Consider the group process skills you will need for the three groups: (1) nursing staff education, (2) interdisciplinary work group, and (3) rapid response team.

Source: American Association of Critical-Care Nurses (AACN). (2006). *Practice alert: Severe sepsis.* Retrieved October 8, 2006, from *http://www.aacn.org/AACN/practiceAlert.nsf/Files/ss/$file/Severe Sepsis 04-2006.pdf*

KEY POINTS

■ A group consists of three or more individuals with some commonality, such as shared goals or interests. Groups to consider in professional nursing practice include professional, work, educational, family, and therapeutic groups, each with specific goals and membership.

■ Group process is described as the dynamic interplay of interactions within and between groups of humans.

■ Groups are classified according to structure (formal or informal), composition, group roles, and focus (professional, work, educational, and therapeutic).

■ The composition of a group may be homogeneous, with the group members sharing similar characteristics, or heterogeneous, with a mix of individuals.

■ The issues to be addressed in establishing a group are the need and objectives for change and basic setup activities, including specifying and aligning the group purpose with the intended membership and determining the appropriate environment and group size.

■ Effective groups are able to accomplish their goals in a manner that allows all members to participate, whereas ineffective groups become fragmented or dysfunctional.

(Key Points continue on page 154)

KEY POINTS (continued)

■ Group leaders structure the sessions to promote communication and participation by all members.

■ Conflict situations can arise in any type of group and conflict resolution is a process that requires problem-solving for effective group process.

■ Groups go through predictable developmental stages: forming, storming, norming, working, and adjourning. The leader modifies her or his approach according to the group's current stage.

■ Traditional group leadership styles are democratic, autocratic, and laissez-faire. Group leaders often use a combination of styles or modify their styles, depending on the group membership or topic being discussed.

■ Functional group roles facilitate the group process and the ultimate effectiveness of the group. They include both functional task roles and functional group-building roles. Nonfunctional group roles are disruptive of group-building, task accomplishment, and progress toward goal attainment.

■ Organizational groups may be interorganizational or intraorganizational, depending on whether they exist between organizational systems or within an organization.

■ Even though technology has provided the opportunity for virtual groups, group process skills are still applicable at a distance in a real-time or asynchronously.

Thought and Discussion Questions

1. Identify at least three groups of which you are a member. Consider the membership, goals, leader, composition, and focus of each group. What are the similarities and differences? Contrast the leadership styles and skills in the three groups.

2. Be prepared to discuss in class the advantages and disadvantages of heterogeneous and homogeneous groups.

3. Observe the members of the next departmental committee or nursing study group you attend.

   - Determine whether the group leader is the designated leader or a member who has assumed this role. If the leader was designated, who made the designation (external or internal designation)? Describe any effect this designation has had on the group function.
   - Describe the roles other members have assumed. Are the group roles different from these individuals' interactions in other settings?
   - Evaluate whether the members appear satisfied with the group's outcomes.
   - Evaluate whether this group or committee meets the characteristics of an effective group.

4. Review the Chapter Thought located on the first page of the chapter and discuss it in the context of the contents of this chapter.

☐ REFERENCES

Arnold, E. (2007). Communicating in groups. In E. Arnold & K. Boggs (Eds.), *Interpersonal relationships: Professional communication skills for nurses* (5th ed., pp. 260-287). Philadelphia: Saunders/Elsevier.

Bailey, J. R., & Yost, J. H. (2004). Role theory: Foundations, extensions, and applications. *BookRags*. Retrieved May 29, 2006, from *http://www.bookrags. com/other/sociology/role-theory-foundations-extensions—eos-04.html*

Berlo, D. K. (1960). *The process of communication: An introduction to theory and practice.* New York: Holt, Rinehart, & Winston.

The Conflict Resolution Network (CRN). (2003). *Conflict resolution skills.* Retrieved May 29, 2006, from *http://www.crnhq.org*

DeWine, S., Gibson, M. K., & Smith, M. J. (2000). *Exploring human communication.* Los Angeles: Roxbury.

Lundin, W., & Lundin, K. (1995). *Working with difficult people.* New York: American Management Association.

McKay, M., Davis, M., & Fanning, P. (1995). *Messages: The communications skills book* (2nd ed.). Oakland, CA: New Harbinger.

Smith, T. E. (2001). *Meeting management.* Upper Saddle River, NJ: Prentice Hall.

Streibel, B. J. (2003). *The manager's guide to effective meetings.* New York: McGraw-Hill.

Tappen, R. M. (2001). *Nursing leadership and management: Concepts and practice* (4th ed.). Philadelphia: F. A. Davis.

Tuckman, B. (1965). Developmental sequence in small groups. *Psychological Bulletin, 63,* 384–387.

Turniansky, B., & Hare, A. P. (1998). *Individuals in groups and organizations.* London: Sage.

Yalom, I., & Leszcz, M. (2005). *Theory and practice of group psychotherapy* (5th ed.). New York: Basic Books.

☐ BIBLIOGRAPHY

Arredondo, L. (2000). *Communicating effectively.* New York: McGraw-Hill.

Barnard, S. (2001). Running an effective meeting. In S. Barnard, P. J. Casella, C. Coffin, T. Hughes, J. W. Hurst, J. S. Rasey, D. Redding, R. J. Robillard, D. St James, & S. C. Ullery, *Writing, speaking, and communication skills for health care professionals* (pp. 293–304). New Haven: Yale University.

Berne, E. (1963). *The structure and dynamics of organizations and groups.* New York: Grove Press.

Blatner, A. (2006) *Role dynamics: An integrative approach to psychology and user-friendly language.* Retrieved May 31, 2006, from *http://www.blatner.com/adam/level2/roletheory.htm*

Corey, M. S., & Corey, G. (2002). *Groups: Process and practice* (6th ed.). Belmont, CA: Wadsworth.

Creighton, J. L. (2004). *Using group process techniques to improve meeting effectiveness.* Retrieved May 29, 2006, from *http://www.effectivemeetings.com/teams/teamwork/creighton.asp*

Dana, D. (2001). *Conflict resolution: Mediation tools for everyday worklife.* New York: McGraw-Hill.

Fisher, R., & Shapiro, D. (2005). *Beyond reason: Using emotions as you negotiate.* New York: Viking Press.

Galanes, G. J., Adams, K., & Brilhart, J. K. (2007). *Effective group discussion* (12th ed.). New York: McGraw-Hill.

Merton, R. K. (1957). *Social learning theory and social structure.* New York: Free Press.

Moss, S. A., & Ngu, S. (2006). The relationship between personality and leadership preferences. *Current Research in Social Psychology.* Retrieved May 31, 2006, from *http://www.uiowa.edu/~grpproc/crisp/crisp11_6.pdf*

☐ ONLINE RESOURCES

Social-Role Theory
http://changingminds.org/explanations/theories/social_role.htm

The Conflict Resolution Network (CRN)
http://www.crnhq.org

EffectiveMeetings.com
http://www.effectivemeetings.com

■ *Genevieve M.* **Bartol**

Critical Thinking

> **"** *The whole of science is nothing more than a refinement of everyday thinking.* **"**
>
> Albert Einstein, Physics and Reality, 1936

Chapter Objectives

On completion of this chapter, the reader will be able to:

1. Explain what the term critical thinking means.
2. Describe some important characteristics of the critical thinking process.
3. Discuss the relationships between the nursing process and critical thinking.
4. Apply the components of critical analysis to a given nursing practice situation.
5. Analyze problem-solving skills needed in nursing practice case studies.

Key Terms

Critical Thinking	Hypothesis Testing	Concept Formation
Reflective Thinking	Moral Reasoning	Interpretation of Data
Reactive Thinking	Induction	Application of Principles
Problem Identification	Deduction	Interpretation of Feelings, Attitudes, and Values
Data Collection	Assumption Identification	

Thinking is quite simply the action of the mind to produce thought. Critical has several connotations. Critical, for example, can be understood as an inclination to find fault, as a time or state on which something depends, as a point at which a crisis or change may occur, as an important or essential element, or as a careful analysis of a problem. What then is critical thinking? What images do these words, when combined, bring to mind? Do you visualize a person who finds fault with everyone and everything? Or do you imagine someone who ponders esoteric and weighty matters in ivory tower aloofness? You may see it as only the latest buzzword in nursing, one that was added to the tiresome emphasis on the nursing process in your undergraduate nursing program.

The proliferation of journal articles, monographs, essays, conference papers, and books devoted to exploring critical thinking in nursing testifies to the current interest but also suggests that a closer look at the term is warranted. We generally recognize that the professional practice situations that nurses encounter daily are characteristically complex, rapidly changeable, ambiguous, particular, and rife with conflict. We increasingly accept the fact that patients are dynamic systems within an energy field that includes family, workplace, environment, culture, and life history. We know that nurses base their practice decisions on a broad pool of knowledge derived from a variety of disciplines. One may then surmise that critical thinking is a special type of thinking essential for delivering holistic nursing care.

The concept of **critical thinking** dates back at least to Socrates in ancient Greece. Dewey (1910/1933) prompted educators to pay attention to how we think and to teach students how to think. Glaser's 1941 and Black's 1952 writings represent efforts to integrate clinical thinking into education (cited in Cassel & Congleton, 1993). Paul (1990) reviewed the efforts to teach reasoning in the 1930s and the 1960s. McPeck (1990) pointed out that before 1980 few schools were concerned with teaching critical thinking, and even fewer theoretical analyses of the concept existed. According to McPeck (1990), he had to search disparate sources to find any sustained published discussions of critical thinking (p. 1) when he researched the topic in 1979–1980. In 1990, Facione (1990) gathered a panel of 48 educators and scholars, including leading figures in critical thinking theory, to work toward a consensus on the role of critical thinking in educational assessment and instruction.

Facione and Facione (1996) reported that the expert researchers and theoreticians described critical thinking as the purposeful, self-regulatory judgment that results in interpretation, analysis, evaluation, and inference, as well as the explanation of the evidential, conceptual, methodological, criteriological, or contextual considerations on which that judgment was based (p. 129). Rubenfeld & Scheffer (1999, 2006) used a Delphi process to arrive at a consensus statement and the components of critical thinking. They determined that critical thinking is "an essential component of professional accountability and quality nursing care" (p. 357). They also identified 10 critical thinking habits of mind and seven critical thinking skills.

As you read this chapter, you will see that despite this statement, the literature is replete with definitions and descriptions of critical thinking. Nevertheless, Paul's (1990) description of critical thinking summarizes it best: "Critical thinking is the art of thinking about your thinking while you are thinking in order to make your thinking better: more clear, more accurate, and more defensible" (p. 44). With that in mind, we will expand upon and detail the context and role of critical thinking in nursing.

CRITICAL THINKING IN NURSING

Nurses have been taught to use the nursing process to guide their practice. The nursing process provides a structure for using knowledge and thinking to provide holistic care for individuals, families, groups, and communities. The process can be used with all theoretical frameworks and clients in all settings. Although its components may be expressed in slightly different ways, the nursing process is basically a problem-solving method that has served nurses well by helping them use empathic and intellectual processes with scientific knowledge to assess, diagnose, plan, implement, and evaluate nursing care and patient outcomes. When used appropriately, the nursing process involves critical thinking. For example, a nurse notices that a patient who underwent surgery two days before has suddenly become agitated. The nurse will consider several possible reasons for the agitation, such as a change in the order for pain medication or bleeding at the surgical site. She will speak with the patient, note anything that occurred prior to the onset of agitation, and gather assessment data, such as vital signs and signs of bleeding at the surgical site. She will determine what intervention is needed and then evaluate if the chosen intervention is effective. Using the nursing process in this manner requires active engagement and cannot just be a matter of filling in the columns. Rather, the person using the process must be able to recognize relationships, connections, and patterns that promote continuous bidirectional movement and openness to new possibilities.

New scientific understandings of living systems show that our former mechanistic view of the world is inadequate (Bartol & Courts, 2005). Human beings are complex, highly integrative systems that are embedded in and supporting other systems. Schuster (2002, p. vii) noted that the commonly used five-column format in nursing care plans were not promoting critical thinking. Care plans using this format were lengthy to write, time consuming, and too often directly copied from a book. Furthermore, the column format seemed to promote linear thinking and failed to address the patterns and connections essential to providing holistic nursing care.

Schuster proposed using a diagrammatic teaching-and-learning strategy to enable students and faculty to visualize the interrelationships among medical diagnoses, nursing diagnoses, assessment data, and treatments. In a three-step process, (Step 1) the major medical diagnoses and the problems that resulted from that diagnosis were identified, (Step 2) the data was organized into a hierarchy of subordinate concepts, and (Step 3) the meaningful associations among concepts were indicated with lines and the nursing diagnoses selected. Schuster called this strategy concept mapping and suggested that it promoted critical thinking. This visual map serves as a personal pocket guide to patient care that can be revised as needed throughout the day. The development of this process illustrates the use of critical thinking to promote critical thinking in students of nursing.

The increasing diversity and complexity of nursing practice and the exponential growth of knowledge require nurses who can think critically. Nurses must master the reasoning skills needed to process growing volumes of information. When nurses assess patients, the data they gather need to be organized into meaningful patterns. Responses to treatment and care need to be evaluated continuously to determine whether or not the nursing diagnosis was appropriate and the intended outcome achieved. Even one additional piece of information related to the patient may change the whole configuration and require redefinition of the problem. In nursing, situations change so rapidly that reliance on conventional methods, procedure manuals, or traditions to guide judgments about the appropriate nursing action required is insufficient.

Critical thinking requires attention to many factors. Complex legal, ethical, organizational, and professional factors are involved in seemingly simple decisions and require critical thinking skills. For example, nurses consider ethical factors (such as keeping patient information confidential) and scheduling factors (such as when to admit visitors) when they decide not to admit visitors to a unit between 10 a.m. and 12 noon because patients are participating in a support group in the commons room. Visitors passing by the commons room may compromise patient confidentiality.

Nurses make inferences, differentiate facts from opinions, evaluate the credibility of the sources of information, and make decisions, all skills that require critical thinking. Because each of these skills can be learned, at least to some extent, an individual can enhance her potential to become an effective critical thinker.

Nursing is sometimes described as a boundary discipline because it draws heavily on knowledge from the sciences and humanities. Using information from one subject to shed light on another subject requires critical thinking skills. Nursing is concerned with human beings who are highly complex integrative systems whose care requires a holistic orientation that attends to cyclic processes, patterns in networks of relationships, and not just signs and symptoms.

Conceptually, it may be argued that general critical thinking skills enhance the ability to make good clinical judgments. Nurses can apply theoretical knowledge to a specific clinical situation, thereby enhancing clinical judgment and decision-making skills. The ability to apply learning from a broad range of disciplines enables nurses to expand and modify existing knowledge to accommodate new situations as well as simplify or speed up the task of learning and performing in new situations. For example, nurses use critical thinking when applying knowledge of physics (principles related to levers, fulcrums, and balance), biology (characteristics of a bone in the early stages of healing), and psychology (ways of helping patients manage the anxiety related to increasing mobilization) when safely transferring a patient recovering from a serious car crash. Because educational programs cannot provide students with all of the clinical experiences and all of the information they need to handle every future nursing situation they will encounter, students must learn to be critical thinkers.

Critical thinking includes analyzing and evaluating the soundness of the written information and expressed opinions we encounter. We cannot assume that because the information is published that it is valid. We need to identify the strengths and weaknesses in the author's argument and the evidence that is

O N L I N E   C O N S U L T

The following website lists a number of questions that may help you critically evaluate what you read: **http://www.services.unimelb.edu.au/llsu/ resources/reading/read2.html** presented. We need to examine any assumptions the author may have made.

Definitions

What is critical thinking? Some nursing educators would argue that it is really the same as the nursing process (Jones & Brown, 1993; Kintgen-Andrews, 1991; White, Beardslee, Peters, & Supples, 1990; Woods, 1993). Others insist that although the nursing process requires critical thinking, critical thinking is much more. It is generally maintained, however, that critical thinking is a valuable skill or set of skills capable of being learned and enhanced (Facione & Facione, 1996, 2000; Rubenfeld & Sheffer, 2006; Schuster, 2002; Smith, 1990; Wilkinson, 2001).

Still, critical thinking is often considered a special, even rare, skill. Because the characteristics of critical thinking match those of sound clinical judgments (Case, 1994), critical thinking is viewed as a highly desirable skill. A review of the nursing literature indicates that there is no general agreement

about what critical thinking is. Definitions abound in the nursing literature; Table 9–1 gives a sampling. The definitions have common elements. Critical thinking is viewed as engaging in a purposeful cognitive activity directed toward establishing a belief or map of action. Each definition speaks to the need for a person to process and evaluate information actively, to validate existing knowledge, and to create new knowledge. Each echoes Dewey's (1933) urging to use **reflective thinking** of the kind that turns a subject over in the mind and gives it serious and consecutive consideration (p. 3). All are consistent with Dewey's definition of reflective thinking as active, persistent, and careful consideration of any belief or supposed form of knowledge in the light of the grounds that support it and the further conclusions to which it tends (Dewey, 1933, p. 9). All suggest using a thought chain (Dewey, 1993, p. 4) that aims at conclusions. Critical thinking is a process that is not engaged in for itself, but rather for the purpose of providing quality patient care. A thought chain refers to the process of moving methodically from one

Table 9.1

Definitions and Descriptions of Critical Thinking

Definition	Source, Date
"The rational examination of ideas, inferences, assumptions, principles, arguments, conclusions, issues, statements, beliefs, and actions" (p. 5).	Bandman and Bandman, 1995
"Reflective and reasonable thinking about nursing problems without a single solution and is focused on deciding what to believe and do" (p. 352).	Kataoka-Yahiro and Saylor, 1994
"A process and cognitive skill that functions in identifying and defining problems and opportunities for improvement; generating, examining, and evaluating options; reaching conclusions and decisions, and creating and using criteria to evaluate decisions" (p. 101).	Case, 1994
"Reasonable and reflective thinking that is focused on deciding what to believe or do" (p. 152).	Kingten-Andrews, 1991
"A process that encompasses a holistic perspective of the entire person—composed of skills, abilities, beliefs, attitudes, goals, emotions, and experiences. In addition, critical thinking involves the ability to view the situation from a holistic perspective" (p. 377).	Thurmond, 2001
"Critical thinking is the process of purposeful, self-regulatory judgment. This process gives reasoned consideration to evidence, contexts, conceptualization, methods, and criteria" (ERIC Document Reproduction No. ED 315).	Facione, 1990

thought to another while remaining open to multiple possibilities. Quite simply, one considers, reflects, decides, and yet remains open to change, always keeping in mind that one additional piece of data can change the whole configuration and send the process in a new direction.

Different elements are also evident in the definitions and descriptions offered in the nursing literature. Some seem to equate critical thinking with reactive thinking (Kataoka-Yahiro & Saylor, 1994; Kintgen-Andrews, 1991). **Reactive thinking** implies a response to what is, and not to what may yet be. Most view critical thinking as a focused, rational analysis of existing knowledge with very specific steps (Bandman & Bandman, 1995; Kataoka-Yahiro & Saylor, 1994; Kintgen-Andrews, 1991). One refers to creating new knowledge (Case, 1994), whereas another implies that only existing knowledge is uncovered (Bandman & Bandman, 1995). Jones and Brown (1993) examine alternative views on critical thinking, arguing that it is both a philosophical orientation toward thinking and a cognitive process characterized by reasoned judgment and reflective thinking (p. 72). Woods (1993) insists on the importance of recognizing the role feelings and attitudes have in critical thinking.

The discussion about critical thinking continues. The many definitions and descriptions suggest that consensus on the role of critical thinking in nursing has not been reached.

Descriptions

The following statements gleaned from the literature and the author's own thinking is an attempt to provide a fuller description of the role of critical thinking in nursing.

- Critical thinking is directed toward taking action. Although it is often associated with scientific reasoning, which includes **problem identification**, **data collection**, and **hypothesis testing**, it is not limited to that activity. Critical thinking also includes the affective processes of **moral reasoning** and development of values to guide decisions and actions (Woods, 1993).
- Critical thinking presumes a disposition toward thinking analytically. Uncritical acceptance of all data is antithetical to critical thinking. An attitude that welcomes intellectual skepticism and honesty is essential. Separating or breaking the whole into parts to uncover the nature, function, and relationships is helpful as long as one maintains a sense of the whole.
- Critical thinking embraces thinking about how we think. We need to monitor our approach to the problem and our reasoning process. An error in

reasoning may be as serious a barrier to finding a solution as a miscalculation in determining a proper drug dose. We should critique the process as well as the proposed solution. Bandman and Bandman (1995) identify fallacies or errors in thinking that one should identify, expose, and resist. To illustrate: A nurse reports that all the laboratory tests for a patient came back negative and implies, therefore, the patient's symptoms must be "all in her head." The fallacy of the appeal to ignorance consists in arguing that in the absence of proof against a diagnosis establishes proof that the patient's symptoms are imaginary.

- Critical thinking assumes maturity. Psychology reminds us that our thinking styles evolve as we grow and develop. We think concretely before we think abstractly. The ability to think abstractly is requisite to critical thinking. We accept many beliefs as children simply because an adult told us they were true. Only as we grow do we question and examine those beliefs. We need to reach the place where we have confidence in our reasoning abilities.
- Critical thinking requires knowledge. A broad educational foundation and a healthy intellectual curiosity are prerequisite. A solid educational foundation needs to be informed by common sense and experience as well as knowledge of one's own biases and limitations (Alfaro-LeFevre, 2003). A zealousness in seeking knowledge and understanding through careful observation and deliberate questioning with openness to possibilities is essential (Rubenfeld & Scheffer, 2006).
- Critical thinking requires skills. We need to know how to gather and evaluate data. We need to distinguish facts from opinions and probe the assumptions behind a line of reasoning. We need to know how to draw inferences from facts and observations, evaluating them as tenable or not. Precision is key. Knowing a fact is insufficient; we need to know how that fact was obtained and from where it was derived. We need to identify what data is missing. Throughout the process, we need to suspend judgment until all the evidence is weighed, even as the situation requires tentative action. There are many ways to view a problem. The way we view a situation influences our proposed solutions.
- Critical thinking, however, is more than a set of skills. Syllogistic thinking, inductive and deductive reasoning, analysis, and synthesis are used, but other styles of thinking are also needed. According to Lonergan (1977), the imagination is the highest function of the intellect and precedes all other thinking activities. Certainly, critical thinking uses imagination. Using a metaphor such as a computer or a holograph to

describe a function of the brain, for example, can provide additional insight into the process. Critical thinking is creative. We reach original solutions by drawing from past experiences and making creative applications to new situations.

- Critical thinking includes feelings because they are inseparable from all thinking and behavior. Feelings cannot be eliminated or viewed as an inconvenience that complicates the activity of critical thinking, but are an integral part of all we do. Our feelings can alert us to possibilities and lead us to creative solutions. To illustrate: A busy staff nurse realized that she could not take time to listen to an elderly patient who began to tell her about his career as a pilot beginning in the 1930s. He was describing in detail the early planes he piloted. Anxious to meet the needs of her other patients, she told the patient that she had to take care of her other patients, but that she knew someone who would very much like to hear what he had to say. With his permission, she dialed her teenage son who aspired to become a pilot and handed the patient the phone. The patient and her son talked for almost two hours to the benefit of both.

- Critical thinking frequently involves finding fault. Questions, disagreements, and even arguments may be included in the process. Critical thinking always challenges the status quo. Seeking the truth, even if the consequences are contrary to one's assumptions and beliefs, is essential.

- Critical thinking considers the complexity and ambiguity of issues. At the same time, critical thinking seeks to identify the essential elements and exclude whatever is irrelevant to the matter being considered. Valid conclusions cannot be drawn or appropriate action taken unless one knows what is to be considered.

- Critical thinking is a contextual activity. We must be aware of our own context and how it influences our thinking. Our social environment, past and present, may bias our thinking, and we must be aware of how this occurs and deal with it appropriately. We do not think in a vacuum.

- Critical thinking is inseparable from language because it is applied to language and expressed through language (Smith, 1990). Attention should be directed to the meaning of words. Words often acquire connotative meanings that over time may differ radically from their original meanings.

- Critical thinking is not always a self-conscious activity. We may not be aware of being engaged in critical thinking, or even alert to its absence. Moreover, we often unconsciously work on problems and reach solutions without knowing precisely how we arrived at them until we reflect on the process. Intuition is frequently an invaluable guide in highly stressful situations.

- Critical thinking is not an esoteric activity. It is something everyone does to some degree at least some of the time. Written guidelines, decision trees, algorithms, and critical pathways formalize the critical thinking process but cannot contain it wholly. Thinking critically is not just a solitary activity. We expose our beliefs and actions, and the thinking that helped us arrive at those beliefs and actions, to the scrutiny of others. We invite this criticism in different ways, for example, by sharing with colleagues in a discussion or writing a report. We often need others to help us see our errors.

- Critical thinking is a habit that improves with proper use and withers with disuse. In the beginning, we use structure to guide our practice. As we gain proficiency, structure diminishes, but we must continue practicing to improve or even maintain our ability to think critically. Following established protocols in a crisis situation may be helpful, but can interfere with recognizing new data.

- Critical thinking includes reflection or contemplation. That is, it requires giving serious thought to a situation with the clear knowledge that even one small additional piece of data may change the whole configuration.

All of these characteristics of critical thinking are present during the process of critical thinking. We may be more conscious of one particular characteristic at a specific point during the process, but the others remain in the background, influencing the outcome.

Measures of Critical Thinking

How do you know if you are thinking critically? Evaluation takes into account the purpose for which the information is gathered, and then a suitable technique is chosen. Many paper-and-pencil objective tests have been designed to measure generic competency in critical thinking, but not specifically in nursing. The Watson-Glaser Critical Thinking Appraisal (W-GCTA), the California Critical Thinking Inventory, and the Cornell Critical Thinking Tests, Level X and Z, are the most widely known and used (Norris & Ennis, 1989). The central aspects of critical thinking—**induction, deduction,** and **assumption identification**—are included in all three, but only the California Critical Thinking Inventory (Facione, Facione, & Sanchez, 2000) attempts to measure the disposition toward critical thinking. These tests, however, are limited and are used mostly for research and not primarily to measure achievement. Probably the best way to increase your critical thinking ability is to critique how you are thinking and practice critical thinking.

DEVELOPING CRITICAL THINKING SKILLS

Critical thinking skills can be developed. Nursing is a practice discipline. A body of knowledge is gained from classes and study and applied in the clinical setting. Information drawn from personal experience in the clinical setting informs this body of knowledge. None of the knowledge in either setting is obtained automatically. Information must be cultivated, organized, and conscientiously arranged by using critical thinking.

Raingruber and Haffer (2001) suggest four strategies that nurses can use to develop critical thinking skill. First, nurses can reflect on accounts of other nurses' clinical experiences. The narratives may be in the form of oral or written accounts and may include anything from a simple story of a clinical event to a detailed case study. Such activities enable you to reach across time and space to broaden your base of knowledge before you encounter those experiences in your clinical practice.

Second, nurses can develop critical thinking skills by applying Brookfield's (1995) three critical thinking processes:

- Securing contextual awareness and determining what needs to be observed and considered
- Exploring and imagining alternatives
- Questioning, analyzing, and reflecting on the rationale for decisions

Third, use mind maps as a visual learning tool. Associations that play a major role in nearly every mental function help you to identify the key elements in a situation and prompt you to generate solutions. For example, you anticipate an assignment in a clinical setting in which you have not previously worked. You are experiencing some anxiety prior to the assignment. You recall being in a similar situation in the past and take steps to reduce your anxiety. You may call a friend for support, review appropriate material in a nursing text, imagine several scenarios that you may encounter during the assignment, and visualize successfully providing quality care to your patients. Briefly, you would rehearse caring for your patients in your mind in anticipation of providing actual care.

Fourth, you can keep a journal of your clinical experiences, noting your concerns about how you coped with particular situations and your reflections about what you could do to improve the care you delivered. Opportunities to reflect in writing help to clarify meanings and promote increased understanding. Examining your reasoning and actions in writing reinforces learning and enables you to draw on knowledge gleaned from this activity in future clinical situations. Even a brief recording of the verbal exchange you had with a patient can help you gain insight into your style of communication and what you can do to improve.

Critical thinking can also be enhanced through the arts. In their psychiatric mental health textbook, Frisch and Frisch (2006) used literary excerpts, movie clips, and classic art pieces to stimulate critical thinking and self-exploration. In doing so, the authors encourage readers to enter the client's world to understand the process and effects of psychiatric disturbances on an individual's overall health and functioning.

Readers are encouraged to examine how their own personal views and feelings influence their delivery of care.

THE NURSING PROCESS AND CRITICAL THINKING

Nurses can also develop a meaningful concept of information and material needed to practice nursing by using logical steps of the nursing process. Taba (Maleck, 1986) identifies four teaching phases necessary for developing critical thinking. Three phases—concept formation, interpretation of data, and application of principles—focus on the cognitive domain. The fourth phase speaks to the affective domain, and entails interpretation of feelings, attitudes, and values.

1. **Concept formation**: Concept formation is similar to the nursing process. First, the nurse needs to identify known data, determine common characteristics, and prioritize data.
2. **Interpretation of data:** Next, nurses are encouraged to differentiate between pieces of information, determine cause-and-effect relationships among variables, and extract meaning from what they observed. These first two logical phases or steps in thinking prepare nurses for the third phase:
3. **Application of principles:** Nurses analyze the nature of the problem or situation. It is important to note that nurses do not ask the analytic "why" questions until this application phase. The premature use of "why" questions produce deductive conclusions, rather than inductive alternatives. The question, "Why does an infection cause an elevated temperature?" tends to lead to a rote response culled from classroom lectures or the textbook. Conversely, a thought-producing question such as *"What factors related to an elevated temperature suggest infection?"* encourages nurses to sift and combine cognitive knowledge to understand an important clinical concept. Only after defining the problem are nurses able to isolate the relationship among the data. Once these relationships are

established, nurses can apply factual information to predict an outcome based on cognitive principles. This approach is not unlike the nursing process. Avoiding "why" questions and asking "what factors," however, helps the nurse avoid the trap of drawing premature conclusions.

4. **Interpretation of feelings, attitudes, and values**. The fourth phase involves principles of interpersonal problem-solving and analysis of values. This activity, although less concrete than the other three phases, is imperative for determining the nature of attitudes and perceptions developed through one's life experiences. For example, a nurse's concern about a rising temperature in a patient taking haloperidol (Haldol) may be provoked by a past experience with a patient who was taking the drug and developed neuroleptic malignant syndrome. At this point, the nurse needs to gather additional data to confirm or rule out the possibility that the rising temperature is a sign of malignant hyperthermia in the present patient, and not leap to a premature conclusion. Additionally, the nurse must be open to other possible explanations for the elevated temperature. Appropriate action is then taken, including gathering additional data when indicated. Once again, this approach helps prevent the common pitfall associated with using the nursing process, which is drawing conclusions based on a formula that does not allow for different possibilities. In other words, it avoids the trap of fitting the patient into the textbook model.

These phases have been described in terms of steps, but they can occur almost simultaneously. Sequencing and pacing questions are essential in critical thinking. Sequencing questions is important because the processes of thought evolve from the simple to the complex. Clinical instruction should follow a carefully sequenced set of experiences and questions. As mentioned earlier, asking "why" questions prematurely would only bring premature closure. The principle of pacing allows nurses to match questions to their levels of readiness and cognitive ability. To accommodate pacing, nurses must pursue each question long enough to permit a variety of responses. In this way, they become active participants in the thinking process, and not simply vessels for facts.

A closer look at the nursing process shows that following it appropriately involves critical thinking. The five steps of the nursing process are:

1. Assessment
2. Diagnosis
3. Planning
4. Implementation
5. Evaluation

This process provides a framework for identifying and treating client problems. The nursing process is an ongoing and interactive cycle that results in flexible, individualized, and dynamic nursing care for all clients. Assessment is the foundation of the process and leads to the identification of both nursing diagnoses and collaborative problems. Nursing diagnosis provides the primary focus for developing client-specific individualization of client goals. The planning process allows for individualization of client goals and nursing care within the context of managed-care guidelines. Implementation involves providing nursing actions to treat each diagnosis. Ongoing evaluation determines the degree of success in achieving the client goals and the continued relevance of each nursing diagnosis and collaborative problem.

The implementation of the nursing process requires complex clinical and diagnostic knowledge and application of critical thinking skills. One needs to be able to think outside of the box, rather than apply readymade formulas gleaned from textbook information. Textbook information is often based on the mythical average and can only serve as a general guide; individuals are much more varied. Learning and applying these skills is a continuing challenge for the nurse and requires much practice. If the nurse uses the diagnostic reasoning process appropriately, the result will be effective nursing interventions leading to desirable patient outcomes.

Nurses must be critical thinkers because of the nature of the discipline and their work. Nurses are frequently confronted with problem situations; critical thinking enables them to make sound decisions. During the course of a workday, nurses are required to make decisions of many kinds. These decisions often determine the health of patients and even their very survival, so it is essential that the decisions be sound. Critical thinking skills are needed to assess information and plan decisions. Nurses need good judgment, for example, to decide what they can manage and what should be referred to another health-care provider. Nurses deal with rapidly changing situations in stressful environments. Treatments and medications are modified frequently in response to a patient condition. Routine behaviors are often inadequate to deal with the complex circumstances. Familiarity with the routine for giving medications, for example, does not necessarily help you intervene appropriately with a client who is afraid of injections. When unexpected complications arise, critical thinking ability helps nurses recognize important cues, respond quickly, and adapt interventions to meet specific needs.

Nurses use knowledge from other subjects and fields. Using insight from one subject to shed light on another subject requires critical thinking skills.

BOX 9.1 Critical Thinking with the Nursing Process

Assessment

- List the significant assessment findings: Objective and Subjective.
- Cluster the significant assessment data by functional health patterns.
- What general problem areas does the patient have?
- Develop data clusters for each of the general problems identified.

Nursing Diagnosis

- From the clustered data, develop at least two diagnostic hypotheses using accepted nursing diagnosis labels.
- Evaluate each of the diagnostic hypotheses by writing and comparing the definitions and applicable defining characteristics of each diagnosis.
- Write complete nursing diagnosis statements, by priority.

Planning

- Plan appropriate nursing interventions.

Implementation

- Implement appropriate nursing interventions.

Evaluation

- Evaluate the outcomes.

EVIDENCED-BASED PRACTICE: CONSIDER THIS . . .

*U*se of critical thinking in nursing involves careful and effective assessment skills. One of the NGC (2002) guidelines calls for a detailed health assessment and personal history for the person with chronic constipation. Following this, planning and intervention activities are recommended to address toileting habits, position, facilities, lifestyle considerations, and pharmacological factors.

Question: How will you use your critical thinking skills in concept care mapping for this individual?

Source: National Guideline Clearinghouse. (NGC) (2002). Practice guidelines for the management of constipation in adults. Retrieved October 7, 2006, from *http://www.guideline.gov/summary/summary.aspx?doc_id=3687&nbr=2913*

Because nurses deal holistically with human responses, they must draw meaningful information from other subject areas to understand the meaning of client data and plan effective interventions. Nurses need knowledge from neurophysiology, social sciences, psychology, and nutrition, for example, to assist patients effectively who are severely depressed.

Case studies offer us excellent opportunities to use critical thinking. The following case study contains data about Mr. Jones, a patient admitted to the same-day surgery unit for repair of a right inguinal hernia. The nurse must use critical thinking in determining appropriate data collection, assessment, nursing diagnoses, and interventions for the care of the patient and his family. Clearly, critical thinking is used in every step of the nursing process as nurses collect, cluster, and analyze data and formulate nursing diagnoses. Critical thinking enables the nurse to provide high-quality care that is appropriate, individualized, creative, sensitive, and comprehensive. In determining the appropriate care for Mr. Jones, it would be helpful for the nurse to organize her thoughts and actions as illustrated in the case study at the end of the chapter.

INTERACTIVE EXERCISES

Go to the Intranet site and complete the interactive exercises provided for this Chapter.

| CASE STUDY | Mr. Jones |

𝓕ollowing is a case study on which you can practice your critical thinking. An analysis of the case study is located on the book's Intranet site.

Case Study

Health History and Range of Symptoms

Mr. Jones is a 45-year-old, married man, employed as a supervisor with Parrish Construction Company. He is brought by his wife to the same-day surgery unit for a presurgery assessment the day before his scheduled surgery. His breath smells of alcohol.

Chief Concern: "I need to get this surgery over with. We have a big job to do at work, and it will be my butt if it is not completed on schedule. I plan to cut down on my drinking. I know I drink too much sometimes, but it's because of the pain from this thing." (Patient points to area of hernia.)

History of Present Illness: Mr. Jones was sent by the nurse, from the construction company to the surgeon, Dr. Judge. Mr. Jones had experienced periodic pain and swelling in his right groin area for at least five years and several times has seen the employee health physician, who told him he had a right inguinal hernia that should be repaired. He admits to experiencing decreased appetite and insomnia for the past 10 days.

Social and Family History

Mr. Jones's father died of cirrhosis at the age of 52 years. His mother is 80 years old and has a history of diabetes. Mr. Jones is the youngest of six children. One brother died at birth, another died at age six of a tumor, and a third brother was a heavy drinker. Two sisters are alive and well.

Mr. Jones has been married to his second wife for nine years; they have no children. His second wife has three boys, aged 12, 14, and 16 years, who live with her first husband and have no contact with Mr. and Mrs. Jones.

Mr. Jones has five children by his first marriage; all are alive and well, living with his first wife. He pays $50 a week for child support for each child. The children visit him every other weekend.

There is no family history of tuberculosis, hypertension, epilepsy, or emotional illness.

Review of Systems

General: No current change in weight and usually feels good, except when the hernia acts up.
Skin: No symptoms.
Eyes: He wears glasses for reading.
Ears: No symptoms.
Nose: No symptoms.
Mouth and Throat: Experiences recurrent episodes of hoarseness. Denies dysphagia.
Neck: No symptoms.
Respiratory System: Denies pain, dyspnea, palpitations, syncope, and edema.
Gastrointestinal System: Reports eating only three "good meals" during the past 10 days. Appetite is good when not drinking. Denies food intolerance, emesis, jaundice, flatulence, diarrhea, constipation, and melena.
Genitourinary System: No symptoms.
Neurological: See "History" and "Interview with Significant Other."

(case study continues on page 166)

CASE STUDY Mr. Jones (continued)

Physical Examination

Mr. Jones is a 45-year-old white man with dark complexion and a ruddy face who appears chronically ill. He is mildly intoxicated and appears anxious. Weight is 136 pounds; height is 5 feet, 10 inches; temperature is 98.8°F, pulse is 92; and regular respirations are 20 and unlabored; blood pressure is 160/90.

Skin: Well hydrated and without lesions.

Head: Normocephalic.

Eyes: PERRLA. Vision corrected with glasses. Visual acuity decreased to 3 mm print at 18 in. on the left and 4 mm print at 18 in. on the right. Extraocular movements full; no nystagmus is noted. Visual fields are intact as tested per confrontation. Conjunctivae are slightly injected. Sclerae clear. Lenses are without opacities bilaterally. Funduscopic examination reveals the discs normally cupped, and no vascular changes bilaterally.

Ears: External ears symmetrical, without lesions. Otic canal is clear. Tympanic membrane pearly gray bilaterally. Hearing is within normal limits per watch tick at 6 in.

Mouth and Throat: Lips, tongue, and buccal mucosa are pink and moist. Teeth are brown, crooked. Gingivae are atrophic. No inflammation of posterior nasopharynx.

Nose: Nasal septum in the midline. Nares are patent bilaterally. Sinuses not tender.

Neck: Full mobility and no significant lymphadenopathy. Thyroid not enlarged, without nodules.

Chest: Bony thorax is without deformity or tenderness. Respiratory movement is full, and diaphragmatic excursion is adequate bilaterally. Lungs are clear to percussion and auscultation.

Cardiovascular: The PMI is in the fifth intercostal space of the LMCL. NSR without murmurs or gallops.

Abdomen: Abdomen is soft and flat. Bowel sounds are heard in four quadrants. Liver is descended 5 cm below the costal margin. No splenomegaly, tenderness, or mass. Surgical scar present in right lower quadrant.

Genitourinary: Normal male genitalia. No hernia palpated.

Rectal: Internal and external hemorrhoids noted at 5 and 7 o'clock. Normal sphincter tone. Anal canal free of tenderness. Prostate is in the midline, firm without nodules, not enlarged.

Extremities and Back: Muscular development symmetrical. Normal in appearance, color, and temperature. Peripheral pulses palpable and symmetrical. Free of varcosities or edema.

Neurological: Speech is slurred, sensorium somewhat cloudy. Cranial nerves II through XII are intact as tested per gross screen. Moderately tremulous. Biceps, triceps, brachioradialis, patella, and Achilles reflexes are symmetrical but brisk. Babinski's are down bilaterally.

Significant Laboratory Findings

Blood alcohol level: 0.29 U/L; Stool guaiac: negative; ECG: sinus tachycardia, otherwise WNL; Chest x-ray: no active chest disease; Coulter-S: Hgb 16.0 g/dL (H), HCT 48.2% (H), MCV 101 m3 (H); CL 92 mEq/L (L); Uric acid 8.04 mg/dL (H), SGOT 90 U/L (H); Liver panel: GGT 66 IU/L (H); and urine: bacteria 21, WBC 8–12

Interview with Significant Other

According to Mrs. Jones, Mr. Jones works out of town from Monday morning to Thursday evening. When he returns home, he begins to drink. He does not drink during the workweek. Mrs. Jones related the following incidents of the past 10 days, which occurred when her husband was intoxicated: ran all of the children out of the home into the rain, scuffled with brother-in-law, and brandished a shotgun after an argument. Mrs. Jones reports that she left her husband in June but returned to him about four weeks ago. She has never attended Al-Anon, but has reviewed information from the Alcoholism Information Center. This is the second marriage for Mrs. Jones; her first husband and her father were alcoholics. ■

KEY POINTS

■ Critical thinking has been defined and described by many scholars. It is multifaceted and involves a combination of logical, rhetorical, and philosophical skills and attitudes that promote the ability to determine what we should believe and do.

■ Critical thinking is essential for professional nursing practice. The need for critical thinking in nursing has greatly increased with the diversity and complexity of nursing practice. Reflective thinking is "active, persistent, and careful consideration of any belief or supposed form of knowledge in the light of the grounds that support it and the further conclusions to which it tends" (Dewey, 1933, p.9).

■ Reactive thinking implies a response to what is, and not to what may yet be.

■ Critical thinking is often associated with scientific reasoning, which includes problem identification, data collection, and hypothesis testing, but it is not limited to these activities.

■ The central aspects of critical thinking are induction, deduction, and assumption identification.

■ Concept formation is similar to the nursing process. First, the nurse needs to identify known data, determine common characteristics, and prioritize data.

■ Interpretation of data occurs when nurses differentiate between pieces of information, determine cause-and-effect relationships among variables, and extract meaning from what they have observed.

■ Application of principles occurs when nurses analyze the nature of the problem or situation and apply factual information to predict an outcome based on cognitive principles.

■ Interpretation of feelings, attitudes, and values requires interpersonal problem-solving and analysis of values.

Thought and Discussion Questions

1. Give an example from your clinical practice for five of the descriptive statements of critical thinking.

2. Select a nursing issue, such as an open visiting policy in the surgical intensive care unit or family presence during a code, and engage in a debate with a peer.

3. Select a problem at your place of work. Explore a solution to the problem with the help of a peer with whom you work. Analyze the problem-solving process you used to address the problem.

4. Review the Chapter Thought located on the first page of the chapter and discuss it (online or in class) in the context of the contents of the chapter.

REFERENCES

Alfaro-LeFevre, R. (2003). *Critical thinking and clinical judgment: A practical approach* (3rd ed.). Cambridge, MA: Elsevier Science.

Bandman, E. L., & Bandman, B. (1995). *Critical thinking in nursing* (2nd ed.). Norwalk, CT: Appleton & Lange.

Bartol, G. M., & Courts, N. F. (2005). The psychophysiology of bodymind healing. In B. M. Dossey, L. Keegan, & C. E. Guzzeta, *Holistic nursing: A handbook for practice* (4th ed., pp. 111–133). Sudbury, MA: Jones and Bartlett.

Brookfield, S. (1995). *Becoming a critically reflective teacher.* San Francisco: Jossey-Bass.

Case, B. (1994). Walking around the elephant: A critical thinking strategy for decision making. *The Journal of Continuing Education in Nursing, 25*(3), 101–109.

Cassel, J. F., & Congleton, R. J. (1993). *Critical thinking: An annotated bibliography.* Metuchen, NJ: Scarecrow Press.

Dewey, J. (1933). *How we think.* New York: D. C. Heath. (Original work published 1910)

Facione, P. (Project director). (1990). Critical thinking: A statement of expert consensus for purposes of educational assessment and instruction. *The Delphi Report: Research findings and recommendations prepared for the American Philosophical Association* (ERIC Doc. No. ED 315 423). Washington, DC: ERIC.

Facione, N. C., & Facione, P. A. (1996). Externalizing the critical thinking in knowledge development and clinical judgment. *Nursing Outlook, 44,* 129–136.

Facione, N. C., & Facione, P. A. (2000). *Critical thinking assessment in nursing education programs: An aggregate data analysis.* Millbrae, CA: Academic Press.

Facione, N. C., Facione, P. A., & Sanchez, C. A. (2000) *Test manual: The California critical thinking skills test.* Millbrae, CA: California Academic Press.

Frisch, N. C., & Frisch, L. E. (2006). *Psychiatric mental health nursing* (3rd ed.) United States: Thomson, Delmar Learning.

Jones, S. A., & Brown, L. N. (1993). Alternative views on defining critical thinking through the nursing process. *Holistic Nursing Practice, 7*(3), 71–76.

Kataoka-Yahiro, M., & Saylor, C. (1994). A critical thinking model for nursing judgment. *Journal of Nursing Education, 33*(8), 351–356.

Kintgen-Andrews, J. (1991). Critical thinking and nursing education: Perplexities and insights. *Journal of Nursing Education, 30,* 152–157.

Lonergan, B. (1977). *Insight, a study of human understanding.* New York: Harper & Row.

Maleck, C. J. (1986). A model for teaching critical thinking. *Nurse Educator, 11*(6), 20–23.

McPeck, J. E. (1990). *Teaching critical thinking.* New York: Routledge.

Norris, S. P., & Ennis, R. H. (1989). *Evaluating critical thinking.* Pacific Grove, CA: Midwest Press.

Paul, R. W. (1990). Critical thinking: Fundamental for a free society. *Educational Leadership, 41,* 44.

Raingruber, B., & Haffer, A. (2001). *Using your head to land on your feet: A beginning nurse's guide to critical thinking.* Philadelphia: F. A. Davis.

Rubenfeld, M. G., & Scheffer, B. K. (1999). *Critical thinking in nursing: An interactive approach.* Philadelphia: Lippincott Williams & Wilkins.

Rubenfeld, M. G., & Scheffer, B. K. (2006). *Critical thinking tactics for nurses.* Sudbury, MA: Jones and Bartlett.

Schuster, P. M. (2002). *Concept Mapping: A critical-thinking approach to care planning.* Philadelphia: F. A. Davis.

Smith, F. (1990). *To think.* New York: Teachers College Press.

Stafford, J. (1953). The interior castle. In *The children are bored on Sunday* (pp. 205–217). New York: Harcourt, Brace.

Thurmond, V. A. (2001). The holisim in critical thinking: A concept analysis. *Journal of Holistic Nursing, 19*(4), 375–389.

White, N. E., Beardslee, N. Q., Peters, D., & Supples, J. M. (1990). Promoting critical thinking skills. *Nurse Educator, 15*(5), 16–19.

Wilkinson, J. M. (2001). *Nursing process and critical thinking.* Saddle River, NJ: Prentice-Hall.

Woods, J. H. (1993). Affective learning: One door to critical thinking. *Holistic Nursing Practice, 7*(3), 64–70.

☐ BIBLIOGRAPHY

Adams, B.L. (1999). Nursing education for critical thinking: An integrative review. *Journal of Nursing Education, 38*(3), 111–119.

Barnet, S., & Bedau, H. (2004). *Critical thinking, reading and writing: A brief guide to argument.* New York: Bedford/St. Martins.

Beckie, T. M., Lowry, L. W., & Barnett, S. (2001). Assessing critical thinking in baccalaureate nursing students: A longitudinal study. *Holistic Nursing Practice, 15*(3) 18–26.

Birx, E. C. (1999). Critical thinking and theory-based practice. In J. W. Kenney (Ed.), *Philosophical and Theoretical Perspectives for Advanced Nursing Practice* (2nd ed., pp. 309–314). Boston: Jones and Bartlett.

Bitner, N. P., & Tobin, E. (1998). Critical thinking: Strategies for clinical practice. *Journal for Nurses in Staff Development, 14,* 267–272.

Brown, J. M., Alverson, E. M. (2001). The influence of a baccalaureate program on tradition, RN-BSN, and accelerated students' critical thinking abilities. *Holistic Nursing Practice, 15*(3), 4–8.

Browne, M. N., & Keeley, S. M. (2003). *Asking the right questions: A guide to critical thinking.* Upper Saddle River, NJ: Person Education.

Castillo, S. L. (2005). *Strategies, techniques, & approaches to thinking: Critical thinking cases in nursing* (3rd ed.). Cambridge, MA: Elsevier Health Sciences.

Chafres, J. (2005). *Thinking critically.* Boston: Houghton Mifflin Company, College Division.

Duchscher, J. E. B. (1999). Catching the wave: Understanding the concept of critical thinking. *Journal of Advanced Nursing, 29,* 577–583.

Gladwell, M. (2006). *Blink: The power of thinking without thinking.* Essex, England: Little, Brown & Company.

Green, C. J. (2000). *Critical thinking in nursing: Case studies across the curriculum.* Upper Saddle River, NJ: Prentice Hall.

Jones, D. (1998). *Exploring the Internet using critical thinking skills.* New York: Neal-Schuman.

Locsin, R. C. (2001). The dilemma of decision-making: Processing thinking critical to nursing. *Holistic Nursing Practice, 15*(3), 1–3.

Nelms, T. P., & Lane, E. B. (1999). Women's way of knowing in nursing and critical thinking. *Journal of Professional Nursing, 15*(3), 179–186.

Nosich, G. M. (2004). *Learning to think things through.* Upper Saddle River, NJ: Prentice-Hall.

Nugent, P. M. (2004). *Fundamentals success: A course review applying critical thinking to test taking.* Philadelphia: F. A. Davis.

Porter, K. A. (1930). The jilting of Granny Weatherall. In *Flowering Judas and other stories* (pp. 80–89). New York: Harcourt, Brace.

Smith-Stoner, M. (1999). *Critical thinking activities for nursing.* Philadelphia: Lippincott Williams & Wilkins.

Spelic, S.S., Parsons, M., Hercinger, M., Andrews, A., Parks, J., & Norris, J. (2001). Evaluation of critical thinking outcomes of a BSN program. *Holistic Nursing Practice, 15*(3), 27–34.

☐ ONLINE RESOURCES

Maricopa Community College
http://www.mcli.dist.maricopa.edu/forum/fall01/tl.html

Prince George's Community College
http://academic.pg.cc.md.us/~wpeirce/MCCCTR/

The Foundation for Critical Thinking
http://www.criticalthinking.org/

■ *Rose* **Kearney-Nunnery**

Teaching-Learning Process

> **❝** *To achieve a lasting change in observed behavior, the value of that change and the intellectual capacity to understand and process the information must first be present.* **❞**
>
> Author

Chapter Objectives

On completion of this chapter, the reader will be able to:

1. Discuss the components of teaching and learning.
2. Examine differences in the ways people learn.
3. Describe methods to assess learning readiness and motivation.
4. Propose different teaching methods for a variety of learning needs.
5. Devise a plan for client education that contains behavioral objectives, a content outline with appropriate teaching methods, and methods for evaluating learner outcomes.

Key Terms

Behaviorist Perspective	Andragogy	Psychomotor Domain
Classical Conditioning	Transformative Learning	Learning Environment
Operant Conditioning	Multiple Intelligences	Cognitive Learning Styles
Gestalt Theory	Teaching	Readiness
Cognitive Theories	Learning	Motivation
Social Cognitive Theory	Affective Domain	Behavioral Objectives
Humanism	Cognitive Domain	

Teaching and learning are integral parts of contemporary nursing practice. Client or patient teaching has long been an expected nursing role. As a process, teaching and learning are much more than sharing and accepting information. There are many components to consider in order for teaching and learning to be effective.

NURSING PROCESS APPLIED TO TEACHING-LEARNING PROCESS

Consider the steps in the nursing process: assessment, diagnosis, outcome identification and planning, implementation, and evaluation. These same steps are applicable to the teaching and learning process.

Assessment

Think about both the learner and the teacher. They represent more than simply the provider and receiver of information. Communication—verbal, nonverbal, and written—is a vital component in the teaching and learning process. It is a mutual process in which critical thinking is essential for both teacher and learner. Both teacher and learner obtain information, use reasoning skills, make analyses based on the data, and then move to decision-making or problem-solving on the learning need. The learner learns from the teacher. But the teacher also gains awareness and skill from each interaction with learners. In the assessment stage, there is essential information we need to know for an effective teaching-learning process. Some of the following questions arise:

- What are the attributes of each individual teacher and learner?
- Are there literacy, bilingual, or information processing issues to be addressed?
- What are the learning needs of the learner?
- How does he or she learn?
- What is the readiness for and motivation to learn?
- What changes in behavior or attitude are perceived as being needed by both the teacher and the learner?
- What individual characteristics will enhance or inhibit learning?
- What is the teacher's teaching style?
- What is the cognitive style of the learner?
- What environmental factors will enhance or inhibit learning?
- What activities and resources will enhance learning?
- How can both the teacher and the learner evaluate the effectiveness of the learning process?

Assessing for a learning deficit or teaching need incorporates many factors. Notice that the concentration of the assessment is on the process of teaching and learning, not on specific content to be included in a presentation of information. Determining content is a discrete task performed later in the process, on the basis of specific attributes and needs of the people and environment. Using this assessment information can lead to a *Diagnosis* about the learner's particular teaching need.

Outcome Identification, Planning, and Implementation

Next, developing behavioral objectives gives direction for a teaching plan and evaluation of the learning. Teaching strategies, methods, and resources to meet the diagnosed learning need, with specific content. Then, plan and implement.

Evaluation

The outcomes of the teaching-learning process are evaluated. The evaluation component focuses on how the learner met the objectives and the specific outcome behaviors from the experience. Outcome objectives should be assessed by both the learner and the teacher. Evaluation is focused on the behavioral objectives specified for the learner earlier in the process. Although the nursing process provides a frame of reference for client teaching, teaching and learning theories provide direction in the process.

TEACHING AND LEARNING THEORIES

Educators have studied learning theories for many years to understand and improve on the teaching-learning process. There are several schools of learning theories. Major examples of these theories applicable to professional nursing practice are behaviorism, gestalt, social cognitive theory, humanism, andragogy, transformative learning, and multiple intelligences (Box 10–1).

Box 10.1 Selected Theories of Learning

- Classical conditioning
- Operant conditioning
- Gestalt theory
- Cognitive development
- Social cognitive theory
- Humanism
- Andragogy
- Transformative learning
- Multiple intelligences

Behaviorism: Classical Conditioning

In introductory psychology courses, classic stimulus-response conditioning and operant conditioning are taught, providing a **behaviorist perspective** on learning. Pavlov's pioneering research with dogs led to our understanding of **classical conditioning**, in which the reflexive responses in behavior result from some stimulus. In classical conditioning, we saw that the pairing of food (the unconditioned stimulus) with the sound of a bell as a neutral (conditioned) stimulus led to salivation in dogs as an unconditioned response—first as an unconditioned response for the sight of the food, and ultimately as a conditioned stimulus with the sound of a bell alone. Using classical conditioning with infants, John Watson provided further insight on learning with his focus on the environment and emotional responses. Watson was a true behaviorist, looking at the development of the emotions of fear, love, and rage through classical conditioning and desensitization in his research with children.

Use of classical conditioning in nursing practice is limited. One situation may be in teaching clients to intervene as needed in response to physiologic or emotional cues, auras, or triggers before an allergic, metabolic, or neural response. The individual with diabetes, a severe allergy, or epilepsy can be taught to perceive and make the association with early signs or symptoms that could lead to a larger physiologic reaction. Classical conditioning is useful for early intervention to circumvent the reaction chain. Reflexes are important in this scenario to ensure that the individual is in a safe environment and has the resources for prompt treatment. Another example is the use of distraction, focusing, and breathing in certain reflexive situations—for clients in labor, in pain, or experiencing fear, for example.

Behaviorism: Operant Conditioning

Operant conditioning provides further clues to learning, with a focus on purposive behaviors and the role of reinforcement. In Thorndike's law of effect, reinforcement of a behavior is more likely to lead to repetition of that behavior. B. F. Skinner's research with rats and reinforcers for learned behaviors provided much additional information. In **operant conditioning**, the behavior is affected by the consequences (reinforcer), but the process is not trial and error (Skinner, 2003, p. 1). This theory introduced positive and negative reinforcers and reinforcement schedules to learning. The work of Skinner led to behavior modification programs and programmed instruction with shaping, reinforcement, and generalization of behavior.

Behavior modification programs are widely used in health care and education. They have been used effectively in certain nursing situations, such as nutritional programs that require a lifelong change in behavior. In such situations, old patterns are broken, stimuli are introduced to effect positive outcomes, responses are generalized to specific dietary items, positive and negative reinforcements are applied, and behavior is shaped over time. Another use for behavioral techniques is with adult clients who have urinary incontinence. One method of treatment includes bladder retraining with the components of education, scheduled voiding, and positive reinforcement.

Behaviorism focuses on observation and measurement of actions in response to some association or conditioning. Rigorous use of the scientific process in the laboratory setting was a major factor in this perspective. Dissatisfaction with the emphasis on conditioning and reinforcement led to the evolution of other perspectives, including gestalt theory, cognitive theories, social learning theory, and humanism. In these later perspectives, we see an increased focus on the human intellect and human emotions.

Gestalt Theory

Gestalt theory focuses on meaning and thought, holding that learning occurs through perception. In the German tradition, a "gestalt" is perception of a whole form rather than its component parts. More than 100 laws on this perspective evolved with the identification of major principles concerning the way we perceive objects related to organization, proximity, similarity, direction, simplicity, background, and closure. Gestalt theorists view learning as based on perception of and completion of patterns. Patterns are perceived and reorganized by the person. In terms of learning, this perspective focuses on how the learner perceives the information and her environment. Kurt Lewin's field theory provided a major influence in this perspective with the emphasis on the importance of the environmental field. The perception of this environmental field by the person influences how that person, as a system, responds within the larger environmental system.

The classic principle in the gestalt perspective is that the whole is not merely the sum of the parts. This principle is consistent with the holistic view of human beings in professional nursing practice. Consider the importance we place on understanding how the person views the information to be learned. This involves teaching materials that are used in addition to perceptual values. Further consider the learning environment and the importance we place on client teaching in an unrushed, private, and comfortable setting when teaching (or promoting change for) specific health practices, as opposed to the hectic clinic environment where the person is distracted by children playing in the waiting room.

Cognitive Theories

Cognitive theories of learning focus on the intellect and the development of knowledge. Recall the example of Piaget's theory of cognitive development from Chapter 3. Schemas were seen as patterns of thought or behavior that become more complex with the addition of more information. *Assimilation* is the acquisition of this information and incorporation into the individual's existing cognitive and behavioral structures. *Accommodation* is the change in the individual's cognitive and behavioral patterns based on the new information acquired. This acquisition of information is learning with the comprehension of concepts, memory, and analysis.

There are many different cognitive theories, mostly focusing on information processing. In nursing practice, use of cognitive theory is readily apparent with our focus on the level of cognitive development and acquisition of health-care knowledge. We use principles of cognitive development to tailor a teaching plan to the client's level of development, whether the client is an elderly diabetic or a child. We are also concerned about the way learners process information, so that we can tailor our teaching strategies to suit their learning styles. In addition, the use of behavioral objectives with our clients provides a focus for developing cognitive skills, moving from recall of knowledge to understanding, application, analysis, evaluation, and creation, as we will see later in the revised taxonomy table (Anderson et al., 2001) that stemmed from the classic work of Bloom's (1956) taxonomy.

Social Cognitive Theory

Cognitive learning through observation and imitation was the basis of Bandura's early theory known as the Social Learning Theory. Through the research of Bandura and his associates, aggressive and socialization behaviors of children were documented after observation of both symbolic and actual models. An important aspect of Bandura's work is the modeling of behavior with television and the effect of visualizing vicarious reinforcement and punishment for behavior. A humanistic, rather than mechanistic, orientation is apparent in this theoretical focus. Bandura (1977) explained the emphasis of vicarious, symbolic, and self-regulatory processes on how humans learn and influence their own destiny. Building on this broader focus on the person, behaviors, and the environment with the concept of self-regulation, Bandura proposed the expansion to the **Social Cognitive Theory** in the 1980s. Since that time, Bandura has incorporated self-efficacy, a theory important to clients in the health-care setting as well as in normal activities. "Efficacy beliefs influence how people think, feel, motivate themselves, and act" (Bandura, 1995, p. 2). Bandura (1995) further identifies four sources of efficacy beliefs: mastery experiences,

vicarious experiences, social persuasion, and physiological and emotional states (pp. 3–5). Efficacy can have a powerful effect as individuals take ownership of their individual learning needs.

Nursing applications of the social cognitive theory are prevalent in the development of psychomotor skills in clients, such as self-administration of medications, procedures, and treatments. We often demonstrate skills to clients in person and expect them to return the demonstration. We provide positive reinforcement in the coaching function during the process, by making comments such as, "That's good," "That's the way," and "What a nice job." We promote healthful practices with encouragement and the hope for positive results as a reinforcement for the behavior. We show clients videos on a procedure in which they see modeling and reinforcement through a case scenario. These nursing behaviors focus on the individual in the environment as a thinking, feeling, and reacting being. Further, the concept of self-efficacy has long been used in nursing research and practice as we strive for the client to move toward independence and positive health-care outcomes. The identified sources of efficacy are consistent with nursing practice with a greater focus on the individual as we promote mastery of skills, use of vicarious experiences in teaching, social persuasion in health promotion activities, and in all cases of practice, have the physiologic and emotional states of clients integrated in the plan of care.

Humanism

Humanism has provided a major perspective on learning and one that has led to revision of older models. In this perspective, the focus is totally on the person. Abraham Maslow and Carl Rogers were major influences on this learning theory. As Maslow (1971) stated:

> The humanistic goal . . . is ultimately the "self actualization" of a person, the becoming fully human, the development of the fullest height that the human species can stand up to or that the particular individual can come to. In a less technical way, it is helping the person to become the best that he is able to become. (p. 169)

The full range of human experiences is considered, as personally experienced and interpreted. Maslow's humanistic focus included motivation as a vital concern. Humanism is the basis of Carl Rogers's person-centered counseling. As described by his daughter, Rogers "above all, valued the worth and dignity of the individual and trusted their capacity for self direction if given the proper environment" (Rogers & Freiberg, 1994, p. iii). Personal growth and autonomy are key to the humanistic perspective.

The humanistic perspective is consistent with the concepts of professional nursing. We focus on the person and assist in empowering him for health (whether an emerging state or to a higher level), therefore focusing on the consumers of health care and advocating for their active involvement in the health promotion process. The environment should be considered in terms of the person and his unique environmental setting and culture. Self-direction and insight into personal beliefs, attitudes, lifestyle, and behaviors are fundamental to the learning process. Culture, literacy, and learning or information processing deficits are also vital considerations with this perspective. As viewed in the health models in Chapter 5, cultural perspectives as a way of life must be included in any useful and humanistic teaching-learning plan. In addition, for effective teaching and learning to occur, deficits in learning or information acquisition or processing are humanistic factors that must be discovered, along with an understanding of adaptive patterns. Most consumers of nursing care are adults: parents, couples, individual adult or aging clients, families, community groups, and even professional peers with unique learning needs and characteristics.

Adult Learning Theories

Learning in adults requires the teacher to make adjustments to meet the different characteristics of learners. Adult learners differ from children in that they have past experiences, good and bad, with both teaching and learning.

Malcolm S. Knowles, who was a major force in adult learning in the United States, focused on **andragogy**. The term *andragogical model* was borrowed from European education (Knowles, 1990; Knowles et al., 1985). Expanding the traditional pedagogical learning models used with children to incorporate learning characteristics and needs of adults, this developmental model proposes that the accumulated life experiences of adults give them different teaching and learning needs from younger learners. In the pedagogical model, learners are generally dependent or passive, have few prior experiences to build on, and have external pressures from parents and others to learn something (Knowles et al., 1985, pp. 8–9). Adult learners are self-directing, have experiences that have shaped their identity, have experienced life events or a learning need that triggers their readiness to learn, have internal motivators, and demand an available, knowledgeable resource to assist them with practical problems and identified needs (Knowles et al., 1985).

As Knowles and associates (1985) have pointed out, adult learners often initially assume the comforting and passive learner roles of pedagogy, but then an inner conflict develops with their self-directing nature. The adult's ego system is based on his self-concept and accumulated knowledge and experiences, whereas a child is gratified by impressing a parent, teacher, or peer. Knowles's developmental focus is demonstrated further with his identification of life problems by age group in early, middle, and later adult life groups. He specified life problems in the areas of vocation and career, home and family life, personal development, enjoyment of leisure, health, and community living (Knowles, 1990). Recall Bandura's (1995) sources of self-efficacy (mastery experiences, vicarious experiences, social persuasion, and physiologic and emotional states) that are consistent with this view.

Adult teaching and learning depend on both physical and psychological climates. Physical climate relates to the learning environment. The set-up of the room should not replicate a stilted lecture setting and should promote comfort so that the learners can focus on learning needs and problem-solving. Knowles emphasized the need for adults to feel at ease in the learning environment, which leads to the psychological climate for the adult learner. Knowles identified seven characteristics of the psychological climate conducive to adult learning: mutual respect, collaborativeness, mutual trust, supportiveness, openness and authenticity, pleasure, and humanness (Knowles et al., 1985, pp. 15–17). Knowles viewed the teacher as the catalyst and facilitator. A common thread running through teaching and learning strategies for adults is mutuality, mutuality in diagnosing, planning, learning, and evaluating. One key to successful teaching and learning in adults is their active involvement throughout the process.

On the basis of Knowles's work, Vella further identified 12 principles for effective adult learning. Then, she further considered six concepts from quantum thinking (relatedness, holism, duality, uncertainty, participation, and energy) and reinforced the following 12 principles with adult education, especially in the use of dialogue to promote optimal learning:

- Participation of the learners in their needs and resources assessment
- Safety in the environment and the process
- Sound relationships between teacher and learner
- Careful attention to sequence of content and reinforcement
- Praxis: action with reflexion or learning by doing
- Respect for learners as decision makers
- Holistic ideas, feelings, and actions
- Immediacy of the learning (relevancy)
- Clear roles and role development (participation in the search for meaning)
- Teamwork and use of small groups
- Engagement of the learners in all domains of what they are learning

- Mutual accountability for the learning. (Vella, 2002, pp. 30–35)

These principles are consistent with our holistic view of clients as unique individuals with respect for their environment. It is critical to promote their empowerment to address their distinctive health-care learning needs. The actions must be meaningful to them for learning to occur.

Transformation Theory

The basis for transformative learning is meaningfulness of experiences, especially for adults who have accumulated knowledge, cultural and environmental patterns, and experiences. Think about the last time you said to yourself, "I'm not going to do that again!"

One of the major theorists in this area is Mezirow (2000) who defines **transformative learning** as follows:

> . . . the process by which we transform our taken-for-granted frames of reference (meaning perspective, habits of mind, mind-sets) to make them more inclusive, discriminating, open, emotionally capable of change, and reflective so that they may generate beliefs and opinions that will prove more true or justified to guide action. (pp. 7–8)

Transformative learning involves three stages: critical reflection of the situation, changing and integrating the new perspective and understanding, and acting on that new understanding. The key is the active and rational process of reflective thinking on past experiences and personal assumptions of the situation. Mezirow (2000) describes this process as reflective discourse: that specialized use of dialogue devoted to searching for a common understanding and assessment of the justification of an interpretation or belief" (pp. 10–11). This use of dialogue with adult learners is similar to the one described by Vella and can be used effectively in individualized or small group learning environments as adults are actively challenged to find meaningfulness of the information.

Critical reflection involves challenging one's assumptions and beliefs. Do they still hold true, or perhaps there is a better way and one that is acceptable to the adult learner in his or her context? This active and thoughtful process is personally determined. This theory of learning has been described as a "theory in progress" as further research evolves. In addition, a current nursing model has evolved from this theory (Fawcett, 2006, p. 504). Transformation theory is consistent with nursing's view of the person as a thinking, feeling, rational being with past experiences and attributes that influence behavior. But notice, the learners are the active ones in the process. They are assisted with the information for critical reflection, but they must challenge their "habits of mind" and "resulting points of view" that Mezirow (2000) refers to as the two components of one's "frame of reference" (p. 17). Then the person must decide whether to take action on the revised perspective as the transformation.

Adult learning theories have evolved from a humanistic philosophy, focusing on the unique combinations of talents and abilities possessed by an individual based on prior learning, skill sets, and contextual factors.

Multiple Intelligences Theory

Another theory of learning focused on the person proposes **multiple intelligences** (Gardner, 1993a, 1993b, 1999), all of which are considered equally important and are most often found in combination in individuals to differing degrees. This theory looks beyond cognitive capacity and encourages a view of the individual's cognitive profile. The basis for the theory is Gardner's observations of and work with children, adults, prodigies, and gifted, normal, autistic, brain-damaged, and autistic savant individuals. Gardner (1999) has characterized the seven different multiple intelligences as shown in Table 10–1 according to eight criteria, two each derived from the biological sciences, logical analysis, developmental psychology, and traditional psychological research. From his original work, Gardner (1999) refined his definition of an intelligence as:

> A biopsychological potential to process information that can be activated in a cultural setting to solve problems or create products that are of value in a culture. (pp. 33–34)

The theory of multiple intelligences allows a greater focus on the individual and her unique talents and combinations of abilities in their contextual setting. As Gardner (1999) points out, "what matters is the use of intelligences, individually and in concert, to carry out tasks valued by a society" (p. 208). In addition, "owing to hereditary, early training, or in all probability, a constant interaction between these factors, some individuals will develop certain intelligences far more than others; but every normal individual should develop each intelligence to some extent, given but a modest opportunity to do so" (Gardner, 1993a, p. 278). Gardner has thought about additional intelligences but, considering his criteria, has not yet definitively added to the list of seven. He does emphasize the importance of values and that "any intelligence can be put to a constructive or a destructive use" (Gardner, 1999, p. 45).

Consider for a moment that you will be caring for two clients following hip replacement surgery and are planning discharge teaching. One client is an architect who designs custom homes and meets with his customers for at least an hour before he develops the house plans to ensure that he truly understands their desires and

Table 10.1

Seven Intelligences (Gardner, 1999, pp. 42–43)

Intelligence	Description	Example(s)
Linguistic	Language and verbal	Poets, writers, speakers
Logical-mathematical	Mathematical cognitive skills in logic, mathematics, and science	Mathematicians, scientists
Spatial	Use of mental models of spatial world; manipulation of patterns	Sailors, engineers, artists, pilots, architects
Musical	Innate musical sense and talent in performance, composition, and appreciation	Musicians, composers
Bodily kinesthetic	Use of body or parts of the body in problem-solving	Dancers, athletes, craftspeople, mechanics
Interpersonal	Understanding intentions, motivation, and desires of others	Politicians, salespeople, teachers, clergy
Intrapersonal	Understanding of self and one's life course	Self-awareness

ideas. The other is a retired English professor who is concerned about the rehabilitation schedule and the completion of a collection of essays that he must submit to the publisher in six weeks. Your approach to each will differ on the basis of their unique talents and abilities.

The perspective of multiple intelligences is humanistic, focusing on the unique combinations of talents and abilities possessed by an individual. These unique individual abilities are consistent with the practice of nursing dealing with the individual and environmental influences. Given the variety of learning theories, however, application may involve selecting a more eclectic approach. Specific teaching guides involve our

ONLINE CONSULT

Gardner at
http://pzweb.harvard.edu/Pls/HG.htm

Maslow at
www.maslow.com

Skinner at
www.bfskinner.org

Or for more information on the different theories, visit:
http://tip.psychology.org

consideration of human beings and the environment, given the particular health focus in contemporary nursing practice. Certain principles provide direction in this process.

TEACHING AND LEARNING PRINCIPLES

The philosophical and theoretical structures of any discipline reflect how the teacher and learner are viewed. In nursing, we view both the teacher and the learner as thinking, reasoning, active participants involved in the teaching-learning process. We believe individuals are influenced by and influence their environment. These environmental influences, including persons, events, and tangible surroundings, must be taken into account when any teaching behavior is considered. In terms of health, teaching in nursing reflects information to promote or maintain the highest level of health attainable. The teacher's and the learner's definitions of health and wellness influence physical, psychological, emotional, and spiritual health as personal determinants of behavior.

Teaching

Although the teaching-learning process is an interactive communication process, its component parts must be considered. With this in mind, several processes can be seen readily as inherent in the teaching-learning process, such as communication and critical thinking. **Teaching** is more than the transmission of information. The information must be received, understood, and evaluated by the learner. Teaching has been described as "an intentional and reasoned act" (Anderson et al., 2001). Benner (1984) has identified the teaching-coaching function of the expert nurse working with acutely ill patients:

1. Use timing to capture learning readiness and motivation
2. Assist with integration of learning into lifestyle
3. Demonstrate an understanding of client's own interpretation of the situation
4. Provide interpretations of situations and rationales for new behaviors
5. Show, through example, coaching behaviors in culturally sensitive issues. (pp. 77–94)

These characteristics demonstrate the active roles of both teacher and learner in the process. Readiness and motivation must be present for both the teacher and the learner during the process. The best teachers are those who truly believe in the information they are sharing and can communicate this belief. They provide the excitement, or at least some reinforcement, for the learner, who wants to know more. The active role of the learner in the process is vital, because passive learning rarely results in persistent change in attitudes or behaviors. The motivation of teacher and learner are also important, as the teacher demonstrates an understanding of the learner's unique characteristics and perspective on the subject or situation. Providing information is the traditional role of the teacher, but doing so in the context of the learner's reality helps provide a rationale for behavior changes. Finally, coaching through example, with sensitivity, is the essence of expert teaching and nursing.

Teaching is an interactive process, not a unidirectional transmission of information. As Benner demonstrates in her examples of expert nurses, we also learn from those we teach.

Learning

Learning is the perception and assimilation of the information presented to us in a variety of ways. Learning contains the following characteristics:

- Perception of new information
- Initial reaction to the information
- Ability to recall or repeat the information (simple knowledge level)
- Rejection or acceptance of the information (understanding)
- Use of the information in a similar situation (application)

An increasing complexity emerges here as the learner moves from receiving and recalling information through:

Understanding

⇓

Application

⇓

Analysis

⇓

Evaluation of the knowledge acquired and *creation* of new applications

- Critical analysis of the information
- Incorporation of the information into the value system (evaluation)
- Use of the information in various situations and combinations (creation)

We see this process in the client who accepts information on the importance of breast familiarity, is able to perform the self-examination, does so on a regular basis in combination with mammography and clinical examinations, teaches her daughter or mother the process, and is now investigating regular screening for colon cancer for herself and family members. This client has moved from simple knowledge to incorporation of knowledge into the value system and behaviors of herself and other family members.

Learning can be enhanced with specific strategies or approaches with learners. Gagne views learning in a hierarchy of complexity that leads to nine instructional events and corresponding learning:

- Gaining attention
- Informing learners of the objective
- Stimulating recall of prior learning
- Presenting the content
- Providing learning guidance
- Eliciting performance
- Providing feedback
- Assessing performance
- Enhancing retention and transfer (Gagne & Medsker, 1996)

Note that this appears to be a linear process, but it fails to take into account the client in her environment and culture, and the various domains of learning. Consider the difference between the knowledge and the consistent demonstration of behaviors. We may "know" something but either consciously or subconsciously decide not to demonstrate that behavior. For example, a client may have been prescribed a low-fat diet and can tell you all about foods with high fat content, but may also decide that ice cream is a part of the diet, ignoring its fat content.

Domains

A domain is merely a category. There are three domains of learning or knowledge: affective, cognitive, and psychomotor.

The **affective domain** includes attitudes, feelings, and values. For example, how the client feels about the importance of or the positive effect on his life of a needed dietary change will influence whether he will make the change. Often, the nursing goal is to incorporate the value of the diet into the person's belief system. Cultural influence, cultural differences in the individual, family, or group, and the nurse's professional influences can all either positively or negatively affect whether the goal is achieved, however.

The **cognitive domain** involves knowledge and thought processes within the individual's intellectual ability. Using the same example of the client and the low-fat diet, the cognitive domain involves understanding the information received about nutrition, diet, health conditions, and indications. The ability to conceptualize types of foods, gram counts, and dietary needs involves comprehension, application, and synthesis at an intellectual level before the client performs the actual behaviors.

The **psychomotor domain** is the processing and demonstration of behaviors; the information has been intellectually processed, and the individual is displaying motor behaviors. To continue with the example, psychomotor skills are demonstrated by how the client has performed on the changed diet, as seen in food diary reporting, preparing and ingesting appropriate foods, and even laboratory reports evaluating bodily functions.

It is important to consider these three domains in the teaching-learning process. Behavioral objectives, teaching content and methods, and evaluation of learning can be very different for the three domains and should be distinct. Remember, to achieve a lasting change in observed behavior (psychomotor domain), the value of that change (affective domain) and the intellectual capacity to understand and process the information for behavioral changes (cognitive domain) must first be present.

Consistent with the philosophical focus of nursing, the **learning environment** is important in any teaching or learning activity. Physical comfort as well as respect and acceptance of the learner are humanistic factors. The consumer of health care may also have physical, sensory, or psychological deficits that can interfere with comfort in the learning environment or in the teaching-learning process, as seen in the physiologic and emotional source

of self-efficacy proposed by Bandura. Comfort measures should be validated with the client before and during the process. Physical comfort can include such things as the temperature of the room and the height or firmness of the chairs, in addition to specific effects of acute or chronic health problems. Sensory concerns include the extraneous sensory stimuli perceived by the teacher or learner in the learning environment, such as sounds, smells, and sights. In addition, the client may have sensory deficits—such as visual, hearing, or information processing problems—that may interfere with learning or may require more resources. Psychological deficits, including fear, problems with cognition, attention span, effects from medications, and worry, can be major inhibitors to teaching and learning. Receptivity of the learner to new and different ideas is vital. Creative measures taken by the teacher to provide for an environment conducive to learning are essential.

To achieve a lasting change in observed behavior (psychomotor domain) the value of that change (affective domain) and the intellectual capacity to understand and process the information for behavioral changes (cognitive domain) must first be present.

COGNITIVE LEARNING STYLES

The *cognitive learning process* is a broad area that examines how meaning is perceived, evaluated, remembered, reinforced, and demonstrated. Piaget gave us information on childhood cognition through observations of his own and other children and provided us with the concepts of assimilation and accommodation. Recall that assimilation is the acquisition and incorporation of new information into the individual's existing cognitive and behavioral structures, and accommodation is the change in the individual's cognitive and behavioral patterns based on this new information. Cognitive learning styles have been discussed with varied research for over 50 years in an attempt to improve teaching and learning outcomes.

In the mid-1980s, Kolb (1981) identified specific learning styles as concrete experience, reflective observation, abstract conceptualization, and active experimentation. And the research and the discussion continue as we seek to understand better how individuals acquire meaning and knowledge. Increasingly we are concerned with the active involvement of the learner in the process, for learning to truly occur. **Cognitive learning styles** or preferences are simply the ways learners perceive, think, organize, use, and retain knowledge. To understand this concept, merely recall colleagues in the same learning environment—those who took copious notes, those who just listened, and those who made notes or drawings on what they interpreted the message in the lecture to be. Understanding the differences in cognitive styles can help teachers and learners make more informed decisions about which learning activities will be useful or productive to learners as individuals and as members of learning groups or communities.

Stemming from a basis in Jung's theory of the unconsciousness and personality, the Myers-Briggs Inventory was developed and has been used widely in education and business applications for learning styles. This personality inventory uses the following four scales to identify 16 personality types that can be further classified for learning preferences:

- Introversion–Extroversion
- Sensing–Intuition
- Thinking–Feeling
- Judging–Perceptive

Check your style with a similar inventory at
**http://www.humanmetrics.com/
cgi-win/JTypes2.asp**

Teaching and learning strategies have developed to match the learner with the teaching resources most effective for his learning style or to develop strategies to adjust to the prevalent teaching style. The main types of learning styles look at preferences for visual learning (reading or watching), auditory (listening or talking), and kinesthetic (doing or participating). For example, some learners are highly visual in the way they perceive information and derive meaning. For these learners, a structured lecture with few visual aids is a less desirable learning environment than one enhanced by visual aids. Others learn better through the written word, either by reading or note-taking. Learners who are highly auditory in their learning preference derive greater meaning from just listening to the information. The theory of multiple intelligences can be useful in this situation, to tailor the learning further to the individual's talents.

Assessment data on learning style may be obtained from the client in a nursing interview rather than formal testing inventories used with larger groups. In essence, good assessment of the learner is vital to ensure the most effective teaching and efficient and enjoyable learning.

READINESS AND LEARNING

Readiness is an important concept in learning, regardless of the learner's chronologic age. **Readiness** relates to the developmental needs and tasks of individuals. Consider the views of two developmental theorists: Erikson (1963) described readiness as critical periods, whereas Havighurst (1972) referred to readiness as sensitive periods or the "teachable moment." For teaching to be effective and learning to take place, the readiness of the learner must be a prime consideration. A good example is the issue of compliance and noncompliance in the client group.

Compliance is an often misused and misunderstood concept. We talk about patients being noncompliant when they do not follow their discharge or health-care teaching. The reasons and background for the behavior in the client group must first be realized and understood, not assumed. Compliance is yielding to the desire of others, possibly as a result of threats or force. But as we see later in the change process, threats and force do not bode well for a permanent change in behavior. Human behavioral change is more effective when one is personally involved in the process. Specifically, how do learning and readiness apply to receiving and accepting information for a change in lifestyle? Consider the teenager undergoing dialysis who carefully monitors his sodium intake after dialysis but fills up on fast food the day or morning before the scheduled dialysis. Is this truly noncompliance or developmental maneuvering with peer pressure and dietary restrictiveness? Now consider the adult cardiac client with a strict dietary sodium restriction. Is noncompliance by this individual due to a stubborn adherence to food preferences, culture, or custom, or perhaps failed health teaching for change because of a failure to achieve learning readiness?

The learner must be willing to change and accept the learning need. When this occurs, readiness for learning is apparent. This can be seen in terms of King's (1981) theory of goal attainment: Both the nurse and the client must be focused on and sensitive to the same goal. Readiness for the learning and teaching is then present. Ultimately, the effectiveness of the teaching methods and content is evaluated on the basis of the learning that did or did not take place. Learning readiness involves the following factors: human motivation, understanding or cognitive level, and applicability or acceptability.

Literacy and language issues are an additional consideration in readiness. For the individual with a low literacy level, years of adaptive behavior may disguise the inability to read basic information. Likewise, an individual who speaks English as a second language may perceive information differently. In each situation, the individual may be unwilling to indicate to the nurse that he did not fully understand or accept the information presented. The readiness to learn is inhibited by additional factors in these cases.

Motivation

Motivation in humans is a manifestation of internal and external personal and environmental factors that cause people to respond to a situation in the way that they do. Motivation has been classically viewed as needs, drives, and impulses that cause behavior. One view of motivation in humans is Maslow's Theory of Human Motivation, based on the hierarchy of basic needs. Maslow (1954) identified 16 propositions about human desires or motivation that implied a complex interrelationship in human motivation based on internal and external factors as personally interpreted by the individual. Maslow's work indicated that the hierarchy of human needs is based on motivation. But motivation is as intricate as the person, not merely inherent impulses and drives. And even more focused on the individual, Bandura (1995) proposes that efficacy beliefs play a key role in the self-regulation of motivation in that people motivate themselves and guide their actions anticipatorily by the exercise of forethought and they form beliefs about what they can do (p. 6).

The concept of motivation, then, considers the person's interpretations of the situation and her ability and willingness. Readiness, therefore, involves motivation and understanding. *Understanding* is the cognitive ability to perceive and intellectualize the content and consequences of information. Bandura believes that most actions are under anticipatory control, as humans use symbolic representation to envision future outcomes of behavior. The way the person views these future consequences of behavior becomes the motivation to behave or proceed in the present. This concept relates well to health teaching, in that the client can be motivated to learn with a realistic anticipation of the situation and consequences. Nurses can recognize client anticipation in the assessment phase, through interview data, diagnosis of the teaching and learning needs, and development of behavioral objectives. During this process, motivation can be assessed and stimulated by the client as well as by the professional nurse.

Cognitive Level

A person's cognitive level is a component of understanding; the content provided must be at the person's level of understanding. Piaget's theory of cognitive development describes the differences in learning levels between the sensorimotor infant developing object permanence and the older child who is able to learn abstract mathematical skills through formal operations. Information must be available to the person at his cognitive level for processing and development of knowledge. The person may require concrete examples to envision future consequences or may be able to handle more abstract or even philosophical examples. An important consideration here is the client's state of health. Current physiologic or psychological functioning and medications may interfere with reasoning and understanding as well as the attention span. Readiness for health teaching in this instance may be at different levels, depending on physical and emotional functioning.

Applicability and Acceptability

Another component of readiness for the teaching-learning process is applicability and acceptability of the information. The person must perceive that the information is applicable to him, as an individual, a member of the family, or a member of a group. If the person denies that a health problem exists, he will not be ready for health teaching in that area. The information is not perceived as personally applicable. *Acceptability* means that the information must be within the person's worldview. Cultural influences are important, because values and belief systems influence understanding and acceptability of information. The health problem and readiness must be seen in the context of the individual's belief system. This is an important relationship, as we see in the health belief model. Cultural assessment data provide important information on the client's belief system that should be incorporated into the teaching-learning process.

PRACTICAL TEACHING TIPS

Developing behavioral objectives sets the stage for the teaching-learning process. Objectives lead to the planning phase with selection of appropriate teaching strategies and methods, and evaluation of both the learning outcomes and the teaching process.

Writing Behavioral Objectives

The purpose of writing **behavioral objectives** is to provide a frame of reference for the intended outcomes of the teaching-learning activity for both the teacher and the learner. The use of behavioral objectives gives us a focus on learners and evaluation of their experiences with specific measures for behaviors. Behavioral objectives are the intended outcomes of the learners, not teacher's goals for the activity.

Think of behavioral objectives in terms of the learner's "who, what, where, when, and how." In viewing the individual components of behavioral objectives, consider those listed at the start of this chapter. Initially, there is the stem statement, "On completion of this chapter, the reader will be able to . . ." This provides the "who"—the reader of the chapter, and the "when"—after completion of the chapter. The "what" and "how" are the action-oriented outcomes that the learner will demonstrate in the listed behaviors.

Behavioral objectives do not address all of the content that will ultimately be included in the teaching plan. Rather, the "what" in the behavioral objectives is the outcome we wish to evaluate after the teaching has occurred. Consider the chapter objectives to determine the "how" and "what" information:

1. Discuss (how) the components of teaching and learning (what).
2. Examine (how) differences in the ways people learn (what).
3. Describe (how) methods to assess learning readiness and motivation (what).
4. Propose (how) different teaching methods for a variety of learning needs (what).
5. Devise (how) a teaching activity on a topic that contains behavioral objectives, a content outline with appropriate teaching methods, and a plan for evaluating learner outcomes (what).

This example focuses on the learner at the end of the prescribed learning activity, with action verbs—discussing, examining, describing, proposing, and devising—as their outcome ability, describing "how" they should be able to perform.

The next focus is on the complexity you as the evaluator (whether learner or teacher) wish to see demonstrated at the end of the activity. This is the degree that can be measured, or the "where." The type and complexity of the outcome behavior are determined by the level of the learning domain.

When developing behavioral objectives, be sure to consider the domains of knowledge. Further, within each domain there is a leveling process, or progress in attainment of increasingly complex skills. From the work of Bloom and other teaching and learning theorists, a revised two-dimensional taxonomy has been developed. The revised taxonomy table considers the interrelationship of two dimensions: knowledge and cognitive processes (Anderson et al., 2001). This is the knowledge or the "what" you wish the learner to acquire, and the cognitive process is the demonstration or "how" the learning is evaluated. The taxonomy table allows objectives to be developed that address both knowledge and processes. Consider that the nursing goal for the client is to be at the procedural knowledge level to apply a dressing change at home but also at the factual knowledge level to evaluate signs of infection or monitor the response to a prescribed medication.

Knowledge Dimension

In this revised taxonomy table, the knowledge dimension represents the four rows of the table with the following knowledge categories:

- Factual, as the basic elements
- Conceptual, or the interrelationships among elements
- Procedural, demonstration of a set of skills
- Metacognitive, as the highest level of awareness of the thought processes. (Anderson et al., 2001)

Consider the difference of these categories in nursing practice, as in the case of a sterile field. "Factual" is simply the knowledge of the components. "Conceptual" would be the understanding of the interrelationship, as with spillage and contamination of the field. "Procedural knowledge" would be in the performance of a dressing change and maintenance of the field. "Metacognitive knowledge" would occur during practice with an unanticipated occurrence and resolution using critical thinking skills. In patient education, we strive for the procedural level, for the return demonstration of a set of skills, as in the dressing change needed at home and the protection of the surgical or wound site.

Cognitive Processes Dimension

In the revised taxonomy table, the cognitive process dimension is represented in the six columns of the table as the following levels of increasing complexity:

- Remember, as recognizing and recalling
- Understand, as interpreting, exemplifying, classifying, summarizing, inferring, comparing, and explaining
- Apply, as executing and implementing
- Analyze, to include differentiating, organizing, and attributing
- Evaluate, or making judgments based on certain criteria
- Create, or developing a new process. (Anderson et al., 2001)

Cognitive processes in this taxonomy build from the simple recall of facts to the extrapolation into a new process. Continuing to use our example, we want the nurse in a preceptor position for a senior student or a new graduate to use cognitive skills through evaluation for the maintenance of the sterile field in all practice applications with the novice nurse or nursing student. In advanced practice, however, the nurse would consistently use all processes in the domain for the specialty area, including the creation of new processes within the selected scope of practice. In the scenario of patient education, the goal would be for the client to be able to remember, understand, and apply specific skills, and to analyze and evaluate when professional intervention is needed, as in the case of potential infection or a complication.

In the cognitive processes dimension, we first have the knowledge received through recall or recognition. Next, we proceed to an understanding of the information. The final levels of the cognitive domain are applying the information, analyzing, evaluating the information, and finally creating for application of the knowledge in other situations. Consider the levels in the cognitive processes domain with the following action words in your behavioral objectives for teaching a client about his or her condition:

1. *Knowledge* implies simply that the learner has perceived the information and can report it back to the teacher. Action verbs such as *identifies, recalls, recognizes,* and *repeats* are useful for behavioral objectives at this knowledge level of the cognitive domains, such as the ability to recall a list of the signs of infection in a learning situation.

2. At the next level, the learner demonstrates *understanding* of the knowledge, based on the four levels of the knowledge dimension. Action verbs for behavioral objectives at this level include *explains* and *compares,* as illustrated by the client who can explain how to look for redness indicating infection in a surgical wound.

3. The third level of the cognitive domain is *application,* demonstrating the ability to relate the learning to a situation. The following action verbs are appropriate for behavioral objectives for the learner's outcomes at this point: *applies, demonstrates, employs,* and *uses.* For example, "the client uses the dressing change skill at home after discharge."

4. Further critical thinking occurs at the next cognitive level of *analysis.* The learner steps back and analyzes the information objectively. Action verbs useful at this level of complexity include *assesses, appraises, organizes,* and *differentiates.* Now the client has determined the need to call the physician's office for evaluation of potential complications from the surgery.

5. *Evaluation* occurs at the next level of cognitive processes in which judgment is an essential component. Action verbs appropriate for this level include *evaluating, testing, monitoring,* and *critiquing.*

6. *Creation* is the highest level of the cognitive domain, in which the learner manipulates the concepts from the learning in new combinations and situations. Action verbs addressing this level of complexity in the taxonomy include *creates, designs, devises, constructs,* and *generates.*

Both the cognitive and psychomotor domains appear in the taxonomy table with the focus on knowledge and the cognitive process. The psychomotor domain is easily apparent in the application of the knowledge. It is important to include behavioral objectives at the various knowledge levels to measure client progress from simple to complex skills. For example, you have taught a newly diagnosed diabetic client to self-administer insulin. As the teacher, you must be able to see how the learner-client has accomplished this task, beyond the simple return demonstration with saline injections you observe. At the next level of manipulation of the psychomotor skill, the learner demonstrates the entire procedure of proper injection of insulin, from filling the syringe to disposing of the supplies. Precision of the psychomotor skill is demonstrated when the learner can perform the injection on schedule with a sense of comfort in her ability in the process, expressed with the phrase "Demonstrates skill in the procedure." Articulation, or full use of the skill, is demonstrated when the diabetic client is able to manage at home with insulin, including testing blood glucose for additional needs during stressful periods. This is reflected in the phrase "Uses results of blood glucose monitoring to regulate. . . ."

The highest level of skill acquisition comes when the individual has a sense of competence and the skill has become a natural part of his routine; the individual can determine signs of hyperglycemia or hypoglycemia and self-test as naturally as he dresses or bathes. The individual has incorporated the process sufficiently to spend a month traveling with a sense of independence, comfort, and control in the process. Action terms reflecting this level include "Independently monitors and effectively regulates administration of insulin." These actions demonstrate Bandura's concept of mastery experiences in self-efficacy.

The affective domain is less apparent in the revised taxonomy table but is inferred in the higher levels of knowledge and cognitive processes. In fact, the creators of the revised taxonomy propose that "nearly every cognitive objective has an affective component" (Anderson et al., 2001). For the affective domain, complexity progresses from receiving to responding, valuing, organizing values, and finally characterizing or standing for certain values transmitted. Consider the newly diagnosed diabetic client. Acceptance of her condition is vital to developing long-range personal care skills. But this is a difficult domain to measure because values and attitudes are more difficult to assess than knowledge or psychomotor skills. Although action verbs for the affective domain include *receiving, responding, valuing, organizing values,* and *characterizing,* this is a difficult domain of learning to evaluate. We must rely on the individual to communicate her attitudes, feelings, and values honestly through verbal and nonverbal behaviors.

Behavioral objectives are the intended action-oriented outcomes of an educational process. These objectives are tools for teaching, learning, and evaluating. Evaluation data can provide useful feedback on whether the learner has achieved the objective or requires repetition, reinforcement, or revision.

Planning for Learning

Once the assessment of learners and teachers takes place and the behavioral objectives have been developed, we must plan for the specific content and how it will be transmitted to the client group. But this sounds very directive and controlling. Recall, with the adult learner, the focus is on the holistic individual based on the assessment data and the mutually acceptable objectives.

The assessment data obtained earlier in this process have been used to define and describe the client, including characteristics, attributes, learning assets and deficits, readiness, and specific needs to be addressed. This procedure was conducted with the client as an individual, family, or group to diagnose the learning needs and prepare for continuation of the process. Next, behavioral objectives were identified to guide the process and plan for the evaluation of outcomes. Now we must plan the content, teaching strategies and methods of delivery, learning resources, and specific evaluation procedures.

Traditional lesson plans are frequently prepared in a column format. The first column contains the behavioral objectives developed for the learning activity. Subsequent columns contain learning content, teaching strategies or principles, learning resources, evaluation methods, and timing, which all can be viewed easily in relation to the behavioral objectives. A sample format is posted on the Intranet site for this text. This format is actually the plan for the teacher to ensure that the behavioral objectives are addressed with appropriate content, methods, materials, and evaluation methods. It may have to be more flexible based on client needs.

The learning content is the specific content outline designed to meet the objective. Teaching strategies relate to the objective and the specific content, including variations for the learning setting and clients. Suggested learning resources and materials, perhaps identifying the appropriate "tear-sheet" or learning module, are proposed to enhance the teaching strategy and meet the learner's cognitive style, especially if a group or lecture presentation is appropriate for the general audience but may not meet the needs of individual learners.

All of the planning so far is the proposal for the teaching-learning activity. Before implementing it, one must specify evaluation methods along with a proposed time frame for the process. Implementation of the teaching-learning process can then proceed using the strategies identified in the plan. Evaluation of the teaching-learning process is essential and is designed to address the behavioral objectives at the level of the taxonomy specified for acquisition of affective, cognitive, and psychomotor behaviors.

Consider the simple example of a 56-year-old female outpatient with unstable hypertension without angina. She has come to the health clinic after being denied health insurance last week because of the prepolicy examination requirement. Blood pressure measurements ranged from 210/105 to 185/100 on the two consecutive visits. She has had no serious illness or hospitalizations, but she is leaving town in five weeks to visit family abroad for a month. Today, her doctor prescribed daily antihypertensive medication and a low-sodium diet. The client has verbalized the need to lower her blood pressure for insurance purposes. She also reported that she has used a salt substitute for the past three days and has continued to play tennis three times a week. Her descriptions of nutritional intake indicate high dietary fat and sodium content in meals prepared at home and selected in restaurants. She volunteers much information about cooking for her family as well as attending gourmet cooking classes at the local college, which she signed up for because she wanted to watch the teacher and ask questions rather than just read the cookbooks.

The assessment data indicate a teaching deficit, learning readiness, and the motivation to adhere to a treatment plan within a confined time frame. You and the client determine that you will schedule individualized teaching sessions with her for her next four weekly visits. Behavioral objectives for this teaching-learning process might include the following:

1. Explains food selection and preparation techniques to maintain a low-sodium diet.
2. Monitors blood pressure regularly.
3. Uses Sular as prescribed, monitoring for side effects, adverse effects, and toxicity.
4. Uses appropriate food choices and preparations for maintenance of a low-sodium diet.
5. Organizes activities including maintenance of her exercise program.
6. Reapplies for health insurance coverage.

The objectives should be mutually acceptable to both you and the client.

The learning content addresses the behavioral objectives by teaching food selections and revisions needed with food preparation, periodic assessment of blood pressure, administration of medication, monitoring for side effects and toxicity, and maintenance of a healthy nutritional and exercise program. Teaching strategies are then selected for the individualized cognitive style of the client, using resources such as videos and written information to take home. Evaluation methods are proposed to address each of the behavioral objectives at the following four weekly visits, specifying the time frame for each activity.

Teaching Strategies and Methods

Teaching strategies and methods are geared toward accomplishing the behavioral objectives in light of the audience. Selection is also based on how the content can best be delivered and addresses the affective, cognitive, and psychomotor domains of learning. Teaching methods generally are lecture presentations, demonstrations, discussions, modeling, role-playing, individualized instruction, programmed instruction, computer-assisted instruction (CAI), other simulations, and group activities. As Bastable (2003) has described, the instructional or teaching strategy is the overall plan for the learning experience whereas instructional methods are the techniques or approaches to bring the learner into contact with the content to be learned (p. 356).

Selection of a teaching strategy and some combination of teaching methods depends on the client. For a client group of 24, a lecture format followed by breaking out into four small groups to apply the lecture content may be quite appropriate for presenting information on child development and wellness practices. For a group of three new mothers on the postpartum unit, a lecture would be impersonal and less effective than a small-group discussion on plans for returning home with their healthy neonates. In our example of the client with hypertension, individualized teaching would be most effective, because the client prefers the interaction with a teacher and has a limited time frame to accomplish the behavioral outcome objectives. The characteristics of the client group and the intended outcomes, therefore, guide the selection of appropriate teaching methods. For further information on selected instructional methods, refer to Table 10–2.

Enhancing the delivery of content and improving learning on the basis of the cognitive style of the client require careful selection of learning resources. Teaching aids and instructional technology are frequently used in

Table 10.2

Sample Teaching Methods

Method	Characteristics	Strategies
Lecture	Large group Controlled by the teacher	▪ To make more learner-centered, provide time for questions/discussion or break-out sessions for discussion ▪ Must address mixed audience of visual, auditory, and kinesthetic learners ▪ Focus on important concepts and provide aids for application of knowledge by learners
Group discussion	Small group Learner-centered as long as it does not revert to a mini-lecture	▪ Requires good skills in group dynamics by the teacher to keep on the topic and focus the learning ▪ Allows opportunities for application of critical thinking skills, problem-solving, and teamwork by the group ▪ Ideal method for transformative learning ▪ Mixed audience of visual, auditory, and kinesthetic learners is still a consideration on a smaller scale ▪ May include demonstrations for active learning
Programmed or computer-assisted instruction	Learner-centered, independent, and self-paced activity	▪ Requires careful design to maintain interest ▪ Requires motivation and persistence by learner ▪ Design promotes individual learner feedback but limited teacher-learner interaction

(Table continues on page 185)

Table 10.2

Sample Teaching Methods (continued)

Method	Characteristics	Strategies
Simulated environments, games, activities, and role-playing	Learner-centered, with an individual or in small groups	■ Requires environmental staging and engaging activity ■ Role-play may be done with descriptive scripts or be more flexible ■ Requires development of rapport and group skills ■ Actively engages learners when the situation is presented in a nonthreatening and nonpersonal manner and viewed as "what if . . ."

client teaching situations to enhance the content and actively involve the learner in the teaching-learning process. Using assessment data, consider how the client told you he best learned information in the past. When preparing for larger group presentations, consider how smaller group activities or assignments will address the needs of learners who do not do their best in the large group setting. Remember, adults learn best when actively involved in the process, both intellectually and physically. Think of ways to move the client from a passive to an active learning situation.

A major consideration is how to enhance the content for the learner's own cognitive style. Some learners are highly perceptive in one or several senses in learning information. They may be highly visual, auditory, tactile, or perceptive in some combination of these senses. Recall the usefulness of understanding multiple intelligences. When you select teaching resources, consider whether the learners are highly visual and obtain and process information mainly through observation of the world around them. These learners do well with visual aids that enhance the content presented in the teaching strategy, such as with presentation graphics or with information presented through pamphlets, handouts, and online searches.

Compare a visual style to the learner whose auditory sense is the most perceptive. Effective auditory teaching aids include videos, audiotapes, and recordings with well-developed sound presentations. In addition, this learner may do well using a recorder to take notes and reinforce learning through review later. For the individual who prefers to touch and manipulate new information, plan for active involvement in the teaching and learning through demonstrations, models, and samples.

Adults learn best when actively involved in the process. Think of ways to move the client from a passive to an active learning situation.

Another consideration is whether the learner prefers to be an individualist or to have other people in the learning environment for interaction and stimulation. Some people learn in a very individualistic way. They prefer to obtain information and then go their own way to process, analyze, and synthesize the material. Having a group discussion to evaluate and apply information directly after it is presented in a lecture is stressful, if not torture, to this individual, who needs time before she can share thoughts or apply the information. Alternatively, some learners enjoy interactions and learning in a stimulating group environment. A large, impersonal lecture is deadly boring to this learner, who thrives on group discussion to work on questions posed in a case study. But learners are generally not easy to classify; these characteristics can be combined over a wide range. Pure types are rare, and the challenge is to find those teaching strategies and resources that enhance the teaching content and promote learning. Resources for different cognitive styles are presented in Table 10–3.

In addition to client teaching, contemporary nursing practice consists of collegial teaching and learning opportunities such as educational programs, lectures, demonstrations, group discussions, professional and clinical conferences, case studies, clinical receptorships, grand rounds, and chat rooms, just to mention a few. The same steps are involved in this process as with assessment, diagnosis of learning needs, development of behavioral objectives, preparation of a plan with selection of teaching strategies and resources, and evaluation methods. The difference generally lies in the size of the group, which can range from a one-to-one collegial or the unit staff to a large interdisciplinary group of professionals who are interested in the latest research on a selected topic. With the larger group, it is essential to assess the prevalent characteristics of the learner population. This includes the overall learning need that will become the topic for the presentation. Behavioral outcomes should address what

Table 10.3

Teaching Methods and Resources to Address the Cognitive Style of the Learner

Cognitive Style	Teaching Methods	Teaching Resources
Highly visual	Small-group discussion, role-playing, simulations, demonstrations, programmed instruction, computer simulations	Multimedia presentations, videos, charts, posters, models, photographs, white/bulletin boards, publications, handouts, reading lists, computer-assisted instruction (CAI) with effective graphics, e-mail, chat rooms
Highly auditory	Lecture and discussion, role-playing, simulations, demonstrations	Videos, recordings (prepared audios or self-recorded tapes made during teaching), CAI with auditory reinforcers, telephone follow-up
Highly tactile	Small-group activities, individualized teaching, role-playing, simulations, demonstrations, games, programmed instruction, computer simulations	Models, bulletin boards, samples, books, pamphlets, prepared handouts, CAI requiring responses to cues, chat rooms, e-mail
Highly interpersonal	Small-group discussion, role-playing, simulations, demonstrations, some computer simulations	Videos, audios, charts, posters, models, photographs, pamphlets, CAI, teleconferencing, chat rooms, e-mail
Highly individualistic	Lecture, simulations, demonstrations, programmed instruction, computer simulations, computer searches	Multimedia presentations, videos, audios, charts, posters, models, photographs, books, handouts, paper and pencils for note-taking, CAI, e-mail

the learners are expected to have gained as knowledge and skills at the end of the program or teaching session, because they will be the ones providing the evaluation data. Teaching strategies may include an interdisciplinary team approach, especially for presentations across disciplines to foster the development of knowledge and collaboration. Although active learning in small groups is highly effective with professional colleagues, this can effectively occur as a small-group breakout phase after the basic information has been presented in a large group presentation format. Highly effective learning resources in this case include multimedia presentations with presentation graphics, videos, posters, models, photographs, pamphlets, handouts, and reading lists. A word of warning with presentation graphics: Do not read the entire presentation from the screen. Present the pertinent points graphically to engage the audience rather than lose their attention (Box 10–2). After the program or presentation, the teacher or program coordinator receives completed evaluation forms from the program participants and then develops an overall analysis based on the evaluation data the participants provide.

Evaluation of Outcomes

Evaluating outcomes is a vital component of the teaching-learning process. It may be ongoing and may lead to important information for revisions needed in subsequent sessions. Although evaluation strategies focus on both the teaching and the learning that occurred, the primary focus is on the learner. Is the learner able to demonstrate the outcomes envisioned at the beginning of the process? As in the nursing process, the evaluation phase of the teaching-learning process is used to assess the effectiveness of the process and whether the client has resolved a knowledge deficit.

Clients are more difficult to evaluate than traditional student learners. Cognitive domain learning activities of students are easily measured with paper-and-pencil tests and computer-adaptive testing that assesses knowledge and cognitive processes. In the client teaching situation,

BOX 10.2 Tips For Presentations

- Do not read from the screen. Presentation graphics should be used to engage the audience. Use the information on the screen as talking points to keep you on track, not to keep the audience distracted.
- Do not use all capital letters—they imply shouting and are not visually engaging.
- Use a clear font, not a fancy script that is hard to read and distracting for the audience.
- Limit the information on a slide or screen; for example, use only four or five lines on the screen that must be legible from the back of the room.
- Keep it simple. Limit the graphics and displays to important information without distracting background colors or graphics.
- Consider the essential number of slides or displays, in terms of content, allotted time, essential information, and printing costs if you are planning on handouts.
- Carefully proofread to avoid spelling and grammatical errors without reliance on the spell-checker function (e.g., *three*, *their*, and *there* are all in the dictionary).
- If you plan on distributing copies of your presentation as handouts or electronically, make sure the copies are readable, have the same information as your presentation, and include appropriate citations, if applicable.
- Remember your highly auditory learner—speak to her, while assisting your visual learner, who is watching the display rather than you.
- For the active learner, consider a follow-up activity to reinforce the content you presented.

such tests are rarely used except in research or large group situations. Client evaluation can be complex, with problems related to timing, access, continuity, measurement, and other factors. In addition, recall that adult learners should be involved in evaluating their own learning. Normally, client evaluation is done with methods such as return demonstrations, observation, diaries, rating scales, discussion, and electronic communication.

We used different action verbs to address the three domains of learning and levels, or taxonomy, within each. Capturing evaluation data requires specificity in the behavioral outcome objective. The objectives should indicate how you are measuring the outcomes of the teaching-learning process.

The affective domain consists of attitudes, feelings, and values. Evaluation data should show how the learner progressed from receiving to internalizing the values mutually agreed on for the learning. In the case of a newly diagnosed diabetic client, the teacher and the learner must be able to measure or see attitudinal or value changes through verbal and nonverbal behaviors. The action verbs in the affective domain are *receiving*, *responding*, *valuing*, *organizing values*, and *characterizing specific values*. We need the individual to communicate her attitudes, feelings, and values in verbal and nonverbal behaviors. Methods of evaluation in this area include interviews, discussions, and observations that demonstrate certain beliefs and values. Another means of evaluating affective learning is a diary in which the client can record feelings and problems that arise between teaching sessions. Analyzing the content of the diaries can provide useful information on the affective domain as well as knowledge gaps in cognitive processes. And with the availability of

electronic communication, cognitive and affective domains can be evaluated via e-mail or electronic postings.

In the cognitive domain, knowledge builds from simple recall to understanding, application, analysis, evaluation, and synthesis or creation of information. Interviews and discussion with clients can be used to evaluate whether the learner can repeat or report back the information as knowledge gains. For understanding, the client describes, explains, and compares information during the interview. Application of the information can be evaluated as the client demonstrates and uses the information, providing specific examples of how this was done. Critical thinking and analysis take this one step further, as the client explains problems and difficulties that arose and steps taken to solve problems without the presence of the teacher. Evaluation by the learner occurs when the client determines which method worked best. Creation involves manipulating the learning in new combinations and effectively applying the information to a similar problem or situation. The learner has devised a new way of handling a situation on the basis of information obtained in another area. Occasionally, post-tests are used in client teaching, but test anxiety is a major deterrent to their use for some clients. The evaluation strategies most useful for both teachers and client-learners to gauge cognitive learning are discussion, questioning, and allowing for description, whether through face-to-face or by electronic means.

Evaluating client outcomes in the psychomotor domain is easiest through direct observation of skill attainment. At the simplest level of psychomotor skill attainment is the client's ability to imitate, as seen in a return demonstration. This allows one to assess understanding and the ability to perform a specific skill, such as testing one's blood glucose. But demonstration of a skill in a clinical setting can be artificial, because the client's own environment often has additional factors not present in the health-care agency, such as shared bathrooms or medication storage problems in a home with toddlers. Flowcharts, diaries, and check sheets are easy for clients to use as reminders and reinforcers in the home, and they can then be discussed at the next clinic visit or teaching session interview. The level of psychomotor skills can be assessed with a checklist or flowchart in terms of following instructions to proper scheduling, precision, and problem-solving in the procedure. The client can be encouraged to note problems encountered and how they were handled, to demonstrate skills in both cognitive and psychomotor domains. Consider the use of electronic calendars or personal digital assistants (PDAs) in some client situations. This will provide evaluation data for both the client, as the learner, and the nurse, as the teacher.

In our example of the client with hypertension, we implemented an individualized teaching strategy within a limited time frame to accomplish the outcome objectives aimed at the cognitive and psychomotor domains. One method of evaluation would be for the client to maintain a diary, including daily food intake and exercise, and list daily blood pressure measurements, medications taken, and effects on a check sheet. This evaluation method provides visual data that address the initial five behavioral objectives agreed on by both the client and the nurse. At each of the four client visits or teaching sessions, the information in the diary is reviewed and discussed. When both the learner and the teacher are satisfied that these objectives have been met, control of the hypertension problem may be present. A health certificate can then be provided by the primary care provider so that the last objective, reapplication for health insurance coverage, can be attempted with an outlook for success. At the final teaching visit, the client and the nurse discuss the strategies and resources used during the four-week process, to evaluate the teaching that took place. Electronic communication provides an additional resource for follow-up and evaluation.

Evaluation data can provide useful feedback that objectives have been met or that repetition, reinforcement, or revision is needed. Teaching strategies, like methods and resources, should be evaluated by both the teacher and the learner. Discovering what worked and what may have worked better helps the learner view the process and reinforce the learning while sharing with the teacher ways to improve and strategies for the future. Important factors here are encouragement and openness for honest and constructive evaluation data from both teacher and learner.

ONLINE CONSULT

Health information and toll-free numbers at
http://www.health.gov/nhic/

Literacy Information at
http://www.nifl.gov

INTERACTIVE EXERCISES

Go to the Intranet site and complete the interactive exercises provided for this Chapter.

EVIDENCED-BASED PRACTICE: CONSIDER THIS . . .

*T*he National Association of Orthopedic Nurses submitted information on the management of clients following insertion of skeletal pins. One of the recommendations with the highest level of evidence was that in addition to providing written instructions on signs and symptoms of infection, clients and their families should be taught and be able to demonstrate pin site care prior to discharge (NGC, 2005, p. 1).

Question: How will you use this information as part of discharge planning and in client teaching activities? Remember to consider your clients individuals and families and their learning needs.

Source: National Guideline Clearinghouse. (NGC). (2005). Skeletal pin site care. Retrieved October 7, 2006, from *http://www.guideline.gov/summary/summary.aspx?doc_id=7420&nbr=4379*

KEY POINTS

- There are several schools of learning theories. Major examples of these theories are behaviorism, gestalt, social cognitive, humanism, andragogy, transformative learning, and multiple intelligences.

- Teaching is more than transmitting information. The information must be received, understood, and evaluated by the learner.

- Learning is the perception and assimilation of the information presented to us in a variety of ways.

- Characteristics of learning include:
  - Perception of new information
  - Initial reaction to the information
  - Ability to remember or repeat the information
  - Rejection or acceptance of the information (understanding)
  - Use of the information in a similar situation (application)
  - Critical analysis of the information
  - Incorporation of the information into the value system (evaluation)
  - Use of the information in various situations or combinations (creation)

- The three learning domains are:
  - Affective—attitudes, feelings, and values
  - Cognitive—knowledge and thought processes
  - Psychomotor—demonstration of behaviors

- Cognitive learning styles look at how information is interpreted, influences from others, and reasoning methods. Teaching and learning strategies can then be developed to match the learner's needs and resources.

- Readiness occurs when the learner is willing to change and view the learning need. Learning readiness includes human motivation, understanding, and applicability or acceptability. Motivation in humans is a manifestation of internal and external personal and environmental factors that cause people to respond to a situation the way they do. In addition, to achieve learning readiness, the person must perceive the information at his level of cognitive functioning, and it must be applicable and acceptable to the person as an individual, a member of the family, or a member of a group.

- The purpose of writing behavioral objectives is to provide a frame of reference for the intended outcomes of the teaching-learning activity for both the teacher and the learner. The focus of the objective is on the learner and the knowledge and cognitive process demonstrated as learning outcomes.

- Teaching strategies are geared toward accomplishing the behavioral objectives in light of the audience.

- Evaluating learning outcomes of the teaching-learning process is essential and is designed to address the behavioral objectives at the taxonomic level specified for the acquisition of affective, cognitive, and psychomotor behaviors.

- Evaluation of teaching strategies by the learner provides a further view of the process and reinforces the learning.

Thought and Discussion Questions

1. Explain which theory of learning and learning style is applicable to the way in which you learn best.

2. Remember those two clients following their hip replacement surgeries? One is an architect who designs custom homes and meets with his customers for at least an hour before he develops the house plans to ensure that he truly understands their desires and ideas. The other is a retired English professor concerned about the rehabilitation schedule and the completion of a collection of essays that must be submitted to the publisher in six weeks. Plan for their individualized discharge teaching using the theory of multiple intelligences.

3. Develop a staff conference as a seminar presentation on a clinical topic, with appropriate content for a unit staff of 10 registered nurses, six licensed practical nurses, and 15 certified assistive personnel. Propose assessment data on the learners and ways to match cognitive styles and teaching strategies for the group. Be prepared to participate in an online or class discussion, to be scheduled by your instructor.

4. Read the case studies in the Case Study Bank on the Intranet Site and be prepared to discuss them in class.

5. Review the Chapter Thought located on the first page of the chapter, and discuss it in the context of the contents of the chapter.

☐ REFERENCES

Anderson, L. W., Krathwohl, D. R., Airasian, P. W., Cruikshank, K. A., Mayer, R. E., Pintrich, P. R., Raths, R. E., & Wittrock, M .C. (Eds.) (2001). *A taxonomy for learning, teaching, and assessing: A revision of Bloom's educational objectives* (abridged ed.). New York: Longman.

Bandura, A. (1995). Exercise of personal and collective efficacy in changing societies. In A. Bandura (Ed.), *Self-efficacy in changing societies* (pp. 1–45). Cambridge, UK: Cambridge University Press.

Bandura, A. (1977). *Social learning theory.* Englewood Cliffs, NJ: Prentice-Hall.

Bastable, S. B. (2003). *Nurse as educator: Principles of teaching and learning for nursing practice.* Boston: Jones and Bartlett.

Benner, P. (1984). *From novice to expert: Excellence and power in clinical nursing practice.* Menlo Park, CA: Addison-Wesley.

Bloom, B. S. (Ed.). (1956). *Taxonomy of educational objectives.* New York: Longman.

Erikson, E. H. (1963). *Childhood and society* (2nd ed.). New York: Norton.

Fawcett, J. (2006). Nursing philosophies, models, and theories: A focus on the future. In A. M. Tomey & M. R. Alligood (Eds.), *Nursing theory: Utilization and application* (3rd ed., pp. 499–518). St. Louis: Mosby.

Gagne, R. M., & Medsker, K. L. (1996). *The conditions of learning: Training applications.* Belmont, CA: Wadsworth.

Gardner, H. (1999). *Intelligence reframed: Multiple intelligences for the 21st century.* New York: Basic Books.

Gardner, H. (1993a). *Frames of mind: The theory of multiple intelligences* (2nd ed.). New York: Basic Books.

Gardner, H. (1993b). *Multiple intelligences: The theory in practice.* New York: Basic Books.

Havighurst, R. J. (1972). *Developmental tasks and education* (3rd ed.). New York: David McKay.

King, I. M. (1981). *A theory for nursing: Systems, concepts, process.* New York: John Wiley & Sons.

Knowles, M. S. (1990). *The adult learner: A neglected species* (4th ed.). Houston: Gulf.

Knowles, M. S., & Associates (1985). *Andragogy in action.* San Francisco: Jossey-Bass.

Kolb, D. (1981). *Learning style inventory.* Boston: McBer and Company.

Maslow, A. H. (1971). *The farther reaches of the human mind.* New York: Viking Press.

Maslow, A. H. (1954). *Motivation and personality.* New York: Harper.

Mezirow, J. (2000). Learning to think like an adult: Core concepts of transformation theory. In J. Mezirow and Associates, *Learning as transformation: Critical perspectives on a theory in progress* (pp. 3–33). San Francisco: Jossey-Bass.

Rogers, C., & Freiberg, H. J. (1994). *Freedom to learn* (3rd ed.). New York: Merrill/Macmillan.

Skinner, B.F. (2003). A brief survey of operant behavior. Retrieved June 26, 2006, from *http://www.bfskinner.org/operant.asp*

Vella, J. K. (2002). *Learning to listen, learning to teach: The power of dialogue in adult education.* San Francisco: Jossey-Bass.

☐ BIBLIOGRAPHY

Blanton, B. (1998). The application of cognitive learning theory to instructional design. *International Journal of Instructional Media, 25,* 171–175.

Canobbio, M. M. (2006). *Mosby's handbook of patient education* (3rd ed.). St. Louis, MO: Mosby.

Fitzpatrick, J. J., Romano, C., & Chasek, R. (Eds.). (2001). *The nurses' guide to consumer health web sites.* New York: Springer.

Flynn, J. P., & Stack, M. C. (Eds.) (2005). *The role of the preceptor: A guide for nurse educators, clinicians, and managers* (2nd ed.). New York: Springer.

Guinee, K. K. (1978). *Teaching and learning in nursing: A behavioral objectives approach.* New York: Macmillan.

Ginsburg, H. P., & Opper, S. (1988). *Piaget's theory of intellectual development* (3rd ed.). New York: Prentice-Hall.

Glanz, K., Rimer, B. K., & Lewis, F. M. (Eds.) (2002). *Health behavior and health education: Theory, research, and practice* (3rd ed.). San Francisco: Jossey-Bass.

Imel, S. (1998). Transformative learning in adulthood. ERIC Digest No. 200. Retrieved June 26, 2006, from *http://www.ericdigests.org/1999-2/adulthood.htm*

Knowles, M. S. (1980). *The modern practice of adult education: From pedagogy to andragogy* (Rev. ed.). Chicago: Follett.

Mezirow, J. (1991). *Transformational dimensions of adult learning.* San Francisco: Jossey-Bass.

Rankin, S.H., Stallings, K.D., & London, F. (2005). *Patient education in health and illness* (5th ed.). Philadelphia: Lippincott Williams & Wilkins.

Redman, B. K. (2001). *The practice of patient education* (9th ed.). St. Louis, MO: Mosby.

Stephenson, P. L. (2006). Before the teaching begins: Managing patient anxiety prior to providing education. *Clinical Journal of Oncology Nursing, 10,* 241–245.

Sternberg, R. J., & Zhang, L. (2001). *Perspectives in thinking, learning, and cognitive styles.* Mahwah, NJ: Lawrence Erlbaum Associates.

☐ ONLINE RESOURCES

Ageless Learner
http://www.agelesslearner.com

Jung
http://www.cgjungpage.org

Gardner
http://pzweb.harvard.edu/PIs/HG.htm

Malsow
http://www.maslow.com

Myers & Briggs Foundation
http://www.myersbriggs.org/

Psychology
http://tip.psychology.org

■ Theresa M. **Valiga**   ■ Sheila C. **Grossman**

Leadership

> ❝ *Do not go where the path may lead.*
> *Go instead where there is no path,*
> *and leave a trail.* ❞
>
> Anonymous

Chapter Objectives

On completion of this chapter, the reader will be able to:

1. Differentiate between leadership and management.
2. Compare and contrast three leadership styles: democratic, authoritarian, and laissez-faire.
3. Distinguish among various theories of leadership: great man theory, traitist theory, situational theory, transformational theory, and leadership task theory.
4. Analyze the interdependence of leaders and followers.
5. Explain how each of the nine tasks of leadership as outlined by Gardner and the concept of stewardship relate to nursing practice.
6. Analyze nursing practice situations in terms of the extent to which leadership was exercised.
7. Identify your own leadership abilities or potential leadership skills.

Key Terms

Leadership Style
Authoritative Leaders
Laissez-Faire or Permissive Leaders
Democratic or Participative Leaders
Great Man Leadership Theory

Traitist Leadership Theories
Situational Leadership Theories
Transformational Leadership Theory
Leadership Tasks Theory

New Science Leadership Theory
Management
Stewardship

*L*eadership is a word that is often used, has tremendous appeal, and evokes images of greatness. When people are asked to think about individuals who have demonstrated leadership, there is likely to be agreement about individuals like Martin Luther King, Jr., Mother Teresa, Gandhi, Jesus Christ, Eleanor Roosevelt, and even Florence Nightingale.

What is it about certain individuals that prompt others to perceive them as leaders? What is it about their character, their style, their manner of interacting with others, or the goals toward which they were striving that makes them leaders? What is it that sets them apart from ordinary citizens, politicians, and managers?

In this chapter, we explore the nature of leadership. We examine some of the hundreds of definitions of the phenomenon, explore selected leadership theories and leadership styles, analyze the concept of transformational leadership, look at leader-follower relations, analyze various components of leadership, and discuss the kind of leadership that is needed, particularly by professional nurses in the 21st century. We assert that each of us has the potential to exercise leadership in our workplaces, professional organizations, and communities.

DEFINITIONS OF LEADERSHIP

The concept of leadership has been studied extensively. As Bass (1990) notes, "There are almost as many different definitions of leadership as there are persons who have attempted to define the concept" (p. 11). Leadership has been conceptualized as a set of traits, a role that needs to be played in any group, a particular position, an art, the exercise of influence, a form of persuasion, a power relation, and a way to attain goals (Bass, 1990). After analyzing 100 years of leadership research, Van Fleet and Yukl (1989) concluded, "Where once we thought of leadership as a relatively simple construct, we now recognize that it is among the more complex social phenomena" (p. 66) in our world. Bennis and Nanus (1985) spoke to the complexity of leadership and how little we truly understand about it when they wrote:

> Decades of academic analysis have given us more than 350 definitions of leadership. Literally thousands of empirical investigations of leaders have been conducted in the last seventy-five years alone, but no clear and unequivocal understanding exists as to what distinguishes leaders from nonleaders, and perhaps more important, what distinguishes effective leaders from ineffective leaders. (p. 4)

In a critique of leadership studies undertaken over the years, Rost (1991) suggested that perhaps the reason we know so little about this phenomenon, even

after so much analysis, is that these studies have missed the "essential nature of what leadership is [and] the process whereby leaders and followers relate to one another to achieve a purpose" (p. 4). Indeed, many of the studies of leadership have focused more on management styles or the person of the leader and ignored or minimized the role of followers in the equation, or the interactions among the leader, the followers, and the vision or goal at hand. Because of the increasingly complex nature of our world, any exploration of leadership for the 21st century must attend to this interrelationship and interdependence.

Although it is true that leaders "cause ripples," "rock the boat," "disturb the status quo," and take risks, they are effective as leaders only when those ripples inspire others to take action, make change, and realize goals. But because leadership is more an art than a science, there is no single or simple way to go about inspiring others; instead, the leader needs to use a number of styles to mobilize a group to achieve great things.

LEADERSHIP STYLES

Style can be thought of as the way in which something is done or said or as a particular form of behavior associated with an individual. Leadership style can be viewed as a set of behaviors that characterize individuals as they perform their leader role. These styles differ in terms of how power is distributed among those leading and those following, how decisions are made, and whose needs are of primary concern.

Factors Influencing Style

One's style reflects forces within oneself, the group, and the situation. Forces within the leader include her value system (as influenced by culture, background, and family context), expectations of self and others, prior experiences in a leadership role, self-confidence, and tolerance for ambiguity and uncertainty. Forces within members of the group include their need for independence, readiness for responsibility, commitment to a common goal, expectations about sharing in decision-making, and ability to deal with the group task. These "forces" often are influenced by the culture and background of the followers, factors that must be taken into consideration when one examines leader and follower behaviors and discusses leadership styles.

Style is also determined by forces within the situation itself. These forces include the traditions and values of the organization, its size and structure, the nature of the task at hand, the time available to accomplish a goal, and the history of the relationships among members of the group.

Types of Leadership Styles

Depending on the mix of these factors, one's style can range from highly structured (or authoritative), to moderately structured (or participative), to minimally structured (or permissive). **Authoritative leaders** maintain strong control over the people in the group, give orders and expect others to obey, dominate the group, and motivate others with fear or rewards. With this style, work often proceeds smoothly, productivity is often high, and procedures are usually well defined; however, creativity, autonomy, and self-motivation are stifled, and the needs of group members go unrecognized.

Laissez-faire or **permissive leaders** use a nondirective style. In addition, they are generally inactive and passive. In fact, one may question whether they are leaders at all because they do not work actively to move the group forward. With this style, group members have a great deal of freedom and self-control. Nevertheless, group members can become disinterested and apathetic, goals may remain unclear, group members receive little or no feedback on their contributions, and often there is confusion about the procedures that guide the work of the group. This style of leadership results in group activity that is usually unproductive, inefficient, and unsatisfying for group members.

Perhaps the most effective style is that practiced by **democratic** or **participative leaders.** Democratic leaders talk about "we" rather than "I," ask stimulating questions, make suggestions rather than issue commands, provide constructive criticism, and are egalitarian. The participative leader has confidence in the ability of group members and actively stimulates and guides them to use their abilities to achieve the group's goals. In this situation, the leader and the followers are mutually responsive, communication is multidirectional, and any member of the group is expected to assume the role of leader as the situation requires (Box 11–1).

Situational details also affect the type of leadership style that is most appropriate. In times of crisis, an authoritarian style may be the most appropriate one for a leader to use. On the other hand, when there is no time pressure to complete a task and the group is a mature one, the permissive style may be most effective. Finally, when one is working to implement changes in a system, using the participative style is apt to yield the best results. Keys to effective leadership are:

- Using the style most appropriate to the group and the task or situation at hand
- Using it at the right time
- Being flexible enough to attend to the needs of the followers
- Using the talents of all group members
- Meeting the goals of the group

The participative approach to leadership reflects some of the more current theories of leadership.

THEORIES OF LEADERSHIP

Several theories of leadership have been advanced over the years. Each of these theories reflected the thinking of the time, and each has some value in helping us consider the complex nature of leadership. As we realize the limitations of each theory, we are building a new foundation to strive continually to understand the phenomenon of leadership.

Great Man Leadership Theory

One of the earliest theories of leadership was the "great man" leadership theory, which asserted that the individual who is born into the proper class and circumstance

Box 11.1 Leadership Styles

These different leadership styles are illustrated beautifully in the novel *Watership Down* (Adams, 1972). This is a story of a group of rabbits that, at the urging and insistence of one member, risk leaving their familiar warren to find a safer place to live. The "leader" of the rabbits' warren of origin is authoritarian in his style; he does not listen to advice, is very efficient, is closed to new ideas, does not adapt to new situations, and is unaware of or not concerned about the needs of the followers. Along the way, the rabbits encounter a warren with a totalitarian regime and another warren that has no "chief rabbit." In the latter warren, everyone does whatever he wants to do, there is no common goal, and the entire warren is rather passive, with little joy evident. Finally, in the community created by the rabbits that left their warren of origin and took the journey described in this book, the unique gifts of each member are recognized and used fully, and the group works together toward common goals. In addition, the leader of this group of rabbits seeks advice from others and encourages initiative, a sense of trust exists among members of the community, and all group members feel that they own the decisions that are made because they are involved in making those decisions. There are many lessons about leadership to be learned from this classic children's story.

is the one to lead the people. This theory, which was consistent with rule by monarchs, lacks relevance for more current, complex, democratic societies.

Traitist Leadership Theories

In an attempt to acknowledge that individuals born outside a royal lineage also provided leadership, theories were developed to outline the ideal mix of traits or characteristics that make the most effective leader—traitist leadership theories. Traits such as height, energy level, socioeconomic status, level of education, gender, decisiveness, and articulateness were related to effectiveness in a leader and offered some useful insights. Despite extensive research within this theoretical framework, however, no single mix of traits emerged to predict, determine, or ensure who would be the best leader in a certain situation. In essence, these theories failed to acknowledge the role of the followers, the situation, and the task at hand in determining leader effectiveness, and they also have been shown to be of little help in understanding leadership in our ever-changing, unpredictable world.

Situational Leadership Theory

Situational theories (like the one proposed by Hersey and Blanchard in 1977) clearly recognized the significance of the environment or situation as a factor in the effectiveness of a leader. They asserted that the leader was the one who was in a position to initiate change when a situation was ready for change. In addition, situational leadership theories acknowledged that leadership is a dynamic process that involves an interplay among (1) the personalities and maturity levels of the leader and followers, (2) the task to be accomplished, (3) the goals to be attained, and (4) the conditions within the environment.

Transformational Leadership Theory

Perhaps one of the most contemporary leadership theories is transformational leadership theory (Barker, 1990, 1991; Barker & Young, 1994; Marriner-Tomey, 1993). This theory asserts that leadership is longer lasting and more far-reaching than had been thought previously. With this type of leadership, the leader engages the full person of each follower and transforms each to move beyond individual needs and interests toward higher-level concerns. The leader raises the consciousness of the followers, heightens their aspirations, and intimately involves them in determining the course of action for the group. The transformational leader operates out of a deeply held personal value system, is visionary, has strong convictions, and interacts significantly with followers to see that the vision is realized.

Leadership Tasks Theory

Among the more recent and scholarly approaches to explaining the universal, multidimensional, and complex phenomenon known as leadership is the work of John Gardner, a noted expert in the field. Gardner (1990) proposed the leadership tasks theory, which embodies the components of effective leadership. He asserts that individuals who consistently engage in tasks of leadership are exercising true leadership and should be recognized for their contributions to their organizations, professions, and communities. These tasks are discussed in detail later.

New Science Leadership Theory

Consistent with the interactive concepts inherent in transformational leadership theory and leadership tasks theory is what is referred to as new science leadership theory. This theory, proposed initially by Wheatley (1992, 2006), asserts that to understand leadership and to function as effective leaders, we must focus on relationships, connections, and holism. We also must appreciate the value of chaos and unpredictability in our world, because chaos helps us create systems that are flexible, accepting of change, attentive to the values of all members, without boundaries, constantly growing and evolving, self-renewing, and organic. Wheatley's ideas are gaining support as individuals examine ways to make organizations increasingly effective and the work of individuals in those organizations increasingly meaningful.

COMPONENTS OF EFFECTIVE LEADERSHIP AND TASKS OF LEADERSHIP

Because Garner's (1990) is one of the newer theories of leadership and because it provides a framework for thinking about what leaders do, we will use his leadership tasks theory to address components of effective leadership:

- Envisioning goals
- Affirming values
- Motivating
- Managing
- Achieving a workable unity
- Explaining
- Serving as a symbol
- Representing the group
- Renewing

Each of Gardner's tasks is explained and related to the practice of professional nursing as a way to illustrate how nurses can and do provide leadership in their organizations, professional associations, and communities.

Envisioning Goals

One of the most significant tasks of leadership is envisioning new goals and possibilities. In fact, leaders are often distinguished from nonleaders by their ability to see a different future, articulate their vision, communicate it to others in such a way that it is accepted by others, and energize others to invest the energy needed to realize the vision and create the desired future.

Does it take special training or mystical insight to envision goals? Is this a leadership task reserved for only a few elite individuals? Of course not. Each and every one of us—if we care enough about our jobs, our professions, and our communities—has some idea of how things could be done better or how "our little corner of the world" could be a better place. The leader, however, is the person who does something with or about that dream. This is the leadership task of envisioning goals. Consider the example in Box 11–2 illustrating this point.

Affirming Values

All groups and organizations are characterized by a set of values that may be clearly stated or may be inferred from the observed behaviors of members of the group. Those values may include such things as family-centered care, helping others develop to their fullest potential, and making the largest profit possible. The individuals who run organizations assume that members of the group accept the organization's values and act in concert with them.

It is all too clear, however, that explicitly stated values, such as providing individualized, high-quality care or respecting the dignity and worth of all individuals, often conflict with the values inferred from approved policies and ongoing practices, such as a drastic reduction in the size of the professional staff. The nurse who exercises leadership serves to remind group members of the values they share, as Box 11–3 illustrates.

As Gardner (1990) notes, "Values always decay over time, however, groups that keep their values alive do so not by escaping the processes of decay but by powerful processes of regeneration" (p. 13). Leaders, such as the nurse described in Box 11.3, initiate and help sustain those processes of regeneration when they fulfill the task of leadership known as affirming values.

Motivating

Although it is critical that a leader envision new goals and help a group affirm the values underlying its existence, those tasks alone will not help organizations progress. A leader is nothing without followers, and if individuals are not motivated to choose to follow a leader, then little forward movement takes place. A leader cannot "go it alone." Thus, another important task of leadership is motivating others.

As individuals, we are motivated by internal forces, such as the desire to learn and grow and the satisfaction of knowing we did the very best we could in a situation, regardless of the outcome. We also are motivated by external forces, such as the praise we might receive from someone else, good grades, and a promotion. Both sources of motivation are valid, and both are important. It is the task of leadership to "unlock or channel" (Gardner, 1990, p. 14) the motives that drive individuals so that they can work to their fullest potential and help the group achieve its goals.

This concept is illustrated in Box 11–4. The nurse manager in this situation was most effective in getting staff to participate in activities that added new skills and new responsibilities even though they already felt overworked. Her use of incentives served to motivate the staff to learn this advanced and time-consuming

Box 11.2 Envisioning Goals

Several RNs are working in a community health center that provides care to a poor, underserved, multicultural population. They frequently comment to one another how discouraging it is to see women have to return to the center several times before they have all their family's health needs addressed, such as immunizations, dental care, gynecologic examinations, vision screenings, and hypertension management. These nurses also recognize that after a while the women fail to keep appointments because it is too difficult to get back and forth to the center.

Although most of these nurses are well aware of the problem and acknowledge the serious implications of it, only one nurse begins to talk about a new approach to making appointments and scheduling visits. She envisions a "one-stop shopping" arrangement whereby the family can come to the center on one day and everyone's needs can be addressed. This nurse begins to talk about this idea to the other nurses, her supervisor, and the center's director. She develops a proposal describing how it can work; and she is willing to spearhead the effort to change the appointment scheduling process. This nurse has envisioned a goal and exercised leadership.

Box 11.3 Affirming Values

Nurses working in the local long-term care facility have always prided themselves on the caring environment they provide for residents and families. Elderly residents are respected, treated with dignity, and involved in their own care as much as possible. However, in recent months, one nurse has noticed that she and her colleagues seem to be spending more time complaining about their workloads, criticizing management, and "cutting corners" in their interactions with residents and families as a way to deal with the increased stresses they are feeling.

Rather than continuing to allow herself to be pulled in this direction, the nurse begins to reflect on why she has chosen to work in this kind of setting and what she finds rewarding about caring for the elderly. She then thinks about what is missing and how some of those basic values of respect and dignity seem to have eroded recently. This nurse exercises leadership when she begins to talk to her colleagues about what values they share that are related to caring for the elderly and how they can refocus their behaviors to reestablish that kind of commitment.

Box 11.4 Motivating

In the last three months, the Intravenous Therapy Department at the local community hospital has been decentralized. This means that staff nurses will have to be educated and responsible for starting their own patients' peripheral lines. Many of the nurses are already feeling overworked and are, in their own words, "not excited about having to do such a time-consuming skill that they do not yet feel confident doing." The nurse manager of one renal medical unit decides to provide an incentive—a complimentary continuing education unit offering on intravenous therapy management—for every nurse who enrolls in the educational program during the first phase of training. The manager further motivates the staff with a complimentary family pack movie pass at the local movie theater after the nurse has successfully started 20 intravenous lines.

This nurse manager is quite creative in motivating the staff initially with tangible awards. Interestingly, since so many of the unit's nurses sign up for the first phase of IV Insertion Training, this unit's staff becomes recognized as Resource IV Starters for the rest of the hospital. Soon the staff is so motivated to be experts on intravenous insertion and management, they start a hospital-wide committee for protocol development and are considered the experts.

skill, and they eventually became recognized as experts in the institution, serving to motivate them even further. The person who acts to inspire, encourage, and energize others is fulfilling an important task of leadership, namely, motivating.

Managing

Management is as much a part of effective leadership as the other tasks described, because if one cannot manage a situation to "make things happen," visions will not be realized, and motivated individuals will soon become frustrated. According to Gardner (1990), the managing task of leadership involves a number of dimensions:

- Planning and setting priorities
- Creating processes and structures that will allow a vision to be realized
- Providing resources, delegating, and coordinating the group's activities
- Making decisions, even difficult ones

We often think that managing functions are the responsibility only of the person who holds some administrative position in an organization. Such persons do need good management skills, but the individual who is providing leadership within a group—and who may not occupy any hierarchical position of authority—also must be able to plan, organize, delegate, and so on. This is the managing task of leaders, as illustrated in Box 11–5.

Achieving a Workable Unity

There is no doubt that when a number of individuals come together in the context of complex organizations to face difficult challenges, conflict is likely to arise. That conflict can come from differences in values, miscommunication or lack of communication, uncertainty, incompatible demands placed on individuals, competition for scarce resources, poorly defined responsibilities, change, and normal human drives for success, power, and recognition. Indeed, there is rarely only one source of conflict. Traditionally,

Box 11.5 Managing

Several weeks ago, the staff on the oncology unit decided they wanted to implement self-staffing, and the nurse manager of the unit agreed that they should pursue the idea. The nurses were excited about this new opportunity, and the nurse manager was pleased with the initiative shown by the staff. Since the time this decision was made, however, no progress has occurred toward implementing the new model. Staff members thought that the nurse manager would guide them in making this change, and the nurse manager assumed that, because the idea came from and is enthusiastically endorsed by the staff, the nurses themselves would work on a plan to "make it happen."

As time goes by, some nurses become discouraged, and they convince themselves that the idea was not a good one after all. Other nurses become angry with the nurse manager, thinking she is "dragging her feet" in an attempt to sabotage the new model. Still others sit passively by, waiting for the nurse manager to tell the staff what to do and when and how to do it. But one nurse realizes that if the group is to do its own staffing, several steps must be taken to make that happen.

This nurse asks the hospital librarian to gather a few recent articles on self-staffing projects that have been implemented elsewhere, and she reviews the notes on change from the leadership/management course she took while in school. She then thinks about the steps that need to be taken on the unit and at higher levels of the hospital before their dream can become a reality. Finally, she reflects on her own talents and those of her colleagues in an attempt to match everyone's strengths with the tasks that need to be done. She then writes all this up as a two-page "proposal," asks the nurse manager for time on the agenda of the next staff meeting to discuss it, presents the proposal to the group as a starting point, and succeeds in getting the group to implement self-staffing within the next two months. As a result of fulfilling the managing task of leadership, this nurse emerges as a leader and helps her peers reach a much desired goal.

conflict has been viewed as bad and something to be avoided at any cost. In the past, the emphasis had been on resolving or getting rid of conflict. Contemporary perspectives on conflict, however, acknowledge that it can be healthy. Because moderate amounts of conflict serve as an incentive to develop, excel, change, and grow, a task of the leader is to manage conflict but not necessarily resolve it. In other words, instead of trying to eliminate conflict altogether, the effective leader works to ensure that the normal conflict that exists in most situations serves to stimulate ideas and new perspectives but does not escalate to a point

where members of the group become immobilized or unproductive.

One of the important tasks of leadership, therefore, is to serve as a unifying force within the group to achieve "some measure of cohesion and mutual tolerance" (Gardner, 1990, p. 16), so that the group can move forward to achieve its goals. The leader needs to try to minimize polarization and the formation of cliques by building teams and creating a sense of community among the group. The example in Box 11–6 illustrates how a nurse can fulfill the leadership task of achieving a workable unity.

Box 11.6 Achieving a Workable Unity

Two years ago, the local medical center merged with two other acute care institutions and downsized its staff. Many of the clinical nurse specialist positions were eliminated, experienced nurses were transferred out of the inpatient setting or resigned because of the poor staffing, and units were staffed heavily with unlicensed assistive personnel. During the last six months, the medical center has begun hiring nurses, most of whom are relatively new graduates. On one unit, there is much unrest among staff, and there seems to be little effort among staff to work collaboratively or to support and encourage one another.

One seasoned nurse, who has experienced major changes many times in the past, is troubled by the lack of cooperation among her nursing peer group. She notices that nurses are unwilling to help one another, rarely comfort one another when someone had a particularly difficult patient assignment, are quick to point out one another's faults, and seem to make more of an effort to build alliances with physicians than with their fellow nurses. All of these, she concludes, are signs of the lack of unity and cohesion on the unit. She is concerned

(box continues on page 199)

BOX 11.6 Achieving a Workable Unity (continued)

that, not only are the nurses dissatisfied with the work they are doing but also patient care might eventually suffer. Thus, she decides to try to do something to coalesce the group.

This nurse makes an effort to compliment her colleagues on the work they are doing. She makes a point to ask others for advice and suggestions on different patient situations, even though she is quite able to manage those situations on her own. She invites a colleague to lunch and takes time to reflect on why she went into nursing and what keeps her excited about her job. She muses about the many times throughout her career when the autonomy and practice of nurses were threatened, how the nurses always thought that the immediate crisis was going to be the one to sound their demise, and how the resilient nurses always came through stronger than ever.

This nurse also talks with the nurse manager about ways she can keep the staff better informed. She asks the nurse manager to allow time on a staff meeting agenda for discussion of concerns and to consider contacting the advanced practice psychiatric nurse to meet with the staff. Finally, she agrees to be the first to talk at the staff meeting about the very real fears and concerns experienced by the nurses, thereby taking the risk of speaking up, a risk she thinks her colleagues might not be willing to take. As a result of these small but focused actions by this nurse, the nurses on the unit start to open up to one another, work together more as a unit, and support one another—through discussion, humor, and other means. In addition, some of the more seasoned nurses begin to mentor the less experienced ones.

Explaining

If individuals opt to follow a leader and work with that leader to achieve a goal or realize a vision, they need to understand what the goal is, what is being expected of them, and why they are being asked to do certain things. An important task of leadership, therefore, is explaining things to followers, teaching them, and being sure they are making an informed choice to follow in the first place.

The nurse described in the situation illustrated in Box 11–7 fulfills this task of leadership in an effective way. This nurse manager explained, taught, and supported his staff. He anticipated their needs and planned, in advance, to meet them or minimize their potentially

Box 11.7 Explaining

After extensive study and consultation, the nursing management team of the nearby rehabilitation center decides to institute computerized bedside charting throughout the institution within the next six months. The system has been selected, the infrastructure has been laid, the hardware has been ordered, and all nurse managers have been trained in the new system. The management team has outlined a plan for implementation, on a unit-by-unit basis, that begins in one month and ends five months later. All nurse managers have been directed to plan to bring their staff members "up to speed," and the heads of all other departments (e.g., Pharmacy, Medicine, Physical Therapy) have been directed to do the same.

Knowing that his unit will be among the first ones to go online, that many of his staff members are not convinced that computerized bedside charting is "the way to go," and that many are not comfortable with computers in general, the nurse manager of one unit formulates a plan to prepare his staff appropriately.

First, he arranges for some nurses from his graduate program classes, who are in institutions that have recently implemented computerized charting, to meet with his staff to talk about what the experience was like for them and how they "survived" it. The nurse manager also gathers a few articles about computers and their use in health care, and he shares these with the staff. He gains approval for his staff to go to the local university school of nursing to practice patient-care documentation in its computer lab and arranges schedules so they have the time to go. In addition, he plans time during several upcoming unit staff meetings to talk about the difficulty of dealing with change, the need for the new computer system, the benefits to patients and staff of such a system, and individuals' fears and concerns about their new responsibilities. Finally, he plans for ongoing resources and opportunities for the staff to raise questions, make suggestions, express fears, and receive support throughout the implementation process and until they feel comfortable with the new system.

negative effect. In essence, he exercised effective leadership in relation to the specific task of explaining. As Gardner (1990) notes, "Leaders teach. . . . Teaching and leading are distinguishable occupations, but every great leader is clearly teaching—and every great teacher is leading" (p. 18).

Serving as a Symbol

One of the most significant roles leaders play and one of the most important tasks they perform is serving as a symbol for the group they lead. In other words, when those outside the group observe, listen to, and interact with the leader, they see, hear, and experience all that the group is attempting to do or be. For example, Martin Luther King, Jr., preached nonviolence, and he acted in a nonviolent way when confronted with charges and challenges from others. Jesus Christ had a vision of a world in which people loved and respected their fellow human beings regardless of who they were or how much or little they had; he lived his life among the poor and persecuted, shared what he had with those in need, and held no king above any peasant. Likewise, Florence Nightingale asserted that a healthy environment was critical to the recovery and well-being of the soldiers wounded in battle, and whenever she had the opportunity to speak to health officials, supervise a hospital, or write about the care of the ill, she was consistent in her message.

No less can be expected of the nurse who is providing leadership in today's world. Consider the nurse who serves as a symbol described in Box 11–8. Serving as a symbol means reflecting the group's values and collective identity in whatever one says and does. Admittedly, this is a serious responsibility for a leader to assume, but it is one that will make her more effective in helping a group achieve its goal.

Representing the Group

A leader often must serve as the spokesperson for the group, argue on its behalf, and represent its wishes and desires to others. When we think of "representing a group," we may conjure up an image of the corporate chief executive officer or the president of the United States giving his "state of the union" address to an audience. This leadership task, however, occurs at all levels and in all types of areas, as Box 11–9 illustrates. The nurse described in this account is an excellent example of the task of leadership that Gardner (1990) refers to as representing the group. She exhibited that "distinctive characteristic of the ablest leaders [namely, that she did not] shrink from external representation. [She saw] the long-term needs and goals of [her] constituency in the broadest context, and [she acted] accordingly" (Gardner, 1990, p. 20).

Renewing

Perhaps most significantly, "leaders must foster the process of renewal" (Gardner, 1990, p. 21). They must constantly provide members of the group with new challenges, reinforce the importance of the goal toward which all are striving, encourage and help group members reach their fullest potential, be willing to change the course of action when it no longer serves the intended purpose, and provide opportunities for members of the group to assume the role of leader. Such actions keep the group stimulated, excited, and energized.

Box 11.8 Serving as a Symbol

Nurse educators teach students about the value of research, the need to base their practice on research findings, the importance of participating in professional organizations, and the significance of lifelong learning, among other things. Additionally, they expect students to internalize these values as they begin or pursue new directions in their professional nursing careers. How many of these educators, however, "practice what they preach" and serve as symbols of that kind of behavior?

Often the educator who is thought of as a leader by her students and her peers is the one who lives these values and integrates them into her teaching. The teacher who tells students about what she learned from a conference, the book she read, or the research presentation she heard is conveying to students that she, too, must continue to learn. By supporting her class presentations with research findings and helping students identify gaps in nursing knowledge and areas in need of further study, the nurse educator is not merely telling students how important research is, she is living that value. Finally, the nurse educator who continually revises the teaching strategies she uses because the latest pedagogic research has shown a certain strategy to be effective in facilitating student learning demonstrates to students how one's practice needs to change continually in response to new knowledge.

Box 11.9 Representing the Group

The nurses who work in the outpatient clinics at the medical center feel they are spending more time on paperwork and clerical duties than on patient care. They are angry, frustrated, and feeling abused.

One nurse in this group—who shares the feelings of anger and frustration—begins to keep track of specific incidents that she and others experience rather than just the vague, general complaints that are often expressed. She also makes an effort to talk with her colleagues about what they think are ways to avoid negative incidents and use their professional expertise better. When she has collected a number of such ideas, she shares them with her peers to validate whether her accounts are accurate and fair. She then asks the group if they want her to speak with the clinic director about their concerns and their suggested solutions, and she asks for their commitment to invest the time and energy needed to make changes in how the work gets done if the clinic director challenges them with that charge.

With the support of her peers, this nurse makes an appointment with the clinic director, calmly and rationally presents specific complaints, offers reasonable and well-thought-out solutions to solving these problems, and suggests that the nursing staff prepare a more comprehensive proposal of ways to deal with these issues. The clinic director is so impressed by the nurse's approach and her ability to speak confidently on behalf of the entire group that he enthusiastically supports the efforts of the staff to explore operational changes that will use their expertise better.

An illustration from the perspective of involvement in professional organizations (Box 11–10) helps illustrate the process of renewal and its positive impact on a group and an entire organization. Although the process of renewal should be a continuous one to keep a group alive and healthy, leaders often must implement strategies to revitalize a group that has been allowed to stagnate, as was the case here. Once that renewal starts, however, the task of leadership may become keeping the energy focused and reasonably controlled.

Box 11.10 Renewing

A staff nurse who works for the visiting nurse service that serves an inner-city community has recently been elected president of a local professional nursing organization. From her involvement in the organization to date, she has observed that in recent years, those who held office and served on committees repeated programs from previous years, "recycled" the same people from one position to another, and structured all meetings in the same way. Additionally, she notes that there has been little, if any, reflection on the purpose of the organization or discussion of where the organization wants to be in the next five to 10 years.

Because this nurse believes so strongly in the purposes of this organization and in the value of organizational work itself, she launches a personal campaign to revitalize the group during her term of office. She goes back to the organization's mission statement and bylaws to note what its stated purpose and goals are. She then asks her friends, work colleagues, and members of the organization to share their ideas about what those goals might suggest in terms of programs and activities they could sponsor in the current health-care climate.

This nurse approaches some of the new graduates who are working at her agency, and she speaks to the faculty member who has students at the agency for clinical experiences. In each instance, she extends an invitation to them to come to the next meeting of the organization and to consider joining the organization and serving on a committee.

She then reflects on the kinds of health-care and patient-care problems she sees in practice every day and reads about in newspapers and professional journals, and she looks at all the flyers posted on the bulletin boards at work announcing conferences, programs, and community projects. This gives her a whole repertoire of possible program topics, speakers, and brochure formats.

Armed with these ideas, she approaches the executive committee of the organization and presents them with a variety of ways to revitalize themselves. She makes sure to acknowledge how the expertise of those on the executive committee matches some of the ideas suggested, recognize the valuable contributions made by members over the years, ensure the group that it does not have to take on many new things all at once, and commit her time and resources to work with others to "make it happen."

Stewardship

Although Gardner (1990) does not include it among his tasks of leadership, a discussion of the concept of leadership would be incomplete without considering the leader's responsibility for sound stewardship. Stewardship involves serving others and advancing their best interests, rather than advancing one's own interests. Block (1993) describes stewardship as a desire and willingness to be accountable for the well-being of the overall group or organization by "operating in service to, rather [than] in control of, those around us" (p. xx). It comprises the following principles (Block, 1993, p. xxi):

- Power is balanced and everyone is involved in decision-making.
- The primary commitment is to the group, organization, or larger community, not to an individual's or small group's own "agenda."
- The organizational culture and overall vision are defined by everyone, not by a select few.
- A more "balanced and equitable distribution of rewards" exists.

Thus, leaders have responsibility for keeping "the big picture," the good of the group or organization, and the ultimate goal or vision in mind. Leadership, in essence, is broadly focused and externally oriented.

NURSING LEADERSHIP IN THE 21ST CENTURY

It is obvious from this discussion of the tasks of leadership that leadership and management are not the same phenomenon. One hopes that an effective manager will also be a leader and carry out all nine of the tasks of leadership as well as be an effective steward, but this is not always the case. One should not assume that everyone in a position of authority—a nurse manager, the vice president for nursing, the dean of a school of nursing, or the president of a professional organization—is automatically a leader.

By the same token, and perhaps more significantly, leadership is not limited to those in positions of authority. Each of us has the potential to exhibit leadership at various points in our professional careers, regardless of our title, position, or academic credentials. The only barrier to our exercise of leadership is our own unwillingness to take on the challenge. There is no doubt that leadership is hard work; it takes time and sustained energy, and the rewards for those efforts often are not immediate. But if nurses and nursing are to assume the kind of position in the health-care delivery system of the 21st century that

we deserve and can manage, each of us must be willing to take on the risk of being a leader.

> Leadership is not limited to those in positions of authority. Each of us has the potential to exhibit leadership at various points in our professional careers, regardless of our title, position, or academic credentials.

Leaders must be aware of the four kinds of futures (Valiga, 1994) that are available to each of us. The *probable future* is what is likely to happen if current situations and directions remain unchanged. For example, it is quite probable that there will continue to be concern primarily for the "bottom line," with only "lip service" given to concerns for quality care. The *possible future* refers to what might happen with only minimal changes. For example, it is possible that more and more unlicensed health-care workers will be created and used to provide direct care, and nurses will hold only oversight and coordinator positions, being minimally involved in the direct care of patients and families. The *plausible future* refers to what could occur if focused efforts are made to accomplish specific goals. For example, it is quite plausible that nurses will be expected to take the lead in interdisciplinary team efforts because of their holistic perspective on patient care. Finally, leaders must attend to—and, indeed, create—the *preferred future*, the state of affairs we want to exist. For instance, nurses should be significant participants in shaping health-care policy to ensure that quality patient and family care takes priority over cost containment and that nurses hold positions of influence in designing that care.

Nursing leaders in the 21st century will have to create our preferred future. In order to do this, they will need a clear vision of what will best serve the profession and the individuals, families, and communities for whom nurses care. They must be proactive, fight for excellence, and be unwilling to accept mediocrity. They must be flexible, willing to change, and able to deal with uncertainty and ambiguity in order to prevent blind-sided reactions to change (Clampitt & DeKoch, 2001).

The nurses we will look to for leadership in the 21st century must be self-assured and self-confident but always open to new ideas and interested in growth and self-improvement. They must be collegial in their interactions with other nurses; acknowledge the strengths, capabilities, and achievements of others; mentor others; and help others take advantage of opportunities to facilitate their own growth. If nursing is to be a powerful force in health care in the 21st century, we will need leaders who are articulate, whose actions are consistent with their words, who are competent and credible, and who can work collaboratively within an interdisciplinary team. Leaders will be needed who are visionary, can ignite followers to join in the effort to turn visions into realities, and can sustain and continually challenge a group as it strives to implement change and face the challenges presented along the way.

Such leaders now exist among our students, staff nurses, professional association staff, nurse educators, nurse administrators, nurse scientists, and nurse entrepreneurs. Each of us must incorporate the tasks of leadership into our professional practice repertoire and perform those tasks as needed (Grossman & Valiga, 2005). This kind of behavior on the part of many nurses will ensure the profession's strong future, and nursing will be a significant player in the health-care arena of the 21st century.

INTERACTIVE EXERCISES

Go to the Intranet site and complete the interactive exercises provided for this Chapter.

EVIDENCED-BASED PRACTICE: CONSIDER THIS . . .

*I*n their position paper on leadership and leadership development priorities, Sigma Theta Tau (2005), the International Honor Society for Nursing, has recognized the importance of clinical leadership in the practice environment, which includes "advocacy for evidence-based nursing practice" (p. 2).

Question: How will you further develop your skills to demonstrate this advocacy for EBP in your practice setting?

Source: Sigma Theta Tau. (2005). Resource paper and position statement on leadership and leadership development priorities. Retrieved October 1, 2007, from *http://www.nursingsociety.org/aboutus/Documents/position_leadership.doc*

KEY POINTS

- Leadership is not the same as management, nor is it tied to a position of authority. Leadership is more an art than a science.

- The relationship between leaders and followers is interactive and mutually beneficial.

- Keys to effective leadership include the use of the appropriate style at a particular time and flexibility to attend to the needs of the followers, use the talents of the group members, and meet the goals of the group.

- Leadership style can be viewed as a set of behaviors that characterize individuals as they perform their leader role. These styles differ in terms of how power is distributed among those leading and those following, how decisions are made, and whose needs are of primary concern.

- There is no single widely accepted definition or theory of leadership.

- Leaders "cause ripples," "rock the boat," "disturb the status quo," and take risks.

- Leaders are visionary. They envision goals and possibilities.

- Leaders help members of a group reflect on their shared vision when they fulfill the leadership task known as affirming values.

- Leaders motivate others to work toward group goals. Motivation includes attending to both internal and external forces that drive individuals to achieve their fullest potential and help a group accomplish its goals.

- Leadership involves managing situations to achieve goals: planning carefully, using creative processes, providing resources, and making decisions.

- Leaders help a group coalesce as a unified whole so that it can move forward to achieve its goals.

(Key points continue on page 204)

KEY POINTS (continued)

- Effective leaders teach and explain so that followers can make informed choices.

- Leaders serve as symbols and spokespersons for a group by reflecting the group's values and collective identity and by representing the group.

- The effective leader exercises good stewardship, a combination of accountability and partnership that best serves the clients (patients), the group, and the profession.

- A group or organization must constantly be renewed to remain viable and strong.

- The role of the follower is critical, for without followers there can be no leaders.

Thought and Discussion Questions

1. Read the children's story *The Little Engine that Could* (Piper, 1961), or Rudyard Kipling's poem "If." How does the little engine or "being a man" relate to leadership and the challenges inherent in the role of leader?

2. Review the Chapter Thought located on the first page of the chapter, and be prepared to discuss its meaning in the context of the contents of this chapter.

☐ REFERENCES

Adams, R. (1972). *Watership down*. New York: Avon.

Barker, A. M. (1991). An emerging leadership paradigm: Transformational leadership. *Nursing & Health Care, 12*(4), 204–207.

Barker, A. M. (1990). *Transformational nursing leadership: A vision for the future*. Baltimore: Williams & Wilkins.

Barker, A. M., & Young, C. E. (1994). Transformational leadership: The feminist connection in postmodern organizations. *Holistic Nursing Practice, 9*(1), 16–17.

Bass, B. M. (1990). *Bass & Stogdill's handbook of leadership: Theory, research, and managerial applications* (3rd ed.). New York: The Free Press.

Bennis, W., & Nanus, B. (1985). *Leaders: The strategies for taking charge*. New York: Harper & Row.

Block, P. (1993). *Stewardship: Choosing service over self-interest*. San Francisco: Berrett-Koehler.

Clampitt, P. G., & DeKoch, R. J. (2001). *Embracing uncertainty: The essence of leadership*. Armonk, NY: M. E. Sharpe.

Gardner, J. W. (1990). *On leadership*. New York: The Free Press.

Grossman, S., & Valiga, T. M. (2005). *The new leadership challenge: Creating a preferred future for nursing* (2nd ed.). Philadelphia: F. A. Davis.

Hersey, P., & Blanchard, K. (1977). *Management of organizational behavior: Utilizing human resources* (3rd ed.). Englewood Cliffs, NJ: Prentice-Hall.

Marriner-Tomey, A. (1993). *Transformational leadership in nursing*. St. Louis, MO: Mosby.

Piper, W. (1961). *The little engine that could*. New York: Platt & Munk.

Rost, J. C. (1991). *Leadership for the twenty-first century*. Westport, CT: Praeger.

Sigma Theta Tau. (2005). Resource paper and position statement on leadership and leadership development priorities. Retrieved October 1, 2007, from *http://www.nursingsociety.org/aboutus/Documents/position_leadership.doc*

Valiga, T. M. (1994). Leadership for the future. *Holistic Nursing Practice, 9*(1), 83–90.

Van Fleet, D. D., & Yukl, G. A. (1989). A century of leadership research. In W. E. Rosenbach & R. L. Taylor (Eds.), *Contemporary issues in leadership* (2nd ed., pp. 65–94). Boulder, CO: Westview Press.

Wheatley, M. J. (1992). *Leadership and the new science: Learning about organizations from an orderly universe*. San Francisco: Berrett-Koehler.

Wheatley, M. J. (2006). *Leadership and the new science: Discovering order in a chaotic world* (3rd ed.). San Francisco: Berrett-Koehler.

☐ BIBLIOGRAPHY

Bennis, W. (1989). *On becoming a leader*. Reading, MA: Addison-Wesley.

Bennis, W., Spreitzer, G. M., & Cummings, T. G. (Eds.). (2001). *The future of leadership: Today's top leadership thinkers speak to tomorrow's leaders*. San Francisco: Jossey-Bass.

Boman, L., & Deal, T. (1995). *Leading with soul: An uncommon journey of spirit*. San Francisco: Jossey-Bass.

Bruderle, E. R. (1994). The arts and humanities: A creative approach to developing nurse leaders. *Holistic Nursing Practice, 9*(1), 68–74.

Burns, J. M. (1978). *Leadership*. New York: Harper Torchbooks.

Cassidy, V. R., & Kroll, C. J. (1994). Ethical aspects of transformational leadership. *Holistic Nursing Practice, 9*(1), 41–47.

DePree, M. (1989). *Leadership is an art*. New York: Dell Publishing.

DiRienzo, S. M. (1994). A challenge to nursing: Promoting followers as well as leaders. *Holistic Nursing Practice, 9*(1), 26–30.

Greenleaf, R. K. (1977). *Servant leadership: A journey into the nature of legitimate power and greatness*. New York: Paulist Press.

Kelley, R. E. (1992). *The power of followership: How to create leaders people want to follow and followers who lead themselves*. New York: Doubleday Currency.

Keirsey, D. (1999, December 20). The four temperaments. Retrieved October 1, 2007 from *http://keirsey.com/matrix.html*

Koestenbaum, P. (2002). *Leadership: The inner side of greatness*. San Francisco: Jossey-Bass.

Kouzes, J. M., & Posner, B. Z. (2002). *Leadership challenge* (3rd ed.). San Francisco: Jossey-Bass.

Nanus, B. (1992). *Visionary leadership: Creating a compelling sense of direction for your organization*. San Francisco: Jossey-Bass.

Rosenbach, W. E., & Taylor, R. L. (Eds.). (2006). *Contemporary issues in leadership* (6th ed.). Boulder, CO: Westview Press.

Rost, J. C. (1994). Leadership: A new conception. *Holistic Nursing Practice, 9*(1), 1–8.

☐ ONLINE RESOURCES

Sigma Theta Tau International
http://www.nursingsociety.org

Keirsey Temperamant Sorter Web site
http://www.keirsey.com

■ Rose **Kearney-Nunnery**

Management in Organizations

> **❝***I am where I am because*
> *I believe in all possibilities.***❞**

Whoopi Goldberg

Chapter Objectives

On completion of this chapter, the reader will be able to:

1. Apply systems theory to an organizational scenario.
2. Examine the goals, structure, functions, and culture of selected organizations.
3. Analyze factors included in motivational and humanistic management theories.
4. Examine the various managerial roles for and skills of nurses in a health-care organization.
5. Apply methods for appropriate and effective delegation in a health-care scenario.

Key Terms

Organization	Organizational Functions	Theory Z
Organizational Structure	Management	Executive
Centralization	Motivational Theories	Organizational Culture
Decentralization	Theory X	Power
Flat Organizational Structures	Theory Y	Negotiation
Tall Organizational Structures	Hygiene Factors	Delegation
	Motivational Factors	

Max Weber (1947), the renowned German sociologist, described an organization in economic and social terms as "a system of purposive activity of a specified kind" (p. 151). An **organization** is simply an arrangement of human and material resources for some purpose, as in the creation of some institution or agency to meet a stated aim. Organizations range from the single-purpose association to multipurpose, monolithic institutions. They have been studied for years in an effort to improve on outputs as the intended mission or purpose. Organizations can be viewed in terms of their structure, function, and people. Most simply, they can be envisioned as the open system described in Chapter 3, with inputs, throughput or transformations, and outputs. But understanding organizations, especially health-care organizations, becomes more complex as organizations expand, contract, and redefine themselves. Changes in organizations are particularly relevant in light of the need for more operational transparency that occurred following recent and highly visible management scandals, along with the view of the global economy.

This chapter examines how organizations are structured and how they are managed to meet their intended mission. Nursing management in an organization must have a broad environmental, interpersonal, and dynamic vision, beyond patients and equipment in an isolated hospital or agency.

Principles of scientific management and management theory have undergone continued investigation and change. Many writers have defined management, but no one definition of management has been accepted universally. They discuss the leader and the manager, sometimes interchangeably. Buckingham (2005) looks at the difference, being the individual's focus: the leader on the future, the manager on staff, and outcomes for the organization. Use of management theories and effective management skills are critical components of professional practice. Communication, negotiation, and delegation are important factors, as are the leadership concepts described in the previous chapter. Applying these concepts to contemporary nursing practice is vital for the operation of a successful organization and an effective health-care system.

ORGANIZATIONS AS SYSTEMS

Systems theory provides a useful perspective for viewing the internal and external influences with any organization. In fact, Bertalanffy (1968), who provided the foundations of general systems theory, stated that the only meaningful way to study an organization is as a system (p. 9). The actual selection of a particular systems model depends on the complexity and uniqueness of the organization. It requires careful assessment of the organization, examining mission and goals, present structure, and the prevailing leadership and management styles being used to guide practice and address organizational goals. Interestingly, Hall and Tolbert (2005) conclude that because organizations are so complex, organizational theories must be used in combination to address the complex phenomena (p. 207).

Health-care delivery systems are complex open environmental systems. Agency administrative policy and operational structures internally influence and guide the system. The surrounding environmental system of the organization is the health-care arena that provides the professional, specialization, economic, and additional value structures for the organizational unit and its members. The broader social environment reflects societal norms and values through the real and potential needs of health-care consumers. Direct or indirect linkages among all system parts are assumed to be essential for effectiveness and continuity. But look further at this complex system and the internal environment.

Intricacies of an Organization

A useful perspective for viewing the intricacies of a health-care organization is to envision it as a system affected by other systems and within the larger health-care and societal systems (environment or suprasystem). In addition, health-care organizations focus on people and have the dynamic influence of emerging technology. As a review, consider the principles of systems theory and organizational characteristics in Table 12–1. To understand the organizational system, a careful assessment is needed of the organization's goals and values, hierarchical structure, leadership and management, interpersonal and communication systems, resources and technology, boundaries, and external environments.

Goals and Values

Goals and values are implied in a statement of purpose or philosophy and are the basis of the organization's existence. The institutional mission statement and original or revised incorporation papers contain valuable information on values—how people within the organization are viewed as customers, staff members, and administrators. Humanistic versus mechanistic values are apparent in these statements of mission, philosophy, and purpose. Organizational values, as the reasons for existence, are provided in vision or goals statements.

Hierarchical Structure

The *hierarchical structure* is the institutional design and lines of authority, as demonstrated by a bureaucratic or

Table 12.1

Systems Theory Components and Organizational Characteristics of a Health-Care Agency

Systems Theory	Organizational Characteristics of a Health-Care Agency
Wholeness	Organizational components of the agency or units and their interactions with each other and their environments, including the health-care system, community, client base, external payors, and corporate system (if applicable). The components cannot stand alone.
Hierarchical Order	The organizational structure as defined through functional and reporting hierarchy and demonstrated by the leadership.
Exchange of Information (Openness)	Boundaries among the different organizational units internally and with external boundaries and environments. This includes communication internally and externally.
Progressive Differentiation	Self-organization and the system become increasingly complex to meet the stated organizational goals for the health care of individuals and groups. This is the area of rules and management procedures to meet the goal for positive health-care outcomes.
Equifinality	Client needs and conditions, as well as provider differences, determine system outcomes. These are the interpersonal relationships and the technology to meet the organizational goals but they may be met in different ways with individual circumstances in a dynamic open system.
Teleology	The behaviors in the internal environment with an arrangement of human and material resources is directed to meet the intended aims. The actions and the behaviors in the organization are directed at the goal for optimal health-care outcomes. These outcomes are defined in the organizational mission, values, and goals statements and demonstrated by the membership.

organic structure. The system structure is described in formal documents and further interpreted in operation through informal sources, such as technical staff, to determine how tasks are actually accomplished in the organization. The structural design is intended to accomplish the system's mission to provide the intended services through leadership and management practices. This structure may be further characterized as complex or simple, centralized or decentralized, tall or flat.

Leadership and Management

Leadership and management styles vary among organizations. As seen later in this chapter, these styles may be directed from the topmost governing board or corporate officers downward, as in a bureaucratic organization operating under Theory X. Alternatively, it may be more flexible and participatory, as in Theory Z organizations. The management style pervasive in the organization should be meeting the organizational goals.

Communication Systems

The *interpersonal and communication systems* are the psychosocial and interdisciplinary relationships unique to the organization—role relationships, attitudes, and values of people and groups within the system. Examine the expected behaviors of each member of the organization and the interrelationships, in both formal and informal interactions. The organizational culture is a vital consideration here.

Resources and Technology

Resources and technology are the physical resources and collaborative human resources. Physical resources include operating and investment capital, equipment, information systems, services, and tangible assets. Collaborative resources are the additional skills and expertise to provide added input to system functions; this includes the resources for evidence-based practice.

External Environments

Once the system itself is characterized, move outward into the environmental layers of the open system, or the suprasystem. To understand the external environment, we must first reevaluate the organization's mission. As in any business, this provides us with market forces. Is a product being produced or a service being delivered, and to whom? Consider the differences between the environments of local organizations focused on a specific community and those of national or multinational conglomerates. To understand an organization's initial environmental layer, focus first on the immediate output of the system. Suppose we are looking at a home-care agency. Such an agency provides home care within specific specialty parameters to an identified service area. In the environment, we initially have the local community with a specific geography, client population, health-care provider groups, payment streams, resources, and health-care needs. This local agency has additional environmental influences from state and federal regulatory bodies and agencies, professional disciplines, and the larger health-care system.

Now, consider these factors with a larger health-care agency, which offers more services to a larger clientele, such as a teaching hospital with a broader service menu and service area. We have to consider the geography, client population, health-care provider groups, payment streams, resources, and health-care needs across the state or perhaps across several states. Services may include not only acute and chronic care but also multispecialty clinics, research, and outreach programs. We have more care providers, including students, faculty, and visiting specialists from various health-care disciplines. There are more requirements and regulations from state and federal regulatory bodies and agencies and professional disciplines, just by virtue of the expanded services, funding streams, and service expectations. Coordination with the broader health-care system must also be considered, as people come from and return to their local areas. External forces also include inputs of energy, information, materials, and myriad technologies received from the environment, transformed, and returned to the environment as outputs.

In an open system, all boundary influences must be identified and relationships evaluated to discover interrelationships and effects. All external layers and interrelating systems are important factors for a true understanding of the influences on any particular open system, as with community support for a local nonprofit agency. They may be positive when speakers at public hearings to support county funding. These environmental influences can have unanticipated repercussions on the system, when this previous support interferes with management decisions.

The health-care environment can easily be seen as highly complex, dynamic, and uncertain. Changes occur constantly. Change is influenced by consumers, technologic advances, government, and third-party payers. The external forces in the broader environment provide inputs into the system and affect internal operations and resultant outputs, such as client outcomes. Health-care organizations must respond to external forces in a rapid, dynamic, and innovative manner and cannot remain static. A humanistic philosophy, with its focus on the people in an organization, is needed for a contemporary and innovative health-care organization. It is the people of the organization that create, define, and fulfill organizational goals. This brings us to an examination of the various structures of organizational systems.

ORGANIZATIONAL STRUCTURES

Mintzberg (1983b) has defined **organizational structure** as "the sum total of the ways in which its labor is divided into distinct tasks and then [how] coordination is achieved among these tasks" (p. 2). Generally, when we think of an organizational structure, we conceive of some type of hierarchy that tells us about positions or roles, responsibilities, status, channels of command or reporting relationships, and tasks to be accomplished. The picture that comes to mind is usually a bureaucratic structure with a multitude of "red tape" with which to contend. This is not always the case. The appropriateness of the structure depends on the organization's purposes (goals and values), how outcomes are best accomplished (leadership and management), the people in the organizational system, the resources and technology used or available, and influences from the external environment(s). These system influences provide us with information on the size and complexity of the organizational structure.

The structure demonstrates the relationships among an organization's components and presents us with its design. Looking at health-care organizations, we find two general structures: bureaucratic and organic. Mintzberg (1983b) places these two organizational designs at opposite ends of a continuum of standardization (Fig. 12–1). This range gives us a way of viewing organizational structures. At one extreme is the controlled, mechanistic, and standardized classic bureaucracy; at the opposite extreme, there is the humanistic organization that contains no standardized processes, outputs, or skills across the structure. Health-care organizations generally fall somewhere between the two extremes, depending on their mission.

Bureaucratic Structure	Organic Structure

High standardization of processes, outputs, and skills	Absence of standardization

■ **Figure 12.1** Mintzberg's continuum of standardization in organizations. (Adapted from Mintzberg, H. [1983b]. *Structure in fives: Designing effective organizations.* Englewood Cliffs, NJ: Prentice-Hall.)

Bureaucratic Organizations

The most recognized and traditional organization is the bureaucratic structure. A bureaucracy is a mechanistic model focused on outcomes. Weber (1864–1920) provided the original bureaucratic model, with a high degree of efficiency and control. His work has been translated and interpreted frequently in research on organizations and organizational theory. Merton (1957) further defined a bureaucratic organization as "a formal, rationally organized social structure involving clearly defined patterns of activity in which, ideally, every series of actions is functionally related to the purposes of the organization" (p. 195). The bureaucratic organization has a hierarchical structure with designated lines of authority and control. The mission of the organization is all-consuming. Actions to meet the purposes and directives are taken in lower layers, whereas policy-making, authority, and control reside primarily in the upper layers of the organization. Specific characteristics of a bureaucratic organization are as follows:

1. A clear-cut division of labor
2. Differentiated controls and sanctions
3. Roles assigned on the basis of qualifications and technical efficiency
4. Clearly stated rules and conformity to regulations
5. A premium placed on precision, speed, expert control, continuity, discretion, and optimal returns on input
6. Strict devotion to regulations
7. Depersonalized relationships. (Merton, 1957, pp. 195–196)

Examples of bureaucratic health-care organizations are depicted in Figures 12–2 and 12–3. In these examples, management and control flow downward from the hospital board through the chief executive officer (CEO) or chief operating officer (COO), who is appointed by the board and is responsible for the organization's mission,

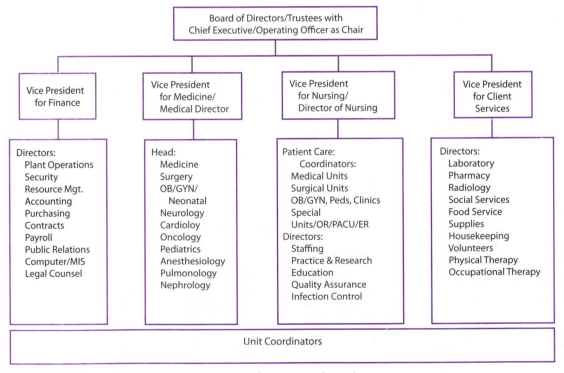

■ **Figure 12.2** Example of flat bureaucratic structure of a community hospital.

■ **Figure 12.3** Example of tall bureaucratic structure of a community hospital.

whether for-profit or not-for-profit. To accomplish these aims, the executive layer is responsible to the CEO or COO. The executives receive mandates and strategic initiatives from the board through the CEO or COO and decide on priorities, plan implementation, and regulations. Executives, in turn, direct their administrative staffs, and on down the line. Titles and functional areas may vary among organizations but each employee has a specific role in carrying out the organization's mission.

A bureaucratic organization is structured, standardized, controlled, and in many instances, authoritarian. Written and unwritten policies and regulations are prevalent, as are specified channels of command. Efficiency and effectiveness in achieving the organizational mission are organizational values. Bureaucratic organizational structures are seen in the older, traditional, and large authoritarian settings in which control and the ultimate mission of the institution are all-consuming. External influences should be predictable to obtain the most efficient functioning of the organization. Channels of command and productivity are important components of the system. But in recent years, a move toward more flexible and humanistic organizational structures, focusing on environmental influences along with employee involvement and job satisfaction for higher productivity, has led to a transformation to more innovative practices.

Organic Organizations

Organic organizational structures, or adhocracies, have evolved to meet the needs of organizations composed of humans in dynamic and sometimes complex environmental settings. The term *adhocracy* implies that the structure is a design that has been developed to meet the organizational mission and specific goals. Hall and Tolbert (2005) characterize these organizations as closely linked to their environments with a network structure of control, continual adjustment and redefinition of tasks, and a communication context of information and advice replacing the traditional supervisory lines (p. 31). These organizations represent a movement from the standardized, mechanistic bureaucracies to humanistic forms arising out of behavioral organizational research and management theories.

Mintzberg (1983b) proposed that this structure is the most useful in a complex and dynamic environment in which experts, managers, and staff from different disciplines cooperate on decentralized project teams to meet a system output goal innovatively. Several organic designs are seen in health-care organizations. The most prevalent organic or adhocratic designs are functional, product, and matrix forms.

Functional Structure

A functional structure, like the bureaucracy, focuses on organizational outcomes; but unlike a bureaucracy, it has control and responsibility spread horizontally across the system to meet specific organizational functions. Daft (2007) notes that this structure is most effective when in-depth expertise is critical to meeting organizational goals and the focus is on efficiency. But, the main weakness "is a slow response to environmental changes that require coordination across departments" (p. 102). A functional form can therefore be used in an organization with a specific function, such as a rehabilitative facility. The function of the rehabilitative care across specialty lines is the organization's purpose. The people in the organization have the decision-making authority for their services in the organization. Functional units are thus arranged in specialty areas, as illustrated in Figure 12–4.

The organization is designed to focus on the function of delivering rehabilitative care to the consumer. Two distinct functions are apparent in our example of this functional form: (1) finance and administration of the agency, and (2) delivery of rehabilitative health care. An executive director or president oversees the organization with the assistance of two directors. The main

organizational function of rehabilitative care delivery is structured as specialty units under the direction of the health-care director. Fragmentation, duplication of services across specialties, and poor coordination limit this design. This limitation becomes more severe as the organization grows in size and complexity—for example, when services increase and the service area is enlarged.

Product Structure

A product or divisional structure is similar to the functional structure except that the organization is focused on the product as the outcome, and not also on the means to the outcome. The people and processes in the product structure are grouped accordingly to meet the intended aim with the goals of coordination and client satisfaction. The product structure promotes flexibility and change with decentralized decision-making, a focus on product goals, and coordination across functions (Daft, 2007, p. 104). Consider the example of a large home-care agency (Fig. 12–5). The product is home-care services, with attention being given to the needs and desires of the home-care client. The product units are organized in terms of nursing services, physical therapy, and speech therapy. Each unit has a director responsible to the president of the agency for the home-care product. Vice presidents are responsible to the president for general functions of health-care referrals, contractual services, personnel, and marketing. Product units are thus arranged in specified areas (nursing, physical therapy, and speech therapy), with each being directed toward service coordination, referrals, contractual services, and marketing to meet consumer needs.

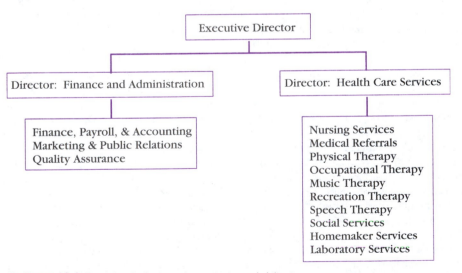

■ **Figure 12.4** Example of a functional organization: rehabilitative agency.

■ **Figure 12.5** Example of a product form organization: home-care agency.

The product structure works well with an organization whose services and marketing are directed at the consumer. This design is flexible in a dynamic or unstable environment, because consumer needs and satisfaction are of prime concern. Divisions are separated by product—nursing care, physical therapy, and speech therapy. But duplication of services is an immediate problem, especially in health care, in which coordination of therapeutic regimens is vital for the consumer.

Matrix Structure

To address the need to coordinate consumer services, another adhocratic design combines the functional and product forms. Multidimensional decision-making and responsibility are the features of a matrix organization. In a health-care agency, this can refer to the product of state-of-the-art care and the function of provision of services to the client as the consumer. An example of the matrix design is an organization whose mission is directed at research and development and provision of care. Research managers in interdisciplinary areas, such as aging, acute infectious processes, mental health, rehabilitation, and health promotion, are located on one side of the matrix, with specialized health-care providers on the other side (Fig. 12–6). People as leaders, managers, and workers, along with tangible resources in the environment, are all represented in the matrix cells. Although this design is challenging, it is consistent with the core competency for health professionals identified in Chapter 1 for working in interdisciplinary teams.

Consider the example of home care for an elderly client following a hip fracture. Care for the client and the family along the continuum would move from acute care to short-term rehabilitation to home care, with interdisciplinary care providers—including home care coordinators, therapists, and specialists—all contributing to the decision-making and service provision. The complexity of this system is initially breathtaking. Both functions and products must be considered in coordination of the services needed by the client. This is a collegial structure with integrated functions and products that require multilayered decisions. The number of people involved in the matrix for decisions varies. Larger organizations may involve only managers in the matrix, with traditional departmental structures evolving under each manager. Smaller organizations, such as the earlier example of a home-care agency, could realistically involve managers and providers in the matrix according to the scope of services (product) and resources (human and material as functions).

The matrix design promotes innovative practices as a result of a consumer focus, in the context of current technology, emergent practice problems, research information, and specialty practice. Research and development issues are directed at current practice, with experts from each area represented for problem-solving and decision-making. This matrix design is seen more frequently in health settings with a dual focus, such as education and service or research and service. The complexity of the design and problems with integration of all appropriate people and resources are the main disadvantages of the matrix form. Daft (2007) describes its disadvantages more fully as follows:

1. Participants experience dual authority, leading to confusion and frustration.
2. Good interpersonal skills and extensive training of participants are needed.

■ **Figure 12.6** Example of a matrix organizational structure.

3. It is time-consuming, with frequent meetings and conflict resolution sessions.
4. Participants must understand and adopt collegial rather than vertical-type relationships.
5. Dual pressure from the environment is required to maintain a balance of power. (p. 111)

Coordination problems are a definite disadvantage of adhocratic designs. Experts and project teams or divisions are focused on innovation and targeting of specific outcomes. This focus may represent only one piece of the mission of the organization, however. Thus, good communication and coordination are critical. But

coordination problems are many times outweighed by the advantages of flexibility, innovation, and human involvement.

As an additional note, the organization may have more than one organizational structure, either embedded or mixed. Recall Mintzberg's (1983b) continuum of standardization in Figure 12–1. The health-care agency may have a formal organizational structure leaning toward a bureaucracy as seen in Figure 12–3. But client services may have a distinct rehabilitative service with a functional structure seen in Figure 12–4. This will add to the complexity of decision-making and management.

Structural Components for Decision-Making and Management

Organizations are also categorized by how the components are arranged, as centralized or decentralized and flat or tall. Centralized and decentralized organizational structures relate to the lines of control and decision-making within the organization. **Centralization** occurs when the span of control or management is in the classic bureaucratic style, governed from the top downward. Authority, control, and decision-making occur in upper management, with less participation from the lower levels. **Decentralization** distributes authority downward in an organization, allowing decision-making and control at local levels. Reasons suggested for decentralization are to establish a more collegial and participatory model, resulting in employee involvement, performance, and satisfaction. Also, the people who are actually involved in the service are making the decisions about it.

Organizations can also be described as having flat or tall structures, depending on the layers of differentiation for authority, decision-making, and coordination. **Flat organizational structures** have a wide base and few layers or tiers for decision-making and authority. Decisions, controls, and governance are widely spread across the organization in a horizontal differentiation. **Tall organizational structures** have more tiers and lines of command, with less local decision-making at the lower levels. Tall organizations have more management levels, with lines of command resulting in a vertically differentiated hierarchical structure. Compare the organizational structures in Figures 12–2 and 12–3. Both are bureaucratic structures, but decisions and work functions are spread more widely across the organization in flat structures.

Deciding whether a centralized or decentralized, tall or flat structure is best depends on the characteristics of the specific organization. As Hall and Tolbert (2005) have observed, high levels of centralization mean greater coordination, but less flexibility and overloaded communication channels as communications flow up and down the hierarchy (p. 62). Many organizations have changed from centralized, tall structures to encourage more employee involvement. But problems can arise when communication, coordination, and monitoring of activities in the organization demand integration for effective functioning. As in his continuum of organizational standardization (see Fig. 12–2), Mintzberg (1983b) suggests that centralization and decentralization be viewed as opposite ends of a continuum rather than absolutes (p. 98). The degree of centralization or decentralization actually should depend on the organization's size, structure, technology, people, and mission to determine where decisions are made best.

ORGANIZATIONAL FUNCTIONS

The purpose or function of the organization is to meet the pre-established goal as outputs from the system. The goals and values described in the institutional mission and purposes statement are the basis for the organization's existence. The mission statement is the overall purpose of the organization, including whether the organization is a for-profit organization or a not-for-profit organization. Stockholders or shareholders expect to see some return on their investment in a for-profit (or proprietary) organization, and this expectation is reflected in organizational goals. Not-for-profit organizations receive funding from various sources, but there is no sense of ownership. In a not-for-profit organization, profits are generally reinvested in the organization to keep it financially competitive.

Once the mission is understood, the targets to achieve this mission become the issue. Organizational goals are specified for effective and efficient functioning. Mintzberg (1983a) has identified four types of goals that demonstrate intent and consistency of behavior in organizations: ideologic, formal, shared, and system.

- *Ideologic goals* relate to the values people in the organization share. An example of an ideologic goal in a health-care organization is access to and provision of high-quality health care for people of all ages.
- *Formal goals* are those authorized through the hierarchy from people with authority who have a power base in the organization.
- *Shared goals* are those set and pursued by a particular group in the organization. Involvement of family members in caregiving is an example of a shared goal that a specialty group favors and implements in the organization.
- *System goals* are those set to maintain the system. Mintzberg (1983a) has identified system goals as survival, efficiency, control, and growth. System goals relate to continuity of the organization and contain a strong economic component. These survival system goals are driving many health-care organizations. These may also be the strategic initiatives or priorities for the organization and specified for action within a certain time frame.

Organizations are now recognizing that goals that are too broad can deplete the resources and effectiveness of the intended outcomes and the system goals. We hear of companies and major industries streamlining and getting "back to basics." They seriously consider examining what they know best, and refining and focusing it, rather than diversifying. Linkages with other organizations that can handle the diversifications better may be more beneficial to both the organization and the consumer group. This development has been seen with restructuring in health-care organizations.

There are three basic reasons for the changes in health-care structures: environmental influences, changes in the provider system, and changes in consumer needs and demographics. First, external environmental influences have had a major effect on health-care organizations, as with diagnosis-related groups (DRGs), the prospective payment system (PPS) for health-care reimbursement, and the safety initiatives. Second, specialization and changes in the health-care provider system have confused consumers and legislators. Disciplinary lines between health-care providers necessarily have some overlap as we implement cross-training, interdisciplinary practice, and focus on humanistic and holistic values for persons and groups. An example is the core competency of working in interdisciplinary teams. Coordination and collaboration are essential attributes in contemporary practice settings. Third, changes in consumer needs related to increased longevity, chronicity, personal involvement, and health promotion must drive the system to provide safe and effective health-care services.

Health-care organizations are now seeing the wisdom of a lesson learned in industry: Not every community hospital needs to have every specialty service. Community hospitals can offer services that are complementary rather than duplicated and meager. Regionalization can be accomplished by having maternal and infant or pediatric services in one agency and cardiac diagnosis, surgery, and rehabilitation in another. This arrangement prevents duplication and fosters quality. The population and the health-service needs must drive the goals of the organization. A needs assessment provides the information for revision of organizational goals. Important considerations include the specific operations of the organization and the available technology.

Specialized knowledge and expertise of professionals and nonprofessionals are represented in formal and informal functions. Formal functions are those defined by the organizational structure. Compare the different functions for a unit manager in a vertical, bureaucratic organization with decision-making in the upper levels of the hierarchy with those for the unit as a cost and decision center in a more horizontal adhocratic structure. This comparison demonstrates a difference in formal operational functions. Informal functions facilitate goal accomplishment and include effective communication channels and how the organizational plans and tasks are actually accomplished in relation to the available resources. It is essential also to be aware of the human factor, or the individuals who coordinate the people and resources to meet the goals of the organization, the managers.

MANAGEMENT

Management, the coordination of resources to achieve organizational outcomes, involves critical thinking, problem-solving, and decision-making. Management should not be confused with leadership. As seen in the previous chapter, a leader mobilizes a group to achieve great things, whereas a manager focuses on directing the group to meet the desired outcomes for the organization through thoughtful and careful planning, direction, monitoring, recognition, development, and representation.

An effective manager must be a good leader, and the combination of effective leadership and management skills provides the nurse with the attributes to face the multitude of challenges in the current health-care system and the various organizational structures. Understanding the foundation of effective management is essential to developing one's own management style.

Management Theories

Management has been studied extensively, with the development of several major theories that are still used to guide current practices. During the 20th century, the major themes were a focus on management science, the process, the people, and even the activities and the intended objectives. Other theories and models are evolving as we attempt to understand and apply the best approaches to "getting things done" efficiently and effectively with the best possible outcomes. The concept of outcomes is an important component in the current view of management, especially in the health-care arena.

The origins of management theory are often attributed to Frederick Taylor (1911), an engineer who used time-and-motion studies to investigate and then apply efficiency principles with the bottom-line focus on productivity. In this early industrial period, training the right people for the task at hand was vital, and these people were rewarded monetarily as productivity levels rose. The focus was one of efficiency, effectiveness, and quality control. This approach was viewed as "working smarter." These principles have been used effectively with production lines, as in the early days of the automotive industry. Taylor's efficiency and productivity principles persist to this day, with the focus on organizing the proper number of trained people and activities to get a job done in the shortest time. These principles have been followed in the use and examination of nurse-patient staffing ratios and skill mix in hospitals.

In the early 20th century, Henri Fayol (1949) looked further at the process of management and the role and functions of the manager. His universal approach highlighted 14 principles including authority, unity of command (one boss and a chain of command), and communication. The role of the manager in this approach encompassed five functions: planning, organizing, commanding, coordinating, and controlling. During the same period, Max Weber (1947) was addressing organizational structure and the need for consistent rules and tasks in the hierarchical structure of the bureaucratic organization.

Other managerial theories evolved, focused on individuals and the goals of organizations. **Motivational theories** are used to identify and describe the forces that motivate individuals toward a goal. Guided by these theories, an effective manager motivates individuals, thus enhancing their productivity and achieving organizational goals. Classic motivational theories have been proposed by Maslow, McGregor, and Ouchi.

As seen previously, in Chapters 3 and 10, Maslow's (1954, 1970) theory of a hierarchy of human needs was based on his 16 propositions on motivation. Motivation in humans is a manifestation of internal and external personal and environmental factors that cause people to respond to a situation in the way that they do. In these principles, the focus is on the individual in a dynamic, complex, and changing environment. Motivation is as intricate as the person, and an individual's personal basic needs must be satisfied before he or she can focus on higher needs, such as self-esteem in one's position and organizational goals. Understanding individual motivation is as important as understanding the skills the individual brings to the task at hand.

McGregor (1960) critically reviewed motivation in *The Human Side of Enterprise*. He proposed his classic two "theories" about human nature. The focus during this time continued to be on the human factors of the worker and how to get the work done. In **Theory X,** individuals are viewed as lazy, needing motivation, avoiding responsibility, and needing constant direction and control by a manager to fulfill their job responsibilities and meet the organizational goals. Rewards and reinforcement are necessary for the individuals, along with a set of rules they must follow. This theory of human nature fits well with the centralized, tall, bureaucratic organizational structure. The role of the manager is one of direction and control.

Alternately, McGregor (1960) postulated **Theory Y,** in which individuals are motivated, self-directed, interested in working toward meeting organizational goals, and willing to accept responsibility without the need for constant direction and supervision. In fact, this constant "management" by the supervisor could deter workers from reaping inner rewards from the job. The role of the manager in this situation should be one of coordination, guidance, and support.

Herzberg's (1966) two-factor theory organizes the individual's motivation for his work according to hygiene and motivational factors. **Hygiene factors** are maintenance factors in the workplace, such as salary, supervision, company policy, working conditions, status, job security, and the job's effect on personal life; these hygiene factors in the workplace can lead to satisfaction or dissatisfaction and are related to the organizational climate. **Motivational factors** are satisfiers within the job that motivate people to higher levels of performance. Motivational factors include achievement, recognition, the work itself, responsibility, and advancement. The manager helps improve job performance by ensuring that both hygiene and motivational needs of the employees are met at some level for both job satisfaction and incentive to achieve the organizational goals.

In the later part of the 20th century, the Japanese style of collaborative management received much attention, with the economic successes viewed within a participatory approach. Ouchi (1981) described this style, **Theory Z,** as an approach in which employees are trusted, empowered, and actively involved in decision-making. The components of Theory Z include collective values and decision-making, long-term or lifetime employment, slower but predictable promotions, indirect supervision, and a holistic concern for employees (Ouchi, 1981). This participatory style involves indirect supervision with the focus on the group. Ouchi (1981) believes that more creative decision-making and more effective implementation occur with the full involvement and consensus of the group (p. 43). There is a "buy-in" by all team members, who are valued as individuals and as important members of the organization. Important values of this theory are trust, fairness, commitment, and loyalty to the organization, which lead to long-term employment and reduced turnover. The use of "quality circles" and "group think" emerged from this theory. Competitiveness in some American organizations is inconsistent with this style of management.

Management-by-objectives (MBO) and the role of the knowledge worker evolved in the business world from the work of Peter Drucker. Originally from Austria, Drucker profoundly influenced American businesses through his many books and observations on organizations and how they are managed. Drucker focused on the people (both managers and work force), the organizational functions, and the results achieved in the process in line with the organizational mission. He believed that the manager's job is "to direct the resources and the efforts of the business toward opportunities for economically significant results" (Drucker, 1998, p. 67). He proposed that management comprises a few essential principles; the first is that "its task is to make people capable of joint performance, to make their strengths effective and their weaknesses irrelevant. This is what an organization is all about, and the reason that management is the critical, determining factor" (Drucker, 1998, p. 172). Later, Drucker (2002) described the requirement in modern organizations for a manager to be a *knowledge worker* or "**executive,** if by virtue of his position or knowledge, he is responsible for a contribution that materially affects the capacity of the organization to perform and to obtain results" (p. 5). The focus is on making a contribution to the organization by virtue of one's intelligence, imagination, and knowledge. Recall that applying quality improvement is one of the five core competencies for all health professionals (Greiner & Knebel, 2003). Drucker's works on management covered a wide range of businesses, including hospitals, and looked at achievement and contributions of individuals within the framework of organizational settings.

Nursing Management

The core competencies for health professionals are essential characteristics in nursing management. The focus of the nurse manager or nurse *executive* must be on the provision of client-centered care while fostering the use of evidence-based practice and quality improvement. The complexity of the interdisciplinary team and the use of informatics will depend on the organizational system. All of these tasks involve people and managing resources for the provision of safe and effective care and positive client and organizational outcomes.

Buckingham (2005) identified four key skills of managers, as picking good people, setting clear expectations, praising excellence, and showing you care for your people—but above all, the manager must discover what is unique about each person and capitalize on it (pp. 81–83). But recall that Fayol (1949) identified management functions as planning, organizing, commanding, coordinating, and controlling. The question becomes one of the consistency of these functions with the humanistic view of nursing and care of clients.

Planning and organizing are indeed talents of the nurse manager. This is an outcome of the steps of assessment and planning in the provision of nursing care in any organizational context. It is setting clear expectations and requires an in-depth understanding of the organization and the people, the true culture of the organization. At times, it will also involve leading the culture, as with incorporation of evidence-based practice in a particular client situation and planning for the efficient and effective use of resources.

Commanding in the context of nursing management involves ensuring that the job is done through delegation and supervision, as in the provision of care to clients. It is picking the right people and capitalizing on their talents and requires knowledge of the care requirements, the clients, and external system influences. It also involves recognition of individual talents and "a job well done." All levels of staffing are a vital consideration, including assistive personnel. Delegation is a skill that grows and evolves, as the nurse manager grows from novice to expert. This is an area that needs careful and ongoing professional development.

In a nursing education program, students focus on "total patient care" as they learn the interpersonal, technical, and clinical judgment skills needed in nursing practice. In the final phase of the educational program, they are engaged in obtaining leadership or management skills. This includes assignment and delegation of activities to other health-care providers, both licensed and unlicensed. Often, these activities are performed with other students rather than within the interdisciplinary team in the acute care setting. Upon graduation and initial licensure, however, nurses are expected to manage the health-care team effectively and to delegate activities and functions to others for the provision of efficient care to clients. Challenges in the workplace, such as economics, constantly add new twists. This leads to the need for coordination of resources, including health-care providers, for accomplishment of the organizational goals and the provision of safe and effective care for clients.

Coordinating is another talent of the nurse manager, as skills in coordination of care have continued to be a component of the practice scope and setting. Controlling in nursing management is ensuring that the care to clients has been provided effectively. Recall, however, that management is the coordination of resources to achieve organizational outcomes and involves critical thinking, problem-solving, communication, and decision-making skills. In addition, remember that Drucker (2002) identified the executive's vital talents of intelligence, imagination, and knowledge. To coordinate health care and the various providers effectively, the nurse must have a thorough understanding and appreciation of the organizational culture.

ORGANIZATIONAL CULTURE

The **organizational culture** is perceptible as the culmination of the norms, attitudes, and values imbedded in the organizational mission and in the expected behaviors of the employees. Daft (2007) views organizational culture as having two dimensions: visible observable symbols (e.g., ceremonies, stories, slogans, behaviors, dress, physical settings) and the underlying values, assumptions, beliefs, attitudes, and feelings of the people (p. 361).

Scrutiny of the organizational culture can provide a sense of the prevailing level of humanism present in the organization—in other words, how people are viewed as employees and consumers. New organizational values and behaviors have emerged as we redefine and recreate organizations for functioning in today's world. We moved from the belief that humans in organizations are lazy and need direction, in McGregor's (1967) Theory X, to the age of humanism. The humanistic perspective is a more positive one that considers the importance of the people in the organization. Still, during times of cost-cutting, a humanistic perspective and recognition of contributions can quickly disappear when the focus turns to head counts or full-time equivalents (FTEs).

Important clues on the involvement, satisfaction, and effectiveness of the people in the organization are reflected in both management styles and the behaviors and attitudes of those in the environment. In health care, the organizational culture includes both the consumers and the providers in the agency. The organizational culture is also influenced by the environment—the immediate institutional or agency environment as well as societal expectations and mandates.

As with any set of cultural expectations, the employees are expected to enculturate (adapt and adopt) and espouse the prevailing principles. Failure to enculturate results in being ostracized or terminated. These cultural expectations are the customary ways of thinking and behaving shared by members of the organization, as a form of socialization and allegiance to the norms of the organization. Incorporation of the specific expectations encompasses this organizational socialization process. An example is adopting and using a specific theory that guides the operation of the organization. At the most ideal level, if the nurse cannot view or provide care for clients in accordance with the specific model used at that agency, such as self-care, the best remedy would be to seek employment at another agency more consistent with the nurse's own worldview.

An understanding of the importance of the organizational climate is apparent from professional groups and associations. In their white paper on the hallmarks of professional nursing practice settings, the American Association of Colleges of Nursing (2002) identified eight key characteristics of the environment that should be evaluated in the organizational climate. Based on a study in 2002, the American Organization of Nurse Executives (McManis & Monsalve Associates, Inc., & AONE, 2003) proposed six critical factors for achieving work environment excellence (p. 5). In 2005, the American Association of Critical-Care Nurses (AACN)

ONLINE CONSULT

American Association of Colleges of Nursing at **http://www.aacn.nche.edu**

American Association of Critical-Care Nurses at **http://www.aacn.org**

American Organization of Nurse Executives at **http://www.aone.org/aone/keyissues/home.html**

Magnet Recognition Program at **http://nursingworld.org/ancc/magnet/index.html**

also started a multi-year *Healthy Work Environment Initiative* that includes six standards also applicable to the organizational culture. And consider the value placed on the organizational culture by the Magnet Recognition Program (American Nurses Credentialing Center [ANCC], 2006). Go to the Online Consult and find the 14 "Forces of Magnetism" in this program and evaluate their contribution to the organizational culture of a hospital system. What these positions and initiatives have in common is the focus on the organizational culture that includes positive leadership, communication, participatory management and local decision-making, and collaboration and interdisciplinary relationships. The concepts are particularly appropriate to understanding the people as individuals and groups in health-care organizations.

Leadership

Chapter 11 presented selected leadership styles and traits. The cultural climate generally supports the predominant leadership style. That is why it is so critical that environments have strong nursing leadership. This is emphasized by American Organization of Nurse Executives (AONE) as "the importance of forging a supportive, empowering work environment that values and nurtures continuous organizational learning and innovation" (McManis & Monsalve Associates, Inc., & AONE, 2003). In addition, part of the requirements for Magnet Status is that the Chief Nursing Officer meets minimal education requirements, has been in a high-level leadership position for at least a year, has been active in the application process, and has implemented the ANA Scope and Standards for Nurse Administrators (ANCC, 2006).

The leadership style is a major influence on the organizational culture. Nurse leaders and managers must have the qualities to envision the future and assist others in the organization to meet the goals of quality health-care outcomes for clients. The American Association of

Critical-Care Nurses (2006) emphasizes that nurse leaders function as role models in skilled communication, for true collaboration, effective decision-making, meaningful recognition, and authentic leadership (p. 38). But, as Leininger (2006) points out, nurse administrators "as leaders need to make their practices congruent with changing cultural values, beliefs, and the lifeways in their local workplace, but must also reasonably fit with societal and world-wide trends" (p. 367). These talented managers must constantly be attuned to both the internal and external environments of the organization.

Communication

Communication of ideas and views is vital in the organizational context. But the prevailing organizational culture may dictate the communication channels and styles. Being able to communicate with clients is quite different from having your ideas heard, considered, and implemented at the organizational level. Portraying yourself as an expert and as a colleague is necessary in both client and professional interactions within the organization. Whether by ensuring that all committee or group members have the opportunity to express their opinions or by making special efforts to demonstrate recognition and give credit for another's ideas, attention to cultural differences is important. It can make the most of the talents, abilities, and skills of the human resources in the organizational system, especially in management of interdisciplinary teams. We will look further at communication in organizations later in this chapter.

Participatory Management and Local Decision-Making

Closely related to leadership style is management focus, whether on individualism and achievement or on collectivism or teamwork as the norms, attitudes, and values of the organization. Management styles have an important influence here. Consider the differences in management with Theory X, which is focused on individual performance, versus Theory Z, which emphasizes collectivism and cooperation. The organizational focus on individualism or collectivism is apparent in promotion and evaluation structures. Administrative policies and procedures provide important clues to the organization's official position. Subgroups or minority groups within the organization may create factions, however. These subgroups may set certain expectations for collectivism and cooperation in behavior or function. For example, the organization may be highly bureaucratic, with expectations and rewards valuing individual performance, competition, and task accomplishment; but if cooperation is the prevailing value in the nursing department, it will be translated into accomplishing outcomes at the upper level of management.

Think about the need for participatory management and decision-making. The American Organization of Nurse Executives (McManis & Monsalve Associates, Inc., and AONE, 2003) have described this *empowered collaborative decision-making* as follows:

> Nurse empowerment combined with collaborative multidisciplinary decision-making is an essential attribute of a work environment that values nurses as professionals and provides policy development roles for nursing leaders and staff. (p. 5)

Participatory management and decision-making are also a requirement for Magnet Status institutions. For eligibility, decentralized, shared decision-making processes must be apparent with nurses in both direct-care and managerial roles involved in decision-making bodies and organizational policy (ANCC, 2006).

Collaboration and Interdisciplinary Relationships

One of the core competencies for all health professionals is to work in interdisciplinary teams. As noted in the Institute of Medicine (IOM) report, "teams tend to reduce the utilization of redundant or duplicate services, and they also tend to develop more creative solutions to complex problems because of their members' diverse academic backgrounds and experience" (Greiner & Knebel, 2003, p. 54). Collaboration is a challenge among professionals, especially when scope of practice issues arise, time is limited, and workloads increase. But teamwork is apparent in some organizational climates that foster interdisciplinary practice.

In 2004, the IOM focused on the safety and work environment of nurses. They identified two necessary precursors to collaboration: individual clinical competence and mutual trust and respect (Page, 2004, pp. 212–213). These two characteristics seem quite basic, but personalities, a challenging and demanding environment, and incorporation into the organizational culture are issues. The IOM report further identified the characteristics of collaboration, including shared understanding of goals and roles, effective communication, shared decision-making, and conflict management (Page, 2004, p. 213). All of these characteristics must be given heed in the culture of a health-care organization.

Other Concepts in Organizational Culture

In addition to understanding the people and groups in the organizational system, other factors provide information on the organizational culture and the operational climate. The organization's history provides a lasting influence. Discovering the critical decisions made in founding the organization reveals the original intent for the organization and views for the future. Closely related to the founding decisions are the current guiding ideals and mission. The guiding ideals and mission relate to the service orientation. Consider the difference between missions and the intended consumer groups in not-for-profit and for-profit organizations. This could range from elected fee-for-service care in the for-profit setting to a not-for-profit agency focusing on health care to the indigent. The philosophy of the organization provides important information about the current ideals and mission. If revisions have been made over the years, it can be quite helpful to look back at old versions to determine whether the philosophy changed in response to environmental factors.

Looking into the community can also influence the organizational culture. Although nurses are quite mobile and no longer tied to a geographic area, community ties with a rural hospital may provide a profound influence. Remembered history and symbolism of the organization contribute additional information, for example, about an institution designed to provide hospital care for a county that has evolved into a regional referral and tertiary-care center. Remembering the traditions of personalized obstetric care, a local woman's group may provide funding for a special prenatal program for indigent pregnant teenagers.

Finally, institutional arrangements and linkages, such as consortia and cooperating or referral agencies, are frequently quite complex but provide essential information on organizational relationships and interrelationships. These facts are necessary for understanding the culture and influences on the organization. But, as Hall and Tolbert (2005) point out, "culture is not a constant . . . values and norms change as the events affect the population involved" (p. 183). The potential for change in the organizational culture requires diligent assessment and communication skills on the part of the nurse manager or executive.

COMMUNICATION UNIQUE TO ORGANIZATIONS

Communication is vital in complex, highly technologic, and dynamic organizations. As was illustrated with organizational functions, the structure of the organization plays an important role in communication channels. Formal channels are easily apparent in highly bureaucratic structures, as dictated by the organizational diagram. But informal communication channels ("grapevines") are sometimes less evident and can be highly effective in such a structure. Consider the need for supplies in some areas of an agency. Ordering can easily be handled through the computerized entry system. But what if some urgently needed item is

unavailable through the system? An informal channel may be used to locate a supply from which the item may be "borrowed," to be replaced as soon as the official order is fulfilled. The departmental secretary who has an informal chain of communication may be able to use her knowledge of these informal systems effectively in such a procurement process.

Communication channels are important considerations for effective decision-making to achieve quality outcomes. Organizational goals and values must be translated, transmitted, and reinforced throughout the system to meet the institutional mission. The specialized knowledge, skills, and resources represented by people require excellent communication within the system and from external environments to be current and responsive to changes in the knowledge base and technology. Communication is the action component of interpersonal and interdisciplinary roles, behaviors, and relationships in the organization system. The formal and informal communications and interactions are the essence of the organizational culture. The organizational structure is the formal design—with its hierarchy or lines of authority—for the communication channels. Communications may be formally dictated in a linear manner by the bureaucratic structure, or they may be flexible and circular in adhocratic matrix designs. Informal communications must be identified to reveal the actual flow of information, decision-making, and goal accomplishment. Communication of information and expectations stems from the pervasive leadership and management styles. Evaluation of the appropriate channels is vital for effective functioning in the organizational setting.

Organizations routinely use methods of communication in addition to the verbal and nonverbal interpersonal communication techniques. Consider the informatics available in organizational settings. We have computer networks, fiber optics, satellite, and teleconferencing technology. Computers manage information storage, inventory, and rapid retrieval, data processing, data analysis, and report generation. The information we compile and the methods we use to transmit it vary with the nature of the communication channel we are using. For example, a general rule in an organization is to limit memos to one page or less and disperse them to the appropriate parties; however, the sender must consider the available and appropriate technology, such as interoffice paper copies or electronic mail or messaging.

Considering the purpose of communication in an organization is indispensable. Whether we are communicating with clients or assistive personnel, both the sending method and the receiver of the information are important. Clear, concise, and timely transmission of information is necessary for an effective management process. Recall from Chapter 8 the "five rights" of organizational communications: (1) the right information or

EVIDENCED-BASED PRACTICE: CONSIDER THIS . . .

*Y*ou are reading an online news article about a study in Australia that found that significant numbers of older hospitalized individuals had problems eating relative to opening preparations, using cutlery and condiments, and reaching or pouring items. Environmental detractors and disturbances were problems (Medical News Today, 2006, p. 1) and almost one-third of these individuals leave most of their meal unfinished (Medical News Today, 2006). You start thinking about the acute care unit where you work and the increased number of geriatric clients. You know staffing is an issue and that dietary aides deliver the trays.

Question: How will you use this information as a nurse-manager to implement a nutritional assessment and assistance program on your unit?

Source: Medical News Today. (2006). *58% of older hospital patients have problems eating and 31% leave most of their meal.* Retrieved October 3, 2006, from http://www.medicalnewstoday.com/medicalnews.php?newsid=52688

content, (2) the right communication channel, (3) the right format, including use of correct grammar, terms, and language, (4) the right level of understanding, and (5) the right technology. The appropriate communication channel must be selected, using the appropriate chain of command to convey your message.

NURSING: POWER, NEGOTIATION, DELEGATION

In the past two decades, health-care organizations have undergone radical change and restructuring. We are now focused on outcomes, customer satisfaction, safety, adequacy of reimbursement for services provided, and the need to address health disparities.

Systems theory fits well with changes going on in health-care organizations. But as the system becomes more and more multilayered, the focus shifts to the openness and flexibility of the system boundaries, greater attention to environmental forces, and expanding relationships among organizations. Special attention to external influences is essential for effective planning and organizing. This includes a focus on the organization, considering its human resources, information systems, and governance structures for delegation and coordination. Ongoing feedback and evaluation become essential. Professional nurses have major roles in all steps of this process as we now focus on strategic initiatives.

Administrative nursing positions in health-care systems have been expanded at all levels. Director and supervisor roles, when still apparent in an organizational chart, have been greatly expanded. As we have seen in the chapter on leadership, nurses have major responsibility in health-care organizations. Nurses influence many different types of colleagues. Nurse managers have knowledge of people and the environmental influences

on health-care needs. This is the domain of nursing. In addition, nurses are now well prepared in organizational theory, finance, and policy. We have entered the administrative arena as interdisciplinary care managers, coordinators, and leaders. Strategic planning, public relations, and cost containment have become essential skills. Nurses who have this knowledge have legitimate power in health-care organizations. But along with this power comes responsibility, accountability, and the need for effective negotiation and delegation skills.

Power

Max Weber (1947) defined **power** as "the probability that one actor in a social relationship will be in a position to carry out his own will despite resistance, regardless of the basis on which this probability rests" (p. 152). More specific to organizations, Mintzberg (1983a) defines power as "the capacity to effect (or affect) organizational outcomes" (p. 4). This latter definition has much relevance for professional nursing practice, because nurses in health-care organizations are positioned to effect or affect positive health-care outcomes. These outcomes can be viewed as outputs from the health-care system, such as clients with improved health status. *Legitimate power* is the authority to effect change within one's position. The professional relationship provides the opportunity for legitimate power, and many nurses now have legitimate power by virtue of their position, role, and expertise. *Informal power* is the assertion of one's will over a situation to achieve a goal without formal or "vested" authority.

Mintzberg (1983a) identified five general bases of power (Box 12–1). These power bases are applicable to professional nursing, especially in organizational settings. First, nurses have demonstrated effective management of resources in decentralized and vertical organizations. They are being vested with responsibility especially with regard to decisions and resources needed

BOX 12.1 The Five General Bases of Power

- Control of resources
- Control of a technical skill
- Control of a body of knowledge
- Exclusive rights or privileges to impose choices (legal prerogatives)
- Access to people who have and can be relied on for the other four

Data from Mintzberg, H. (1983a). *Power in and around organizations.* Englewood Cliffs, NJ: Prentice-Hall.

Box 12.2 Attributes of a Skilled Negotiator: CAVEAT

- **C**ommunication and interpersonal skills
- **A**ssessment skills
- **V**ision and application of needed resources
- **E**ndurance
- **A**wareness
- **T**rustworthiness

for effective organizational functioning. Second, care of clients involves technical skills that must be performed or supervised by nurses. Third, nursing continues to develop its unique body of knowledge needed for evidence-based practice and the health of clients. The fourth base of power involves the legal prerogatives granted and implied under the practice acts, licensure, certification, and professional codes described in Chapter 1. And finally, nurses in interdisciplinary practice have access to colleagues, clients, and influential people on whom they rely for access to the other bases of power. To effect positive health-care outcomes, skills in negotiation are often necessary.

Negotiation for power must first be related to the goals of the organization. Nurses have the ability and responsibility to negotiate for legitimate power in organizations. Nurses certainly have access to these power sources if developed, effectively negotiated, and used.

Negotiation

As discussed in Chapter 8, conflict situations can easily arise in a group setting. And the health-care organization provides the potential for many groups with different compositions, all with the potential for conflict situations to arise. The manager frequently encounters conflict among individuals or groups that necessitates artful use of interpersonal and negotiation skills. Effective conflict resolution by the manager requires negotiation, and ultimately, coming to some compromise. This compromise is most effective when the end result is acceptable at some level to all parties involved.

Koerner and Huber (2006) define **negotiation** as "a process of give-and-take exchange among persons aimed at resolving problems, conflicts, or disputes" (p. 408). The best scenario is a "win-win" situation with collaboration. In this situation, the solution is satisfying to both sides, who have collaborated, and each side senses some satisfaction and feeling of a "win" situation. Alternately, one side prevails ("win-loss" situation) or both sides experience a compromise that is not really satisfying to either side, thus a "loss-loss" situation.

An effective negotiator should consistently refine and nurture negotiation skills (Box 12–2). First, the negotiator must have excellent *communication and interpersonal skills*. The negotiator must be a skilled communicator, for understanding the concerns of both sides and promoting awareness and collaboration. He or she must focus on the facts (verbal and nonverbal) and try to diffuse emotions with effective communication. As Dana (2001) describes negotiation, a smart manager avoids power contests and rights contests, and focuses on finding ways to resolve conflicts through reconciliation of interests (p. 41).

As with any nursing care situation, *assessment skills* are needed to understand the interpersonal and situational influences from all sides. For example, consider a conflict situation that arises in the intensive care setting as the group of physicians and nurses attempt to implement a collaborative practice model. The ultimate goal is for the effective care of the client; the negotiator must have an understanding of all of the facts in order to uncover the common ground for all, physicians, intensivists, Advanced Practice Registered Nurses (APRNs), staff nurses, technicians, therapists, associated service providers, and the clients. The skillful negotiator must understand what is being said and what is actually occurring in the setting, and should be sensitive to all behaviors, nonverbal and expressed cues, and views. The skillful negotiator must assess not only content but also context, culture, behaviors, and players involved.

The ability to envision what potential outcomes could be and how they would affect each side, individually and collectively, is key. The *vision* of the potential outcomes must be framed for the individuals involved, on the basis of the facts of the situation and the resources available. *Endurance* is a definite prerequisite throughout the process and during the inevitable peaks, valleys, and stalemates that can occur. There are times when the negotiation process must be halted to allow the various individuals or groups to refocus on facts and dilute emotions.

The acute *awareness* of the negotiator must prevail throughout the entire process, from identification of conflict, alertness to all behaviors and actions throughout, to the levels of satisfaction of both parties once the resolution has been agreed upon. This awareness of behavior and situation will have to be restated to all parties on an ongoing basis to focus on the facts continually.

Another important characteristic of the negotiator is *trustworthiness*. All parties must sense the fairness of the negotiator in the process. Building trust is a necessary skill, not only to gain the cooperation of both sides during the negotiation but also to help build trust in the process and the ultimate resolution. The process is often not a smooth, linear activity when one is dealing with people, partiality, and conscious or unconscious behaviors.

Marquis and Huston (2006) identify destructive or manipulative negotiating tactics as the use of ridicule, inappropriate questioning, flattery, demonstrating a sense of helplessness, and aggression or taking over the situation (p. 540). These tactics are ineffective and may delay resolution or even escalate the conflict. Such tactics inhibit the building of trust and negate the collaborative process. The end result of the negotiation process must be a compromise acceptable to all at some level of satisfaction. If a compromise cannot be reached, an impasse results. In this situation, the conflict will escalate at some later point, perhaps in a different form or with different players.

Ideally, the negotiation process should take place on neutral ground, or at least in a secure environment acceptable to both parties. Specific terms are used in negotiation tactics, like "reaching a stalemate" (an impasse) and "tradeoffs" (concessions), of which the negotiator must be aware. Marquis and Huston (2006) recommend further that upon resolution of the conflict, the negotiator send a follow-up letter to both parties describing the agreed terms (p. 539). This is a follow-up as reinforcement for both recognition of individual involvement and the results of the process. The correspondence can take the form of a formal memo or an electronic communication commending the participation of both sides in the resolution and restating the agreed-upon conditions. The attributes of a successful negotiator are also essential in delegation activities.

Delegation

Delegation is defined as the "transfer of responsibility of the performance of an task from one individual to another while retaining the accountability for the outcome" (American Nurses Association [ANA], 2005, p. 4). Further, the National Council of State Boards of Nursing (NCBSN) (2005) views delegation as "a skill requiring clinical judgment and final accountability for client care" (p. 1).

Delegation activities occur when the novice nurse enters practice on the first day of professional practice. But as mentioned, educational preparation provides the concepts for the process, although seldom the opportunity to truly develop these critical skills, especially when the new nurse is confronted with long-term interdisciplinary staff who may be entrenched in a certain way of providing care. The new nurse is responsible for the care of a group of clients and works with assistive personnel necessary for the provision of quality care. But delegation is a difficult activity for the novice whose skills are being developed and refined. And the accountability for the delegated act is not consistently internalized, as simple tasks are performed by others for the delivery of care. It is not a matter of simply "assigning" a list of tasks or relying on a nurse manager to make these assignments. Consider the standard practice of routine vital signs taken by assistive personnel like Certified Nursing Assistants (CNAs) or Unlicensed Assistive Personnel (UAPs). We have lost the concept of "monitoring" vital signs when the nurse assumes that the readings will be reported by the assistive personnel in a timely manner. Consider the problems with this arrangement:

- Skill of the assistive personnel
- Accuracy of readings according to a prescribed schedule
- Report on the findings
- Interpretation of readings
- Nursing judgment on readings, their accuracy, and other variables in the client's condition
- Alternate comfort measures that could have an effect on readings

And the list goes on.

Delegation is not the "hand-off" of a routine task. Application of the principles of delegation is essential to effective management as well as for client safety.

Principles of Delegation

In 2006, the ANA and the NCSBN announced a joint statement on delegation. Basic principles of delegation involve awareness of the differences between assignment, delegation, responsibility, and accountability. Assignment is the distribution of work that each staff member is responsible for during a given work period (ANA, 2005, p. 4). Delegation "is the transferring to a competent individual the authority to perform a selected nursing task in a selected situation; the nurse retains accountability for the delegation" (NCSBN, 2007, p. 2). The responsibility for completion of the task has been delegated, but not the accountability for ensuring that the task has been completed correctly by the right person who has been supervised appropriately. Recall from Chapter 1 that according to the Code of Ethics for Nurses, responsibility is defined as accountability for performance of the duties associated with the professional role, and accountability is being answerable to oneself and others for one's judgments and actions in the course of nursing practice, regardless of health-care organization policies or provider directives (ANA, 2001, pp. 16–17). The nurse maintains both the responsibility and the accountability for the delegated action. The skillful manager must nevertheless delegate some activities for necessary care of the client and to ensure patient safety.

Process of Delegation

The NCSBN (2007) envisions delegation as a four-step process: assessment and planning, communication, surveillance and supervision, and evaluation and feedback. The importance of delegation as a process is based on good assessment of the client, the environment, and providers who are capable and able to be delegated to provide appropriate care for the client. The process does not stop with the delegation. The delegation of a responsibility must be based on this assessment and must be made to the correct person, with monitoring by the nurse, who maintains the accountability for the function. The NCSBN (2007) has further provided decision trees in their position paper located on their public website, one as a tool to assist in the process of delegation to assistive personnel and one for accepting assignment to supervise assistive personnel. (See Online Consult.) These decision trees are also available in Appendix B of the Joint Statement on Delegation by the ANA and NCSBN (NCSBN, 2006). Both of these decision trees provide specific questions to be addressed for safe practice with delegation. The delegation model developed by the ANA (2005) clearly illustrates that the nurse assesses the client, the delegate, the setting, and the task but that the nurse retains the accountability for the delegation and the client outcomes. Nursing judgment plays a role in the entire process through the evaluation phase. It is vital to remember that nursing judgment cannot be delegated.

In their classic work on delegation, the NCSBN (1998) identified five "rights" of delegation (Box 12–3). These five rights have been further endorsed in the 2006 ANA/NCSBN Joint Statement. First, the *task* must be the right one for the client. The nurse must use clinical judgment, not merely assign a CNA a group of rooms

BOX 12.3 The Five Rights of Delegation

The RIGHT
- Task
- Circumstances
- Person
- Direction/Communication
- Supervision/Evaluation

From National Council of State Boards of Nursing. (1998). *The five rights of delegation*. Chicago: Author.

for taking vital signs. The *circumstances* must be right for the particular client and her care needs—again a nursing judgment—as well as for delegation. The right *person* means the right person for the care activity, nurse, technician, or assistive personnel. This person who will be delegated the care of the client must clearly understand what is involved with the care to be given (*direction*). Two-way communication skills are critical. The fifth right is the provision of the correct *supervision* and evaluation of the care and the person who was delegated to provide the care. Once again, supervision and evaluation require the use of nursing judgment.

Where is the client? Consider the patient fresh from surgery who has just arrived on the floor: The nurse first makes the assessment of the client to determine status and care needs. The nurse then decides what type of monitoring of vital signs is needed for the client's well-being. The assistive person has been trained to take vital signs and has demonstrated this skill (certified to perform it). But does this nurse know that the vital signs will be taken accurately and as directed; in other words, is this the right person for the job? If this assistive person is the correct person, then the nurse gives clear, understandable directions, including the reporting cycle back to the nurse for the nurse's clinical judgment. Along with this, the nurse provides the appropriate supervision and evaluation of the care given.

Delegation involves giving responsibility but not abdicating the accountability for the task or activity.

The manager's knowledge of her staff is critical to successful delegation. The education, experience, prior performance, willingness, and expertise of the person should be considered before appropriate delegation can occur. It is the responsibility of the delegator to make an adequate assessment, which should include how long the individual will need supervision and what type of supervision. Individual Nurse Practice Acts in some states provide specific language and requirements for appropriate delegation by nurses. Be aware of both the provisions in your state practice act and the agency policies and procedures. You must abide by the legal authority in your practice act.

Delegation errors can jeopardize the client. The correct balance is the key. Delegation is necessary to provide effective care for clients. The nurse must be the one involved with the clinical judgment for the client's well-being but cannot perform all tasks involved in this process. Delegation is an essential skill of the nurse. Delegation is one of the nine provisions in the Code of Ethics for Nurses (ANA, 2001) and, specific to nurse managers and executives in the interpretative statements, it is the manager's "responsibility to provide an environment that supports and facilitates appropriate assignment and delegation" (p. 17). This environment includes appropriate orientation, mentoring, and protections for clients. Once again, we have the core competencies for the nurse as providing client-centered care that is based on evidence of efficacy and quality improvement, provided in an interdisciplinary team, and communicated with the assistance of informatics.

Change for the good of clients or the health-care industry can be a result of applying principles of management in health-care organizations. As we will see in the next chapter, professional nursing practice has an integral role in the change process.

INTERACTIVE EXERCISES

Go to the Intranet site and complete the interactive exercises provided for this Chapter.

ONLINE CONSULT

Access delegation resources from the following Web sites:

ANA Principles for Delegation at **http://nursingworld.org/MainMenuCategories/ HealthcareandPolicyIssues/ ANAPositionStatements/joint.aspx**

ANA/NCSBN Joint Statement on Delegation at **https://www.ncsbn.org/pdfs/ Joint_statement.pdf**

NCSBN Delegation Documents at **https://www.ncsbn.org/cps/rde/ xchg/SID-53EFFC2A-0A259009/ncsbn/ hs.xsl/323.htm**

KEY POINTS

- An organization is simply an arrangement of human and material resources for some purpose, such as creating an institution or agency to meet a stated aim. Organizations can be viewed in terms of their structure, function, and people.

- Organizational structure is the design of the organization, including the type of hierarchy that tells us about positions or roles, responsibilities, status, channels of command or reporting relationships, and tasks to be accomplished. The major organizational structures are bureaucratic and organic (adhocratic).

- Centralized versus decentralized organizational structures involve the lines of control and decision-making within the organization.

- Organizations are also described according to the layers of differentiation for authority, decision-making, and coordination. Flat organizational structures have a wide base and few layers or tiers for decision-making and authority, whereas tall organizational structures have more tiers and lines of command, with less local decision-making at the lower levels.

- Organizational functions include goals and operations to fulfill the mission of the organization.

- Management is the coordination of resources to achieve organizational outcomes and involves critical thinking, problem-solving, and decision-making.

- From a focus on the organization and increasing productivity, humanistic theories of management emerged, including the classic motivational theories proposed by Maslow, McGregor, Herzberg, and Ouchi.

- Drucker (2002) proposed that a manager is an executive who is focused on contributing to the effectiveness of organization by virtue of intelligence, imagination, and knowledge (p. 2).

- The organizational culture involves the culmination of the norms, attitudes, and values related to the organizational mission, accompanied by the expected behaviors of people.

- The organizational communication process can also be thought of as containing five "rights": (1) information or content, (2) communication channel, (3) format, including use of correct grammar, terms, and language, (4) level of understanding, and (5) technology.

(Key points continue on page 227)

KEY POINTS (continued)

■ Power is the ability to effect change in people's behavior or in the organization. Legitimate power is the authority to effect change within one's position. Power bases are built on control of resources, technical skills, and a body of knowledge as well as exclusive rights and access to other people with power.

■ Effective conflict resolution requires negotiation or coming to a win-win solution.

■ Delegation is the "transfer of responsibility of the performance of an activity from one individual to another while retaining the accountability of the outcome" (American Nurses Association, 2005, p. 4).

■ The five "rights" of delegation are the right task, the right circumstances, the right person, the right direction or communication, and the right supervision or evaluation (NCSBN, 1998).

Thought and Discussion Questions

1. Characterize the organization of the institution where you work. Describe the structure, functions, lines of decision-making, communication patterns, and sources of power relative to the organizational mission. Be prepared to participate in a discussion (online or in class) to be scheduled by your instructor.

2. Considering what you have learned from this chapter and the previous one, differentiate between management and leadership. Where do the two concepts overlap?

3. Interview a member of the administrative team from a large health-care facility on the various positions held by nurses. Describe their roles, changes that have occurred, areas of legitimate power, and the skills professional nurses need in this setting. Be prepared to participate in a discussion to be scheduled by your instructor.

4. Observe the start of a shift on a nursing unit. Describe the differences between assignment and delegation. Be prepared to participate in a discussion to be scheduled by your instructor.

5. Review the Chapter Thought located on the first page of the chapter, and discuss it in the context of the contents of the chapter.

☐ REFERENCES

American Association of Colleges of Nursing. (2002). *AACN white paper: Hallmarks of the professional nursing practice environment.* Retrieved June 12, 2006, from http://www.aacn.nche.edu/publications/positions/hallmarks.htm

American Association of Critical-Care Nurses (2006). *AACN's standards for establishing and sustaining healthy work environments: A journey to excellence.* Retrieved June 12, 2006, from http://www.aacn.org/aacn/pubpolcy.nsf/Files/HWEStandards/$file/HWEStandards.pdf

American Nurses Association (ANA). (2001). *Code of ethics for nurses with interpretive statements* (Publication No. CEN21 10M 08/01). Washington, DC: American Nurses Publishing.

American Nurses Association (ANA). (2005). *Principles for delegation.* Retrieved June 21, 2006, from http://nursingworld.org/staffing/lawsuit/PrinciplesDelegation.pdf

American Nurses Association (ANA) and National Council of State Boards of Nursing (NCSBN). (2006). *Joint statement on delegation.* Retrieved on November 29, 2006, from https://www.ncsbn.org/pdfs/Joint_statement.pdf

American Nurses Credentialing Center. (2006). *The magnet application and appraisal process.* Retrieved June 12, 2006, from http://nursingworld.org/ancc/magnet/index.html

Bertalanffy, L. V. (1968). *General system theory: Foundations, development, applications.* New York: George Braziller.

Buckingham, M. (2005). *The one thing you need to know ... about great managing, great leading, and sustained individual success.* New York: Free Press.

Daft, R. L. (2007). *Organizational theory and design* (9th ed.). Mason, OH: Thompson South-Western College Publishing.

Dana, D. (2001). *Conflict resolution: Mediation tools for everyday worklife.* New York: McGraw-Hill.

Drucker, P. F. (2002). *The effective executive revised.* New York: Harper Collins Publishers.

Drucker, P. F. (1998). *Peter Drucker on the profession of management.* Boston: Harvard Business Review.

Fayol, H. (1949). *General and industrial management* (C. Storrs, Trans.). London: Pittman & Sons.

Greiner, A. C., & Knebel, E. (Eds.). (2003). *Health professions education: A bridge to quality.* Washington, DC: Institute of Medicine.

Hall, R. H., & Tolbert, P. S. (2005). *Organizations: Structures, processes, and outcomes* (9th ed.). Upper Saddle River, NJ: Pearson Prentice-Hall.

Herzberg, F. (1966). *Work and the nature of man.* Cleveland, OH: World Publishing.

Koerner, J., & Huber, D. (2006). Communication, persuasion, and negotiation. In D. Huber, *Leadership and management in nursing* (3rd ed.). Philadelphia: Saunders.

Leininger, M. (2006). Culture care theory and uses in nursing administration. In M. Leininger & M. R. McFarland, *Culture care diversity and universality: A worldwide nursing theory* (2nd ed., pp. 365–379). Boston: Jones and Bartlett.

Marquis, B. L., & Huston, C. J. (2006). *Leadership roles and management functions in nursing: Theory and application* (5th ed.). Philadelphia: Lippincott Williams & Wilkins.

Maslow, A. H. (1970). *The farther reaches of the human mind.* New York: Viking Press.

Maslow, A. H. (1954). *Motivation and personality.* New York: Harper.

McGregor, D. (1967). *The professional manager.* New York: McGraw-Hill.

McGregor, D. (1960). *The human side of enterprise.* New York: McGraw-Hill.

McManis & Monsalve Associates, Inc., and American Organization of Nurse Executives. (2003). *Healthy work environments, Vol. 2: Striving for excellence.* Retrieved June 14, 2006, from http://www.aone.org/aone/keyissues/hwe_excellence.html

Merton, R. K. (1957). *Social theory and social structure* (Rev. ed.). Glencoe, IL: Free Press.

Mintzberg, H. (1983a). *Power in and around organizations.* Englewood Cliffs, NJ: Prentice-Hall.

Mintzberg, H. (1983b). *Structures in fives: Designing effective organizations.* Englewood Cliffs, NJ: Prentice-Hall.

National Council of State Boards of Nursing. (1998). *The five rights of delegation.* Chicago: Author.

National Council of State Boards of Nursing (NCSBN). (2007). *Delegation.* Retrieved October 1, 2007 from https://www.ncsbn.org/cps/rde/xchg/SID-53EFFC2A-0A259009/ncsbn/hs.xsl/323.htm

Ouchi, W. G. (1981). *Theory Z: How American business can meet the Japanese challenge.* Reading, MA: Addison-Wesley.

Page, A. (ed.). (2004). *Keeping patients safe: Transforming the work environment of nurses.* Washington, DC: Institute of Medicine.

Taylor, F. W. (1911). *The principles of scientific management.* New York: Harper & Row.

Weber, M. (1947). The fundamental concepts of sociology (A. M. Anderson & T. Parsons, Trans.). In T. Parsons (Ed.), *Max Weber: The theory of social and economic organization* (pp. 87–157). New York: Oxford University Press.

☐ BIBLIOGRAPHY

American Nurses Association. (2004). *Scope and standards for nurse administrators* (2nd ed.) (Publication No. 03SSNA). Washington, DC: American Nurses Publishing.

Bridges, W. (2000). *The character of organizations: Using personality type in organization development.* Mountain View, CA: Davies-Black.

Chait, R. P., Ryan, W. P., & Taylor, B. E. (2005). *Governance as leadership: Reframing the work of nonprofit boards.* Hoboken, NJ: John Wiley & Sons.

Locke, E. A. (1982). The ideas of Frederick W. Taylor: An evaluation. *Academy of Management Review, 7*(1), 14.

Spangle, M., & Isenhart, M. W. (2002). *Negotiation: Communication for diverse settings.* Thousand Oaks, CA: Sage.

Tappen, R. M. (2001). *Nursing leadership and management: Concepts and practice* (4th ed.). Philadelphia: F. A. Davis.

Wink, P. (2003). *Negotiate your way to riches: How to convince others to give you what you want.* New York: Barnes and Noble.

Wywialowski, E. F. (2004). *Managing client care* (3rd ed.). St. Louis, MO: Mosby.

Zimmermann, P. G. (2002). *Nursing management secrets: Questions and answers about nursing management.* Philadelphia: Hanley & Belfus.

☐ ONLINE RESOURCES

American Nurses Association
http://nursingworld.org

American Association of Colleges of Nursing
http://www.aacn.nche.edu

American Association of Critical-Care Nurses
http://www.aacn.org

American Organization of Nurse Executives
http://www.aone.org/aone/keyissues/home.html

Magnet Recognition Program
http://nursecredentialing.org/magnet

National Council of State Boards of Nursing
http://www.ncsbn.org

Peter F. Drucker
http://www.peter-drucker.com

■ *Rose* **Kearney-Nunnery**

Change

13

> ❝ *We must always change, renew, rejuvenate ourselves; otherwise we harden.* ❞
>
> Johann von Goethe 1749–1832

Chapter Objectives

On completion of this chapter, the reader will be able to:

1. Differentiate among the theories of change.
2. Apply the stages of change to a client situation.
3. Given a practice situation, describe the roles and characteristics of an effective change agent.
4. Discuss differences needed in the change process for use with individuals, families, and groups.
5. Describe the process and strategies for effective organizational change.
6. Evaluate your personal change quotient.

Key Terms

Change
Planned Change
Change Agents
Restraining Forces
Driving Forces
Unfreezing
Moving

Refreezing
Transtheoretical Approach
Transitions
Internal Influences
External Forces
Change Quotient

Change is a part of normal daily life. We talk about changing our hair color, our attitude, someone else's mind, and so on. **Change** can be defined as a process that results in altered behavior of individuals or groups. Change that is accidental, spontaneous, or haphazard is caused by outside forces. On the other hand, intentional or **planned change** involves conscious effort toward some goal as a deliberate and collaborative process. Change is an integral and essential component of professional nursing practice with nurses as change agents in health-care settings.

In today's world, change must be viewed as affecting both the individual and the group. One example of planned change would be an individual going on a diet. The result (the change) is a decrease in weight. Such a change may also come about unintentionally, through outside influence. A family crisis or a bout of depression may lead to weight change. Or suppose the individual was eating chocolate. Gaining weight was not the intention—eating chocolate was—but weight gain was an unintended consequence. In contrast, as a planned change process, the same individual may have gone to Weight Watchers. Improved nutrition and eating practices also influence other family members through food selections and meal preparation in the home, and even may influence friends and colleagues through the individual's example.

Change is a daily occurrence in society. Think about the number of times you have read or heard of global relations, changes in political forces, and changes in health-care organizations. More people are beginning to embrace change since Johnson (2002) published his now classic *Who Moved My Cheese?* comparing the mice and the *Littlepeople* doing the simple things that can either work or immobilize the situation when things change. Still, making change is not an easy process for individuals or organizations.

In professional practice, we need to focus on the process of planned change, being proactive rather than reactive. Planned changes for individuals or groups in the environment require structural shifts or altered behaviors for improved functioning. Improved functioning involves new (changed) behaviors, attitudes, and relationships. Professional nurses are **change agents** for people and health. Their role is to move for needed, planned change for individuals, families, community groups, and society. Such practice should occur in individual practice as well as on an organizational level.

THEORIES OF CHANGE

Understanding the theories of change applicable to individuals, families, groups, and society is the first step in moving from being reactive to unintended change to becoming proactive in creating positive, planned change.

Chinn and Benne (1976) described three classic change philosophies: (1) the empirical-rational nature of man, (2) normative-educative philosophy, based on human motivation and norms (attitudes, values, skills, and relationships), and (3) power-coercive philosophy, based on leadership and the application of power (p. 23). The change models that follow reflect the empirical-rational philosophy and the normative-educative. These two philosophical orientations focus on the nature of the person or the group in the context of the environment.

Lewin

The classic change theorist was Kurt Lewin with his normative-educative model based on human motivation and norms in the group. Lewin (1951), who developed a model based on his Field Theory, a method of analyzing causal relationships and building the scientific constructs for change (p. 45). The mathematical model in his theory merely indicates that human behavior is based on the human being (or group) and his environment at that point in time. Lewin (1951) focused on social change, pointing out that "group life is never without change, merely differences in amount and type of change exist" (p. 199). In groups and organizations, multiple influences from individuals and their reactions to the environment cause group behaviors and norms. This Field Theory proposes that the status quo, or a state of equilibrium, is maintained when restraining forces and driving forces balance each other. To achieve change, the restraining forces must be weakened and the driving forces strengthened. Consider the illustration of change in Figure 13–1.

Restraining forces in society resist change; they include norms, values, relations among people, morals, fears, perceived threats, and regulations. In essence, these restraining forces are the "old guard" that maintains the status quo. **Driving forces,** on the other hand, support change and include the desire to please or the desire for more novel, effective, efficient, or merely different activities. System imbalance becomes the impetus for change. The process involves weakening the restraining forces and strengthening the driving forces. To do this, Lewin proposes three methods: unfreezing, moving, and refreezing of group standards.

Unfreezing involves disequilibrium, discontent, and uneasiness. Lewin (1951) states that "to break open the shell of complacency and self-righteousness, it is sometimes necessary to bring about deliberately an emotional stir-up" (p. 229). The restraining and driving forces are identified, and comparisons are drawn between the ideal and the actual situation. To bring about change, participants must make the need for change apparent and accepted. In many situations, making individuals uneasy and discontented with the environmental system is the initial step in the process. Malcontents want

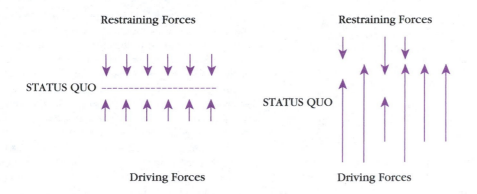

Restraining Forces   Restraining Forces

STATUS QUO   STATUS QUO

Driving Forces   Driving Forces

(Equilibrium)   *(Unequilibrium; setting for change)*

■ **Figure 13.1** Illustration of restraining and driving forces in the change process.

change, whereas individuals who are satisfied and comfortable with the current state of affairs resist changes that will create disequilibrium. Activities are centered on unfreezing the existing equilibrium.

Moving occurs when the previous structure is rearranged and realistic goals are set. The system is moved to a new level of equilibrium. Choices must be made about accepting the change agent and the roles of the group members in the change process. At this stage, group decisions are preferable for moving toward permanent change. This represents the distribution of power among the group members to make them driving forces engaged in the process. The individual involved in the change process acts as a member of a group in which new social values and norms are being established.

A new status quo is established with **refreezing.** Refreezing describes the new level of equilibrium and reinforcement needed for the new patterns of behavior. The focus is on maintaining the goal achieved and highlighting the present benefits over past practices.

Consider Lewin's model with a client population. The individual with heart disease who is started on a low-salt, low-fat diet has a teaching need to bring permanent change to his diet. You discover through interviews with the client and family members that the diet at home is highly seasoned and high in animal protein and fats. *Restraining forces* in this situation are cultural values, family traditions, individual and group (family) preferences in food selection and preparation, attitudes toward diet, foods, or food preparation, fears of further illness with changes in diet, and attitudes toward restrictions on personal lifestyle.

Now consider each of these factors in relation to all members of the household and the client's work, recreation, and social environments. Think about the *driving forces:* fear of further illness without the dietary changes, respect for advice given, support network, educational presentations, role models, and so forth. *Unfreezing* involves the identification of the restraining

and driving forces, motivating the client toward change, and assessing readiness for teaching. *Moving* consists of supporting a positive attitude toward change and providing nutritional information, including food selection, preparation, and presentation options. *Refreezing* would occur with the client's stabilization, evidenced through subjective reports (e.g., food diary), objective observations (e.g., health assessment), and laboratory findings in the rehabilitation phase. Valuable nursing theories to support nursing actions include King's Theory of Goal Attainment and Orem's Self-Care Agency. Supporting attitudinal and behavioral changes could occur through follow-up telephone or e-mail service after discharge or interviews at clinic appointments. A similar application could be developed for group change using Lewin's Field Theory or the Health Belief Model. See Chapter 5 for more information.

Lippitt

As an outgrowth and expansion of Lewin's theory, Lippitt (1973) pointed out that "if we want to understand, explain, or predict change in human behavior, we need to take into account the person and his environment" (p. 3). He identified several complex factors of human behavior that must be considered: motivation, multiple causation, and overrationalized habits. Looking at both individual and organizational change, he focused further on the change agent and defined seven specific phases (Figure 13–2) within an idea, similar to Lewin's change model. Thus, Lippitt described more specific activities that are still applicable to the three steps of unfreezing, moving, and refreezing.

Unfreezing, Moving, Refreezing

For *unfreezing,* there is the need to collect data and diagnose the problem and the key people. The driving and restraining people, environmental, and organizational forces are identified, defined, and targeted. Second, the

7. Terminating the Relationship
6. Maintaining the Change
5. Choosing the Change Agent's Role
4. Selecting Change Objectives
3. Change Agent's Motivation and Resources
2. Assessment of Motivation and Capacity for Change
1. Diagnosis of Problem

■ **Figure 13.2** Lippitt's (1973) seven stages of planned change.

motivation and resources are assessed to identify the desire and capacity for change. This includes resistance and readiness of the people in the environment. In the third step, the change agent's motivation, commitment, and resources must be assessed for the potential success of the change activity. The skills, efforts, and responsibilities are critical planning pieces in this phase of change.

For *moving*, change objectives must be selected with consideration of activities for progressive change. Lippitt used the leverage point concept as the starting point at which receptivity for change is apparent and the objectives are initiated. Planning and evaluation are primary activities in this step. Then, following the development of an action plan with evaluation criteria, the change agent and group roles are selected and assigned. Acceptance and selection of an appropriate role is critical in defining the power, outcomes, and strategies of the change agent.

Refreezing, or maintaining the change, occurs through ongoing training, communication, and support of the people in the environment. Communication by both sides, the driving and the restraining forces, advertises the success of the change using actual evaluation results. In many cases, the loudest and most visible of the restraining forces become the change agent's greatest supporters when they accept the merits of the process with evaluation. How many times have you heard someone say, "I never thought it could be done but . . ." or "I was behind that all along but I did not want to show it"? Finally, terminating the helping relationship is necessary on the part of the change agent and major players for the change to become part of the people and the environment, and not just the activity of a select individual or group. Rather, it becomes the new norm of the people or the organization.

Role of Change Agent

A major piece of Lippitt's (1973) model involves the roles for the professional change agent. He proposed four major roles for the change agent:

- Specialist
- Coordinator
- Fact finder and information link
- Consultant

Lippitt views the selection of the appropriate role for the change agent as essential in the moving phase of change. As a *specialist*, the change agent is the expert in the environment on methods and strategies for change. As a *coordinator*, the change agent functions as manager, who plans, organizes, and coordinates efforts and programs for the change. The change agent as a *fact finder and information link* serves as a seeker, clarifier, synthesizer, reality-tester, and provider of information, as well as a communications link among all participants in the system (Lippitt, 1973, pp. 60–61).

The consultant role is viewed as the most important role for the change agent, both inside the system and with external individuals, groups, and environments. In fact, Lippitt (1973) developed a model of eight specific activity roles within this consultant role, which are viewed along a continuum from advocate through expert, trainer, alternative identifier, collaborator, process specialist, fact finder, and reflector (p. 63). The correct role for the change agent depends on the people, the environment, and how much direction is needed from the agent to implement the change. As the advocate, the change agent as a consultant is highly directive in leading the group toward change. Conversely, the change agent is the least directive as a reflector, helping the group clarify and evaluate their efforts. The change agent must have knowledge, skill, and perseverance in the work-intensive process of change.

Consider, again, our example of the client who must change to a low-salt, low-fat diet. Under Lippitt's model, first, you need to collect data on meals, food preferences, and preparation at home. You identify, define, and target the environmental forces—family, friends, and cultural and collegial (work or recreational) forces. Second, you assess the motivation, resistance, readiness, and resources of the client and his family to identify the desire and capacity for change in dietary habits. In the third step, your motivation, commitment, and resources must be realized as the nurse-change agent. Your skills, efforts, and responsibilities are critical in this planning phase. Lippitt's concept of leverage point occurs when the client and his family are receptive to change and the action plan is initiated with evaluation criteria. Your role as change agent is defined specific to the client and his needs. Consider the applicability of Orem's three modes of nursing, especially the supportive-educative mode, in relation to his continuum of consultant activities. Your role as change agent may alter rapidly as the client moves from the hospital setting to the home and clinic settings. Empowerment of the client and his significant others is critical for success in this type of change. And with the maintenance of the change in diet and health status that occurs through ongoing training in dietary management, communication, support, and reinforcement during the follow-up period, the client and family are moved into the termination phase. The helping relationship is no longer necessary and the dietary changes have become part of the person and family in their environment.

Havelock

Havelock (1971) used a system and process model to depict an organization with the following major concepts: role, linkages, and communication for transfer and use of knowledge. Using the three major perspectives of problem-solving, research-development-diffusion, and social interaction, Havelock further examined the linkage process to view the change in the broader system (Havelock & Havelock, 1973). His model reflects the empirical-rational nature of humans.

Building on Lewin's stages of change, Havelock added steps, highlighting communication and interpersonal activities in these steps:

- Perception of need
- Diagnosis of the problem
- Identification of the problem
- Devising a plan of action
- Gaining acceptance of the plan
- Stabilization
- Self-renewal. (Havelock & Havelock, 1973)

Unfreezing, Moving, Refreezing

For *unfreezing*, the perception of a need for a change in the system is followed by diagnosis and identification of the problem. At this time, a reciprocal relationship develops between the user (client) system and a resource system. Linkages with needed resources are made in this initial stage before moving on the change. Havelock and Havelock (1973) stress that the problem-solver must be "meaningfully linked to outside resources" (p. 23).

Moving toward change requires devising a plan of action and gaining acceptance of the plan in the system. This is a stage of searching for a solution and applying that solution to the identified problem, using resource linkages in the environment.

In the final step, *refreezing*, stabilization and the need for self-renewal are specified. First, stabilization in the system is specified to sustain the change (refreezing). Havelock describes self-renewal as being needed to sustain the client system in the future. This sense of self-renewal is the empirical-rational nature of people where the new values, goals, and activities of the system become the norm.

Role of Change Agent

The importance of and roles for the change agent are also key components of Havelock's model, which lists four roles for the change agent:

- Catalyst
- Solution giver
- Process helper
- Resource linker. (Havelock & Havelock, 1973, p. 60)

These roles become increasingly complex. The catalyst serves as the impetus for change. The resource linker brings people, environments, and resources together at the system and macrosystem levels (Havelock & Havelock, 1973, pp. 60–64). For effective functioning within these roles, Havelock further developed a training program for preparing effective change agents.

Havelock's model can also be used with the example of dietary change for our client with heart disease. Communication and interpersonal activities are core ingredients in the nurse-client relationship. Identifying the need for altering dietary salt and fat relates to the client's medical condition. The personal, environmental, social, cultural, and dietary habits are assessed through interview, to define the problem. A reciprocal relationship between the client system and a resource system occurs through linkages, including meeting with a nutritionist for food selection and preparation options. Informational lists on cookbooks, restaurants, and community associations advocating healthy eating with low-fat, low-salt meals are provided. Using this model, the nurse encourages linkages with outside resources such as the American Heart Association, American Association of Critical-Care Nurses, and collegial relationships with nutritionists, rehabilitation specialists, and cardiologists. The plan for dietary change is devised in collaboration with the client system and includes linkages with community resources acceptable to the client and his family. Recall the concept of cultural competence from Chapter 5 and how it is necessary in this model. Linkages must be retained with the client after discharge, in the home, clinic, or rehabilitation setting. This follow-up is necessary for stabilizing the diet, given the client's physiologic and psychosocial system influences. The role of the nurse-change agent has moved from catalyst and solution giver in the initial phase of problem identification, to process helper in the planning phase, and then to resource linker. The changes in diet must become a part of the client's value system. The nurse-change agent then terminates the relationship with the client while linkages with external resources provide the client with self-renewal.

Rogers

As an outgrowth of the change model, Rogers developed the Diffusion of Innovations model. In 1971, Rogers and Shoemaker stated the following:

Although it is true that we live more than ever before in an era of change, prevailing social structures often serve to hamper the diffusion of innovations. Our activities in education, agriculture, medicine, industry, and the like are often without the benefit of the most current research knowledge. The gap between what is actually known and what is effectively put to use needs to be closed (p. 1).

This is still true today, more than 35 years later. We live in a time of even greater social change. This model was used in nursing in the 1980s to promote research-based practice and is quite appropriate today with the imperative for evidence-based practice.

Rogers and Shoemaker (1971) focus on communication and view *change* as the effects of a new idea or innovation being adopted and put into use or rejected. Change may occur at the level of the individual, group, organization, or society. The model was first proposed with four major steps in the process of social change: knowledge, persuasion, decision, and confirmation (Rogers & Shoemaker, 1971, p. 25). Rogers (1983) then extended the Innovation-Diffusion process to five stages:

- Knowledge
- Persuasion
- Decision
- Implementation
- Confirmation

The interest and commitment of key people and policy-makers are critical in this model.

Unfreezing, Moving, Refreezing

Developing a sequence of knowledge, persuasion, and decision-making is the key activity in the *unfreezing* stage. To develop knowledge, key people and policy-makers are introduced to the innovation to gain understanding. Then comes persuasion to develop attitudes on the innovation. Rogers (1983) uses persuasion to focus on the individual whose attitudes change, either positively or negatively toward the innovation, not on the external force that changes one's mind. The decision to adopt or reject an innovation is the bridge between the unfreezing and moving stages in Rogers' model.

Implementation applies to the stage of *moving*. Revisions, potential adoption, or rejection of the innovation occurs in this implementation phase. Rogers' fifth step, when the innovation changes from being novel to being part of the routine or norm, involves *refreezing* the equilibrium. He calls this step *confirmation*, in which reinforcement is sought and the key people and policy-makers decide to maintain or discontinue the innovation. Rogers (1983) admitted that the research evidence shows no clear distinction between the implementation and confirmation steps. This may be related

to the idea of a flexible time span between implementation and confirmation, when the process of refreezing for the innovation occurs. Rogers (1983) describes the final confirmatory stage as "routinization" of the innovation.

Throughout the entire process, five attributes determine the rate of adoption of an innovation by members of a social system:

- Relative advantage
- Compatibility
- Complexity
- Trialability
- Observability. (Rogers & Shoemaker, 1971, p. 39; Rogers, 1983, pp. 238–240)

These attributes should be included in all evaluation plans and data on the change. Relative advantage is determined through comparison of the innovation with what was done in the past. The advantage may be effectiveness as well as efficiency, and the process has been described as weighing economic advantages or the cost-effectiveness. Compatibility with the values, beliefs, and needs of the group is the second factor. The complexity (difficulty in use), trialability (experimental trials), and observability (visible evidence) are all considered in the implementation stage and have a direct effect on adoption, revision, or discontinuation of an innovation.

Role of Change Agent

Rogers' model also highlights the roles of the change agent, which occur in the following sequence:

1. Develops the need for change
2. Establishes the relationship with the client system
3. Diagnoses the problems
4. Motivates the client system for change
5. Translates intent for change into the actions needed
6. Stabilizes change in system and "freezes" new behavior
7. Terminates the relationship. (Rogers, 1983, pp. 315–317)

Like Lippitt, Rogers views the change agent as a professional, skilled in change for effective functioning in the role.

We take a slightly different approach with the application of Rogers' Innovation-Diffusion process model to our example of the client who needs to change his diet. You have found research studies on effective dietary compliance in cardiac rehabilitation. You now wish to bring this innovation into practice in your organization to use in client teaching programs. During the initial development of knowledge, key people and policy-makers in nursing service and cardiology are introduced to the teaching program content and methods, along with the results from use with clients in other settings. Next, you need to persuade people of the effectiveness and applicability of this approach—the organization and its resources as well as the client population. The decision is made whether to adopt or reject the new teaching program. If it is decided to try the teaching program with a client population, the phase of implementation is entered. The teaching program may be revised, adopted, or rejected on the basis of its specificity and acceptability to the client group and the organization. If the teaching program is found to be applicable and advantageous, it is "confirmed" as the agency procedure or organizational norm. If the procedure is not adopted, the key people and policymakers must confirm the decision to discontinue the program. These are the steps toward implementing evidence-based practice at the organizational level.

The Transtheoretical Approach

Another model of change arose from a behaviorist perspective and psychotherapy. Prochaska, DiClemente, and Norcross (1992) describe their program of research focused on how people as "self-changers" intentionally change their behavior, both with and without psychotherapy (p. 1102). This led to the emergence of their **Transtheoretical Approach** to change, which they describe as an eclectic model that does not dictate adherence to a specific type of psychotherapy. The empirical basis for this theory provides a broad range of studies on individuals and groups (both inpatients and outpatients), from family therapy to addictive conditions and health-promotion activities. One of the original core concepts of this theory is that people who change or who recover from an addictive condition experience an invariant series of stages for the change to occur (Prochaska & DiClemente, 1984, p. 21). Key components of this model are stages of change and processes for intentional change to occur. Developmental and environmental changes can also occur, but unless individuals see this as an intentional change, they will feel coerced and reversion to the prior behavior may occur (Prochaska & DiClemente, 1984, p. 80).

Originally, the Transtheoretical Model included five linear stages (precontemplation, contemplation, decision, action, and maintenance) but was then modified based on statistical analysis to four stages, because the individual's decision to make a change included both contemplation and action. The four stages of change—precontemplation, contemplation, action, and maintenance—were envisioned as a revolving door with the potential for relapse (Prochaska & DiClemente, 1984, p. 23).

Further research provided the basis for the refinement of the model, as a spiral with five stages of change, in which relapses were the norm resulting in regression and the potential for later progression through the five stages (Prochaska et al., 1992, p. 1104). Consider these five stages as described in Table 13–1. Termination with the firm establishment of the changed behavior does not occur until the individual no longer has to make any conscious efforts to avoid a relapse to the prior behavior (Prochaska & DiClemente, 1984, p. 29). The research has indicated that most "self-changers" will "recycle several times through stages before achieving long-term maintenance" (Prochaska et al., 1992, p. 1111).

In addition to the stages of change through which the individual progresses, the model proposes that certain behaviors or processes are more apparent and effective in selected stages of change. A behaviorist philosophy to change is apparent in the 10 proposed processes that occur in the different stages of change as follows:

- Consciousness raising with education and information
- Self-reevaluation as with values clarification
- Self-liberation with a commitment to action
- Counter-conditioning as with alternatives to the behavior
- Stimulus control or counteracting negative stimuli
- Reinforcement management or self-rewards for positive behaviors
- Helping relationships, both social and therapeutic support systems
- Dramatic relief or expressing feelings
- Environmental reevaluation as with the effect of the problem on the environment
- Social liberation and advocacy. (Prochaska et al., 1992, p. 1108)

Subsequent research has identified that the most frequently used processes across the various types of intentional change were helping relationships, consciousness raising, and self-liberation, except in the case of overweight individuals who used more self-liberation and stimulus control (Prochaska et al., 1992, p. 1107). These change processes focus on cognitive, affective, and psychomotor behaviors. In the early precontemplation and contemplation stages of change, the cognitive change processes can lead to preparation for change. Active behavioral change processes are critical in the action and maintenance stages, however (Prochaska et al., 1992, p. 1112).

Unfreezing, Moving, Refreezing

The five stages of change are also consistent with Lewin's stages of change. Unfreezing occurs in the stages of precontemplation, contemplation, and preparation, especially with the cognitive change processes.

Table 13.1

Transtheoretical Model and the Stages of Change

Stage of Change	Behavioral Characteristics	Changes Processes
Precontemplation	Satisfaction with the current situation. The individual indicates no intention to change and may deny the existence of a problem.	↓ Consciousness raising ↓ Dramatic relief ↓ Environmental reevaluation
Contemplation	Acknowledges that a problem exists but has not made a commitment to change the negative behavior. Important clues for this stage are a lack of readiness for the change despite thoughtful consideration of the positives and negatives of the situation.	↓ ↓ ↓ Self-reevaluation
Preparation	In this stage the commitment to change is made and the individual is intending to take action in the near future.	↓ ↓ Self-liberation
Action	Positive actions are now taken for a change in behavior. Individuals in this stage have altered their behavior for a period from one day to six months (Prochaska et al., 1992, p. 1104)	↓ Reinforcement ↓ management ↓ Helping relationships ↓ Counter conditioning ↓ Stimulus control ↓
Maintenance	The new behaviors have now replaced the prior ones. The individual is committed to the change on an ongoing basis. The theorists describe the "hallmarks" of this stage as stabilizing behavioral change and avoiding relapse, which can last from six months to a lifetime (Prochaska et al., 1992, p. 1104).	

Source: Prochaska, J.O., DiClemente, C. C., & Norcross, J. C. (1992). In search of how people change: Applications to addictive behaviors. *American Psychologist, 47*, 1102–1114.

Moving starts with the stage of preparation for the change and then into action. Recall that in the action stage of the Transtheoretical Model, the individual has implemented a changed behavior from one day to six months. Refreezing occurs in the maintenance stage with the stabilization of the behavior.

The Individual as the Change Agent

In this theory, the individual is the agent of change, with external assistance of "helping relationships" in

the change process. The focus is clearly on the individual and the potential for relapse and is applicable for individuals as "self-changers," especially given a situation for client teaching.

Applications of the theory have been noted in the case of both addictive behaviors and for promoting healthier lifestyles. For use with groups, effectiveness depends on whether the individuals are at the same stage of change (Prochaska & DiClemente, 1984). For example, for effectiveness, group members must be homogeneous in terms of their readiness for change as opposed to a group with individuals in the precontemplation stage (and satisfied with the status quo) and those in the action or maintenance stages.

The focus of the Transtheoretical Approach is on the individual and the potential for relapse is consistent with the focus of nursing on human beings in their unique environment and with their unique characteristics and needs. They may need additional time to succeed in the changed behavior. As previously noted by the theorists, many need to "recycle" through the stages. As with our example of the client who must change to a low-salt, low-fat diet, assessment of individual and environmental characteristics is still essential, as is readiness for change. This assessment of readiness will direct your use of change processes to assist the individual through the particular stage of change. For example, with client teaching as a helping relationship, you may be providing informational materials in the precontemplation and contemplation stages as consciousness raising activities. Also consider the use of active behavioral change activities with food diaries and reinforcement management in the active stages of change. A key component of the self-liberation process in change in the Transtheoretical Approach is the concept of choice with the component of decision-making and commitment to the decision (Prochaska & DiClemente, 1984, p. 38). And individual differences, self-esteem, and motivation must be considerations in the case of a relapse.

TRANSITIONS

In the area of organizational change, the concept of **transitions,** as a corporate change phenomenon, has emerged with the move to more humanistic organizational theories as these same organizations struggle to survive and thrive in the economic climate. As illustrated in the Harvard Business Essentials (2003), "accepting the necessity and inevitability of change enables [businesses] to see times of transformation not as threats but as opportunities—opportunities for reinventing the company and its culture" (pp. 1–2). Numerous consultants as change agents assist corporations through these transitions. Organizational changes fall generally in the areas of mergers, cost-cutting, customer service, or changes in processes of how things get done (Harvard Business Essentials, 2003). In health care we have seen all of these types of changes, with process changes an imperative as we focus on safety initiatives and evidence-based practice. Two particular change models reflect the humanistic focus of organizations in transition.

Bridges' Making Transitions

Rather than focusing on change as a situation like relocation, Bridges (2003) looks at the psychological processes in stages of transition (Box 13.1) where people must "come to terms with the details of the new situation that the change brings about" (p. 3). These three stages of transition are interacting and nonlinear and may be occurring at the same time at different parts of the organization and with different people.

In the initial stage, this theory focuses on people who have to first "let go" of the comfortable and safe in their day-to-day lives and experience loss. Resistance is to be expected because Bridges (2003) terms this initial stage as an ending in that "before you can learn a new way of doing things, you must unlearn the old way" (p. 23). He describes a grief and mourning process requiring acceptance of and assistance for the people in the organization.

Bridges (2003) describes the second stage as one of great uncertainty, chaos, and the opportunity for innovation. People have given up the old way of doing things but need support in innovation and assistance in the process. He describes Neutral Zone Management as the "only way to ensure that the organization comes through the change intact and that the necessary changes actually work the way they are supposed to" (Bridges, 2003, p. 42). He even recommends the use of transition teams composed of organizational members to monitor the process, progress, and to be the communication channel to the leadership of the organization.

The third stage is The New Beginning described as a release of new energy in a new direction and with a new identity (Bridges, 2003, p. 57). Again, the humanistic perspective is apparent with celebrations of the new corporate identity and the people in the new culture actively involved and rejuvenated. Bridges actively speaks to leadership and provides examples of successes and pitfalls that occur in the transition. Organizational leadership must focus on the culture with respect for transition to the new beginning. Checklists are provided to address questions on progress throughout the process.

Bridges' three stages of organizational change can parallel the three stages of unfreezing, moving, and

---

Box 13.1 Bridges' Stages for Managing Transitions

- Ending, Losing, Letting Go
- The Neutral Zone
- The New Beginning

Source: Bridges, W. (2003). *Managing transitions: Making the most of change* (2nd ed.). Cambridge, MA: DaCapo Press.

ONLINE CONSULT

William Bridges & Associates Transition Training at
http://www.wmbridges.com

refreezing, but this model focuses on the management and people in the organization for success in the process. As Bridges (2003) points out, "The way change was managed in the past was designed to get warm bodies on the production line" (p. xi).

Four Quadrants of Change

Another organizational change model focuses on the humanistic factors within the organization with important considerations of personal transformation. Although not related to particular stages, the *Four Quadrants of Change* is a circle divided in quarters (see Box 13–2) as interacting and vital considerations for success in the organizational change process. The top two quarters represent the individual in the organization but first with psychological, spiritual, and cognitive attributes that must be considered in the transformation process. Quadrant one focuses on the inner development of people, and the recognition that no substantive change is possible without a change in the consciousness of the people (Anderson, Klein, & Stuart, 2000, p. 32). Quadrant two represents the interpersonal and technical skills for motivation and peak performance in the organization (Anderson et al., 2000, p. 32).

At the bottom of the circle, quadrants three and four represent the organizational influences. Quadrant three is the organizational culture and traditions. Quadrant four is the organizational design with technology, policies, procedures, and workflow that determine performance of the organization (Anderson et al., 2000, p. 33). Consideration of all four quadrants is vital in the change process for an organization, but the theorists caution that the humanistic quadrants are vital for an organizational change to succeed. They consider this as a personal transformation and a conscious choice because "organizational change is not a question of skills and structure alone, but of identity and worldview" (Anderson et al., 2000, p. 34).

Box 13.2 The Four Quadrants of Change

- Quadrant 1: Individual/Internal
- Quadrant 2: Individual/External
- Quadrant 3: Collective/Internal
- Quadrant 4: Collective/External

Source: Anderson, B., Klein, E., & Stuart, J. (2000, January/February). Why change is a consciousness choice. *The Journal for Quality and Participation, 23,* 32–36.

The Role of the Change Agent

In both transitions models, the role of the change agent is the leadership driving the change, with management firmly focused on the organizational culture for reinventing the organization and survival in a humanistic environment. Understanding of human nature and its resistance to change as a loss of the comfortable is necessary for the change agent.

The transitions models are focused on organizational change, but the view of change as a transition with the concepts of loss and rejuvenation are still applicable to our example of the client with a need for a change in diet. The grief, mourning, and loss over past heritage and practices must be considered along with the uncertainty and potential for innovation during the time of transition to the new dietary regime. Perhaps this could be a family cookbook of new recipes and preparations. An important thought is the celebration of the new beginning and whether we help our clients sufficiently celebrate their success with a changed behavior.

The various models of change are summarized in Table 13–2. Selecting an appropriate model to guide practice involves how you look at the world and what is most helpful in driving your skills as an agent in the change process. Moving from the theoretical stages of change to strategies for change brings the focus to the external influence or change agent.

CHANGE AGENTS

Our second step in becoming a major player in the change process is to develop greater understanding of the roles and attributes of a successful change agent. We have seen the importance of the change agent emerge in the models of Lippitt, Havelock, and Rogers. Recall that in the Transtheoretical Approach, your role as an agent of change will be a part of the "helping relationship." Table 13–3 summarizes the roles and activities of the change agent in these models. In Lewin's original model, change in humans is a function of the person and her environment at that point in time. Consider the roles of the change agent in the three general phases of change.

Unfreezing

Good interpersonal and assessment skills are needed to acquire data to weaken restraining forces and enhance driving forces in the present system, and the agent must consider both internal and external system forces. The change agent must then establish a climate that encourages and supports change. Needs assessment, diagnosis, and the establishment of a professional relationship have occurred consistently during the unfreezing phase

Table 13.2

Comparison of the Stages of Change Represented in Theoretical Models

Theorist	Stages						
Lewin (1951) Force Field	[1] Unfreezing	[2] Moving	[3] Refreezing				
Lippitt (1973) Planned Change	[1] Diagnosis of problem	[2] Assessment of motivation and capacity for change	[3] Change agent's motivation and resources	[4] Selecting change objectives	[5] Choosing change agent's role	[6] Maintaining the change	[7] Terminating the relationship
Havelock (1971) Linkages	[1] Perception of need	[2] Diagnosis of the problem	[3] Identification of the problem	[4] Devising a plan of action	[5] Gaining acceptance of plan	[6] Stabilization	[7] Self-renewal
Rogers (1983) Innovation-Diffusion	[1] Knowledge	[2] Persuasion	[3] Decision	[4] Implementation	[5] Confirmation		
Transtheoretical Approach Prochaska et al., 1992	[1] Precontemplation	[2] Contemplation	[3] Preparation	[4] Action	[5] Maintenance		
Bridges (2003) Making Transitions	[1] Ending, Losing, Letting Go	[2] The Neutral Zone	[3] The New Beginning				

Table 13.3

Comparing Roles for the Change Agent from Different Theoretical Models

Stages of Change	Lippitt (1973)	Havelock (1973)	Rogers (1983)	Bridges (2003)

Unfreezing	A specialist in the diagnosis and assessment of client system and change agent as:
	■ Information seeker
	■ Clarifier
	■ Synthesizer
	■ Reality-tester
	■ Provider
	■ Problem-solver
		A catalyst in the identification of needs, diagnoses, and all aspects of the problem within the roles of:
		■ Clarifier
		■ Synthesizer
		■ Reality-tester
		■ Provider
		■ Problem-solver
			Range of roles from support to consultant for sharing knowledge, building persuasiveness, and leading the group toward decision making on innovation through activities of:
			■ Needs identification
			■ Establishment of professional relationship with client system
			■ Diagnosis of problems
			■ Motivation of client system
				The critical ingredient is the match or at least a working understanding of the consistency between the character type of the organization and the change agent.
				    Acceptance and acknowledgment of the grief and mourning process for the loss is vital.
				    The need for detailed information on the plan because the transition must be transmitted and reinforced.
				    Good listening and communication skills are essential with a focus on the person as a member of and part of the organization.

Moving	Communication link viewed within one of eight directive to nondirective consultative roles: ■ Advocate ■ Expert ■ Trainer ■ Alternative identifier ■ Collaborator ■ Process specialist	Solution giver and process helper as: ■ Clarifier ■ Synthesizer ■ Reality-tester ■ Provider ■ Problem-solver	Range of roles from support to consultant to translate intent for change into the actions needed	The Neutral Zone is a time of uncertainty and uneasiness in the organization and among the people. Once again, excellent communication skills are vital to keeping people informed, on target, and to avoid the development of damaging coalitions, which can inhibit the transition.

■ Fact-finder
■ Reflector

A transition monitoring team keeps management aware of the progress of the grass-roots members in their transition. Bridges (2003) does point out that role of the team is to monitor progress and should be time limited.

Refreezing

Consultation for:
■ Maintenance of the change
■ Termination of the relationship

Resource linker for stabilization and self-renewal as:
■ Clarifier
■ Synthesizer
■ Reality-tester
■ Problem-solver

Range of roles from support to consultant for:
■ Confirmation of change and stabilizing the adoption to prevent discontinuance and reinforce new behaviors
■ Termination of relationship

The New Beginning is a time of excitement and celebration for members of the organization in the new ways of the organization. Important roles for both the change agent as the manager of the transition and also for the leadership of the organization with the new culture.

in all models. Now consider the similarity of this stage to the assessment and diagnosis activities of the nursing process.

In the nursing process, health assessment data are collected and problems are identified. Assessing the client's characteristics, her current level of satisfaction with her health problem and condition, and her perception of her situation is an essential component of this activity. Diagnostic statements are developed after needs identification. Asking questions and diagnosing the problem for changed client behaviors or responses lead to the planning stage of the nursing process.

Moving

The change agent must help the client group set and strive for clear, realistic goals. A good deal of the change agent's time and energy is needed during this phase for strategies to deal with those who are resisting change. Again, interpersonal and motivational skills are critical. The change agent must constantly assess and evaluate resistance, conflict, readiness for change, and motivation in the client system, and must maintain movement toward the goals and objectives of change.

As in the nursing process, the major activities of the moving stage are implementing plans, goals, and objectives and collecting evaluation data. Client data are analyzed, interpreted, and acted upon. The nurse actively uses critical thinking, decision-making, interpersonal, and evaluation skills. The same skills are necessary to move toward change. This stage will probably be the most comfortable for the nurse functioning as a change agent, because skills in this area are developed through nursing practice.

Refreezing

Providing rewards and reinforcement for the change is a major part of the change agent's role in the third stage. Evaluation data for reinforcement of change must be used as supportive evidence. Activities for the change agent during this stage are supportive, initially, but involvement decreases with the need to terminate and have the client system totally involved in and responsible for the change without external intervention from the change agent. Recall that in the Transtheoretical Approach, the stage of maintenance may last a lifetime until the individual no longer has to make any conscious effort to avoid a relapse and the helping relationships may be the social support system.

In the nursing process, the nurse-client relationship is terminated when objectives are achieved and nursing diagnoses are resolved. The nurse has prepared the person or family for this termination long before discharge orders are written or the person leaves the agency environment. Just as discharge planning starts with admission, this last stage must be planned for and worked toward during the entire change process, with the person, family, or group taking increasing responsibility for the new behaviors.

The interventions of a skilled change agent can make all the difference in the planned change process. The essential skills of change agents include the following:

- Vision for the future and creativity
- Ability to look at a situation narrowly and broadly (assessment and critical thinking skills)
- Good interpersonal skills, including those of communication, motivation, assertiveness, problem-solving, and group process
- Flexibility and a willingness to consider alternative views
- Perseverance and a positive attitude
- Integrity and commitment
- Ability to manage conflict and resistance
- A focus on human beings and celebrating their accomplishments

CHANGE IN INDIVIDUALS, FAMILIES, AND GROUPS

As noted earlier, Chinn and Benne (1976) categorized change strategies into three major types: empirical-rational, normative-reeducative, and power-coercive. Power-coercive strategies are based on the application of power by legitimate authority. Nursing concerns are with human beings and their empowerment for healthy behaviors or the creation of optimal health status. Applying power as "the authority" is inconsistent with empowering people. One can alter practices, procedures, or the environment in organizations as a coercive change by imposing major policy, but think of the upheaval this change creates. Coercive change may be necessary in an emergency situation or when the person or family must have major assistance. The problem is that the change may not persist unless the person or group has internalized it into the value system.

The philosophical basis of nursing is consistent with the empirical-rational or the normative-reeducative strategies for change. The empirical-rational strategy assumes that people are rational and have a self-interest in change. Power for the individual or group occurs through knowledge. The normative-reeducative approach is based on social norms and the person's interaction with the environment. The normative-reeducative philosophy can be viewed as empowerment with an emphasis on interpersonal skills. Both of these philosophical orientations are consistent with nursing, but their applicability differs according to the nursing model selected for practice. For example, King's Theory of Goal Attainment, Orem's General Theory of Nursing, and

Roy's Adaptation Model contain philosophical assumptions similar to the reeducative strategies, with the person viewed as a thinking, feeling, reacting being in the context of his environment.

Because nursing looks at human beings and their interactions within the environment, several factors must be considered in the change process. These include resistance to change, empowerment or involvement of the client, and environmental, cultural, or situational factors.

Resistance to Change

A major concern of the change agent is the person's or group's resistance to change. To handle this resistance, one must evaluate what makes people resist change. People are naturally threatened by change. Change involves loss. It is a threat to their value system and a loss of the comfortable status quo. They feel vulnerable and insecure. Stress is created and must be managed. The need for the change may also be mistrusted or misunderstood. Another innately human characteristic is the fear of failure or being unable to perform the new activities or tasks. This creates more stress. This is the state of relapse in the Transtheoretical Approach in which the individual can then "recycle" through the stages.

Resistance to change can be reduced by several techniques:

- Careful planning
- Allowing sufficient time
- Support and reinforcement
- Involving the person or group

Understanding the full impact of individual or group norms and planning for a change in attitudes can lead to changes in behavior. Recall the adage, "Fools rush in." Allowing sufficient time for the change to occur and persist is essential. A gradual move toward change is more effective than a radical move. The time needed depends on the physical, psychosocial, cultural, and attitudinal characteristics of the individual or group. Patience, persistence, perseverance, and creativity are essential traits of the change agent. Another strategy for decreasing resistance to change is good communication with key and resource people throughout the entire process. In addition, a good deal of support and reinforcement will be needed. This requires excellent interpersonal skills, verbal and nonverbal, with both individuals and groups.

The involvement of the person or group is needed for lasting change. It is essential to build on their readiness, motivation, self-concept, abilities, and resources throughout the process. Involving people in planning and decision-making both reduces resistance to change and creates empowerment. Strategies for involving

people include education, training, socialization and persuasion (not imposing), and facilitation. This is a "helping relationship." It would often be easier to make the change yourself as an external force, but the action by the client system is slower and more enduring. Note that education and training involve enlightenment and preparation rather than preaching. This creates the empowerment and sets the stage for a revision of the norm or value system and self-efficacy.

Environmental Assessment

Looking at the situation or environment is critical in the change process. First, one must understand the past or the personal history of the individual, family, or group. You include a past, personal, psychosocial, family, and environmental history in a health history. These are important basic items of information to obtain before doing the physical appraisal in any health assessment. The same thing is needed in the change process. The following questions will help in understanding the situation and people:

1. What types of change has the person or group faced in the past? Information on experience and success with change is valuable to determine whether this person is a novice with change, has embraced change throughout life, or falls somewhere between these experiential extremes.
2. How has the person or group handled change? Stress and coping factors will emerge with this information. You can then discover how to motivate and support behaviors.
3. What resources have been available or used in previous change activities?
4. What is the person's or group's perspective on the applicability of the resources in the environment to the present situation? Human resources are support systems, and can include family, friends, colleagues, clergy, professionals, and even "ideal" role models. These resources may help the person or group. If these are not available or appropriate, linking the person or group with similar resources may be effective. Some people do well in support groups whereas others need more individualized support.

HEALTH-CARE ORGANIZATIONAL CHANGE

Both internal and external influences in contemporary health care are major considerations for change in health-care institutions. As Hall and Tolbert (2005) propose, "organizational survival, or the avoidance of death, is . . . the ultimate test of an organization, but at any time, unless death is imminent, what goes on in the organization is based on both environmental pressures and goals" (p. 155).

Everyone within an organization has faced organizational change, from minor changes in policy to restructuring of services. Many have experienced or know a colleague who has experienced a radical reorganization, with restructuring and managerial shifts, layoffs, or ownership changes. With organizational change comes tension and conflict as a natural function of stress on the system, its people, and their daily activities and interactions. Transitions and the sense of loss are important considerations.

Systems theory provides a useful perspective for viewing the internal and external forces of any organization. A health-care institution or agency is an open environmental system with great complexity. The organization must be considered in terms of the system, as well as the macrosystem and client system. **Internal influences** come from agency administrative, policy, and operational factors guiding the system. Bridges (2000) describes this as the character of the organization. The surrounding environmental system of the organization is the health-care arena, which provides the professional, specialization, reimbursement, and additional value structures for the organizational unit and its members. The broader social or macroenvironment reflects societal norms and values through the needs and potential needs of consumers of health care. Linkages among all system parts are assumed as necessary for effectiveness and continuity. But look further at this complex system and the internal environment.

When change is proposed for an agency or institutional system, an in-depth look at the organizational environment is needed. Internal sources of change can arise from any one or some combination of these system components. Consider the traditional health-care agency, the hospital. The associated internal forces can be described as follows:

- Goals and values for health care are specified for an organization as a purpose, philosophy, vision, or mission statement. Valuable information on the internal forces is apparent with this organizational view of people, health, and health care before translation into departmental or policy statements. Insight can also be obtained from the historical documents on how the institution evolved into a modern health-care organization.
- The knowledge and skills of the health-care providers and physical resources in the system are vital considerations. Consider internal forces from the specific equipment, services, and expertise of professional and nonprofessional labor forces in the organizational setting.

- Interpersonal and interdisciplinary relationships with role relationships, attitudes, and values of people and groups within the system must also be considered. Nurses are expected to exhibit behaviors related to the roles of health-care provider, manager, teacher, researcher, and advocate and to collaborate with members of other health-care disciplines.
- The organizational design to provide health-care services must also be considered. In addition to organizational charts, position descriptions, and policy and procedure manuals, informal sources, such as technical and clerical staff, can provide valuable information on the organization's daily operations to illustrate how tasks are accomplished in the organization.
- Governance by a governing board and corporate officers may include paid or volunteer board members, required institutional review boards, and the chief executive team or officers.

External environmental influences are the next factors to consider in terms of impact on the system. **External forces** include inputs of energy, information, and materials received from the environment, transformed, and returned to the environment as outputs. One input into the hospital environment is the client system. The client enters the hospital with a health-care deficit and, through the care received while hospitalized (throughput), strives for a higher level of wellness as the intended outcome (output). But environmental influences add more complexity. External forces are the broader environment providing inputs into the system. As with any open system, however, the external forces affect internal operations, and an exchange of information is returned to the environment as outputs.

External forces have a major impact on the function of the traditional hospital. Suppliers to be considered include physicians, drug and equipment companies, volunteers, and educational facilities. Physicians supply patients. Drug and equipment companies compete for contracts, and organizations seek purchasing power with consortia or multiorganizational contracts. Volunteers provide valuable transportation, recreational, and interpersonal services without which many hospitals could not survive. Educational suppliers provide additional health-care services, with trainees as residents, interns, nurses, therapists, and other preparers of ancillary personnel, as well as the future workforce. And national safety initiatives add additional responsibility and complexity. In addition, new staff members bring different ideas and methods into the system.

Customers are generally thought of as the client system: inpatients, same-day surgery clients, and clinic clients. But the concept of customer can be seen more broadly to include community initiatives, educational programming, health contracts with business and industry, health maintenance organizations (HMOs), and physician practice groups. Large corporate entities, intraorganizational agreements, health insurers, and second- and third-party payers are major service and economic influences on the client system. Federal legislation, state laws, local ordinances, regulatory bodies, court precedents, insurers, and professional organizations all have a legal effect on the hospital.

On a broader, macrosystem level, consider changes predicted for the population. The increase in the elderly population, especially frail elders, has a great impact on services that will be needed. The national, state, and local economies, with their associated concerns about costs, are other societal factors that have a profound effect on hospitals and health-care organizations. All of these factors, individually and combined, influence how the hospital markets and cares for its customers and personnel and meets their organizational mandates and mission.

But let us return to the change process and activities in the phases of unfreezing, moving, and refreezing. During *unfreezing,* the major change activities include assessment, diagnosis, and establishment of a professional relationship. Assessment must involve in-depth analysis and synthesis of both internal and external forces. As with individuals, families, and groups, methods for data collection include interviews and observation. But with a larger group of people, methods can include questionnaires or surveys for timely and, at times, confidential collection of data.

Like the past and personal change history obtained on a smaller scale with the person, family, or group, an organizational history provides valuable insights. The organizational history can reveal information on development and problem resolution to this point. Methods for gathering an organizational history require not only skillful interviewing of key people but also a careful review of records and documents of the organization.

Consider all environments, including the constraints, demands, and opportunities present. Resources in the environment—people and physical resources—provide major influences on any organizational change. Identifying the driving forces and individuals in the system is essential to building a base of support. Analyze external environments, especially population trends.

Diagnosis of problems becomes more complex as the volume of information and number of people increase. Whether the change agent is selected from within the organization or is an external consultant, he will need a high level of skill to achieve organizational change. Clear understanding of both internal and external forces will be necessary, along with a good deal of fortitude to survive the experience. And keep in mind the sense of loss members of the organization may experience in this initial stage of transition.

The *moving* phase in organizational change involves developing strategies to match resources with constraints, demands, opportunities, and history as part of the planning process for change to proceed. Changes in goals and values must be reflected in organizational documents. Key work groups will be needed for decision-making and policy formation. People in the organization will need some retraining and educational programs to transmit knowledge of resources and to refine skills. A great deal of time and energy will be needed for the people. Role and status relations will require finesse and great sensitivity. Relating to the variable and altering readiness, resistance, and motivation of many individuals and groups will be quite a challenge.

People must be actively incorporated and empowered in this decision-making and implementation phase. Remember, this may be an opportunity for innovation in moving to a new organizational design or initiative. Involvement of people in the organizational change process necessitates use of excellent leadership and skills in group dynamics, conflict management, and team building. This is especially true when the methods for accomplishment of work activities have undergone major revisions. Communication links with management must be increased and reinforced as organizational members are included rather than alienated from key planners and controllers in the system. Minimizing people's stress and turmoil is a major function of the change agent in this phase.

A formalized evaluation plan must be in place and must be initiated in this moving phase. Data collection and feedback on the process, communicating even small results, are vital and must be ongoing. People in the system need to be continually aware of the result of their efforts. If indicated in the evaluation data, additional resources or linkages must be sought. This is the feedback loop that continues through the phase of refreezing and is essential to any successful organizational change. Evaluation data must be systematically recorded, analyzed, interpreted, and communicated. Evaluation data can be communicated through distribution of short reports, articles, or observations from various sources in newsletters and on bulletin boards, electronically, and in formal and informal discussion groups. Keeping the people on track and moving toward new organizational goals and norms requires stamina and a positive outlook despite the inevitable pitfalls and sidetracking that will occur.

Involvement of people in the organizational change process necessitates use of excellent leadership and skills in group dynamics, conflict management, and team building.

Refreezing the change may take longer than anticipated in the multilevel organizational system. The turmoil and differences that have arisen in the organization environment and the strength of external forces will influence the firm establishment of the change as the new organizational norm. Support and reinforcement are indispensable activities of the change agent, along with ongoing analysis, interpretation, and communication of the evaluation findings. The role will naturally become more consultative as termination approaches. At this point, the change should be a part of the expectations of the organization and its members. Ownership of the change is held by the people in the institutional or agency environment and not by key people or the change agent.

Consider the following example of organizational change, extending services from the traditional hospital into the community. Needs assessment, diagnosis of problems, and motivation in agency subsystems must occur in the unfreezing phase for organizational change. In addition to the traditional hospital, this change may involve outpatient departments and clinics, home-care agencies, rehabilitation or nursing home settings, HMOs, physician groups, and therapy group practices.

Internal restraining and driving forces are important. Organizational goals and values for health care in the mission statement must change with the move from hospital to home, outpatient, or community care. The physical resources, knowledge, and skills of the health-care providers must now be broadened, such as intravenous and other therapies requiring periodic skilled in-home nursing care. Extended interpersonal and interdisciplinary relations are needed with a move into the community, along with coordination of services, role relationships, attitudes, and values of people. Nursing roles of health-care provider, manager, teacher, researcher, and advocate are expanded to include service facilitator and coordinator. The organizational structure is enlarged, with agencies providing both inpatient and community services, or it becomes more flexible and interactive with other environments providing health-care services. Management is similarly broadened to include overseeing corporations, resulting in buying power, larger constituencies, and overriding governing boards. This translates into more complex goals and policies and comprehensive strategic initiatives provided by the governing board in an effort to reach out into the community.

The design for the provision of care has changed from the image of the traditional 120-bed community hospital. The external forces that drove the need for change include health-care needs of the client population, reimbursement policies, provider restrictions, and societal trends. Earlier hospital discharge and high-technology home care in the client system have driven service providers from the traditional hospital setting into the community. A good deal of this has been secondary to the reimbursement and insurance restrictions.

Organizational Change Suggestions

Organizations will continue to change and evolve in response to internal and external forces and the needs of the client system. Nurses have growing responsibility in this area. They function as members of change teams, as change agents, and as developers of organizational systems. This will continue and expand in interdisciplinary practice as their skills in change are recognized and sought. Remember the following steps regardless of the extent of the organizational change:

- *Always do your homework.* Be prepared with the information about and knowledge of the organization. Spend the time and acquire the information and background needed before acting or reacting. Then proceed from a solid theoretical base. Understand the change process and all the steps. Review your talents for change strategies.
- *Know your restraining and driving forces.* Take the time to understand or, at minimum, recognize these behaviors. Share information. Make both sides aware of the situation. Take more time to understand behavioral reactions. Cultivate the driving forces and become viewed as the champion for the cause. Use all your skills in interpersonal relationships, and develop more.
- *Be sensitive to environments.* Increase your awareness of what is occurring in society and health care. Look beyond your immediate environment. Analyze internal and external forces. Imagine how your environment could be affected by these forces. Use intuition and insight as well as foresight. Be both inspired and inspiring.
- *Maintain a positive attitude and refuse to be diminished by negativity.* Negative colleagues and superiors will always be present. They are an environmental hazard. Someone will always be readily available to tell you that something never has or never can be done. If your "homework" background knowledge told you something different, become the agent of change instead of another restraining force. Have courage.
- *Be open and receptive to new ideas.* No matter how you long to keep things as they currently are, be mindful that there may be a better way of doing things. Refuse to be limited by the present, and look to the future and evidence-based practice—a core competency. Remember, conventional wisdom can be a barrier to needed change.
- *Be open to new people.* Venture out of your discipline. View the situation as larger than nursing care. Collaborate with other health professionals. Discuss. Debate. Interact. Try to recognize when turf issues arise, and negotiate on the basis of facts and what will be best for the client system and the organization while maintaining the integrity of your profession.

- *Involve others.* Try not to do it all yourself. Remember that the most successful and enduring changes occur when others are involved. The change has to become the norm and the expectation of the people in the environment.
- *Refine skills.* Cultivate your change agent skills. Recall the skills and roles of the change agent. Continually develop and refine these skills. Make adaptations necessary for the people and the environments. Look at yourself as objectively as you look at others. If assistance or collaboration is needed, get it.
- *Reassess and evaluate.* Remember to evaluate activity and progress continually. Sufficient time for the change to occur and persistence are necessary components of organizational change. Recall Rogers' (1983) attributes in the diffusion of innovations, which determine the rate of adoption by members of a social system: relative advantage, compatibility, complexity, trialability, and observability. Include these attributes in your evaluation process.

- *Persevere, persevere, persevere.* Have fortitude. Use resources to cope with your stress and frustration levels. Organizational change is not easy. Look for small gains as major steps in the process. Strive for the finish line, but do not look for accolades. Terminate the relationship as the organizational norm takes hold and the organization congratulates *itself* on the accomplishment. Celebrate successes.

The philosophical basis of nursing focuses on the health of human beings as individuals, families, groups, and society in a complex environment. And practice must be based on the latest evidence of efficacy and acceptability. In this role, nurses can be highly effective change agents. How comfortable are you with change? Think about your **change quotient** as your ability to address needed change and to help others as a change agent.

INTERACTIVE EXERCISES

Go to the Intranet site and complete the interactive exercises provided for this Chapter.

EVIDENCED-BASED PRACTICE: CONSIDER THIS . . .

St. Pierre (2005) has shown that transforming a hospital-based journal club from a vehicle for information sharing to one with an emphasis on practice implications and action planning can have positive effects on patient care.

Question: How will you use this information and become a change agent to implement EBP?

St. Pierre, J. (2005). Changing nursing practice through a nursing journal club. *MEDSURG Nursing, 14,* 390–392.

KEY POINTS

- The classic change model was developed by Lewin (1951), based on his Field Theory. This model contained three phases in the change process: unfreezing, moving, and refreezing.

- Building on Lewin's work, Lippitt (1973) considered human motivation, multiple causation, and habits. He defined seven specific phases in the change process: diagnosis of the problem, assessment of motivation and capacity for change, change agent's motivation and resources, selecting change objectives, choosing the change agent role, maintaining the change, and terminating the relationship. A focus on the change agent emerged with four specific roles and skills.

- Havelock's change model contains the major concepts of role, linkages, and communication. This adds steps to the three stages of change, with heightened communication and interpersonal activities. Havelock and Havelock's (1973) seven steps in the change process are perception of the need, diagnosis of the problem, identification of the problem, devising a plan of action, gaining acceptance, stabilizing the plan, and self-renewal. Four different roles for the change agent are proposed in Havelock's model.

- Rogers' (1983) Diffusion of Innovations model has a five-stage view of change: knowledge, persuasion, decision, implementation, and confirmation. Rogers also considers five factors that influence the rate of adoption of an innovation and that may be used as evaluation criteria in the change process. Seven roles for the change agent are highlighted in this model of change.

(Key points continue on page 248)

K E Y   P O I N T S   (continued)

■ The Transtheoretical Approach to change focuses on the individual as a "self-changer" and is depicted as a spiral with five stages of change: precontemplation, contemplation, preparation, action, and maintenance, with 10 associated change processes that occur in the different stages of change (Prochaska et al., 1992).

■ Bridges (2003) looks at the psychological processes of change within the stages of (1) ending, losing, letting go, (2) the neutral zone, and (3) the new beginning.

■ The roles and attributes of a skilled change agent are included in the models by Lippitt, Havelock, and Rogers. General roles for the change agent are assessor or evaluator, communicator, translator, encourager, mediator, and consultant.

■ In relation to the activities in the nursing process, the phases of change are consistent with assessment, diagnosis, planning, implementation, and evaluation for resolving the problem or stabilizing the change. They can also lead to the implementation of evidence-based practice in place of traditions from the past.

■ The skills of change agents include having a vision for the future and creativity, good assessment skills, good interpersonal skills, flexibility, perseverance, and a positive attitude, integrity and commitment, the ability to manage conflict, and resistance.

■ Strategies for reducing resistance to change include careful planning and timing, along with good communication and interpersonal skills.

■ Empowerment or involvement of the client is needed for lasting change. Strategies for client involvement include education, training, socialization and persuasion, and facilitation.

■ Environmental or situational factors relative to individuals, families, and groups provide additional information in the change process. Past experience, stress and coping factors, motivational clues, and resources are important data sought by the change agent.

■ To view organizational change, look at internal and external forces with a multisystem approach. And consider the concept of transitions.

■ Suggestions for people involved in organizational change include (1) being knowledgeable about the organization, its restraining and driving forces, and the environments, (2) maintaining a positive attitude and being receptive to new ideas and people, (3) involving other people in the change, (4) continuing to refine skills and reevaluating the situation, and (5) persevering throughout the process.

Thought and Discussion Questions

1. Recall a change that has taken place in your family. Using Lewin's theory, identify the restraining and driving forces.

2. Identify some specific sources of internal change in your organization and name the driving forces.

3. Recall a change that has taken place in your organization. Using Lippitt's theory, identify the seven stages of planned change and the roles of the change agent(s) in the process.

4. List at least six specific environmental factors that could influence change in a health-care organization. Be prepared to discuss these factors in class or online, as scheduled by your instructor.

5. Use Lewin and the Transtheoretical Approach to explain the steps of the process for permanent change to help a new 18-year-old single mother with a normal 7 lb, 9 oz full-term infant (appropriate for gestational age [AGA], Apgar score of 9) develop parenting skills and health care, including prevention and health maintenance.

(Thought and Discussion Questions continue on page 249)

Thought and Discussion Questions (continued)

6. Read *Who Moved My Cheese* by S. Johnson (2002) and determine which character you most resemble and which one you most want to be like. Be prepared to participate in a discussion on your selection of characters, either online or in class as scheduled by your instructor.

7. Review the Chapter Thought located on the first page of the chapter, and discuss it in the context of the chapter.

REFERENCES

Anderson, B., Klein, E., & Stuart, J. (2000, January/February). Why change is a consciousness choice. *The Journal for Quality and Participation, 23,* 32–36.

Bridges, W. (2000). *The character of organizations: Using personality type in organization development.* Mountain View, CA: Davies-Black.

Bridges, W. (2003). *Managing transitions: Making the most of change* (2nd ed.). Cambridge, MA: DaCapo Press.

Chinn, R., & Benne, K. D. (1976). General strategies for effecting change in human systems. In W. G. Bennis, K. D. Benne, R. Chinn, & K. E. Corey (Eds.), *The planning of change* (3rd ed., pp. 22–45). New York: Holt, Rinehart & Winston.

Hall, R. H., & Tolbert, P. S. (2005). *Organizations: Structures, processes, and outcomes* (9th ed.). Upper Saddle River, NJ: Pearson Prentice-Hall.

Harvard Business Essentials (2003). *Managing change and transition.* Boston: Harvard Business School Press.

Havelock, R. G. (1971). *Planning for innovation through dissemination and utilization of knowledge.* Ann Arbor, MI: Institute for Social Research, University of Michigan.

Havelock, R. G., & Havelock, M. C. (1973). *Training for change agents: A guide to the design of training programs in education and other fields.* Ann Arbor, MI: Institute for Social Research, University of Michigan.

Johnson, S. (2002). *Who moved my cheese?* New York: G. P. Putnam's Sons.

Lewin, K. (1951). *Field theory in social science.* New York: Harper & Row.

Lippitt, G. L. (1973). *Visualizing change: Model building and the change process.* La Jolla, CA: University Associates.

Prochaska, J. O., & DiClemente, C. C. (1984). *The transtheoretical approach: Crossing traditional boundaries of therapy.* Homewood, IL: Dow Jones-Irwin.

Prochaska, J. O., DiClemente, C. C., & Norcross, J. C. (1992). In search of how people change: Applications to addictive behaviors. *American Psychologist, 47,* 1102–1114.

Rogers, E. M. (1983). *Diffusion of innovations* (3rd ed.). New York: Free Press.

Rogers, E. M., & Shoemaker, F. F. (1971). *Communication of innovations: A cross-cultural approach* (2nd ed.). New York: Free Press.

BIBLIOGRAPHY

Bandura, A. (1977). Self-efficacy: Toward a unifying theory of behavioral change. *Psychological Review, 84*(2), 191–215.

Family Drug Support. (2004). Submission to the Senate Legal and Constitutional Committee Disability Discrimination Act Amendment Bill. Testimony presented February 3, 2004. Retrieved July 16, 2006, from *http://wopared.aph.gov.au/Senate/committee/legcon_ctte/completed_inquiries/2002-04/disability/submissions/sub19.doc*

Flower, J. (1996). *The four quadrants of change.* Retrieved July 24, 2006, from *http://well.com/user/bbear/quadrant.html*

John, J. H., Yudkin, P. L., Neil, H. A. W., & Ziebland, S. (2003). Does stage of change predict outcome in a primary-care intervention to encourage an increase in fruit and vegetable consumption? *Health Education Research, 18,* 429–438.

Levesque, D. A., Prochaska, J. O., Cummins, C. O., Terrill, S., & Miranda, D. (2001). Assessing Medicare beneficiaries' readiness to make informed health plan choices. *Healthcare Financing Review, 23*(1), 87–104.

Lippitt, G. L., & Nadler, L. (1967, August). Emerging roles of the training director. *Training and Development Journal, 9,* 2–10.

ONLINE RESOURCES

William Bridges & Associates Transition Training
http://www.wmbridges.com

■ *Joseph T.* **Catalano**

Professional Ethics

> **❝** *The time is always*
> *right to do what is right.* **❞**
>
> Martin Luther King, Jr.

Chapter Objectives

On completion of this chapter, the reader will be able to:

1. Analyze and define the key terms used in ethics.
2. Distinguish between the two primary systems used in resolving ethical dilemmas.
3. Apply the steps of the ethical decision-making model.
4. Analyze and discuss the key ethical principles involved in (a) access to care, (b) organ transplantation, (c) euthanasia, (d) AIDS and HIV, (e) advance directives, (f) staffing and delegation, and (g) cloning.

Key Terms

Autonomy	Obligations	Utilitarianism
Justice	Legal Obligations	Deontology
Distributive Justice	Moral Obligations	Rule Deontology
Fidelity	Rights	Act Deontology
Beneficence	Welfare Rights	Code of Ethics
Nonmaleficence	Ethical Rights	Euthanasia
Veracity	Option Rights	Advance Directives
Standard of Best Interest	Normative Ethics	Cloning

s a registered nurse who has been in professional practice for some years, you are aware of the many changes occurring in the current health-care system. You have also likely encountered some of the difficult ethical dilemmas associated with these changes. By definition, ethical dilemmas present problems that defy a simple solution (Catalano, 2006).

For some reason, many nursing education programs presume that students are able to resolve ethical dilemmas from their past experiences and home moral training, and provide little training on professional ethics. As a result, nurses faced with difficult ethical dilemmas sometimes deal with them in several less than satisfactory ways (Salladay, 2006b). They may decide to do nothing at all, with the hope that the problem will resolve itself or someone else will solve it. If that fails, some nurses may use the "it just feels right" technique, choosing the solution that produces the least internal discomfort (Catalano, 2006).

In truth, ethical decision-making is a skill that can be learned just like inserting a catheter, starting an intravenous line, or writing a nursing diagnosis (Curtin, 2006). And as with any learned skill, the more you practice it, the more proficient you become.

ETHICAL PRINCIPLES

No two ethical dilemmas are exactly alike, but when you begin to analyze them, you will find a few key ethical principles that seem to reoccur and serve as the underpinnings for a variety of situations. At the heart of the dilemma is often a conflict between two or more of these basic principles (Davis & Aroskar, 1997). Understanding what the principle is (Box 14–1) and how it relates to the client's situation is the beginning of resolving the dilemma.

Autonomy

Autonomy is the right of self-determination, independence, and freedom. The term refers to the clients' right to make health-care decisions for themselves, even if

Box 14.1 Ethical Principles

- Autonomy
- Justice
- Fidelity
- Beneficence and Nonmaleficence
- Veracity
- Standard of Best Interest
- Obligations
- Rights

you do not agree with those decisions (DeVeaux, 2006). Autonomy, as with most rights, is not absolute, and under certain conditions, limitations can be imposed on it. Generally, these limitations occur when one individual's autonomy interferes with others' rights, health, or well-being. For example, a client can generally use his right to autonomy by refusing any or all treatments. In the case of contagious diseases that affect society, such as tuberculosis (TB), however, the individual can be forced by the health-care and legal systems to take medications to cure the disease (Aiken & Catalano, 1994). The individual can also be forced into isolation to prevent the spread of the disease.

Justice

Justice is the obligation to be fair to all people. The concept is often expanded to what is called social justice, which refers to the individual's right to be treated equally regardless of race, sex, marital status, medical diagnosis, social standing, economic level, or religious belief (Esterhuizen, 2006). The principle of justice underlies the first statement in the American Nurses Association (ANA) *Code for Nurses*: "The nurse in all professional relationships practices with compassion and respect for the inherent dignity, worth and the uniqueness of every individual unrestricted by considerations of social or economic status, personal attributes, or the nature of health problems" (American Nurses Association, 2001). **Distributive justice** sometimes includes ideas such as equal access to health care for all citizens. As with other rights, limits can be placed on justice when it interferes with the rights of others.

Fidelity

Fidelity is the obligation to be faithful to commitments made to yourself and others. In health care, fidelity includes your faithfulness or loyalty to agreements and responsibilities accepted as part of the practice of the profession. Fidelity is the main support for the concept of accountability, although conflicts in fidelity might arise from obligations to different individuals or groups. For example, a nurse who is just finishing a very busy and tiring 12-hour shift may experience a conflict of fidelity when she is asked by a supervisor to work an additional shift because the unit is understaffed. The nurse would have to weigh her fidelity to herself against fidelity to the employing institution and fidelity to the profession and clients to do the best job possible, particularly if she felt that her fatigue would interfere with the performance of those obligations.

Beneficence and Nonmaleficence

Beneficence is a very old requirement for health-care providers. It views the primary goal of health care as doing good for clients under the care of those providers (Catalano, 2006). In general, the term *good* means more than just technically competent care for clients. Good care requires a holistic approach to the client, including her beliefs, feelings, and wishes as well as those of the family and significant others. The main problem you will encounter in implementing the principle of beneficence is determining exactly what is good for another and who can best make the decision about this good.

Nonmaleficence requires that health-care providers do no harm to their clients, either intentionally or unintentionally. In a sense, it is the reverse side of beneficence, and it is difficult to speak of one concept without the other. In current health-care practice, the principle of nonmaleficence is often violated in the short term to produce a greater good in the long-term treatment of the client. For example, a client may undergo a very painful and debilitating operation to remove a cancerous growth that will prolong her life in the long term.

By extension, the principle of nonmaleficence also requires you to protect from harm those who cannot protect themselves. This protection from harm is particularly important in such groups as children, the mentally incompetent, the unconscious, the elderly, and others who may be too weak or debilitated to protect themselves. For example, there are strict regulations in cases of experimentation with groups such as the mentally handicapped, children, and prisoners.

Veracity

Veracity is the principle of "truthfulness." It requires you to tell the truth and not to intentionally deceive or mislead clients. As with other rights and obligations, there are limitations to this principle. The primary limitation is when telling the client the truth would seriously harm (principle of nonmaleficence) his ability to recover or would produce greater illness. You may often feel uncomfortable giving clients "bad news" and may prefer to avoid answering their questions truthfully. Feeling uncomfortable is not a good enough reason to avoid telling clients the truth about their diagnosis, treatments, or prognosis. Clients have a right to know this information (Collis, 2006).

Best Interest

The **standard of best interest** involves decisions made about clients' health care when they are unable to make informed decisions about their own care. The standard of best interest is based on what the health-care providers and the family decide is best for that individual (Rehnsfeldt, 2005). It is very important that you consider the individual's expressed wishes, either formally in a written declaration (such as a living will)

or informally in what may have been said to family members.

The standard of best interest should be based on the principle of beneficence. Unfortunately, in situations in which clients are unable to make decisions for themselves, the dilemma may be resolved by a unilateral decision made by the health-care providers. Unilateral decisions that disregard the clients' wishes, implying that the health-care providers alone know what is best, are examples of paternalism.

Obligations

Obligations are demands made on individuals, professions, society, or government to fulfill and honor the rights of others. **Obligations** are often divided into two categories:

- **Legal obligations** are those that have become formal statements of law and are enforceable under the law. For example, you have a legal obligation to provide safe and adequate care for clients to whom you are assigned.
- **Moral obligations** are based on moral or ethical principles but are not enforceable under the law. For example, you are on vacation and encounter an automobile collision; in many places you may have no legal obligation, but as a nurse you have a strong moral obligation to stop and help the victims.

Rights

Rights are generally defined as something due to an individual according to just claims, legal guarantees, or moral and ethical principles. Although the term *right* is frequently used in both the legal and ethical systems, its meaning is often blurred in everyday usage. Individuals tend to claim things as "rights" that are really privileges, concessions, or freedoms. Several classification systems for rights delineate different types of rights. The following three types of rights are included in most of these systems:

- **Welfare rights** (also called *legal rights*) are based on a legal entitlement to some good or benefit. These rights are guaranteed by laws (such as the Bill of Rights) and their violation can come under the power of the legal system. For example, citizens of the United States have a right to equal access to employment regardless of race, sex, or religion.
- **Ethical rights** (also called *moral rights*) are based on a moral or ethical principle. Ethical rights usually do not have the power of law to be enforced. Ethical rights are, in reality, often privileges allotted to certain individuals or groups of individuals. For example, in the United States and South Africa, the right to health

care is really a long-standing privilege, whereas in many other industrialized countries, it is a legal right.

- **Option rights** are based on a fundamental belief in the dignity and freedom of human beings. Option rights are particularly evident in free and democratic countries, such as the United States, and much less evident in totalitarian and restrictive societies, such as North Korea. Option rights give individuals freedom of choice and the right to live their lives as they choose, but within a set of prescribed boundaries. For example, in the United States, you may wear whatever clothes you choose, as long as you do wear some type of clothing.

TWO ETHICAL SYSTEMS

Every time you interact with a client in a health-care setting, an ethical situation exists. You may not realize it, but you are continually making ethical decisions in your daily practice. This process is known as **normative ethics**. Normative ethical decisions deal with questions and dilemmas requiring a choice of actions in which the rights or obligations of the nurse and the client, the nurse and the client's family, or the nurse and the physician conflict. In resolving these ethical questions, you are probably using one of two, or perhaps a combination of two or more, ethical systems.

The two fundamental systems most used in ethical decision-making related to health care are utilitarianism and deontology (Catalano, 2006). Both systems apply to bioethics—the ethics of life (or death, in some cases). *Bioethics* and *bioethical issues* are terms that are in common use and that have become synonymous with health-care ethics, including questions not only of life and death but also of quality of life, life-sustaining and life-altering technologies, and bioscience in general (Mathes, 2005). The following discussion of these two ethical systems is undertaken in the context of bioethics.

Utilitarianism

Utilitarianism (also called *teleology*, *consequentialism*, and *situation ethics*) is defined as the ethical system of utility. As a system of normative ethics, utilitarianism defines "good" as happiness or pleasure. It is based on two underlying principles: "the greatest good for the greatest number" and "the ends justify the means." On the basis of these two principles, utilitarianism is sometimes subdivided into rule utilitarianism and act utilitarianism. According to rule utilitarianism, you draw on your past experiences to formulate internal rules that are useful in determining the greatest good. With act utilitarianism, the particular situation

that you find yourself in determines the rightness or wrongness of a particular act. In practice, the true follower of utilitarianism does not believe in the validity of any system of rules, because the rules change according to the circumstances surrounding the decision to be made (Aiken, 2003).

Situation ethics is probably the most publicized form of act utilitarianism. Joseph Fletcher, one of the best-known proponents of act utilitarianism, outlines a method of ethical thinking in which the situation determines whether the act is morally right or wrong. Fletcher views acts as good to the extent that they promote happiness and as wrong to the degree that they promote unhappiness. He defines *happiness* as the happiness of the greatest number of people, but the happiness of each person has equal weight (Fletcher, 1966). For example, abortion is considered ethical in this system in a situation in which an unwed welfare mother with four other children becomes pregnant with her fifth child. The greatest good and the greatest amount of happiness may be produced by aborting this unwanted child, for whom this mother cannot provide adequate food or care.

On the basis of the concept that moral rules should not be arbitrary but should serve a purpose, ethical decisions derived from a utilitarian framework weigh the effect of alternative actions that influence the overall welfare of present and future populations. As such, this system is oriented toward the good of the population in general, and the individual as he participates in that population.

Advantages

The major advantage of the utilitarian system of ethical decision-making is that many individuals find it easy to use in most situations. Utilitarianism is built around an individual's own happiness needs, of which she has an immediate and vested knowledge. Another advantage is that utilitarianism fits well into a society that shuns rules and regulations. The follower of utilitarianism can justify many decisions on the basis of the "happiness" principle. Its utility orientation also fits well into Western society's belief in the work ethic and the behavioristic approach to education, philosophy, and life.

For example, the follower of utilitarianism holds to a general prohibition against lying and deceiving because, ultimately, telling the truth will lead to more happiness than lying. Yet truth telling is not an absolute requirement to the follower of utilitarianism. If telling the truth would produce widespread unhappiness for a great number of people and future generations, then it would be better ethically to tell a lie. Although such behavior might appear to be unethical at first glance, the follower of strict act utilitarianism would have little difficulty in arriving at this decision as logical.

Disadvantages

Utilitarianism has some serious limitations as a system of health-care ethics or bioethics. An immediate question arises as to whether "happiness" refers to the average happiness of all or the total happiness of a few. Because individual happiness is also important, you must consider how to make decisions when the individual's happiness conflicts with the larger group's happiness. More fundamental is the question of what constitutes "happiness." Similarly, what constitutes the "greatest good for the greatest number?" Who determines what is "good" in the first place? Is it society in general? The government? Governmental policy? The individual? In health-care delivery and the formulation of health-care policy, the general guiding principle often seems to be the greatest good for the greatest number. Yet where do minority groups, such as African Americans and Native Americans, fit into this system?

The "ends justify the means" principle has also been rejected historically as a method of justifying actions. It is generally unacceptable to allow any type of action to go forward in the hopes that the final goal or purpose is good. The Nazis used this aphorism to justify a variety of actions that were not "good."

The other difficulty with this system is in quantifying such concepts as good, harm, benefits, and greatest. This problem becomes especially acute in dealing with health-care issues that involve individuals' lives. For example, an elderly woman has been sick for a long time, and that illness has placed great financial hardship on her family. It would be ethical under utilitarianism to allow this client to die, or even to euthanize her, to relieve the financial stress created by her illness.

The use of utilitarianism as an ethical system in health-care decision-making requires the additional principle of distributive justice—such as equal access to care—as an ultimate guiding point. Nonetheless, whenever you combine an unchanging principle with this system, you negate the basic concept of pure utilitarianism. Pure utilitarianism, although easy to use as a general decision-making system, does not always work well as an ethical decision-making system in health care because of its arbitrary, self-centered nature. In the everyday delivery of health care, utilitarianism is often combined with other types of ethical decision-making to resolve ethical dilemmas.

Deontology

Deontology is a system of ethical decision-making based on moral rules and unchanging principles. This system is also called the *formalistic system*, the *principle system of ethics*, and *duty-based ethics*. A follower of a pure deontologic system of ethical decision-making believes in the ethical absoluteness of principles, regardless of the consequences of the decisions based on them. This strict adherence to an ethical theory, in which the moral rightness or wrongness of human actions is considered separately from the consequences, is based on a fundamental principle called the *categorical imperative*. It is not the results of the act that make it right or wrong, but the principles on which the act is based. These fundamental principles are ultimately unchanging and absolute and are derived from the universal values that underlie all major religions. The concern for right and wrong in the moral sense is the basic premise of the species and social cooperation. The deontologic system is also divided into rule deontology and act deontology.

Rule deontology is based on the belief that there are standards for the ethical choices and judgments made by individuals. These standards are fixed and do not change when the situation changes. The number of standards or rules is potentially unlimited, but in reality, and particularly when one is dealing with bioethical issues, many of these principles can be grouped together into a few general or "cover" principles. These principles can also be arranged into a type of hierarchy of rules, including such maxims as "Persons should always be treated as ends and never as means," "Human life has value," "One is always to tell the truth," "Above all in health care do no harm," "The human person has a right to self-determination," and "All persons are of equal value." These principles echo such fundamental documents as the Bill of Rights and the Hospital Patient's Bill of Rights (American College of Physicians, 1998).

Act deontology places the highest value on the moral values of the individual. It requires that you make the same decision in any similar situation, regardless of time, place, individuals involved, and external circumstances. Act deontology does not depend on unchanging external rules as rule deontology does. Rather, you obtain all the data you can about the dilemma, and then make the decision. The decision (act) makes it correct simply because it was made. For example, a community health nurse working in a prenatal clinic believes that birth control methods are moral and therefore gives birth control information and pills to a sexually active teenager. The nurse would also give the same types of information to the next sexually active teenager who came into the clinic for care, without regard to the teenager's beliefs or background.

Advantages

Rule deontology is useful in making ethical decisions in health care because it holds that an ethical judgment you make is based on principles that will be the same in a variety of similar situations, regardless of time, location, and the particular individuals involved. In addition, deontologic terminology and concepts are similar to the terms and concepts used by the legal system. The legal system also stresses rights and duties, principles, and rules. But there are significant differences between the two. Legal rights and duties are enforceable under the law, whereas ethical rights and duties usually are not. In general, ethical systems are much wider and more inclusive than the system of laws they underlie.

Disadvantages

The deontologic system of ethical decision-making is not perfect. Some of the more troubling questions are: "What do you do when the basic guiding principles conflict with each other?" "What is the source of the principles?" and "Is there ever a situation in which an exception to the rule applies?"

Although various approaches have been proposed to circumvent these limitations, it may be difficult for nurses to resolve situations in which duties and obligations conflict, particularly when the consequences of following a rule end in harm to a client. In reality, there are probably few followers of pure deontology, because most people consider the consequences of their actions in their decision-making.

Act deontology negates the underlying philosophy of the deontologic system requiring unchanging external rules, because you must obtain all the data you can about the dilemma, and then make the decision. This approach is difficult to use in resolving ethical dilemmas because of its lack of rules. It requires you to judge each situation individually and arrive at the same decision in similar cases. You may not have the time or energy to analyze each situation you encounter thoroughly in providing care to clients.

APPLYING ETHICAL THEORIES

Ethical theories do not provide cookbook solutions for resolving ethical dilemmas. Instead, they give you a framework for decision-making, which you can apply to individual ethical situations. At times, you may find ethical theories too abstract or general to be of much use in specific ethical situations. Without them, however, ethical decision-making often becomes an exercise in personal emotions. Many nurses attempting to make ethical decisions use elements from both of the two theories, as presented here.

The Decision-Making Model in Ethics

Nurses, by definition, are problem-solvers, and one of the important tools regularly used in problem-solving is the nursing process. The nursing process is, if nothing else, a systematic, step-by-step approach to resolving problems that deal with a client's health and well-being.

Although you routinely deal with problems related to the physical or psychological needs of clients, you may feel inadequate when dealing with their ethical problems. No matter what the health-care setting, however, you can develop the decision-making skills necessary to make sound ethical decisions if you learn and practice using an ethical decision-making model.

An ethical decision-making model provides a method for answering key questions about ethical dilemmas and organizing your thinking more logically and sequentially. Although several ethical decision-making models exist, the problem-solving method presented here is based on the nursing process. It should be a relatively easy transition for you to move from the nursing process used in resolving clients' physical problems to the ethical decision-making model to resolve ethical problems.

> Nurses, by definition, are problem-solvers, and one of the important tools regularly used in problem-solving is the nursing process

The chief goal of the ethical decision-making model is to determine right from wrong in situations with no clear or readily apparent demarcations. This process presupposes that a system of ethics exists, that you know what the basic ethical principles are, and that the system applies to similar ethical decision-making problems despite multiple variables. At some point, you need to undertake the task of clarifying your own values, if you have not done it already (Fig. 14–1). You also need an understanding of the possible ethical systems that may be used in making decisions about ethical dilemmas (Catalano, 2006).

The following five-step ethical decision-making model is presented as a tool for resolving ethical dilemmas (Box 14–2).

Step 1: Collect, Analyze, and Interpret the Data

Obtain as much information as possible concerning the particular ethical dilemma you are facing. Among the

---

Box 14.2 *Steps of Ethical Decision-Making*

1. Collect, analyze, and interpret the data.
2. State the dilemma.
3. Consider the choices of action.
4. Analyze the advantages and disadvantages of each course of action.
5. Make the decision.

PART I — Rank the following from 1 to 5, with 1 being the item with the highest priority and 5 being the item with lowest priority.

A. A hospital must cut back its budget or go bankrupt. Which of the following clients should be given priority for care?
_____ A newborn with multiple birth defects who is likely to be retarded for life.
_____ A 47-year-old male scientist with an acute MI who has just discovered a new medication that might cure HIV.
_____ An 88-year-old retired female grade-school teacher who was recently diagnosed with liver cancer.
_____ A 17-year-old runaway who is addicted to cocaine and is pregnant.
_____ A 58-year-old construction worker who has severe emphysema due to his 2¹/₂-pack-a-day smoking habit.

B. The nurse assigned to a client who has a bleeding ulcer secondary to stress. Which aspects of his care would receive highest priority?
_____ Give him pain medications to make him comfortable.
_____ Explain the relationship between stress and ulcers.
_____ Involve him as much as possible in his self-care.
_____ Encourage him to talk about his job and family, etc.
_____ **Teach him about diet and medication to control ulcers.**

PART II — Rate the following statements on a scale of 1 to 5.
(1 = strongly support; 2 = support; 3 = no opinion; 4 = reject; 5 = strongly reject).
_____ 1. Abortion is always wrong, no matter what the circumstances.
_____ 2. People who receive the death penalty, deserve it.
_____ 3. Life support should be terminated for clients when they are not likely to live.
_____ 4. Street drugs should be made legal.
_____ 5. Prisoners, genetically defective, mentally retarded persons should be sterilized.
_____ 6. Premature, drug-addicted newborns should be allowed to die.
_____ 7. Condoms should be given out in high schools to prevent pregnancy and HIV.
_____ 8. All hospitalized clients should be routinely screened for HIV and AIDS.
_____ 9. Scientists should be allowed to use aborted fetuses for fetal tissue research.
_____ 10. All newborn infants should be genetically screened for inherited diseases.

PART III — Complete the following sentences.

1. The one thing I have always wanted to do is _____
2. If I just inherited 5 million dollars, I would _____
3. As president of the United States, I would _____
4. If I died today, I would like my obituary to say _____
5. If I could control the world and its destiny, I would _____

PART IV — Below is a partial list of things people value. Complete the list, then rank each item from 1(highest value) to ? being the lowest value.

___ family _____
___ career _____
___ religion _____
___ honor _____
___ material possessions _____
___ health _____
___ recreation _____
___ professionalism _____

■ **Figure 14.1** Values clarification tool.

issues important for you to know are the client's wishes, the family's wishes, the extent of the physical or emotional problems causing the dilemma, the physician's beliefs about health care, and your own orientation to life-and-death issues.

For example, many nurses must deal with the question of whether or not to initiate resuscitation efforts when a terminally ill client is admitted to the hospital. Physicians often leave verbal instructions indicating that you really should not resuscitate the client but merely go through the motions to make the family feel better. Your dilemma becomes whether to attempt seriously to revive the client or to let her die quietly.

Important information that would help you make the best decision includes the mental competency of the client to make a no-resuscitation decision, the client's desires, the family's feelings, and whether the physician sought input from the client and family before leaving the orders. Many institutions have policies concerning no-resuscitation orders, and you should consider these in the data collection stage.

After collecting as much information as possible, you need to bring the pieces of information together into a form that will give the dilemma the clearest and sharpest focus.

Step 2: State the Dilemma

After you have collected and analyzed all the available information, you need to state the dilemma as clearly and succinctly as possible. Recognizing the key aspects of the dilemma helps focus your attention on the important ethical principles. Most of the time, the dilemma can be reduced to a statement or two revolving around key ethical principles. These dilemmas often involve a question of conflicting rights, obligations, or basic ethical principles.

In the question of slow resuscitation versus no resuscitation, the dilemma might be stated as "The client's right to self-determination and death with dignity versus the nurse's obligation to preserve life and do no harm." In general, the principle that the competent client's wishes must be followed is unequivocal. If the client has become unresponsive before expressing his wishes, then the family members' input must be given serious consideration. Additional questions can arise if the family's wishes conflict with those of the client.

Step 3: Consider the Choices of Action

After you have stated the dilemma as clearly as possible, you should attempt to list, without consideration of their consequences, all the possible courses of action that you can take to resolve the dilemma. This brainstorming activity, in which you consider all possible courses of action, may require input from outside sources such as colleagues, supervisors, and even experts in the ethical field. The consequences of the different actions are considered later.

Some of the possible courses of action to consider in the resuscitation example are:

- Resuscitating the client to your fullest capabilities, despite what the physician has requested
- Not resuscitating the client at all, just going through the motions without any real attempt to revive the client
- Seeking another assignment to avoid dealing with the situation
- Reporting the problem to a supervisor

- Attempting to clarify the question with the client
- Attempting to clarify the question with the family
- Confronting the physician about the question

Step 4: Analyze the Advantages and Disadvantages of Each Course of Action

Some of the courses of actions you developed in the previous step are more realistic than others. The unrealistic actions become readily evident during this step in the decision-making process, when you consider the advantages and the disadvantages of each action in detail. Along with each option, you must consider the consequences of taking each course of action. You should evaluate the advantages and disadvantages of the consequences thoroughly.

For example, you should consider whether initiating discussion about the order would anger the physician or cause her to distrust you in the future. Either of these responses might make practicing at that institution difficult. The result might be the same if you successfully resuscitate the client despite orders to the contrary. Not resuscitating the client has the potential to involve you in a lawsuit if no clear order for no resuscitation exists. Presenting the situation to a supervisor may, if the supervisor supports the physician, cause you to be labeled a troublemaker and may have a negative effect on your future evaluations. The same process can be applied to the other possible courses of action.

By thoroughly considering the advantages and disadvantages of each possible action, you should be able to deduce your realistic choices of action. An important factor to include in your deliberations is the ANA's *Code for Nurses* (2001).

Step 5: Make the Decision

The most difficult part of the process is actually making the decision and living with the consequences. By their nature, ethical dilemmas produce differences of opinion, and not everyone will be pleased with your decision.

In the attempt to solve any ethical dilemma, there is always a question of the correct course of action. The client's wishes almost always supersede independent decisions you might make. Collaborative decision-making about resuscitation that involves the client, physician, nurses, and family is the ideal solution and tends to produce fewer complications in the long-term resolution of such questions.

NURSING CODE OF ETHICS

A **code of ethics** is generally defined as the ethical principles that govern a particular profession. Codes of ethics are presented in general statements and do not give specific answers to every possible ethical dilemma that might arise. These codes do, however, offer you guidance in your ethical decisions (see Box 1–2).

Ideally, codes of ethics should undergo periodic revision to reflect changes in the profession and society as a whole. Although codes of ethics are not legally enforceable as laws, consistently violating the code of ethics is taken as an indication of an unwillingness to act in a professional manner and often results in disciplinary actions, ranging from reprimands and fines to suspension and revocation of licensure (Salladay, 2006a).

The ANA Code for Nurses has been acknowledged by other health-care professions as one of the most complete ethical codes. It is sometimes used as the benchmark against which other codes of ethics are measured. Yet a careful reading of this code of ethics reveals only a set of clearly stated principles that you must apply to actual clinical situations. For example, if you are involved in the resuscitation situation described earlier, you will find no specific mention of "no resuscitation" orders. Rather, you must apply general statements, such as "The nurse provides services with respect for human dignity" and "The nurse assumes responsibility and accountability for individual nursing judgments, and actions," to the particular situation.

COMMON ETHICAL DILEMMAS IN NURSING

Although the potential ethical dilemmas you might face in your career are almost unlimited, you are likely to encounter certain issues in your practice. A complete analysis of each of these issues is beyond the scope of this book, but the important ethical features are presented so that you will be able to analyze the dilemma and make an informed decision. Resolving ethical dilemmas is never an easy task, and it is likely that you will displease someone with your decision, no matter how carefully and thoughtfully you have made it.

Access to Care

Although access to health care has been a concern in the United States for many years, it is only with recent proposed changes in the health-care system that it has been pushed into the headlines as an important ethical and social issue. In today's health-care system, some individuals obtain the best care that medicine and technology can provide, whereas others can neither afford to see a physician nor purchase the medications that are prescribed. The underlying ethical principle involved in access to care is that of justice, particularly distributive justice. The basic question is whether health care is a

universal right to be allotted to all citizens, or a privilege limited to those who can pay for it.

On the surface, the current health-care system seems to be based on the belief that health care is a privilege. Yet the government recognizes the needs of some of those who cannot afford health care, such as the elderly, poor, and disabled, and subsidizes their health care through a variety of programs, such as Medicaid. The end result is that the United States spends more on health care than any country in the world, with most of that money coming from the pockets of taxpayers.

Those who support universal access and health care as a basic right of every citizen are faced with the specter of health-care rationing, however. The reality of the situation is that if universal access becomes the law of the land, some form of restricted access to services will be likely to control the flow of money. A system of universal access to health care in the United States means that some health-care goods must be rationed.

Ideally, under the ethical principle of distributive justice, everybody should have open access to every type of health care. Because that type of access is unrealistic, a decision must be made about what health-care services will be restricted to which groups of individuals. All of the current proposals for universal coverage would limit those health-care services that generally fall into the tertiary category—highly specialized diagnostic and treatment regimens, organ and tissue transplantation, and procedures that merely prolong life temporarily.

The group that is most often targeted for rationing of health care is the elderly, because they are a rapidly growing, easily identified group that has high health-care costs. The cost of health-care for the elderly in the last year of their life has amounted to one percent of the total gross national product (GNP) each year since 1984 (Tschudin, 2006). Also, the traditional role of the elderly in society is to care for the young and future generation, not to absorb a large portion of their heritage in the form of expensive resources.

Nevertheless, there is a strong prohibition in this country against using age alone as a criterion for restriction of services. Allocation of health-care services based on need seems to be a more equitable way to arrive at the decision. It would make more sense to restrict the use of expensive technologies by all age groups rather than all sources for the elderly only. The elderly have also contributed a great deal to this country over the years, compared with the younger members of society, and it seems only fair that they receive the care they have earned. Many nurses find it difficult to reconcile their personal and professional codes of ethics with limiting resources for just one group, such as the elderly. It is unlikely that professional groups, such as nurses, would abide by a policy that restricted care to the elderly.

What is the solution to this dilemma? As with most ethical dilemmas, there is no perfect solution, yet nurses can contribute a great deal to resolving this question. Underlying any resolution to the access-to-care problem is the requirement for a fundamental shift in attitude and philosophy about health care. No longer can curing disease and extending life be the primary focuses of health care. Rather, the health-care system needs to adopt caring as a central goal of health care. Nurses understand caring as a mode of treatment. Physicians and other health-care providers can learn it. Caring will refocus the goals of health care toward a more equitable and rational use of health-care resources.

Organ Transplantation

Despite the widespread public and medical acceptance of organ transplantation as a highly beneficial procedure, ethical questions remain. Whenever a human organ is transplanted, a large number of people are involved, including the donor, the donor's family, medical and nursing personnel, the recipient, and the recipient's family. Society in general could also be added to this mix, because of the high cost of organ transplantation, which is usually borne directly by tax monies or indirectly in the form of increased insurance premiums. Each one of these people or groups has rights that may conflict with the rights of the others.

Most institutions that perform transplants, or organizations that are involved in obtaining organs, have developed elaborate, detailed, and involved procedures to help deal with the ethical and legal issues involved in transplantation (McKenney, 2003). Despite these efforts, some ethical issues still arise whenever organ transplantation is considered. Consider the ethical principles involved, such as autonomy, justice, beneficence, and standard of best interest.

One particularly sensitive issue arises when a child is involved. Although parents are legally permitted to give consent for medical procedures for their children, the child must also have some input in the decision, particularly if the procedure poses a risk to her life, such as a kidney transplantation. By legal definition, a child younger than the age of 18 years cannot give informed consent to such a procedure. Yet it seems unethical to coerce the child into donating a kidney if she really does not want to do it. In the case of children, it is important to obtain both parental consent and informed assent, in which the child is aware of decisions and involved in the process.

Despite the best efforts of the medical and legal community to establish criteria for death, ethical questions about when a person is really dead remain (Daly, 2006). Does brain death, the most widely accepted criterion for death, really indicate that a person no longer exists as a human being? Or is there some other criterion that should be examined? Such organs as heart, lungs, and liver must come from a donor whose heart is still beating. Might there be a tendency therefore to declare brain death before it actually occurs?

One of the most difficult ethical issues involved in organ transplantation is the selection of recipients. The number of people who need organs far exceeds the number of available organs. Many potential ethical dilemmas arise from this fact. Should someone receive an organ because he is rich or famous or knows the right people? The national organ recipient list attempts to list and rank all persons who need organs in a nondiscriminatory manner. Some of the important criteria are need, length of time on the list, potential for survival, prior organ transplantation, value to the community, and tissue compatibility.

Nurses can be, and often are, involved in some aspects of the organ donation process. Many states have passed laws requiring that health-care workers ask the family members of potential organ donors whether they have ever thought about organ donation for their dead or dying loved one. Many nurses, particularly those in critical care units, provide care for clients who are potential organ donors. Nurses in operating rooms may help in the actual surgical procedures that remove organs from a cadaver and transplant them into a recipient's body. Many floor nurses provide the postoperative care for clients who have received a transplanted organ. Home health-care nurses give follow-up care to these clients at home.

Nurses working with organ transplantation must be sensitive to the potential for manipulation. Most people who are seeking organ transplantation are desperately ill or near death. They and their families can be either very easily manipulated or very manipulative. On the other side, the families of potential organ donors are usually emotionally distraught as a result of the sudden and traumatic loss of a loved one. They, too, are vulnerable to manipulation. As a general rule, neither the donor nor his family should play any part in selecting a recipient. Nurses must avoid making statements or giving nonverbal indications of their approval or disapproval of potential recipients. For example, a statement such as "I hope the teenager gets the kidney rather than the old lady" may prejudice the whole process.

Euthanasia

The term **euthanasia** generally means a painless or peaceful death. A distinction is often made between passive and active euthanasia. *Passive euthanasia* usually refers to the practice of allowing an individual to die without any extraordinary intervention. Such practices as do not resuscitate (DNR) orders, living wills, and withdrawal of ventilators or other life support are usually included under this umbrella definition (Edwards, 2006). *Active euthanasia*, in contrast, describes the practice of speeding an individual's death through some act or procedure. This practice, also sometimes referred to as *mercy killing*, takes many forms, ranging from using large amounts of pain medication for terminal cancer clients to using poisons, carbon monoxide, guns, or knives to end a person's life.

Assisted suicide, brought to public attention by Dr. Kevorkian, a Michigan physician, is really a type of active euthanasia or mercy killing (Catalano, 2006). The central issue that has been pushed to the fore by Dr. Kevorkian's public practice of assisted suicide is whether or not it is ever ethically permissible for health-care personnel to assist in taking a life. In all states but one the practice is illegal. The definition of *homicide*—bringing about a person's death or assisting him to do so—seems to fit the act of assisted suicide. Yet there is a great deal of hesitation on the part of the legal system to prosecute persons who are involved in assisted suicide for terminally ill clients.

The fundamental ethical issue is the right to autonomy or self-determination (Catalano, 2006; Johnstone, 2006). In almost every other health-care situation, a client, as long as he is competent, can make decisions about what care is acceptable and what care he will refuse. Yet when it comes to the termination of life, this right no longer seems to apply. Supporters of the practice of assisted suicide hold to the belief that the right to self-determination remains intact even in the decision to end life. It is the last act of a very sick individual to control his own fate. Medical personnel, many believe, should be allowed to assist these clients in this procedure, just as they are allowed to assist clients in other medical and nursing procedures.

Those who oppose assisted suicide find these arguments lacking in ethical principle. Legally, ethically, and morally, suicide in American society has never been accepted. Health-care staff go to great lengths to prevent clients from injuring themselves when they are

identified as suicidal. In addition, it would seem that individuals in the terminal states of a disease who are overwhelmed by pain, and depressed by the thought of prolonged suffering, might not be able to think clearly enough to give informed consent for assisted suicide. Also, the termination of life is final. It does not allow for spontaneous cures or the development of new treatments or medications.

Although nurses are unlikely to be employed in assisted-suicide clinics, the reality of active euthanasia has been and will continue to be part of modern-day health care. Nurses need to remember the principle of nonmaleficence. There is a very strong obligation to do no harm to clients. Assisting in or causing the death of a client would seem to be an obvious violation of this principle.

HIV and AIDS

Few diseases have the power to raise the strong opinions that human immunodeficiency virus (HIV) and acquired immunodeficiency syndrome (AIDS) do. Nurses who for years held strongly to the ethical principle that all clients regardless of race, sex, religion, age, or disease process should be cared for equally, now question their obligation to take care of clients with AIDS (Bruton, 2005).

Several ethical issues underlie the AIDS issue. One of the most important is the right to privacy. Some people believe that this issue has been carried to extremes. Many diseases that are highly contagious and sometimes fatal—TB, gonorrhea, syphilis, and hepatitis—must be reported to public health officials. Although there is a general requirement to report infection with HIV or AIDS to the Centers for Disease Control and Prevention (CDC), many states have strict laws regarding the confidentiality of the diagnosis (Simpson, 2006). Revealing the diagnosis of HIV or AIDS even to other health-care personnel brings the possibility of a lawsuit against the health-care provider or institution. It is important to remember that the right to privacy is not an absolute right. If the right to privacy can be violated when the public welfare is threatened by such diseases as TB, syphilis, and gonorrhea, is it not logical to include AIDS in this group? Is it unjust to ask health-care providers to care for clients with this disease without knowing that the clients have it? A parallel question involves the client's right to know when a health-care provider is infected with HIV or AIDS.

Another important ethical issue is the right to care. May a nurse refuse to care for a client with a highly contagious and potentially lethal disease, such as HIV, hepatitis B, or medication-resistant TB? Obviously, a fundamental right of being a client is receiving care, just as a fundamental obligation of a nurse is to provide care. The first statement of the ANA *Code for Nurses*

ONLINE CONSULT

In 1997, Oregon enacted the *Death with Dignity Act*, which legalizes physician-assisted suicide through voluntary self-administration of lethal medications but prohibits euthanasia, in which another person directly administers a medication to end an individual's life. Find more at
http://www.ohd.hr.state.or.us/chs/pas/pas.cfm

states that a nurse must provide care unrestricted by any considerations. There may be some exceptions; for example, if the nurse were pregnant, or receiving chemotherapy, or had other immunity problems, she might be able to refuse an assignment because of safety considerations. But in most situations, the nurse would be obligated to provide the best nursing care possible for all clients, including those with dangerous diseases.

What about the issue of justice, in light of the tremendous cost involved in treating individuals with AIDS? Studies estimate that the medical cost of treating clients with AIDS from the time of diagnosis to the time of death is in the neighborhood of $900,000 per client. In the face of this crisis, governmental agencies that bear the brunt of the cost of AIDS treatment will have to make some hard decisions. With more than 1 million people already infected with this disease, the cost to society is astronomical.

Advance Directives

Advance directives have been used in health care for a number of years. Originally developed as a means for clients to express their wishes about the type and amount of health care they desired if they became unable to make decisions at a future date (right to self-determination), advance directives are now a required part of the health care of all clients. Under the Omnibus Budget Reconciliation Act of 1990, all hospitals, nursing care facilities, home-care agencies, and care providers are required by law to ask clients about advance directives and provide information about them if so desired (Catalano, 2006).

Advance directives can take the form of living wills and medical durable power of attorney (MDPOA). A *living will* is defined as a directive from a competent individual to medical personnel and family members regarding the treatment he is to receive when he is no longer able to make decisions (Briggs, 2002). This directive is ideally in the form of a written document, but it may also take the form of verbal directions to a health-care provider that are documented in the client's health-care record. No standard form is accepted by all states. Some living wills are very specific as to the treatments that can and cannot be used, but other forms provide only general directions, such as "no extraordinary measures."

As a nurse, you can play an important part in identifying potential problems in a client's living will. If a client has already written a living will, you need to make sure it is signed and witnessed properly or notarized. Generally, health-care providers and the client's family members are excluded from witnessing a living will. In addition, if the living will is more than two years old, you should encourage the client to review it and update it if needed. Also, see how clear and detailed the statements are about which treatments are to be used or excluded. Often clients do not understand such modes of treatment as intubation, ventilation, defibrillation, medication administration, and resuscitation. Explain any new modes of treatment that may have been developed since the client first composed the living will. Finally, encourage the client to give copies of the document to his next of kin, primary physician, and attorney. Some states even allow the client to register a living will with certain agencies in the state, such as with the secretary of state (Catalano, 2006).

Although the use of the living will seems to be a relatively simple way to resolve a complicated situation in health care, be aware of a number of ethical pitfalls. One of the most common ethical questions revolves around the client's level of knowledge of potential and future health-care problems he may encounter. Living wills are often composed while the client is in a relatively positive state of health and may be directed toward only a few "common" problems with which he is familiar. For example, the client may anticipate a myocardial infarction (MI) and give specific directions for treatments to be excluded in this condition, such as "no CPR" or "no defibrillation." Suppose the client is in an automobile collision, has a crushed chest, and needs to be connected to a ventilator for proper healing of the ribs. If he is unconscious and cannot give directions to the health-care team, should they not intubate him and attach him to the ventilator because of his living will? Did he really intend to exclude this situation? In general, if there is any indication that the client did not fully understand the implications or use of possible therapies, the validity of the whole living will is in question and can probably be disregarded.

Nurses working with clients who have a living will sometimes encounter ethical questions concerning the principles of beneficence and nonmaleficence. As defined earlier, the principle of beneficence states that your primary duty as a nurse is to do good for the client, and the principle of nonmaleficence requires you to protect the client from any harm. From the perspectives of beneficence and nonmaleficence, you may believe that following a client's living will violates these principles. Some nurses are ethically uncomfortable in situations in which implementing a client's living will involves the termination of life-sustaining treatments already in use. When you "pull the plug" on a ventilator or tube feeding, you seem to be doing definite harm to that client, namely, causing her death (Gastmans, 2006).

A third difficulty that you may encounter with a living will is actually enforcing it. The legal and ethical systems overlap a great deal in this dilemma. Strictly speaking, unless a state has enacted into law a special type of living will called a *natural death act*, the living will is not legally enforceable. Although 44 states have these acts, they vary widely in wording and requirements. Some of these laws recognize the living will only if it is in accord with the physician's plan of treatment. Other states have laws that are so specific in defining "terminal illness" that they require the client to die within a few hours of implementing the living will. Very few of these laws have any provisions to protect nurses and other health-care providers from criminal or civil actions if they do carry out the living will. You need to know not only whether your state has a natural death act but also what it says specifically about living wills.

The other form of advance directive, used less commonly than the living will, is the MDPOA, or health-care proxy. This type of advance directive allows the client to designate another person to make health-care choices if she becomes unconscious or otherwise unable to make decisions. Like the living will, the MDPOA has difficulties. State laws vary widely as to who can be given this power, how long the power lasts, and the legal process involved in verifying the person with the power of attorney. The ethical issues surrounding the MDPOA are very similar to those for living wills. In addition, some clients may designate two or more persons to have MDPOA. Making health-care decisions when these individuals disagree about the care they think the client wants is extremely complicated.

Staffing and Delegation

You have probably already encountered "health-care restructuring" at your workplace. No matter how it may have been presented, all restructuring has cost

containment as its primary goal. Almost all health-care facilities are attempting to find ways to cut their costs while maintaining at least minimal standards of care. You may have been exposed to terms such as *managed care*, *resource allocation*, and *change in provider mix*. Be cautious when these terms are used, because they usually mean that the ratio between professional staff and unlicensed staff is changing, with the potential to produce ethical conflicts that challenge your role as a professional nurse. Consider the ethical principles of autonomy, justice, fidelity, beneficence and nonmaleficence, veracity, standard of best interest, and obligations.

The current trend to use more unlicensed assistive personnel (UAP) poses ethical and legal concerns for you in your attempt to carry out your ethical and professional responsibilities. As a nurse, your main goal is to provide respectful, competent, and compassionate care for your clients using your expertise, knowledge, and professional skill. Professional nurses in most settings have always relied on some type of UAP help, but as the mix of professional to nonprofessional care providers changes, your ethical and legal obligations also change (Watson, 2006).

The professional nurse's primary commitment has always been and should always be to the health, well-being, and safety of the client. Nurses act as advocates for clients and should always be aware of, and take appropriate action regarding, situations in which incompetent, unethical, or illegal practice is performed by anyone providing care. Although it is possible for UAPs to provide safe care within their scope of practice, they may end up carrying out procedures that require skills inappropriate for their level of training. It is your ethical and legal responsibility to identify situations in which client care is adversely affected and to take action to change or eliminate the potential for harm.

Legally and ethically, professional nurses are responsible for the actions taken and judgments made by those they supervise in the provision of care. Neither physician's orders nor the employing agency's policies release nurses from the responsibility for actions taken or judgments made by subordinates (Ward, 2005). Nurses can protect themselves from unethical or illegal situations by constantly evaluating how staffing changes affect the safety and quality of the care being provided. By becoming involved in the formulation of institutional policies through active participation on various in-house committees, nurses can have a major influence on the staffing practices at their institution. It is also ethically permissible, and even desirable, that nurses protest and take appropriate action when they judge that UAPs are being used inappropriately or unsafely in client care situations.

Similarly, nurses are ethically and legally accountable for the appropriate delegation of nursing care activities to other health-care workers. It is important that nurses know the level of training of UAPs assigned to them and evaluate their competency when assigning client care tasks. It is ethically irresponsible to assign a nursing care function to an unlicensed assistant for which he is not prepared or qualified. Employer policy statements do not release the nurse from accountability for inappropriately assigning an unprepared unlicensed assistant to a task that ultimately results in harm to the client. The educator role of the professional nurse now has importance in helping to prepare and instruct UAPs in the work setting. Professional nurses will also be spending more of their time evaluating the competency of other health-care workers as they provide care in order to protect clients from harm.

In our rapidly changing health-care system, the use of UAP-type workers will only increase. Correspondingly, you will need to understand your growing professional and legal obligations regarding these workers. As with most ethical questions, there is no single right answer to the dilemma posed by UAP. You are the professional, and your judgment and accountability are not abdicated through delegation. You, as a professional nurse, must always keep in mind the ultimate goal for all clients: safe and high-quality care.

Cloning and Genetic Manipulation

With the successful birth of Dolly the sheep in Scotland in 1996, the world was awakened to the reality of **cloning** as a viable reproductive method. Since that time, all sorts of animals have been cloned. The concept of cloning, which has existed since the discovery of DNA in the 1950s by Watson and Crick, is based on the fact that every cell in an animal's body contains all the genetic information needed to reproduce every other cell in the body. In the strict scientific meaning of the word, the *cloning process* occurs when any cell in an animal's body is removed, is placed in an appropriate growth environment, and develops into an identical reproduction of the animal from which the cell came. In practice, however, scientists still do not understand what triggers some parts of a DNA strand to become active and reproduce and other parts of the DNA strand to remain dormant. Currently, if a skin cell is removed from a human being and placed in a growth medium, it will grow only new skin, not another identical person.

Although you are probably familiar with the popular term "cloning," the scientific name for the process used to produce Dolly and other animals is *somatic cell nuclear transfer technique*. First, an unfertilized ovum is removed from an animal, and then all the genetic material (DNA) is removed from the ovum. The next step requires the scientists to remove the DNA from a cell in the animal that they wish to clone and to insert it into the unfertilized, DNA-free ovum. The ovum

with the new DNA is then implanted in the uterus of an appropriate animal, and it grows into an identical twin of the donor of the DNA. In the case of Dolly the sheep, the DNA donor was her mother. Therefore, Dolly is an identical twin of her mother, even though she is six years younger.

Another technique that may be referred to as "cloning" is really embryo splitting. After an ovum is fertilized by a sperm, either naturally or with in vitro fertilization (IVF), a single cell results, called a zygote, which contains a combination of genetic material (DNA), half from the father and half from the mother. Left alone to develop, that single cell will eventually develop into an individual who shares some of the inherited features of both parents as a result of the combination of DNA. Within 12 hours after the zygote is formed, it begins to divide into two, then four, then eight, and then 16 identical cells. When it reaches 16 cells, it enters the morula stage.

While the embryo is dividing, up to and including the morula stage, the cells can be divided and separated. Because the cells are all identical, contain all the genetic material necessary to produce a new individual, and have fully active DNA, each cell is essentially a zygote. Once the cells are divided and separated, they can be implanted into several appropriate females and will continue to divide and develop into identical twins, or triplets, or more. Also, when the embryo is in the early four- to eight-cell stage, these cells can be separated, the genetic material removed from them, and new genetic material inserted. The cell with the new DNA will then grow into a twin of the animal from which the DNA was taken. It appears that by using the embryo-splitting procedure, scientists could produce an unlimited supply of ova for somatic cell nuclear transfer procedure.

With the IVF procedure, embryo splitting, and DNA transfer, the fertilization and early development process occurs in a laboratory in a petri dish. After the cells begin to develop, they are implanted into an appropriate female for the remainder of the pregnancy. Although the cloning or embryo-splitting process is relatively simple, its success rate is marginal at best. In order to produce Dolly the sheep, more than 1000 ova were genetically treated. Of those 1000, only 29 actually began to develop, and of the 29 that developed, only one actually produced an animal (Dolly).

Ethical Issues

Shortly after the news of Dolly the sheep reached the U.S., a raging debate developed over whether the cloning of humans was ethical, moral, or even legal (Rapport, 2003). Although other issues have pushed this one from the front burner, from the public standpoint, the three most troubling ethical issues were the loss of uniqueness of the individual, the potential misuse of the technology by diabolical scientists, and the degeneration of society as it now exists. Other, more traditional ethical concerns—such as medical risk to the mother or child (beneficence and nonmaleficence), life status of the embryos produced by the procedure, distributive justice issues of cost and availability of technology, and autonomy issues of using humans as incubators or sources of organs for donation—also remain troubling (Tschudin, 2006).

The belief that genetic determinism will produce individuals who not only look but also act identically is fundamentally flawed. The fact that identical twins are exact genetic copies of each other demonstrates this result. Although every cell in each twin's body is genetically identical to every cell in the other twin's body, experience shows us that they usually develop very individual personalities and character traits. Personality development is influenced by a wide range of environmental and experiential elements, not just genetic composition. If and when human cloning becomes a reality, cloned human babies who are born to mothers who live in different situations, although they may look the same, will likely have very different personality traits.

Similarly, the belief that there is a loss in quality each time an individual is cloned is not supported by experience. In many cases, for example, photocopies may actually be of higher quality than an original paper document. However, cloning is more than making photocopies, because the process is very different. The danger of "bad copies" from cloning that may well result in offspring of inferior quality or with congenital defects arises from the mechanical collection and transfer of the very fragile DNA strands. Scientists know that damaging even one gene sequence can produce birth defects.

In most ethical dilemmas, motive is an important element in determining the rightness or wrongness of an act (Milton, 2006). There are several possible motivations to clone human beings, ranging from egotism to helping an infertile couple have a child. The egotistical motivation conjures up images of the diabolical scientist or political leader who wants to create a "super-race" through the repeated cloning of physically and mentally superior individuals (like himself or herself, no doubt). You can imagine what Hitler might have done with this technology if it had existed at the time of the Second World War. What about cloning great inventors, brilliant leaders, or famous athletes? What owner of a football, baseball, or basketball franchise would not want a team of Terrell Davises or Cal Ripkens or Michael Jordans? Could embryo factories be far behind?

A somewhat more altruistic, although still potentially objectionable motive is the cloning of humans for the purpose of organ donation. Theoretically, the person who needs a heart transplant could donate DNA and, after a period of time, have an individual who has a heart with a perfect genetic match. However, most people have a strong abhorrence for the use of a cloned child as a means to an end, especially if harvesting the organ (as in a heart transplant) would result in the death of the child. However, some scientists in Texas have managed to clone mice without heads, whose organs were then transplanted back into the DNA donor mice. What if human clones could be created without heads? Would these headless beings truly be human, or would they just be biological storage units for organs that could be used for donation when the need arose? Although at first glance this practice might seem abhorrent, is it really that different ethically from the sperm, egg, embryo, or organ banks that exist today?

In the past few years, several parents have decided to have children for the primary purpose of providing bone marrow for an older child who was afflicted with leukemia. In several cases, the children were an identical six-antigen match, and the bone marrow was harvested from the infant and transplanted into the sick child, who recovered completely from the disease. Is having children for this purpose so different from cloning children for use as organ transplants? What if scientists were to learn how to clone just one organ or specific tissue at a time? If a person needed a new liver, the DNA from her liver could be transferred to an ovum, and then a new liver grown in the laboratory. A similar procedure already exists, without ethical objections, for growing new skin used for grafting in burn patients.

Some parents might be motivated to clone a replacement child for one who has died or is going to die. These parents could "set aside" a clone through the embryo-splitting technique that could be stored in an embryo bank and could later be implanted and grown if the original child died. The underlying motivation would seem to be very selfish and self-serving—that is, to create a replacement child for relief of the parent's grief and sense of loss over the death of the first child. In reality, many couples who have lost a child to death have subsequent children to make their lives fuller and more meaningful. In addition, is the cloned child really a replacement for the child who died? Although the child would look the same, as discussed previously, his personality and temperament would likely be much different.

Similarly, the infertile couple who had tried all other methods and were unable to have a child might seek a cloned embryo as a last resort. This motivation may pose the fewest ethical objections. Rather than using ova, semen, or both from unknown individuals, they might opt to use their own DNA, from either the father or mother, to produce a child.

Ethical issues and ethics are a part of your daily practice. In today's world, with rapidly advancing technology and unusual health-care situations, ethical dilemmas are increasing. You can be prepared to deal with most of these dilemmas if you keep current with the issues and are able to use a systematic process for making decisions about them. Hiding from ethical issues is not a solution. At some point, you will have to make difficult decisions. One of the most difficult parts of ethical decision-making is that someone is likely to be unhappy about your decision. But if you have made the decision after analyzing the situation on the basis of sound ethical principles, you should be able to defend it to anyone.

INTERACTIVE EXERCISES

Go to the Intranet site and complete the interactive exercises provided for this Chapter.

EVIDENCED-BASED PRACTICE: CONSIDER THIS . . .

*O*ne of the measurement criteria in the ANA (2004) Scope and Standard of Practice under the Ethics Standard concerns resolving ethical issues and serving on ethics committees.
   Question: What is the record for service on the Ethics Committee at your agency?

American Nurses Association (ANA). (2004). *Nursing: Scope and standards of practice.* Washington, DC: Author.

K E Y   P O I N T S

■ Ethical decision-making is a skill that can be learned and developed through practice.

■ The steps in the ethical decision-making process are to collect and analyze the data; state the dilemma; consider the choices of action; analyze the choices and consider the consequences; and make the decision.

■ Utilitarianism is a system of ethical decision-making based on the principle of the greatest good for the greatest number of people. Deontology is a system of ethical decision-making based on unchanging rules and principles, without consideration of the consequences.

■ The ANA *Code for Nurses* serves as the ethical guidelines for the profession of nursing. It provides the nurse with general statements about nursing ethics, which the nurse needs to interpret and apply to individual ethical situations.

■ The key ethical issues involved in organ transplantation revolve around the ethical principles of distributive justice, informed consent, and determination of death.

■ Ethical questions concerning end-of-life decisions often involve a conflict between the client's right to self-determination and the nurse's obligations of beneficence and nonmaleficence.

■ A number of ethical principles are involved in ethical dilemmas created by the HIV and AIDS issue. These include the right to privacy, self-determination, the right to care, and distributive justice in the form of health-care workers' and society's right to protection from dangerous diseases.

■ Although advance directives are now a legal part of the health-care system, a number of ethical issues still plague their use. The primary ethical concern is that of informed consent. Many clients have only a limited knowledge about the types of treatments possible for various conditions.

■ A relatively new ethical concern for nurses involves current trends in health care for the increased use of unlicensed assistive personnel. Professional nurses are ethically and legally accountable for the care provided by these individuals.

■ Cloning is a new technology with a promising future, but it also raises a number of disturbing ethical questions that nurses are likely to face in the future.

Thought and Discussion Questions

1. Look at the ANA Code of Ethics for Nurses, and identify where the ethical principles come into play in its tenets.

2. Think of a recent ethical decision you have made in practice. Which ethical system do you use when making decisions? What systems do your colleagues use? How would the outcome in your earlier decision differ if you used the other system?

3. Name 10 of your rights and classify them as legal, ethical, or option rights.

4. If you were to update or revise the ANA Code of Ethics for Nurses, what changes would you make so it is more reflective of the current health-care scenario?

5. Should people who have harmed their health by drinking, smoking, and drug use have the same right to health care as people who have taken care of themselves? What ethical issues would come into play in restricting access to care?

6. Review the Chapter Thought located on the first page of the chapter, and discuss it in the context of this chapter.

☐ REFERENCES

Aiken, L. M. (2003). Critical care nurses' use of decision-making strategies. *Journal of Clinical Nursing 12*, 476–483.

Aiken, T. D., & Catalano, J. T. (1994). *Legal, ethical, and political issues in nursing*. Philadelphia: F. A. Davis.

American College of Physicians. (1998). Ethics manual (4th ed.). *Annals Internal Medicine, 128*, 576–594.

American Nurses Association. (2001). *Code for nurses with interpretive statements*. Washington, DC: Author.

Briggs, L. A. (2002). End-of-life decision-making: Having those difficult discussions. *American Journal of Nurse Practitioners, 6*(8), 9–12.

Bruton, J. (2005). Ethical issues in HIV nursing. *HIV Nursing, 5*(4), 3–4.

Catalano, J. T. (2006). *Nursing now: Today's issues, tomorrow's trends*. Philadelphia: F. A. Davis.

Collis, S. P. (2006). The importance of truth-telling in health-care. *Nursing Standard, 20*(17), 41–45.

Curtin, L. (2006, April). The long & short of it: Cutting corners . . . where it hurts. *Healthcare Traveler, 13*(10), 14, 16–17.

Daly, B. J. (2006). End-of-life decision making, organ donation, and critical care nurses. *Critical Care Nurse, 26*(2), 78–86.

Davis, A. J., & Aroskar, M. S. (1997). *Ethical dilemmas and nursing practice* (4th ed.). Stamford, CT: Appleton & Lange.

DeVeaux, T. E. (2006). Non-heart-beating organ donation: Issues and ethics for the critical care nurse. *Journal of Vascular Nursing, 24*(1), 17–21.

Edwards, J. (2006). Maximizing organ donation opportunities through donation after cardiac death. *Critical Care Nurse, 26*(2), 101–115.

Esterhuizen, P. (2006). Is the professional code still the cornerstone of clinical nursing practice? *Journal of Advanced Nursing, 53*(1), 104–110.

Fletcher, J. (1966). *Situation ethics*. Philadelphia: Westminister John Knox Press.

Gastmans, C. (2006). Role of nurses in institutional ethics policies on euthanasia. *Journal of Advanced Nursing, 54*(1), 53–61.

Johnstone, M. (2006). The ethics and practical importance of defining, distinguishing, and disclosing nursing errors: A discussion paper. *International Journal of Nursing Studies, 43*(3), 367–376.

Mathes, M. (2005). Ethics, law, and policy: On nursing, moral autonomy, and moral responsibility. *Medsurg Nursing, 14*(6), 395–398.

McKenney, E. (2003). Legal and ethical issues related to nonheart beating organ donation. *AORN Journal, 77*, 973–976.

Milton, C. L. (2006). Research ethics standards: Are they significant or only symbolic? *Nursing Science Quarterly, 19*(1), 19.

Rapport, F. (2003). Exploring the beliefs and experiences of potential egg share donors. *Journal of Advanced Nursing, 43*(1), 28–42.

Rehnsfeldt, A. (2005). The relevance of the ethics of understanding of life in nursing. *International Journal for Human Caring, 9*(4), 39–44.

Salladay, S. A. (2006a). Natural disasters: Putting your life on the line. *Nursing, 36*(2), 24.

Salladay, S. A. (2006b). Untimely advice: "Rapid response" ethics. *Nursing, 36*(3), 66–67.

Simpson, R. L. (2006). Ethics and information technology: How nurses balance when integrity and trust are at stake. *Nursing Administration Quarterly, 30*(1), 82–87.

Tschudin, V. (2006). How nursing ethics as a subject changes: An analysis of the first 11 years of publication of the journal Nursing Ethics. *Nursing Ethics, 13*(1), 65–75.

Ward, C. W. (2005). Ethics, law, and policy: Registered nurse safe staffing act of 2005. *Medsurg Nursing*, *14*(6), 399–401.

Watson, J. (2006). Caring theory as an ethical guide to administrative and clinical practices. *Nursing Administration Quarterly*, *30*(1), 48–55.

☐ BIBLIOGRAPHY

Alexander, G. L. (2006). Issues of trust and ethics in computerized clinical decision support systems. *Nursing Administration Quarterly*, *30*(1), 21–29.

Breier-Mackie, S. (2006). Ethics connection: Who is the clinical ethicist? *Gastroenterology Nursing*, *29*(1), 70–72.

Callister, L. C. (2006). Perinatal ethics: State of the science. *Journal of Perinatal & Neonatal Nursing*, *20*(1), 37–39.

Catalano, J. T. (1997). Ethical decision making in the critical care patient. *Critical Care Clinics of North America*, *9*(1), 45–52.

Delmar, C. (2006). Caring—ethical phronetic research: Epistemological considerations. *International Journal for Human Caring*, *10*(1), 22–27.

Friedson, J. B. (2005). Flu vaccination—a moral responsibility for nurses: Nurse ethicists weigh the risks and benefits. *Nursing Spectrum*, *15*(26), 22–23.

Grace, P. J. (2006). The clinical use of placebos: Is it ethical? Not when it involves deceiving patients. *American Journal of Nursing*, *106*(2), 58–61, 66.

Lützén, K. (2006). Developing the concept of moral sensitivity in healthcare practice. *Nursing Ethics*, *13*(2), 187–196.

Oberle, K. (2006). Ethical considerations for nurses in clinical trials. *Nursing Ethics*, *13*(2), 180–186

Richardson-Tench, M. (2006). Nursing ethics in practice: Issues for perioperative nursing. *Journal of Perioperative Practice*, *16*(3), 138, 140–143.

Rosell, T. D., & Catlin, A. J. (2006). An ethics conflict and culture: Should this kidney be used? *Pediatric Nursing*, *32*(1), 68–70.

Stanford, K. (2006). The ethical leader. *Nursing Administration Quarterly*, *30*(1), 5–10.

Volker, D. L. (2003). Is there a unique nursing ethic? *Nursing Science Quarterly*, *16*, 207–211.

Wysoker, A. (2005). Psychiatric-mental health nurses and the aftermath of Hurricane Katrina: Fulfilling the ethical responsibilities. *Journal of the American Psychiatric Nurses Association*, *11*(6), 364–365.

☐ ONLINE RESOURCES

Agency for Healthcare Policy and Research (AHCPR)
http://www.ahcpr.gov or contact *info@ahcpr.gov*

National Health Information Center (NHIC)
http://health.gov/nhic
or contact *NHICinfo@health.org*

AIDS Info BBS Database
http://aidsinfobbs.org/
or contact Ben Gardiner at *ben@aidsinfobbs.org*

American Association of Critical-Care Nurses
http://www.aacn.org
or contact *info@aacn.org*

Bioethics Discussion Pages
http://www-hsc.usc.edu/~mbernste/
or contact Maurice Bernstein, MD, at
DoktorMo@aol.com/

Bioethics Online Service
http://www.mcw.edu/bioethics/bos.html
or contact Art Derse at *aderse@its.mcw.edu*

HIV InfoWeb
**http://med-libwww.bu.edu/library/
tutorial/section2hivinfo.html**

National Human Genome Research Institute (NHGRI)
http://www.genome.gov

National Office of Public Health Genomics
http://www.cdc.gov/genomics/

■ Vicki L. **Buchda**

Managing and Providing Care

66 *Indeed, some observers believe that
health-care delivery in this country will inevitably
be facing a 'perfect storm' over the next decade as several
major environmental trends converge.* 99

*McManis & Monslave Associates and the American Organization
of Nurse Executives, 2003*

Chapter Objectives

On completion of this chapter, the reader will be able to:

1. Discuss the current issues that affect planning and provision of health care for clients and groups of clients.
2. Describe the evolution and current concerns of work environments and nursing care delivery systems.
3. Contrast the various models of nursing care delivery.
4. Describe the documentation system and the taxonomy needed for selected care-delivery systems.

Key Terms

Transformational Change

Value

Cost-Effective

Outcomes of Care

Differentiated Nursing
  Practice

Team Nursing

Primary Nursing

Case Management

Critical Pathway

Nursing Minimum Data Set

Health-care management and delivery systems have evolved as health care has experienced rapid and dramatic changes in financing, reimbursement, technology, lengths of stay, and increased numbers of aging and chronically ill individuals. The Pew Health Professions Commission has observed that "over the past 50 years, nursing has changed substantially from a largely supportive role in health care to one with many independent and complex responsibilities in health-care delivery" (O'Neil, 1998, p. 61). The changing role of the nurse is compounded by a shortage of health-care workers (including nurses), scarce resources, and concern about quality (American Hospital Association [AHA], 2002). Nurses are typically the largest segment of an acute care facility's personnel budget, so for economic reasons, nursing has become a target for redesign and restructuring. According to the AHA, many health-care workers, including nurses, are dissatisfied with their work (2002). The work environment and delivery systems can have positive effects on quality, outcomes, cost effectiveness, safety, and work satisfaction. This chapter explores these trends and issues from a historical perspective to lay the framework for understanding where we stand today in health care. While there is no one clear direction emerging for the future, there are road maps, metrics, and measures that will assist nurses in identifying and proactively creating work environments, delivery systems, and communication vehicles that will support safe and effective client care.

ORGANIZING CARE IN TODAY'S CLIMATE

It is true that economics drives health-care reform and therefore has had the greatest impact on how American health care is organized and delivered (Porter-O'Grady & Wilson, 1995). For example, the transition from "health" care to "managed" care has significantly changed practice settings and has brought expanded practice opportunities (American Nurses Association [ANA], 1998). Yet the demand by consumers and payers for safer care is a key component in reform as well. Articles about safety in hospitals appear almost monthly in the popular press, and consumers are being given advice by multiple sources, including their employers, about how to protect themselves. For example, General Motors produced a publication entitled Health Care 101: A Conversation about Health Care (General Motors, 2005). In it, general opinions and concerns about the U.S. health-care system are shared, as well as information to help consumers understand their role in health care. Frequently this

advice involves inquiring about the registered nurse (RN)-patient ratios.

Leaders in health care understand, however, that truly transformational change is required to enhance patient safety. Henricksen, Keyes, Steven, and Clancy (2006) define **transformational change** in health care as "the process of taking an organization or work unit that has probably performed well enough to maintain the status quo but now needs to 'reinvent' or transform itself into an entity that is much better equipped to respond to the challenges of a rapidly changing external environment" (p. 21). This is the type of change that will be required in the future.

Advances in technology are also influencing care delivery. For example, with improvement in diagnostic and therapeutic procedures, more patients are cared for in outpatient settings. In inpatient settings technology allows for innovations such as remote monitoring of ICUs by nurses and intensivists, called eICUs (Garber, 2006). Another emerging technology is that of a microchip, which, when implanted beneath a person's skin, could contain that person's entire medical record. These types of changes will dramatically influence how care is delivered. It has been noted in the past that new skill sets are required of nurses, including participation in continuous improvement as a routine part of clinical care (O'Neil, 1998, p. 41). Nurse involvement in defining and designing care will be even more important in the future.

Ultimately, care is planned, organized, and provided to meet the needs of clients, nurses, and the department or organization. The focus now in planning care has shifted to incorporate not only how the care is delivered but the work environment itself because a link with quality and safety has been established. Moreover, consumers are demanding more client-focused, value-based, and outcome-oriented care.

The Role of the Work Environment

The work environment is the context within which care is delivered. There are a number of reasons why work environment is vital. An unhealthy work environment contributes to the nursing shortage, quality of care issues, and patient safety concerns. For these reasons, the elements of a healthy work environment have attracted more attention recently by various groups, including professional nursing organizations.

Staff nurses have identified several conditions that make a hospital a good place to work, including management style, quality of leadership, organizational structure, staffing, and personnel policies and programs (Schaffner & Ludwig-Beymer, 2003). The Institute of Medicine (IOM) convened a committee to study nurses' work environments and patient safety, and found serious threats "in all four of the basic components of all organizations—organizational management practices, workforce deployment practices, work design, and organizational culture" (Page, 2004, p. 3). According to Aiken and colleagues (2001), nurses are very dissatisfied with their work environments in this country and others, and core problems in work design and workforce management threaten the provision of care. This level of dissatisfaction leads to shortages, and shortages also contribute to dissatisfaction.

A report published by the AHA entitled *In Our Hands* (2002) makes recommendations to address the shortages of health-care workers. Several recommendations involve the work environment and culture. The recommendations are in part:

1. Foster meaningful work by transforming hospitals into modern-day organizations, in which all aspects of the work are designed around patients and the needs of staff to care for and support them.
2. Improve the workplace partnership by creating a culture in which hospital staff—including clinical, support, and managerial staff—are valued, have a sustained voice in shaping institutional policies, and receive appropriate rewards and recognition for their efforts.

Magnet Recognition

These recommendations have themes similar to the original findings of a study conducted in 1982, which studied hospitals that seemed to be able to attract and retain nurses (McClure, Poulin, Sovie, & Wandelt, 1983). These hospitals were dubbed "magnet" hospitals for their ability to attract and retain nurses, and the study noted that nurses who practiced at these hospitals experienced professional and personal satisfaction in their jobs (Box 15–1). Further, the environments supported excellence in nursing services and promoted quality patient care. The Magnet Recognition Program® was developed to recognize health-care organizations that provide excellent nursing care based on quality indicators and standards of nursing practice as defined by the ANA's Scope and Standards for Nurse Administrators (ANA, 2004).

The American Association of Critical-Care Nurses (AACN) identified six guiding principles that are evidence-based and complementary to the Magnet principles. These principles are based on the premise that effective communication, collaboration, and solid organizational systems are essential for establishing and

ONLINE CONSULT

For more detail about the nine elements and the guiding principles refer to
http://www.aone.org/aone/resource/guidingprinciples.html

Box 15.1 Fourteen Forces of Magnetism

Fourteen forces of magnetism (ANCC, 2007)

- Quality of Nursing Leadership
- Organizational Structure
- Management Style
- Personnel Policies and Programs
- Professional Models of Care
- Quality of Care
- Quality Improvement
- Consultation and Resources
- Autonomy
- Community and the Healthcare Organization
- Nurses as Teachers
- Image of Nursing
- Interdisciplinary Relationships
- Professional Development

Refer to the American Nurse Credentialing Center for further information about the Magnet Nursing Services Recognition Program for Excellence in Nursing Services at http://nursecredentialing.org/magnet/ American Nurses Credentialing Center (ANCC). (2007). Forces of magnetism. Retrieved October 5, 2007 from *http://www .nursecredentialing.org/magnet/forces.html*.

maintaining a healthy work environment in which quality care can be delivered (AACN, 2005). In a like manner, the American Organization of Nurse Executives (AONE) also has identified a set of assumptions and guiding principles to assist in conversations about the future of care delivery systems (Thompson, 2006).

Work Environment in Nonhospital Settings

While much of the focus of recruitment, retention, staffing shortages, and the work environment has been on hospitals, the same issues exist in other settings as well. Home health-care agencies are facing many of the same issues, prompting research about the types of environments that will keep nurses working in that area (Flynn, 2005). The bottom line is that the work environment is critical in the quality and safety of care provided in all settings.

Overtime

Working overtime, whether it is mandatory or voluntary, is another key aspect of the work environment. Fatigue contributes to errors, work-related illness, and injuries among nursing staff (ANA, 2001). In the IOM report *Keeping Patients Safe*, Page discusses the effects of fatigue on decision-making, reaction time, and actual errors (2004). More recently, studies have demonstrated a link between the length of work shifts and errors (Scott, Rogers, Hwang, & Zhang, 2006).

Outlook

Hospitals and health-care organizations are responding. According to a recent study, hospitals are implementing short-term and long-term strategies to respond to the nursing shortage. Changing the nurses' work environment was identified by the authors as a long-term strategy to the nursing shortage. Twenty-eight hospitals reported making at least one change to the work environment, primarily through changing staffing levels. The changes "do not involve substantial changes to care delivery" (May, Bazzoli, & Gerland, 2006, pp. 3–4). In a series of reports, Buerhaus and colleagues examined specific aspects of the nursing workforce. One of the conclusions in the final report is that based on surveys of nurses in the U.S., the workforce conditions improved between 2002 and 2005 (Buerhaus, Donelan, Ulrich, Norman, & Dittus, 2006).

The retention of older nurses in the workforce is also extremely important for the sheer numbers of people and for their experience and wisdom. A report by the Robert Wood Johnson Foundation summarizes the impact of the aging of the U.S. workforce and the recruitment and retention of retired nurses. Many of the recommendations are consistent with the principles of those identified in the Magnet study, but with greater attention to the environmental elements such as ergonomics, lighting, and overall ambiance. There is also more focus on harvesting the knowledge and wisdom of experienced nurses and on greater flexibility in design of the work and in work shifts so that all generations of nurses can have their talents and skills maximized in the workplace (Hatcher, 2006).

Client-Focused Care

As providers of care, nurses and other health-care providers recognize the need to shape a system focused on and organized around health-care consumers: clients, their families, and communities. Today an interdisciplinary plan of care is developed and implemented for each client, with goals and interventions mutually agreed on by the care providers and client. The link between clientcentric care and quality and safety has been established (IOM, 2001). Consumers do not have a good way to judge the quality of their health care and so often base their evaluation on clues such as "their care being organized around their needs rather than the doctor's schedules, the hospital's processes . . ." (Berry & Bendapudi, 2003, p. 102).

This shift in values also influences department organization. Historically, hospital services were organized around functions for the convenience of the staff. For example, inpatient and outpatient services were combined, requiring outpatients to navigate through inpatient facilities. In the client-focused paradigm, it is logical to organize and deliver care according to the client's needs. In the 1990s, this involved some models of restructuring and redesigning of roles so that, for example, the admitting department admits the client at the bedside. Another trend is for facilities to form centers for outpatient care, including surgical services, for the convenience of the client.

Value

Another theme driving health-care organizational reform is value. Consumers and payers are demanding **value** in health care, which has two essential components: cost and quality. In addition, appropriateness of care is important (IOM, 2001). Value can be expressed as "quality at a reasonable cost in a milieu of efficacy" (Pinkerton, 2001, p. 684). Understanding this concept is vital because "survival in a reformed health-care industry will require nurses to articulate their value—i.e., nurses must demonstrate how they contribute to improving the quality of desired patient outcomes and reducing costs" (Arford & Allred, 1995, p. 64). The public expects it as well. In a national opinion survey conducted by the American Nurses Association (ANA) (1999), results indicated that when choosing a hospital, 93% of Americans would be more confident if they knew that the hospital had met rigorous quality standards (p. 1). Nurses are in a position to demonstrate their contribution to quality client outcomes and their ability to plan and deliver cost-effective care.

Accomplishing this involves, in part, matching needs with resources, so that the most cost-effective care provider is delivering the care. **Cost-effective** analysis examines the relationship between the cost to provide the service and the outcomes (Arford & Allred, 1995). Less expensive substitutes for professional nurses (referred to by some as "cheaper doers") therefore may not be cost-effective if outcomes are poor. But using professional nurses to perform tasks that could be delegated is not cost-effective either (Box 15–2). As Malloch and Conovaloff (1999) have pointed out, mismatching care providers and clients has been the recurring bane of quality care (p. 50).

○NLINE ○ONSULT

The Institute of Medicine's second report on the quality of health care in America outlines the current concerns of health-care delivery and imperatives for the future in the United States. The report is available online at **http://www.iom.edu/focuson.asp?id=8089**

Box 15.2 Delegation

Many models of care delivery incorporate unlicensed assistive personnel (UAP). Licensed nurses must have competencies in delegation and supervision. *Delegation* is "transferring to a competent individual the authority to perform a selected nursing task in a selected situation. The nurse retains accountability for delegation" (National Council of State Boards of Nursing [NCSBN], 1995, p. 2). The five rights of delegation (NCSBN, 1995) are:

- The right task
- The right circumstance
- The right person delegating and carrying out the right task on the right client
- The right directions or communications
- The right supervision

Proving Value and Demonstrating Outcomes

One of the most important challenges in making care more client-focused and valuable is for nurses to demonstrate clearly their contributions to **outcomes of care**. Porter-O'Grady and Malloch (2003) point out that "in the 20th century, the focus of work was on performing the right processes. In the 21st century, the focus is on obtaining the right outcomes" (p. 5). The 2004 IOM report acknowledged that "research is now beginning to document what physicians, patients, other health-care providers, and nurses themselves have long known: how well we are cared for by nurses affects our health, and sometimes can be a matter of life and death" (Page, 2004, p. 2). Nurses can use outcome evidence to demonstrate their value to clients and to the health-care system.

○NLINE ℂONSULT

For more information about delegation, refer to the following:

National Council of State Boards of Nursing at **https://www.ncsbn.org/introduction.pdf**

American Nurses Association at **http://nursingworld.org/MainMenuCategories/ ThePracticeofProfessionalNursing/ InfoforNurses/ ANANCSBNStatementonDelegationpdf.aspx**

http://nursingworld.org/MainMenuCategories/ HealthcareandPolicyIssues/Reports/ ANAPrinciples/PrinciplesofDelegation.aspx

Documentation of outcomes is key because nurses can demonstrate their value only by defining the link between the quality of nursing care delivered and client outcomes. In addition, only by understanding the link between nursing care and client outcomes can we measure the effect of changing care-delivery systems (ANA, 1995). Nurses need to define their contributions to the complex care delivered to ensure that their unique contributions are recognized, as nursing care becomes even more highly integrated with other interdisciplinary team members.

Although the term "nurse-sensitive outcome indicators" has been used more frequently since the patient safety literature has become more prevalent, work by nurses to link patient outcomes with nursing care began in the 1990s. The ANA began a multi-phase initiative, called Nursing's Safety and Quality Initiative, in 1994. The goal was to "investigate the impact of health-care restructuring on the safety and quality of patient/client care and the nurses who provide that care" (ANA, 2002a, p. 2). A project reported by the ANA (1995) explored many of the links between nursing care and client outcomes in acute care by identifying quality indicators. Called the Nursing Report Card for Acute Care, this report card–type study identified 21 nursing quality indicators that have strong conceptual ties to quality nursing care. Although the study could not link all of the indicators to quality nursing care, the report emphasized the importance of such report cards and identified areas, through a review of current research and literature, where nursing is making a contribution. In 1997, a study was conducted to assess the feasibility of obtaining nurse staffing and outcome measures and to test relationships between nurse staffing and specific outcome indicators (ANA, 1997). Numerous indicators were found to be correlated with nurse staffing: length of stay, pressure ulcers, pneumonia, postoperative infections, and urinary tract infections (ANA, 1997b). Next, the ANA developed nurse-sensitive indicators for community-based, nonacute-care settings (ANA, 2000a). In 1998, the ANA also funded the development of a national database for nursing-sensitive quality indicators, called the National Database of Nursing Quality Improvement (NDNQI). The University of Kansas School of Nursing houses and operates NDNQI. Data on the following structure, process, and outcome nursing-sensitive quality indicators are collected in this database (ANA, 2006):

- Mix of RNs, licensed practical nurses (LPNs), and unlicensed staff caring for patients in acute-care settings
- Nursing care hours provided per patient day
- Pressure ulcers
- Patient falls
- Pain management

- Physical/sexual assault
- Peripheral IV infiltration
- RN education/certification
- Nursing staff satisfaction

Although participation by acute-care organizations in NDNQI is voluntary, over 700 organizations are choosing to report their results (ANA, 2005b). In return, they are given their own data and data from like institutions so they can compare themselves to a national benchmark for each indicator.

More recently, the National Quality Forum (NQF) endorsed 15 voluntary consensus standards for nurse sensitive care. This is the "first-ever set of national standardized performance measures to assess the extent to which nurses in acute-care hospitals contribute to patient safety, health-care quality, and a professional work environment" (National Quality Forum, 2004, Forward). In response to a request for indicators, NDNQI submitted several nurse-sensitive quality indicator definitions to NQF (ANA, 2006). Several measures have been endorsed by NQF, and while there are some similarities between these measures and those collected by NDNQI, data definitions and data-collection methodologies are not alike for all measures. Further, NQF has not yet developed benchmarks. These measures continue to evolve as yet another organization, the Joint Commission on Accreditation of Healthcare Organizations (JCAHO), has become involved in further defining them.

The next logical step is to use evidence to improve practice. The responsibility to structure nursing practice on the basis of outcome data rests with nursing and poses some challenges for nurses who have followed routines for years. Taking and documenting vital signs, for example, is a firmly entrenched practice usually based on routine. Nurses are being asked to examine such practices for their contribution to the outcome. If they cannot establish a link to a positive outcome, the practice should be dropped. A move toward evidence-based practice to achieve the best possible outcomes is critical in order to offer the quality and value demanded by health-care consumers.

Nurse Staffing Levels

Adequate staffing levels and the right type (mix) of staff are key to organizing health organizations effectively and to providing quality care. This was confirmed when the results of a continuing study of nurse staffing and patient outcomes was reported by the ANA in 2000. In that study, the five outcome measures that were piloted in the 1997 study were correlated to the amount and mix of nursing staff. The results of this study came at a time when hospitals were reducing RN staffing in an attempt to save money (ANA, 2000). In

1999, the ANA published a document called the Principles for Nurse Staffing (ANA, 1999). The purpose of this document was to demonstrate "how complex nurse staffing decisions are and to identify the major elements to consider when evaluating the safety and appropriateness of nurse staffing" (ANA, 1999). More recently the ANA published a guide to using the staffing principles (ANA, 2005c).

Needleman, Buerhaus, Mattke, Stewart, and Zelevinsky (2002) demonstrated a link among a higher proportion of care provided by RNs, a greater number of hours of care by RNs per day, and better patient outcomes for hospitalized patients. They studied "Outcomes Potentially Sensitive to Nursing (OPSNs)," which they selected on the basis of the literature as well as exploratory measures. They found, for example, that among medical patients, a higher portion of hours of care per day provided by RNs and a greater absolute number of hours of care per day provided by RNs were associated with a shorter length of stay (LOS) and lower rates of urinary tract infections and upper gastrointestinal bleeding. The proportion of care hours provided by RNs was linked to lower rates of pneumonia, shock or cardiac arrest, and failure to rescue. There were similar findings in surgical patients (Needleman et al., 2002). The discussion about the right number of RNs continues, however, and the debate about whether LPNs can help alleviate the nursing shortage continues. Different perspectives on this topic are presented in an article by Seago and colleagues (2006).

In another study about hospital nurse staffing, Aiken, Clark, Sloane, Sochalski, and Silber (2002) found a relationship between staffing and the nurse-sensitive indicator of failure to rescue. They determined that for each patient in excess of a nurse/patient ratio of 4:1 there was a seven percent increase in the chance of failure to rescue and a seven percent increase in the likelihood of a patient dying within 30 days of admission. As the number of patients cared for by an RN increased, the chances of patient death increased. Higher numbers of patients per RN were

O*NLINE* C*ONSULT*

The ANA (2006) defines terms pertaining to staffing and quality of care that are frequently used interchangeably and sometimes inappropriately. For example, in theory, there is a difference between safe and appropriate staffing (safe staffing is a prerequisite to appropriate staffing). For more information refer to

http://nursingworld.org/MainMenuCategories/ ThePracticeofProfessionalNursing/ PatientSafetyQuality.aspx

also associated with job dissatisfaction and, ultimately, nurse burnout (Aiken et al., 2002).

Matching the right number of caregivers with the right knowledge, skills, and abilities to the patient-care requirements (i.e., staffing) is essential. Yet there is no one right answer to the question: "How many nurses is enough?" Licensure, regulation, and legislation are regarded by some as the answer. Some states now have mandatory staffing ratios. What these ratios fail to address is the complexity of the care environment, the competence of the personnel, and the acuity and workload involved for the patient. Accreditation agencies are interested in this as well. In 2002, the JCAHO added standards addressing the effectiveness of staffing. The purpose is to require accredited agencies to use data to assess staffing effectiveness.

NURSING ROLES

It is clear that nursing contributions to client outcomes are important, but what exactly do these contributions entail? McCloskey (1995) describes two roles for the nurse: provider of care and manager of the care environment. As providers of care, nurses deliver direct and indirect care for individual clients and for groups of clients. *Direct care* is defined as those interventions "performed through interaction with the patient(s)" (Bulachek & McCloskey, 1999). *Indirect care* is performed on behalf of the client to support the direct-care interventions. An example of indirect care is communication with other interdisciplinary team members.

In addition to being the provider of care, nurses play a role in managing the care environment. At the client care level, nurses' care management responsibilities include organizing, directing, and coordinating the care. The responsibility for matching needs with resources, as described earlier, is one aspect of this role. The role may also include talking with payers (including insurance companies), negotiating for client services, and advocating within the organization on behalf of a client.

Nurses also have management responsibilities within the client care unit or department. These responsibilities include delegating and supervising other personnel and unit operations, such as staffing and scheduling. This aspect of the management role varies with the

ONLINE CONSULT

For more information about the Joint Commission on Accreditation of Healthcare Organizations (JCAHO), refer to its Web site at
http://www.jointcommission.org

work environment, but the trend is toward flatter organizations, with direct-care providers assuming more of the traditional management roles in the department (Page, 2004).

Interdisciplinary Care Delivery

In the current system, nurses work closely with other interdisciplinary team members, such as social workers, therapists, and dietitians. The contributions of each of these highly skilled team members is coordinated and integrated into the plan of care for clients by professional nurses. As new models of work organization and structure emerge in practice, care will be delivered to clients by groups of care providers working in highly integrated teams. Cost and quality will continue to be the emphasis, and the *team* will be held accountable for the outcomes of the care.

Interdisciplinary teams, working collaboratively to deliver care, support cost-effectiveness because more often the right person with the right skills is delivering the service. This is an important step in matching needs with resources. The development of highly integrated interdisciplinary teams is not without problems, however. Some of the issues that need to be addressed are defining contributions to care, territoriality, and the shift in power. As discussed earlier, defining the contributions to care by the various providers is one of the greatest challenges facing health-care providers. It is an important step in the process, because matching the person with the knowledge, skills, and abilities to achieve the best outcome cost-effectively is the key to achieving value. The setting (e.g., intensive care unit, home health, or the whole community), the needs of the clients, and economics drive the logical providers and coordinator of care. This may lead to concerns about turf; for example, nurses may give up some responsibilities to social workers, and physicians to nurses. Some may regard this shift in accountability and power as threatening.

A common response to nursing shortages, shortages or other changes in other professions, and the cost of nursing salaries is to redesign roles (Kerfoot, 1997). There are many challenges for nurses inherent in these innovations. Nurses are being asked to delegate to and supervise personnel with various backgrounds and levels of competence.

Differentiated Nursing Practice

The concepts of matching needs with resources and care providers with client needs may seem simplistic, but with the many levels of nursing practice, different curricula, and various education requirements, this task becomes more complex. In order to articulate contributions to care and cost effectiveness, nursing must closely examine its own knowledge and skill sets.

Although there is agreement about the importance of the role of the registered nurse, the debate about educational preparation for professional nursing has been ongoing for almost 40 years. Currently, most nurses (57%) are employed by hospitals (Garber, 2006), and most job descriptions for registered nurses define one set of performance expectations to fulfill the role, regardless of educational preparation. With these blended job descriptions, some nurses' knowledge and skills are being underutilized and others are being asked to perform at levels higher than that for which they were prepared. To be seen as efficient and cost effective in the future, nursing may benefit from differentiated nursing competencies.

The phrase "A nurse is not a nurse" is understood within nursing to acknowledge that nurses are highly skilled professionals, many of whom are subspecialized and not interchangeable with one another. Nurses themselves think of the concept in terms of whether or not they could "float to" or practice in another area. Increasingly, however, the "recognition of the complexities of health care and the rapid expansion of knowledge is increasing the pressure to raise the level of basic education" (Nelson, 2002). It is proposed that, ultimately, "the more educated practitioner will be more cost-efficient" (Joel, 2002).

Levels of nursing practice were first introduced by the ANA in 1965, and **differentiated nursing practice** has been a goal of nursing professionals for several decades (American Association of Colleges of Nursing [AACN], 1995). It was recognized at that time that nurses possess a variety of skill sets, depending on educational preparation and experiential learning, and that clients and the profession would benefit from differentiating the practice. There are two types of differentiated practice: education-based practice, which is delineated according to educational credentials, and assessment-based practice, which incorporates both education and experiential learning.

One model of differentiated practice that defines roles according to educational preparation was proposed by Primm (1986). This model defines major and minor components of nursing practice, and these various components are assigned according to the nurses' educational preparation. *Technical nurses* care for clients and are responsible for meeting identified care goals in a specified work period and within structured health-care settings that provide policies and procedures as well as nursing experts for consultation and support. *Professional nurses* care for families and communities from the time of admission to after discharge, in structured and unstructured settings and in situations that may not have policies and procedures but that require independent nursing decisions (Primm, 1986).

The need for differentiated practice is compounded during times of shortage, and yet the tendency is just the opposite.

The discussion about educational levels for Advance Practice Nurses (APNs) began over 20 years ago and is once again hotly debated. In 2004, the American Association of Colleges of Nursing (AACN) members voted to approve a position paper requiring a Doctorate of Nursing Practice (DNP) for all new APNs by 2015 (Lenz, 2005). The rationale for a practice doctorate for APNs is similar to the rationale for Bachelor of Science in Nursing (BSN) entry into practice for RNs. The need for safe patient care, the increasing complexity of the environment, and parity with other professions are all arguments for both. In addition, visionary leaders in practice are required at tables where high-level decisions are made (Lenz, 2005).

As identified earlier, however, decisions regarding nursing practice should be made based on evidence, and at this time "there is no evidence to suggest that a practice doctorate will contribute to patient safety" (Fullerton, 2005, p. 4). Furthermore, Fullerton (2005) goes on to say that while other disciplines (audiology, physical therapy, and pharmacology) have moved to clinical doctorates, there is no evidence that the additional education has improved patient outcomes.

All differentiated nursing-practice models recognize the contributions of all nurses and pave the way for better delineation of outcomes with clearer job descriptions and expectations. Implementing such models increases efficiency and cost-effectiveness because it "places the highest-quality, lowest-cost provider next to the patient" ("Differentiated Nursing Practice," 1995). The need for differentiated practice is compounded during times of shortage, and yet the tendency is just the opposite. During times of shortage there is a great deal of pressure to reduce educational requirements and change licensure and accreditation standards (Donley & Flaherty, 2002). In addition, the shortage of nurses makes employers shy about offending any group of nurses in the workforce (Nelson, 2002).

DELIVERING CARE

Nursing care delivery systems have undergone tremendous redesign to meet the changing needs of clients, nurses, and the organization. Role redesign is a common response to nursing shortages, changes in other professions, and the cost of nursing salaries (Kerfoot, 1997). There are many challenges and opportunities for nurses inherent in delivery innovations.

To be effective, the nursing care delivery system must be consistent with the mission, vision, and values of the care providers, the department, and the organization (Schaffner & Ludwig-Beymer, 2003). Schaffner and Ludwig-Beymer (2003) have identified other factors to consider by anyone redesigning a care-delivery model or assessing the one being used:

- Number of RNs available in the organization and in the market area
- Fiscal resources available to fund salaries and costs, such as training
- Nursing acceptance of the model
- Expected outcomes, such as risk reduction, fewer medication errors, fewer pressure sores, improved patient satisfaction, and improved pain management. (p. 216)

For these reasons, what may seem to be an ideal care-delivery system in one organization may not work for another organization. Therefore, this section is meant to be descriptive and not prescriptive. In general, however, key factors that define success include:

- Client focus
- Cost effectiveness
- Outcome orientation
- Safety
- Matching of needs with resources
- Documentation of care and outcomes
- Setting (work environment) that supports professional nursing practice

A comprehensive model also involves having the right caregivers available to provide care. Various acuity and/or workload systems have been developed and implemented in efforts to classify or categorize clients by needs to ensure assignment of the right caregivers. It is beyond the scope of this chapter to discuss staffing and scheduling systems, but such systems assist in the process of planning and evaluating models of care delivery.

Models of Care Delivery

Care-delivery models have evolved through the years to meet the demands and challenges of the health-care arena, including safe patient care, optimal patient care outcomes, and an environment that supports the recruitment and retention of nurses.

ONLINE CONSULT

For more information about patient classification, workload, and acuity systems, refer to the Utilization Guide for the ANA Principles for Nurse Staffing at
http://nursingworld.org/MainMenuCategories/ HealthcareandPolicyIssues/Reports/ ANAPrinciples/NurseStaffing.aspx

For the purposes of this discussion, the term *care-delivery model* refers to the delivery of patient care. Some authors consider shared governance or shared decision-making as a care system or model (Anthony, 2004). As identified earlier, the environment in which the care is delivered is critical to nurse satisfaction and patient safety. Shared governance is considered part of the environment or the context in which the care is delivered.

Many factors influence the models of care delivery existing today. This section offers a brief review of generic care-delivery models. In-depth discussions of various delivery models are provided in other sources (Hoover, 1998; Mayer, Madden, & Lawrenz, 1990; Nursing Clinics of North America, 1992; Walker, 1991; Walker et al., 1994). Although care delivery models have undergone many changes, their underlying objectives are to "assess the patient, identify the nursing needs of the patient during hospitalization, and provide the nursing care necessary until the patient is discharged" (Lyon, 1993).

Case Method

The case method was one of the earliest models of care delivery. A nurse was assigned to provide complete care for a client or group of clients for a defined period, usually eight hours. Sometimes referred to as private-duty nursing or total patient care, this method was inefficient and costly because one nurse provided all care to the client (Cohen & Cesta, 1993; Poulin, 1985). While this method was based on the holistic philosophy of nursing (Grant & Massey, 1999) and allowed the nurse to develop a good relationship with the client, it had the disadvantage of high personnel costs (pp. 34–35).

Functional

Functional nursing evolved next, improving on the case method of assignments by using a variety of caregivers to complete the tasks (Cohen & Cesta, 1993). This model allocated tasks or functions. For example, one nurse gave all medications, another performed all treatments, and other caregivers gave all baths. Although a variety of caregivers participated in client care delivery in this model, the functional model has been criticized because it emphasizes task completion over client needs, resulting in fragmentation of care and unmet client needs (Thomas & Bond, 1991). The lack of ongoing personal contact with the client and absence of continuity of care have been cited as distinct disadvantages of this care model (Grant & Massey, 1999, p. 35).

Team

Team nursing emerged after World War II, when there was a shortage of nurses and other personnel were recruited to deliver care (Lyon, 1993). In the team model, other health-care workers—some licensed, such as a licensed practical nurse, and some unlicensed, such as aides and orderlies—were assigned to teams that were responsible for a group of patients and delivered care under the supervision of a registered nurse. The team was led by a team leader, who delegated the tasks and activities, provided some direct care, and coordinated all care. Team nursing provided an advantage over functional nursing by providing professional nurses to more clients, improving continuity of care, and freeing professional nurses from performing nonprofessional tasks (Cohen & Cesta, 1993). Team nursing also provided a higher level of job satisfaction for nurses over the functional method (Grant & Massey, 1999, p. 35).

Team nursing has inherent problems, however. It results in fragmented care, complex channels of communication, and shared responsibility with lack of accountability (Manthey, 1980). Care is fragmented by being divided into components delegated to appropriate caregivers, so that clients are cared for by at least three people during an eight-hour shift (RN, LPN, and nursing assistant) with a total of nine caregivers in a day. Communication is also complex; the caregivers report to the team leader, who relays the information to the next shift's team leader. In some cases, the team leader reports to a charge nurse, who relays the information to another charge nurse, who passes it on to the team leader. The information is subject to misinterpretation by each person in the chain.

Responsibility and accountability are major issues in team nursing. The nursing care plan, for example, is supposed to be completed and updated routinely, usually daily. The team leader bears this responsibility, as does the next shift team leader. What is not completed on one shift is completed on the next shift. According to Manthey (1980), shared responsibility equals no responsibility, and activities like completing care plans are not carried out consistently with this model.

Primary

Primary nursing evolved to meet the needs that were not addressed in the team nursing system. Manthey (1980) described primary nursing as a delivery system designed to "rehumanize" hospital care through decentralized decision-making. Responsibility for one client's care, 24 hours a day, is allocated to a primary nurse who actually provides the care whenever possible. Because one nurse has the responsibility, accountability, and authority to assess clients needs, develop a plan of care, and evaluate the clients' responses to the plan of care, a therapeutic relationship can be established between the nurse and the client (Mathews & Kamikawa, 1994; Wilkinson, 1994). The concepts of 24-hour accountability and RNs directing other RNs

differentiate this model from the case method model of delivery.

The primary nursing model recognizes the contributions of various care team members but relies heavily on RNs, not only for care planning but also for delivery of care. Because of this high reliance on RNs, primary nursing was frequently perceived as a costly model of care delivery. RNs are usually very satisfied with this care delivery model (Schaffner & Ludwig-Beymer, 2003). In Great Britain, Rigby, Leach, and Greasley (2001) report, primary nursing has been credited with pushing "an undervalued occupation towards greater professional recognition," but they also acknowledge that this "theoretical idea that may not be achievable in practice" (p. 530).

Patient-Focused Care

The nursing shortage of the 1980s, the cost of an all-professional staff, and obstacles to implementing primary nursing (such as 12-hour shifts) led some hospitals to examine alternatives to primary nursing. There are many variations of the patient-focused care model, but in general, services are decentralized to the patient care area. The focus is on patient needs rather than staff needs. In this model an RN, along with unlicensed assistants, manages a group of patients (Schaffner & Ludwig-Beymer, 2003). These assistants are cross-trained to perform tasks and skills that traditionally were performed by staff from other areas. For example, these personnel (frequently referred to as technicians) were cross-trained to draw laboratory specimens, perform ECGs, and clean the room. Some of the challenges of these types of models are role design/redesign, delegation and supervision skills of the RN, and varying levels of educational preparation of the assistive person. Because of these challenges, according to Kany (2004), these changes "resulted in injury among patients and health-care workers, demoralized a generation of nurses, and tarnished the profession's image and attractiveness to potential candidates" (p. 8).

Case Management

The forces in health care today have made it necessary to develop care delivery systems that go beyond the industrial model, which emphasized task completion and outputs, to integrated systems that include mechanisms to define the links between nursing care and outcomes and to demonstrate cost effectiveness. In evaluating care delivery systems, many institutions have implemented the case management model because it helps organize care around the client and is in concert with interdisciplinary and intradisciplinary differentiated practice. Because this model addresses many concerns previously identified, it is discussed here is some depth. Entire texts have been written about case management, however, and you are encouraged to refer to these and other sources for further information (Powell, 2000a and 2000b).

Case management is not a new concept. Nurses and members of other disciplines have been providing case management for clients for many years in various settings. Community public health programs have had case management services since the 1900s (Lyon, 1993). Behavioral health nurses have been using many of the concepts in the community since the 1960s. Case management received more attention from other areas of health care, including acute-care settings, when insurance companies began using the model. In recent years, it became one of the most frequently used care models in the country (AHA, 1990). Now the model is not only well recognized but also universally accepted (Powell, 2000b).

Case management is an approach to care. The purpose stays constant regardless of setting: it is to improve patient care, promote efficiency and efficacy in the use of resources, and ultimately improve patient outcomes. This care delivery model is focused on the client, promotes continuity and cost effectiveness, recognizes the contributions of the members of the interdisciplinary team, and allows for differentiation of practice within the nursing profession. In the acute-care setting it is frequently used in addition to, not in place of, the other care delivery models already discussed. While those models provide a methodology for accomplishing patient care on a shift-by-shift or day-by-day basis, case management provides a centralized way to review all patients to ensure that the goals are being met and that a discharge plan is in place. It provides a way to navigate the system on behalf of the patient. In this model, a case manager, typically a nurse, is responsible for the care of a group of patients. In an acute-care setting, a caseload might be made up of all of the patients on one patient-care unit.

There are many definitions of case management. Bower (1992) described case management as a "paradoxically simple yet complex concept" (p. 3). Simply stated, *case management* refers to "patient-focused strategies to coordinate care" (Bower, 1992, p. 2). Case management has also been defined as "an approach that focuses on the coordination, integration, and direct delivery of patient services, and places internal controls on the resources used for care" (Cohen & Cesta, 1993). Gerber (2001) combines the definition of the Case Management Society of America (CMSA) and Smith's definition to provide the following descriptive definition of case management:

> Nursing case management can be defined as the application of the collaborative and interdisciplinary case management process by professional nurses to promote the delivery of high quality,

holistic, cost-effective health and illness care to individuals and groups within communities and complex organizational systems through patient advocacy, communication, and effective management of available resources. (p. 693)

The purposes of case management are to ensure cost effectiveness, quality, and continuity of care.

Case management is a care delivery model focused on the client that promotes continuity and cost effectiveness, recognizes the contributions of the members of the interdisciplinary team, and allows for differentiation of practice within the nursing profession.

Case management is often confused with other concepts, including managed care, because the terms are frequently used interchangeably and because the historical development is similar (Cohen & Cesta, 1993). Refer to Chapter 19 for an in-depth discussion of managed care plans and financing. Case management services are frequently provided by acute-care facilities after clients are admitted, because insurance pays only a designated amount of money, either per day or for the entire period of hospitalization, and the incentive is for hospitals to provide care as cost-effectively as possible. More recently, trends include providing case management in the emergency department (ED). Because more and more patients are covered by some type of managed care plan, many of which have contracts with designated facilities, it is in the client's and the hospital's best interest to make sure that the client's hospitalization will be covered.

Case management can be provided in a variety of settings. Lyon (1993) delineates three categories of case management in health-care settings: hospital-based case management, case management across the health-care continuum, and community case management.

Hospital-Based Case Management

Hospital-based case management began with the introduction of the prospective payment system in 1983 (Lyon, 1993). Since then, professional nurses have been responsible for clients' lengths of stay and for matching needs with resources.

The case management care-delivery model can be implemented in a way that addresses some of the issues identified earlier; the care clients receive is provided by the caregivers with the right knowledge and skills, and in the right setting for the intensity, amount of care needed, and severity of illness. The role of case managers is to facilitate and integrate the contributions of the interdisciplinary team. The case manager's role also lends itself to intradisciplinary differentiation. For these reasons, this model facilitates cost-effective, quality care.

The role of case manager is carried out differently in different models. Case managers, for example, can be staff nurses who, with some additional training and education, incorporate case management activities into the planning and provision of care on a daily basis. Some organizations have designated case managers for groups of clients. Others have case managers who follow clients within the hospital, but also follow select groups of clients through the continuum of care. Some organizations assign case managers to a unit or units with clients who have common diagnoses, whereas others assign case managers to follow clients through the course of the hospital stay. Each model has advantages and disadvantages, and no one model is right for every organization. Some organizations even use case managers differently within the setting, depending on the client type and other identified needs. For example, one case manager in a hospital may be unit-based and another population-based, crossing units.

The case management system can be used with a variety of nursing care delivery systems—primary, team, functional, or combinations of these systems (Lyon, 1993). If it is used with one of these client care delivery systems, the case management system can be overlaid onto the existing structure, or the entire system can be reengineered. Another strength of the case management system is that it can be used with differentiated care models. For example, more experienced or baccalaureate-prepared nurses are assigned to manage a caseload of patients in addition to their other patient care responsibilities. The technical or less experienced nurse, meanwhile, might have a greater direct patient-care load without the case management responsibilities.

There are several levels of complexity in planning and organizing care in case management models. Case managers prioritize for groups of clients, and then address the needs of individual clients. As a part of their role, nurse case managers evaluate practice patterns for appropriateness, timeliness, and medical necessity. A systematic process is used to address overutilization and underutilization of resources, inefficiencies, and delays. Care and services are coordinated and integrated.

The following is an example of a model in an acute-care setting in which a nurse case manager is responsible for a group of clients. These steps represent an approach to a caseload model but they do not have to be carried out in this order:

1. The process used to organize a day or caseload involves reviewing payer status of the clients. Clients who are members of capitated plans, for instance, may be evaluated first, because the case manager often communicates with payers about the clients' status and anticipated length of stay. Health plans commonly need to "authorize" admissions and continued stays.

2. The case manager prioritizes review of medical records. This may be accomplished by talking with other members of the health-care team and responding to potential problems they identify, or answering referrals from other sources.

3. Clients are evaluated, usually daily, according to some criteria for appropriateness of service level, such as intensity of service and severity of illness. This evaluation is key in matching needs with resources, because some levels of care, such as intensive care, are very costly to the organization. If the client no longer meets intensity or severity criteria for the intensive care unit, the case manager facilitates transfer to an appropriate level of care. Sometimes the case manager determines that the resources a client needs are too intense for a particular unit and recommends transfer to a higher level of care. The case manager always keeps in mind the cost-to-quality equation.

4. The case manager also focuses on individual clients, evaluating what the client needs now, what needs are anticipated, and what resources are available. The case manager works through any obstacles to achieve the best outcome, as mutually agreed upon with the client.

5. The case manager helps the team develop and implement the plan. This involves communicating with the client and family, nurses, and other members of the interdisciplinary team.

6. The case manager also has responsibility for evaluating the case management process, including productivity indicators, quality and outcome indicators, and financial information tracking.

7. The evaluation information is used to change practice, for instance, to match the care provider who has the knowledge, skills, and abilities with the care to be given. The case manager usually facilitates development of clinical pathways and ensures appropriate documentation.

Case Management Across the Continuum

Case management services can be episodic—usually initiated and completed during a hospital stay, as described in the previous section—or they can continue as the client moves back into the community. Some models that include services across the continuum report improvement in the quality of care and cost reduction (Koerner & Karpiuk, 1994; Lamb & Huggins, 1990). Sioux Valley Hospital, which uses differentiated case management, saved more than $500,000 in a six-month period through the case management of 35 complex patients (AACN, 1995). The type of service provided depends on the patient population, the goals of the program, and the provider. For example, case management for a group of clients with congestive heart failure (CHF) might be performed by advanced practice nurses such as a clinical nurse specialist (CNS). The CNS would follow the patient in the hospital, ensure that discharge teaching is completed, and then monitor the patient with telephone calls or visits in an outpatient clinic. The goal of case management in this case is to prevent re-admission to the hospital through early detection and intervention in this chronically ill population.

Case Management in the Community

Some case management programs are community-based and begin after clients are discharged from the hospital. These services are provided by nurses and other members of the interdisciplinary team. Clients are assessed, counseled, reminded of appointments for follow-up, and referred to other professionals as needed. These services are frequently provided for behavioral health clients who are reintegrating into the community. These services may be provided by the health maintenance organization (HMO) case manager, who is accountable for coordination of care overall, or by other case managers who manage "crisis and details while that patient resides in their respective level of care" (Powell, 2000b). These case managers specialize in areas such as home health, skilled nursing, and rehabilitation.

Critical Pathways

Some of the case management strategies, such as integrating and coordinating services and tracking outcomes, are not easy to implement. Tools are available, however, to facilitate the processes. One of the tools for supporting this process is a document developed to define the care for a particular client type, commonly referred to as a **critical pathway**, or CareMap™.

Critical pathways are important tools for mapping client care and expected outcomes throughout an acute episode of illness (Gibson, 1996). They define not only care but outcomes as well, and they encourage identification of variances so that new interventions can be planned. Critical pathways are different from nursing care plans, which focus on individual differences; critical pathways define the most usual care for a client type and focus on the similarities of clients. They guide health professionals to the most common ways of treating and responding to a given episode of illness. Critical pathways also allow for documentation of care provided and comparison of clients' actual status with predefined outcomes. Variances from the plan, in either the care the client is to receive or the outcomes achieved, can be tracked and analyzed.

Typical critical pathways identify the care that clients receive during a specific time frame, along with expected outcomes. Critical pathways are developed by interdisciplinary teams through a systematic process. Some maps extend across the care continuum and follow the client into the community, but most are designed for the acute-care period.

Documentation

The shift in care delivery systems has also contributed to a shift in the focus of nursing documentation. In the functional model, documenting task completion was the focus. As the movement into team nursing and then primary nursing emphasized greater continuity of care, the nursing care plan gained importance as a system to document the care.

With the shift to a patient-centered care focus, the use of language in documentation also changed. Client databases, rather than nursing admission forms, are now completed at admission, and client or patient care plans, not nursing care plans, are developed. Classification systems now are increasingly focused on client outcomes.

As the environment, including reimbursement structure, risk management, and the focus on patient safety, continues to change, the emphasis on documentation will also continue to change. For example, under a reimbursement structure in which the provider or health-care institution is reimbursed on the basis of charges, it is extremely important to document all supplies and equipment used. Some plans will not reimburse for the use of a specialized bed, such as a low-air-loss bed, without daily documentation that the client is using the bed. Infusion of every liter of intravenous solution must be documented, or the payer can refuse to pay for the solution, even though it was charged to the client. A payer can refuse to reimburse an entire hospital stay for failure to document administration of an antibiotic. Documentation is also important in traditional quality management monitoring and risk management.

The amount of time consumed by documentation is continually questioned. Health-care professionals are familiar with the saying "If it isn't documented, it isn't done." In a 2002 publication entitled *Principles for Documentation,* the ANA said that conscientiousness by nurses in complying with all of the documentation requirements was pulling nurses away from direct patient care. The implementation of documentation by exception, in which nurses document abnormal or significant findings, has assisted with some of the burden of documentation, but it is noted in the IOM report that 13% to 28% of a nurse's time in acute care is consumed in documentation, and the figure is even higher in home care because of regulatory requirements (Page, 2004, p. 6). This time could be spent actually providing patient care and in patient monitoring. Although automated systems have improved access to information, in general, they have not reduced the time spent in documenting.

On a global level, a "national health information infrastructure is needed (1) to provide immediate access to complete patient information and decision support tools for clinicians and their patients, and (2) to capture patient safety information as a by-product of care and use this information to design even safer delivery systems" (Aspden, Corrigan, Wolcott, & Erickson, 2004, p. 1). At the local level, the implementation of health-care information systems that have features such as physician or provider order entry will ultimately improve patient safety. For example, transcription errors will be reduced. There are risks that come with these systems, however. Although transcription errors are reduced, a physician or provider may place an order for a client and may not even be in the same building when doing so. That may reduce the conversation between the nurse and the physician, which would have occurred in the past. Other risks identified in the literature include 1) the absence of nursing terms in electronic data sets, 2) the substitution of information technology for RNs, 3) documentation that does not reflect nurses' unique contributions to care, 4) a focus on technology and not the client, and 5) physical safety concerns for the nurse who may be asked to use devices placed in spaces that are not ergonomically correct (Milholland, 2001).

NURSING INFORMATION AND DATA SETS

As nursing care delivery has become more complex, so too has documentation. That complexity is further compounded with the use of information systems, both to support the delivery of care and the documentation of care. In 1995, the ANA formed the Nursing Information & Data Set Evaluation Center (NIDSEC) to "review, evaluate against defined criteria, and recognize information systems from developers and manufacturers that support documentation of nursing care within automated Nursing Information Systems (NIS) or within computer-based Patient Record (CPR) systems " (ANA, 2006).

NIDSEC is the only group that has developed standards for nursing data and information systems. NIDSEC recognized the need for standards and developed them to evaluate four dimensions of nursing data sets and the systems that contain them. Standards were developed for nomenclatures (the terms used), clinical content ("linkages" among terms), clinical data repository (how data are stored), and general systems characteristics (performance, security). Organizations can voluntarily submit systems for evaluation. Several systems have met the criteria and are or were recognized by NIDSEC for having met standards.

Standardized nomenclatures are known also as classification systems, taxonomies, and languages. According to Bulachek and McCloskey (1999), the five purposes for classification systems of nursing practice are:

- To link knowledge about diagnosis, treatments, and outcomes
- To facilitate the development of nursing and health-care information systems
- To facilitate teaching of decision-making to nursing students
- To help determine the costs of services provided by nurses
- To articulate with the classification systems of other health-care providers

It is important for nursing to agree upon and adopt standardized nomenclature, because as discussed

EVIDENCED-BASED PRACTICE: CONSIDER THIS . . .

*T*he Agency for Healthcare Research and Quality (AHRQ, 2003) presented evidence from the scientific literature on the effects of health-care working conditions on patient safety. Part of their EBP Program, AHRQ reported the following three findings:

- Strategies to increase staffing levels of licensed and unlicensed nurses in both acute-care hospitals and nursing homes will likely lead to improved patient outcomes.
- Duration of experience of the health professional is associated with better patient outcomes for some types of clinical care.
- Systems to reduce interruptions and distractions will likely reduce the incidence of medical errors. (AHRQ, 2003, p. 2)

Question: How will you use this information as a nurse-manager for client safety?

Source: The Agency for Healthcare Research and Quality (AHRQ). (2003). The effect of health-care working conditions on patient safety. Retrieved October 8, 2006, from http://www.ahrq.gov/clinic/epcsums/worksum.htm

earlier, nurses are being asked to identify what they do and what they contribute to care. This identification requires collection of essential nursing information, including nursing diagnoses, interventions, and outcomes. Without consistent methods of documentation, national databases, or agreement of the language to be used, nurses cannot be sure that they are comparing "apples to apples." The standardized nomenclatures assist us in organizing data; ultimately that data must be "represented and managed so they can be processed using well-designed computer algorithms" (Harris, Graves, Solbrig, Elkin, & Chute, 2000, p. 539) to facilitate patient care and to ensure quality and cost effectiveness.

The ANA recognizes 13 data element sets and terminologies. A sample of some of these sets is discussed below.

Nursing Minimum Data Set

One goal the profession is working toward is to implement the uniform collection of essential nursing information, known as the **Nursing Minimum Data Set** (NMDS) (Moorhead, McCloskey, & Bulechek, 1993). This database will provide large data sets allowing nursing data to be compared across populations, to complement information from other professionals. The ANA (1997c) has supported the development of the NMDS and predicts that the data set will:

- Contribute to the delivery of safe, effective nursing care
- Describe nursing practice
- Provide quality control data
- Facilitate the analysis and evaluation of health policy
- Advance nursing knowledge
- Contribute to the structure of nursing education
- Facilitate the allocation of nursing resources
- Contribute toward payment reform for nursing services
- Assist in determining the cost of nursing care
- Assist in determining nursing's contributions to client care. (p. 2)

Implementation of the NMDS depends on having a standardized language for four essential components: nursing diagnosis, nursing interventions, nursing outcomes, and nursing intensity (Delaney & Moorhead, 1995).

ONLINE CONSULT

For a complete list of the data element sets and their descriptions, refer to the ANA Web site at **http://nursingworld.org/npii/terminologies.htm**

Diagnoses

Classification of client problems has been available for more than two decades through the North American Nursing Diagnosis Association (NANDA) and as a component of the Omaha System. These two systems are very different; NANDA's approach is very broad, but the Omaha System focuses on community health (Delaney & Moorhead, 1995).

Interventions

Several classifications for nursing interventions have been developed, including the Omaha System, the Home Healthcare Classification, and the Nursing Interventions Classification (NIC). A research team at the University of Iowa began work on the most comprehensive classification, NIC, in 1987. Since the initial classification was published in 1992, research has continued. Researchers constructed, validated, and coded a taxonomy. Through clinical field testing, they also identified the need for linkages between NANDA, NIC, and nursing outcomes classifications (NOC—see following). The challenge in the clinical setting is to document both professional knowledge (for research and statistical purposes), and care delivered (for legal and reimbursement purposes). See Appendix B.

Outcomes

A standardized language for nursing outcomes was developed by another research team at the University of Iowa. With the development of Nursing Outcomes Classification (NOC), the nursing process elements of the NMDS are complete. The NOC includes outcome labels, label definitions, indicators for each outcome, and a five-point Likert-type measurement scale (Johnson, Maas, & Moorhead, 2000).

Recently, a new data set was introduced by the American Operating Room Nurses Association (AORN), the Perioperative Nursing Data Set (PNDS). AORN (1999) has stated that the "initial goal in developing the data set was to develop a unified language so that nursing care could be systematically quantified, coded, and easily captured in a computerized format in the perioperative setting" (p. 1). This data set is based on the Perioperative Patient Focused Model that is designed to "delineate the relationships within the domains of nursing concern: nursing diagnoses, nursing interventions, and patient outcomes in continuous interaction with the health-care system" (AORN, 1999, p. 1).

Intensity

The fourth component NMDS requires is standardized language for nursing intensity. Nursing intensity is difficult to define, and even more difficult to measure.

Nursing must be able to document the resources required to provide client care and achieve defined outcomes (Delaney & Moorhead, 1995). Without this language, determining the true cost of care will be difficult, and making it cost effective will be even more difficult.

Although it is extremely important to capture nursing's contribution to care and outcomes, it is also important to acknowledge that as we move to highly integrated interdisciplinary teams, we may not be able to use language that belongs exclusively to nursing. As integrated documentation is developed, and all professionals rely more heavily on communication in records, language that everyone can use is required.

INTERACTIVE EXERCISES

Go to the Intranet site and complete the interactive exercises provided for this Chapter.

KEY POINTS

■ Health-care planning and provision are changing dramatically as a result of shortages of care providers, economics, and changing population.

■ Cost, quality, and safety are the essential components of care.

■ The economic forces and philosophical shifts experienced today are encouraging nurses to demonstrate their contributions to client outcomes.

■ Roles of the interdisciplinary and intradisciplinary care providers should be differentiated by knowledge, skills, abilities, and contributions to client outcomes.

■ Various care delivery models, such as team and primary nursing, are currently used to organize the delivery of care. Models must address the needs of the organization, match the organization's culture and values, and consider the content of care delivered.

■ Case management is one care delivery model that addresses many of the current concerns of care delivery systems. Critical pathways are tools that assist in achieving the goals of case management.

■ Documentation, an essential component of care, is changing as care delivery systems and reimbursement systems change.

■ Nursing is developing taxonomies to assist in identifying what nurses do and what they contribute to care. The Nursing Minimum Data Set will assist in the uniform collection of essential nursing information.

Thought and Discussion Questions

1. Participate in a discussion on the importance of the NMDS. Why would it be helpful for the profession of nursing and health care in general, and what difficulties may be encountered in its use?

2. Analyze the care delivery system on a client-care unit. What model is in place? Are responsibilities differentiated according to knowledge, skills, and abilities?

3. Think of some ways that your organization has made changes to focus more centrally on clients. Think about and be prepared to discuss the model of care delivery used in your organization.

4. Review the Chapter Thought located on the first page of the chapter, and discuss it in the context of this chapter (either online or in class).

☐ REFERENCES

Aiken, L. H., Clarke, S. P., Sloane, D. M., Sochalski, J. A., Busse, R., Clarke, H., et al. (2001). Nurse's reports on hospital care in five countries. *Health Affairs, 20*(3), 43–53.

Aiken, L. H., Clarke, S. P., Sloane, D. M., Sochalski, J. A., & Silber, J. H. (2002). Hospital nurse staffing and patient mortality, nurse burnout, and job dissatisfaction. *Journal of the American Medical Association, 288*(16), 1987–1993.

American Association of Colleges of Nursing. (1995). *A model for differentiated nursing practice*. Washington, DC: American Association of Colleges of Nursing.

American Association of Critical-Care Nurses. (2005). *AACN standards for establishing and sustaining healthy work environments: A journey to excellence* [Electronic version]. Aliso Viejo, CA: American Association of Critical-Care Nurses. Retrieved August 17, 2006, from *http://www.aacn.org/aacn/pubpolcy.nsf/Files/HWEStandards/$file/HWEStandards.pdf*

American Hospital Association. (1990). *Report of the hospital nursing personnel survey—1990*. Chicago: American Hospital Association.

American Hospital Association. (2002). *In our hands: How hospital leaders can build a thriving workforce*. Chicago: American Hospital Association.

American Nurses Association. (1995). *Nursing report card for acute care*. Washington, DC: American Nurses Publishing.

American Nurses Association. (1997a). *Implementing nursing's report card: A study of RN staffing, length of stay, and patient outcomes*. Washington, DC: American Nurses Association.

American Nurses Association. (1997b). Nursing's quality indicators for acute-care settings and ANA's safety and quality initiative. Retrieved November 26, 2006 from *Nursing Facts. http://www. nursingworld.org/readroom/fssafety.htm*

American Nurses Association. (1997c). Position statement: A national nursing database to support clinical nursing practice. Retrieved November 26, 2006 from *www.nursingworld.org/readroom/position/practice/prdatabs.htm*

American Nurses Association. (1999). Press release: Americans support rigorous standards for nursing care. Retrieved November 26, 2006 from *http://www.nursingworld.org/pressrel/1999/pr0507.htm*

American Nurses Association. (2000). *Nurse staffing and patient outcomes in the inpatient hospital setting*. Washington, DC: American Nurses Association.

American Nurses Association. (2000a). ANA identified indicators for community-based, nonacute care. Retrieved November 26, 2006 from *http://nursingworld.org/pressrel/2000/pr0420.htm*

American Nurses Association. (2001). Opposition to mandatory overtime. Retrieved November 26, 2006 from *http://www.nursingworld.org/readroom/position/workplac/revmot2.htm*

American Nurses Association. (2002). Nursing-sensitive indicators for community-based nonacute settings and ANA's safety and quality initiative. Retrieved November 26, 2006 from *Nursing Facts. http://nursingworld.org/readroom/nurssens.htm*

American Nurses Association. (2002). *Principles for documentation*. Washington, DC: American Nurses Association.

American Nurses Association. (2004). *Scope and standards for nurse administrators* (2nd ed.). Washington, DC: American Nurses Association.

American Nurses Association. (2005a). Principles for delegation. Retrieved November 26, 2006 from *http://nursingworld.org/staffing/lawsuit/PrinciplesDelegation.pdf*

American Nurses Association. (2005b). Survey of 76,000 nurses probes elements of job satisfaction. Retrieved November 26, 2006 from *Press Release. http://nursingworld.org/FunctionalMenuCategories/MediaResources/PressReleases/2005/pr04018524.aspx*

American Nurses Association. (2005c). *Utilization guide for the ANA principles for nurse staffing*. Retrieved November 26, 2006 from *http://nursingworld.org/staffing/lawsuit/PNSUtilGuide.pdf*

American Nurses Association. (2006). Nursing information and data set evaluation. Retrieved August 17, 2006, from *http://nursingworld.org/nidsec/prtindex.htm*

American Nurses Association. (2006). The National Center for Nursing Quality Indicators: The national database of nursing quality indicators (NDNQI). Retrieved November 26, 2006 from *http://nursingworld.org/quality/prtdatabase.htm*

American Nurses Credentialing Center (ANCC). (2007). Forces of magnetism. Retrieved October 5, 2007 from *http://www.nursecredentialing.org/magnet/forces.html*

American Operating Room Nurses Association (AORN). (1999). Perioperative nursing data set. Retrieved November 26, 2006 from *www.aorn.org/research/pnds.htm*

Anthony, M. K. (2004, January). Shared governance models: The theory, practice, and evidence. *Online Journal of Issues in Nursing, 19*(1), Manuscript 4. Retrieved November 26, 2006 from *www.nursingworld.org/ojin/topic23/tpc23_4.htm*

Arford, P. H., & Allred, C. A. (1995). Value = quality + cost. *Journal of Nursing Administration, 25*(9), 64–69.

Aspden, P., Corrigan, J. M., Wolcott, J., & Erickson, S. M. (Eds.). (2004). *Patient safety: Achieving a new standard*. Washington, DC: The National Academies Press.

Berry, L. L., & Bendapudi, N. (2003, February) Clueing in customers. *Harvard Business Review*, 100–106.

Bower, K. A. (1992). *Case management by nurses*. Washington, DC: American Nurses Publishing.

Buerhaus, P. I., Donelan, K., Ulrich, B. T., Norman, L., & Dittus, R. (2006). State of the registered nurse workforce in the United States. *Nursing Economics, 24*(1), 6–12.

Bulechek, G. M., & McCloskey, J. C. (1999). *Nursing interventions: Effective nursing treatments* (3rd ed.). Philadelphia: W. B. Saunders.

Cohen, E. L., & Cesta, T. G. (1993). *Nursing case management: From concept to evolution.* St. Louis, MO: Mosby.

Curtin, L. (2003, September 30). An integrated analysis of nurse staffing and related variables: Effects on patient outcomes. *Online Journal of Issues in Nursing.* Retrieved November 26, 2006 from *www.nursingworld.org/ojin/topic22/tpc22_5.htm*

Delaney, C., & Moorhead, S. (1995). The nursing minimum data set, standardized language, and health-care quality. *Journal of Nursing Care Quality, 10*(1), 16–30.

Differentiated nursing practice in all care settings. (1995). *Journal of Nursing Administration, 7*(8), 5–6.

Donley, R., & Flaherty, M. J. (2002). Revisiting the American Nurses Association's first position on education for nurses. *Online Journal of Issues in Nursing, 7*(2).

Flynn, L. (2006). The importance of work environment: Evidence-based strategies for enhancing nurse retention. *Home Healthcare Nurse, 23*(6), 366–371.

Fulton, J. S., & Lyon, B. L. (2005, September 30) The need for some sense making: Doctor of nursing practice. *Online Journal of Issues in Nursing, 10*(3), Manuscript 3. Retrieved November 26, 2006 from *http://www.nursingworld.org/ojin/topic28/tpc28_3.htm*

Garber, K. M. (Ed.). (2006). *The U.S. health care delivery system: fundamental facts, definitions, and statistics.* Chicago: American Hospital Association.

Gerber, R. M. (2001). Case management: Tomorrow's vision. In N. L. Chaska (Ed.), *The nursing profession: Tomorrow and beyond* (pp. 691–700). Thousand Oaks, CA: Sage Publications.

Gibson, S. J. (1996). Differentiated practice within and beyond the hospital walls. In E. L. Cohen (Ed.), *Nurse case management in the 21st century* (pp. 222–244). St. Louis, MO: Mosby-Year Book.

Grant, A. B., & Massey, V. H. (1999). *Nursing leadership, management, and research.* Springhouse, PA: Springhouse Corporation.

Harris, M. R., Graves, J. R., Solbrig, H. R., Elkin, P. L., & Chute, C. G. (2000). Embedded structures and representation of nursing knowledge. *Journal of the American Informatics Association, 7*(6), 539–549.

Henricksen, K., Keyes, M. A., Stevens, D. M., & Clancy, C. M. (2006). Initiating transformational change to enhance patient safety. *Journal of Patient Safety, 2*(1), 20–23.

Hoover, K. W. (1998). Nursing work redesign in response to managed care. *Journal of Nursing Administration, 28*(11), 9–18.

Institute of Medicine. (2001). *Crossing the quality chasm: A new health system for the 21st century.* Washington, DC: National Academy Press.

Institute of Medicine. (2004). Keeping patients safe: Transforming the work environment of nurses. Retrieved November 26, 2006 from *http://www.nsp.edu/openbook/0309090679/html/1.html*

Joel, L. A. (2002). Education for entry into nursing practice: Revisited for the 21st century. *Online Journal of Issues in Nursing, 7*(2). Retrieved November 26, 2006 from *http://www.nursingworld.org/ojin/topic18_4.htm*

Johnson, M., Maas, M., & Moorhead, S. (2000). *Nursing outcomes classification (NOC)* (2nd ed.). St. Louis, MO: Mosby.

Kany, K.A. (2004). Nursing in the next decade: Implications for health care and for patient safety. *Online Journal of Issues in Nursing, 9*(2), Manuscript 3. Retrieved November 26, 2006 from *http://nursingworld.org/ojin/topic24/tpc24_3.htm*

Kerfoot, K. M. (1997, December 22). Role redesign: What has it accomplished? *Online Journal of Issues in Nursing, 2*(4). Retrieved November 26, 2006 from *www.nursingworld.org/ojin/tpc5/tpc5_3.htm*

Koerner, J. G., & Karpiuk, K. L. (Eds.). (1994). *Implementing differentiated nursing practice: Transformation by design.* Gaithersburg, MD: Aspen.

Lamb, G. S., & Huggins, D. (1990). The professional nursing network. In G. G. Mayer, M. J. Madden, & E. Lawrenz (Eds.), *Patient care delivery models* (pp. 169–184). Rockville, MD: Aspen.

Lenz, E. R. (2005, September 30). The practice doctorate in nursing: An idea whose time has come. *Online Journal of Issues in Nursing, 10*(3), Manuscript 1. Retrieved November 26, 2006 from *http://www.nursingworld.org/ojin/topic28/tpc28_1.htm*

Loquist, R. S., & Brady, M. S. (2001). South Carolina statewide articulation model. Retrieved November 26, 2006 from *http://www.sc.edu/nursing/cic/*

Lyon, J. C. (1993). Models of nursing care delivery and case management: Clarification of terms. *Nursing Economics, 11*(3), 163–169.

Malloch, K., & Conovaloff, A. (1999). Patient classification systems, part 1: The third generation. *Journal of Nursing Administration, 29*(7/8), 49–56.

Manthey, M. (1980). *The practice of primary nursing.* Boston: Blackwell.

Mathews, B. P., & Kamikawa, C. (1994). Primary nursing. *Nursing Administration Quarterly, 19*(l), 48–50.

May, J. H., Bazzoli, G. J., & Gerland, A. M. (2006). Hospitals' responses to nurse staffing shortages. *Health Affairs, 25*(4), 316–323.

Mayer, G. G., Madden, M. J., & Lawrenz, E. (Eds.). (1990). *Patient care delivery models.* Rockville, MD: Aspen.

McCloskey, J. C. (1995). Recognizing the management role of all nurses. *Nursing and Health Care: Perspectives on Community, 16*(6), 307–308.

McClure, M. L., Poulin, M. A., Sovie, M. D., & Wandelt, M. A. (1983). Magnet hospitals: Attraction and retention of professional nurses (the original study). In M. L. McClure and A. S. Hinshaw (Eds.) (2002). *Magnet hospitals revisited.* Washington, DC: American Nurses Publishing.

Milholland, D. K. (2001). Information systems technologies: Rewards and risks. *The Nursing Risk Management Series, Article 1. http://nursingworld.org/mods/archive/mod311/cerm2ful.htm*

Moorhead, S. A., McCloskey, J. C., & Bulechek, G. M. (1993). Nursing interventions classification: A comparison with the Omaha system and the home healthcare classification. *Journal of Nursing Administration, 23*(10), 23–29.

National Council of State Boards of Nursing. (1995). Delegation: Understanding the concepts and decision-making process. Retrieved November 26, 2006 from *http://www.ncsbn.org.files/publications/positions/delegate.asp*

National Quality Forum. (2004). National voluntary consensus standards for nursing-sensitive care: An initial performance measurement set. Retrieved November 26, 2006 from *http://www.qualityforum.org/txNCFINALpublic.pdf*

Needleman, J., Buerhaus, P., Mattke, S., Stewart, M., & Zelevinsky, K. (2002). Nurse-staffing levels and quality of care in hospitals. *New England Journal of Medicine, 346*(22), 1715–1722.

Nelson, M. A. (2002). Education for professional nursing practice: Looking backward into the future. *Online Journal of Issues in Nursing, 7*(2). Retrieved November 26, 2006 from *http://www.nursingworld.org/ojin/topic18_3.htm*

Nursing Clinics of North America (NCNA). (1992). *Nursing Clinics of North America, 1*(27).

O'Neil, E. H. (1998). *Recreating health professional practice for a new century: The fourth report of the Pew health professions commission.* San Francisco, CA: Pew Health Professions Commission.

Page, A. (Ed.). (2004). *Keeping patients safe.* Washington, DC: The National Academies Press.

Pinkerton, S. (2001). Organizing nursing in an integrated delivery system (IDS). In N. L. Chaska (Ed.), *The nursing profession: Tomorrow and beyond* (pp. 681–690). Thousand Oaks, CA: Sage Publications.

Porter-O'Grady, T., & Malloch, K. (2003). *Quantum leadership: A textbook of new leadership.* Sudbury, MA: Jones and Bartlett.

Porter-O'Grady, T., & Wilson, C. K. (1995). *The leadership revolution in health care: Altering systems, changing behaviors.* Gaithersburg, MD: Aspen.

Poulin, M. (1985). Configuration of nursing practice. In American Nurses Association (Ed.), *Issues in professional nursing practice* (pp. 1–14). Kansas City, MO: American Nurses Association.

Powell, S. K. (2000a). *Advanced case management: Outcomes and beyond.* Philadelphia: Lippincott-Raven.

Powell, S. K. (2000b). *Case management: A practical guide to success in managed care.* Philadelphia: Lippincott-Raven.

Primm, P. L. (1986). Entry into practice: Competency statements for BSNs and ADNs. *Nursing Outlook, 34*(3), 135–137.

Rigby, A., Leach, C., & Greasley, P. (2001). Primary nursing: Staff perception of changes in ward atmosphere and role. *Journal of Psychiatric and Mental Health Nursing, 8*, 525–532.

Schaffner, J. W., & Ludwig-Beymer, P. (2003). *Rx for the nursing shortage.* Chicago: Health Administration Press.

Scott, L. D., Rogers, A. E., Hwang, W. T., & Zhang, Y. (2006). Effects of critical care nurses' work hours on vigilance and patients' safety. *American Journal of Critical Care, 15*(1), 30–37.

Seago, J. A., Spetz, J., Chapman, S., & Dyer, W. (2006). Can the use of LPNs alleviate the nursing shortage? *American Journal of Nursing, 106*(7), 40–49. *http://nursingcenter.com/library/JournalArticle.asp?Article_ID=650919*

Thomas, L. H., & Bond, S. (1991). Outcomes of primary nursing: The case of primary nursing. *International Journal of Nursing Studies, 28*(4), 291–314.

Thompson, P. (2006). Guiding principles. *Hospitals and Health Networks Magazine*, August 12. *http://www.hhnmag.com/hhnmag/jsp/articledisplay.jsp?dcrpath=AHA/PubsNewsArticle/data/0407HHN_OutBox&domain=HHNMAG*

Walker, D. D., Jones, S. L., Yamauchi, S. S., Lima, C., Archer, S., Mathews, B. P., et al. (1994). The Queen's Medical Center Honolulu, Hawaii. *Nursing Administration Quarterly, 19*(1), 33–65.

Walker, P. H. (1991). Dollars and sense in health reform: Interdisciplinary practice and community nursing centers. *Nursing Administration Quarterly, 19*(1), 1–11.

Wilkinson, R. A. (1994). A more autonomous and independent role: Primary nursing versus patient allocation. *Professional Nurse, 9*(10), 680–684.

☐ BIBLIOGRAPHY

Aiken, L. H., Clarke, S. P., Cheung, R. B., Sloane, D. M., & Silber, J. H. (2003). Educational levels of hospital nurses and surgical patient mortality. *Journal of the American Medical Association, 290*(12), 1617–1623.

Altman, G. D. (1993). Adjusting primary nursing to 12-hour shifts. *Nursing Management, 24*(2), 80–82.

American Nurses Association. (1997). Managed care: Challenges and opportunities for nursing. *Nursing Facts.* Retrieved November 26, 2006 from *www.nursingworld.org/readroom/fsmgdcar.htm*

American Nurses Association. (1997). Position statement: AORN official statement on RN first assistants. Retrieved November 26, 2006 from *www.nursingworld.org/readroom/position/joint/jtassist.htm*

American Nurses Association. (1997). Position statement: The right to accept or reject an assignment. Retrieved November 26, 2006 from *www. nursingworld.org/readroom/position/workplace/wkassign.htm*

American Nurses Association. (1999). Health care and the nursing workforce issues in the United States. *Nursing Trends & Issues, 4*(1), 1–9.

AzNA awarded report card grant. (1996, May). *Arizona Nurse*, 3.

Barry-Walker, J., Bulechek, G., & McCloskey, J. C. (1994). A description of medical-surgical nursing. *MEDSURG Nursing, 3*(4), 261–268.

Bellack, J. P., & Loquist, R. S. (1999). Employer responses to differentiated nursing education. *Journal of Nursing Administration, 29*(9), 4–8.

Brady, M., Leuner, J., Bellack, J. P., Loquist, R. S., Cipriano, P. F., & O'Neil, E. H. (2001). A proposed framework for differentiating the 21 Pew competencies by level of nursing education. *Nursing and Health Care Perspectives, 22*(1), 30–35.

Cohen, E. L. (1996). *Nurse case management in the 21st century.* St. Louis, MO: Mosby.

Daly, J. M., Mass, M., & Buckwalter, K. (1995). Use of standardized nursing diagnosis and interventions in long-term care. *Journal of Gerontological Nursing, 21*(8), 29–36.

Gessner, T. L. (1998). Job design and work processes in patient care. In J. A. Dienemann (Ed.), *Nursing administration: Managing patient care* (2nd ed., pp. 359–378). Stamford, CT: Appleton and Lange.

Havens, D. S., & Aiken, L. H. (1999). Shaping systems to promote desired outcomes: The magnet hospital model. *Journal of Nursing Administration, 29*(2), 14–20.

Hayes, P. (1998). Managed care: Impact and relevance for regulation. *Issues, 19*(3), 1–2. Retrieved November 26, 2006 from *www.ncsbn.org/files/publications/issues/vol193/mcimpact193.asp*

Himali, U. (1995). Managed care: Does the promise meet the potential? *American Nurse, 27*(4), 1, 14, 16.

Hyams-Franklin, E. M., Rowe-Gillespie, P., Harper, A., & Johnson, V. (1993). Primary team nursing: The 90s model. *Nursing Management, 24*(6), 50–52.

Kayuha, A. A. (1996). Organizational systems. In C. Loveridge & S. Cummings (Eds.), *Nursing management in the new paradigm* (pp. 24–57). Gaithersburg, MD: Aspen.

Kerr, M. E., Hoskins, L. M., Fitzpatrick, J. J., Warren, J. J., Avant, K. C., Carpitano, L. J., et al. (1992). Development of definitions for taxonomy II. *Nursing Diagnosis, 3*(2), 65–71.

Loquist, R. S., & Bellack, J. P. (1998). *South Carolina colleagues in caring project: A model for differentiated entry level nursing practice by educational program type.* (Available from the South Carolina Colleagues in Caring Project, University of South Carolina College of Nursing, Columbia, SC 29208.)

Loquist, R. S., & Bellack, J. P. (1999). *Into the future: Recreating South Carolina's nursing workforce for the 21st century.* (Available from the South Carolina Colleagues in Caring Project, University of South Carolina College of Nursing, Columbia, SC 29208.)

Malloch, K., Neeld, A. P., McMurry, C., Meeks, L., Wallach, M., Williams, S., & Conovaloff, A. (1999). Patient classification systems, part 2: The third generation. *Journal of Nursing Administration, 29*(9), 33–42.

Marrelli, T. M. (1997*). The nurse manager's survival guide: Practical answers to everyday problems.* St. Louis, MO: Mosby.

McCloskey, J. C., & Bulechek, G. M. (Eds.). (1996). *Nursing interventions classification (NIC)* (2nd ed.). St. Louis, MO: Mosby.

McManis & Monslave Associates and American Organization of Nurse Executives. (2003, November/December). Striving for excellence: Insights from a key informant survey on nursing work environment improvement and innovation. *Nurse Leader, pp. 13–19.*

Milton, D. (1992). The evaluation of new nursing structures in single or multifacility systems. In C. Wilson (Ed.), *Building new nursing organizations: Visions and realities* (pp. 187–208). Gaithersburg, MD: Aspen.

National Council of State Boards of Nursing. (1998). Nursing supply/demand issue brief from the policy futures panel. *Issues, 19*(3), 1–3. Retrieved November 26, 2006 from *www.ncsbn.org/files/publications/issues/vol193/supply193.asp*

Nooner, K. (2004, May). Bouncing patients? Capacity issues and diversion status toy with efficient throughput. *Nursing Management,* 39–44.

North American Nursing Diagnosis Association. (1992). *NANDA nursing diagnosis: Definition and classification 1992.* St. Louis, MO: North American Nursing Diagnosis Association.

Pila, L. (1999). How the nursing shortage jeopardizes patient care. Retrieved November 26, 2006 from *www.nurses.com/content/news/article asp*

Powell, S. K. (1996). *Nursing case management.* Philadelphia: Lippincott-Raven.

Rundall, T. G., Starkweather, D. B., & Norrish, B. R. (1998). *After restructuring: Empowerment strategies at work in America's hospitals.* San Francisco: Jossey-Bass.

Simmons, F. M. (2005). Hospital overcrowding: An opportunity for case managers. *The Case Manager, 16*(4), 52–54.

Smith, G. (1994). The paradox of collaboration. *Nursing and Health Care, 15*(7), 338–339.

Stevens, K. R., & Weiner, E. E. (2001). Informatics for nursing practice. In N. L. Chaska (Ed.), *The nursing profession: Tomorrow and beyond.* Thousand Oaks, CA: Sage Publications.

Swansburg, R. C., & Swansburg, R. J. (1999). *Introductory management and leadership for nurses* (2nd ed.). Boston: Jones and Bartlett.

Terry, D. (1999). Effective employee relations in reengineered organizations. *JONA's Health Care, Law, Ethics, and Regulation, 1*(3), 33–40.

■ Rose **Kearney-Nunnery**

Healthy Initiatives
for At-Risk Populations

> " *Wherever we look upon this earth, the opportunities take shape within the problems.* "
>
> Nelson Rockefeller, 1908–1979

Chapter Objectives

On completion of this chapter, the reader will be able to:

1. Describe the national initiatives aimed at improving health and reducing health disparities.
2. Identify trends and health needs of our at-risk populations.
3. Discuss strategies for reducing health disparities for at-risk population groups.
4. Discuss the characteristics of the aging population.
5. Examine the issues to address in minority health-promotion activities.
6. Contrast urban and rural community health-care needs and resources.
7. Identify the role for professional nurses in community and public health initiatives.

Key Terms

Healthy People 2000

Priority Areas

Health Promotion
   Strategies

Health Protection
   Strategies

Preventive Services

Healthy Communities

Healthy People 2010

Focus Areas

Leading Health Indicators

Aging Adults

Disability

Chronicity

Minority Health

Urbanized Area

Rural Area

Rural Health

Community Health Nursing

Two major community health initiatives began in the last decades of the 20th century in the United States: Healthy People and Healthy Communities. The focus became one for the health of the nation as a whole through concentration on wellness and healthful initiatives for the next century. A strategic planning process began to create 10-year objectives for disease prevention and health promotion. For *Healthy People 2000* (U.S. Department of Health and Human Services [USDHHS], 1992) "specificity of particular objectives for groups at higher risk had been part of the design . . . [with objectives] delineated far more extensively than were the 1990 objectives according to demographic and socioeconomic dimensions of risk" (p. vii). This focus continued as a national commitment with *Healthy People 2010*, which was introduced to the nation on January 25, 2000. *Healthy Communities* was designed to help implement these objectives in community settings. We now see that healthy behaviors and prevention are vital for individuals, families, and society.

As a corollary to this movement, we have also seen a greater focus on consumer and public protection. In 1998, the President's Advisory Commission on Consumer Protection and Quality in the Healthcare Industry presented a final report with more than 50 objectives identified to address problem areas, including avoidable errors, both underutilization and overuse of services, and variation in services. Measures proposed to strengthen the health-care industry included use of group purchasers, having informed consumers with access to services, accountability, reducing errors and increasing safety, and addressing the needs of vulnerable populations. Sources of vulnerability were identified as economic status and geographic location; health, age, and functional or developmental status; communication barriers; and unexplained vulnerability associated with race, ethnicity, and sex (The President's Advisory Commission on Consumer Protection and Quality in the Health Care Industry, 1998, pp. 130–132). At the end of the 20th century and into the next decade, the focus on patient safety was highlighted further with the subsequent Institute of Medicine (IOM) reports on the current state of health care for consumers and calls for safety improvements.

The nation's population profile is changing. We are older and more diverse. Although we remain a youth-oriented society, the aging of the "baby boomers" has a profound effect on the demographics and the health needs of the population. In addition, we are indeed becoming more culturally diverse and must endeavor to celebrate, respect, and embrace our differences while eliminating health disparities. Professional nursing practice has a vital role in promoting health and health initiatives and in eliminating health disparities.

HEALTHY PEOPLE 2000

In **Healthy People 2000**, three general goals were stated as national health promotion and disease prevention objectives:

- Increase the span of healthy life for Americans
- Reduce health disparities among Americans
- Achieve access to preventive services for all Americans. (USDHHS, 1992, p. 6)

This initiative took a major step in that it did not merely look at the health of the nation, but rather, it devised strategies for improvement. The outcome was the specification of 22 **priority areas** for health promotion and disease prevention. For each priority area, the workgroup formulated objectives with specific targets to measure success in addressing the three major goals. The priority areas were further classified as health promotion, health protection, and preventive services. Recall the discussion on levels of prevention (primary, secondary, and tertiary) in Chapter 5. The terminology from *Healthy People 2000* (USDHHS, 1992) identified **health promotion strategies** as individual lifestyle and personal choices. Health promotion activities are both protective and preventive, but they require consumers to be actively involved in all levels of prevention. **Health protection strategies** consist of environmental or regulatory measures that confer protection on population groups. **Preventive services** comprise counseling, screening, immunization, and chemoprophylactic interventions. The 22 priority areas, along with a summary of the outcomes, are listed in Table 16–1. The initiative also looked at specific age groups (infants, children, adolescents and young adults, adults, and older adults) and special populations (low-income, minorities, and people with disabilities) in order to address specific health promotion and disease prevention efforts within these divergent groups. Consider the trends found with this national health initiative.

Infants

Healthy People 2000 outcomes demonstrated a dramatic decline in the infant mortality rate. This decline placed the United States at a rank of 25th lowest in the ranking among developed nations in infant mortality (National Center for Health Services [NCHS], 1999b). Although maternal and infant health was ranked 14th in importance among the 22 priority areas, continued attention was needed in this area to maintain the decline in infant mortality and morbidity.

Children 1 to 14 Years of Age

Mortality rates in children met the *Healthy People 2000* objective. In fact, the rates surpassed the year 2000 target. Childhood deaths from drowning and fire

Table 16.1

Healthy People 2000: Priority Areas for Health Promotion and Disease Prevention

Category & Priority Area	Findings*
	Health Promotion
1. Physical Activity and Fitness	Decline in coronary death rates *Problem areas:* Overweight prevalence and lack of progress in physical activity
2. Nutrition	Progress toward targets *Problem areas:* Overweight prevalence, calcium consumption, and iron deficiency
3. Tobacco	Progress demonstrated *Problem area:* Smoking cessation attempts decreased among pregnant women
4. Alcohol and Other	Drugs/alcohol-related MVA and cirrhosis deaths decreased *Problem areas:* Marijuana use in adolescents and cirrhosis deaths in selected minority groups increased
5. Family Planning	Pregnancy, birth, and abortion rates for adolescent females declined *Problem area:* Hispanic adolescent pregnancy rates increased
6. Mental Health and Mental Disorders	Decline in suicide rate and increased use of community support services *Problem area:* Increased proportion of people who do not take steps to reduce stress
7. Violent and Abusive Behaviors	Decline in suicide, firearm death, and homicide rates *Problem areas:* Increase in child abuse and neglect
8. Educational and Community-Based Programs	Increase in average number of years of healthy life and greater access for preschool children *Problem area:* Previous declines in healthy life between 1990 and 1994
	Health Protection
9. Unintentional Injuries	Increased use of seat belts and fire and drowning deaths were below baseline *Problem areas:* MVA crash and alcohol-related deaths declined below the baseline data, but remained above the target
10. Occupational Safety and Health	Decline in work-related injuries and injury deaths and cases of hepatitis B *Problem areas:* Leading causes of work-related injury deaths were highway crashes and homicides
11. Environmental Health	Decline in the number of waterborne disease outbreaks *Problem areas:* Increased awareness needed of presence and dangers of radon
12. Food and Drug Safety	Decline in outbreaks of *Salmonella* *Problem area:* Reporting of serious adverse events to the Food and Drug Administration (FDA) declined

(Table continues on page 292)

Table 16.1	

Healthy People 2000: Priority Areas for Health Promotion and Disease Prevention (continued)

Health Protection	
13. Oral Health	Decline in oral cancer mortality rates and increased use of oral health-care system *Problem areas:* Dental caries, gingivitis, and tooth loss in adults and screening of children prior to entry in school
Preventive	
14. Maternal and Infant Health	Decline in infant mortality and hospitalization for severe complications in pregnancy *Problem areas:* Increase in fetal alcohol syndrome, infant neural tube diseases related to low folic acid intake, and low/very low birthweight births
15. Heart Disease and Stroke	Decline in mortality from heart disease and stroke, yet higher among African Americans *Problem areas:* Increase in end-stage renal disease and obesity
16. Cancer	Declines in mortality from lung, female breast, and colorectal cancer *Problem areas:* Data and actions needed on limitations to sun exposure
17. Diabetes and Chronic Disabling Conditions	Declines in activity limitations due to chronic conditions, asthma, and sensory impairments *Problem areas:* Increase in rates of activity limitation due to chronic back conditions and increase in diabetes prevalence and mortality, especially in selected minority groups
18. HIV Infection	Decline in the number of diagnosed AIDS cases and prevalence of HIV *Problem areas:* Increased AIDS incidence rates for African American, female, and Hispanic populations
19. Sexually Transmitted Diseases	Lowest rates for primary and secondary syphilis; repeat gonorrhea rate met Y2K objective; and improvement in pelvic inflammatory disease, gonorrhea, chlamydia, and hepatitis B rates *Problem area:* Clinician counseling is declining
20. Immunization and Infectious Diseases	Vaccination levels in children at the highest level recorded and incidence of vaccine-preventable diseases low *Problem areas:* Continued monitoring and measures of infectious diarrhea incidence
21. Clinical Preventive Services	Increase in the average number of years of "healthy life" and in the number of adults with a specific source of primary health care *Problem area:* Financial barriers to receipt of clinical preventive services
Other	
22. Surveillance and Data Systems	*Impression:* "Public health and surveillance is the systemwide collection, analysis, and use of health information" (NCHS, 1999a, p. 217).* *Problem area:* Consistency in measurement and collection of data nationwide

Key: AIDS, acquired immunodeficiency syndrome; FDA, U.S. Food and Drug Administration; HIV, human immunodeficiency virus; MVA, motor-vehicle accident; Y2K, year 2000.
*Data and quote from National Center for Health Statistics. (NCHS). (1999a). *Healthy People 2000 review, 1998–99.* Hyattsville, MD: Public Health Service.

diminished, as did the incidence of nonfatal poisonings and activity limitations due to otitis media as a result of this national initiative. Another good finding in the progress report was the increased use of child restraint systems in motor vehicles. However, a continued problem area was the asthma hospitalization rate for children, which was still above the baseline rate and was identified as a major cause of morbidity.

Adolescents and Young Adults Ages 15 to 24 Years

Death rates in this age group declined in the 1990s, meeting the year 2000 target. Still, the leading causes of death for adolescents and young adults were motor-vehicle accidents, other unintended injuries, homicide, and suicide. The proportion of students who participated in daily school physical education had not improved despite the potential for obesity implicit in a sedentary lifestyle. In addition, after a marked decline in heavy drinking reported in high school students, there was a slight increase, although the rate was still near the target. Mixed trends were noted for adolescent substance abuse. Rates of suicide, physical fighting, and weapon carrying by adolescents declined and were moving toward the targets. The prevalence of *Chlamydia trachomatis* also decreased in female adolescents and young adults.

Adults 25 to 64 Years

Although the 2000 target was not met, the mortality rate in adults declined. Mortality rates from cancer dropped below the year 2000 target, related to the declines in deaths from breast, colorectal, and lung cancers. Mixed trends were reported for the incidence of nonfatal work-related injuries. Although a decline in nonfatal work-related injuries has been reported in some professions and occupations, the rate for nursing and personal-care workers moved away from the target and was higher than those for all other work areas reported.

The Aging Population

The leading causes of mortality in the aging population were heart disease, cancer, stroke, chronic obstructive pulmonary disease, diabetes, and unintentional injuries or accidents. Although limited data were available, the aging population (70 years and older) demonstrated an increase in difficulty performing two or more personal-care activities, with a 16% increase overall and a 31% increase in African Americans during the 1990s (NCHS, 1999a, p. 17). In 1994, 54 million people in the United States, or roughly 21% of the population, had some level of disability (USDHHS, 2000a, p. 15). In 2004, although 2% of the adult population in the United States (approximately 3.7 million people)

required the help of another person with activities of daily living and 7.6 million (4%) required help with instrumental activities such as household chores or shopping, these percentages in the population aged 75 and older rose to 10% and 19% respectively (Adams & Barnes, 2006, p. 12). Mortality from motor-vehicle accidents and falls rose, especially in the older aging population. Although more of the aging population was involved in health-promotion activities, as with influenza immunizations, mammograms, and Papanicolaou tests, a serious challenge existed in activities of daily living with advanced longevity. Visual and hearing impairments were also documented.

Selected Population Groups

Healthy People 2000 focused also on health disparities and demonstrated that a disparity existed between African Americans and the overall population with respect to average life expectancy (USDHHS, 1995). African Americans were found to have a significantly lower life expectancy (USDHHS, 2000a, p. 12). Disparities also included differential rates in infant mortality, receipt of prenatal care, maternal mortality, homicides, acquired immunodeficiency syndrome (AIDS), lung cancer, breast cancer, coronary heart disease, diabetes complications and related deaths, and immunizations. Elimination of these health disparities became a major initiative in *Healthy People 2010*.

For Native Americans and Alaskan natives, seven health areas were highlighted: alcoholism and substance abuse, child and family violence, diabetes, women's health, the health of the elderly, maternal and child health, and injuries. The report made particular mention of the variable infant mortality rates, with some areas below the national average and some significantly higher. Violence and injuries represented another area of particular risk for these populations, although more than half of the objectives specific to this minority group were progressing toward the year 2000 objective.

Asian Americans and Pacific Islanders were found to have a higher life expectancy than the population as a whole. Several health problems were particularly noteworthy for these groups, however. Although rates of cerebrovascular diseases were rising in this group, cancer was the leading cause of death for Chinese, Korean, and Vietnamese population groups. In addition, tuberculosis incidence demonstrated a slight increase, remaining well above both the year 2000 objective and its prevalence in the total population.

It was estimated that by 2010, Hispanic Americans would be the largest minority group in the United States. This group is also the largest uninsured group. Particular areas of concern included infant mortality rates, prenatal care, and receipt of preventive health screenings and care. Other areas in which this population failed to meet

Healthy People objectives were obesity, adolescent pregnancies, homicides, diabetes, and human immunodeficiency virus (HIV) and AIDS.

People with Disabilities

In 1994, 54 million people in the United States, or roughly 21% of the population, had some level of disability (USDHHS, 2000a, p. 15). The two leading causes of disability (nonfatal head and spinal-cord injuries) declined, whereas other conditions that led to disability increased, including fetal alcohol syndrome, visual impairments, asthma, and complications of diabetes. The study revealed an escalating relationship between lower incomes, limitations in activity, and chronic conditions.

People with Low Income

Several areas were of particular concern in the lower-income population, including prenatal care, birth weight, food security, health-care visits, immunizations, insurance coverage and health screenings, perceived health status, activity limitations, and mortality rates. Higher levels of education were associated with greater levels of prenatal care and higher birth weights of infants. People with low income had lower levels of health insurance, perceived health status, and activity. They also had a higher mortality rate.

HEALTHY COMMUNITIES

The American Public Health Association (APHA) (1991) published *Healthy Communities 2000: Model Standards* to assist planners in adapting the *Healthy People 2000* objectives to the needs and resources of individual communities. The conceptual basis of **Healthy Communities** included the following:

- Emphasis on health outcomes
- Flexibility as a planning tool
- Focus placed on the entire community
- Governmental presence at the local level
- Importance of negotiation to maintain local flexibility
- Standards (uniform objectives) and guidelines (local adaptations)
- Accessibility of services
- Emphasis on programs. (APHA, 1991, pp. xvii–xix)

The *Healthy People 2000* priority areas and objectives were reprinted in the document, accompanied by a model standards goal that provided flexible, practical guidance for achieving the objectives. A table format was used for identification of the focus area, objectives, and indicators for an outcome measurement. Blanks were included in the objectives and guidelines to allow planners to tailor them to their local communities. The indicators promoted consistent measurement across communities. By the final review point for *Healthy People 2000*, most states, the District of Columbia, and Guam had statewide objectives, some with comprehensive strategic plans and assessment projects that addressed the objectives. The strategic planning process continued in 2001 with a look to 2010, and ultimately, the publication of a revised resource to address the newer national initiatives in *Healthy People 2010*.

HEALTHY PEOPLE 2010

The prevention agenda for the nation and the associated objectives for the next decade were introduced in January 2000 as **Healthy People 2010** (USDHHS, 2000a) with two major goals:

- To increase the quality and years of healthy life
- To eliminate health disparities

Notice that these two objectives were more aggressive than the 2000 objectives. For instance, *Healthy People 2000* sought to reduce health disparities, whereas *Healthy People 2010* plans to eliminate them. Building upon *Healthy People 2000*, *Healthy People 2010* specified 28 **focus areas** containing objectives and targets specified for the nation (Table 16–2) to address the specific trends of the decade, such as diversity and the aging population. *Healthy People 2010* used a systematic approach to health improvement guided by a model with four key elements: goals, objectives, determinants of health, and health status. The objectives are to "focus on the determinants of health, which encompass the combined effects of individual and community physical and social environments and the policies and interventions used to promote health, prevent disease, and ensure access to quality health care" (USDHHS, 2000a, p. 7).

Specific objectives in each focus area were designed to address the health initiative as subgoals under the direction of a lead government agency. Objectives were both measurable (with specific set targets for which data are tracked) and developmental (for which no baseline data was available). For example, the focus area of health communications contains six objectives (Box 16–1). The first, "Increase the proportion of households with access to the Internet at home," is measurable because there was baseline information that 26% of homes had Internet access in 2000 (USDHHS, 2000a, pp. 11–13). The

ONLINE CONSULT

Healthy People 2010 at
http://www.healthypeople.gov

Table 16.2

Healthy People 2010: Focus Areas with Midcourse Review

Focus Area	Care Components	Objectives*
Access to Quality Health Services	Clinical preventive care Primary care Emergency services Long-term care & rehabilitative services	3 (Recommended deletion 1-2) 6 5 2
Arthritis, Osteoporosis, and Chronic Back Conditions	Arthritis Osteoporosis Chronic back conditions	8 (Revisions proposed to all 8) 2 1
Cancer	—	15 (One recommended revision)
Chronic Kidney Disease	—	8 (One recommended revision)
Diabetes	—	17 Recommended deletion of 5-8 & 5-9 and revision to 5-11)
Disability and Secondary Conditions	—	13 (Revisions to 6)
Educational and Community-Based Programs	School setting Worksite setting Healthcare setting Community setting and select populations	4 (One recommended revision) 2 3 (Proposed deletion of all 3) 3 (Revisions to 2)
Environmental Health	Outdoor air quality Water quality Toxics and waste Healthy homes and healthy communities Infrastructure & surveillance Global environmental health	4 (One recommended revision) 6 (Revisions to 3) 5 (One recommended revision) 8 (Revisions to 5) 5 (Recommended deletion of 8-28 and revisions to 4) 2
Family Planning	—	13 (Revisions to 4)
Food Safety	—	7 (Recommended deletion of 10-7 and revisions to 4)
Health Communication	—	6 (Revisions to 2)
Heart Disease and Stroke	Heart disease Stroke Blood pressure Cholesterol	6 (Revisions to 4) 2 (One recommended revision) 4 4 (One recommended revision)
HIV	—	17 (Recommended deletion of 13-7,9,10 & 12, and revisions to 5) & objective moved here from STD focus group

(Table continues on page 296)

Table 16.2		

Healthy People 2010: **Focus Areas with Midcourse Review** (continued)

Focus Area	Care Components	Objectives*
Immunization and Infectious Diseases	*Diseases preventable through:* ■ Universal vaccination ■ Targeted vaccination Infectious diseases and emerging antimicrobial resistance Vaccination coverage and strategies Vaccine safety	 5 3 13 (Recommended deletion of 14-15 and revisions to 4) 8 (Revisions to 4) 2 (One recommended revision)
Injury and Violence Prevention	Injury prevention Unintentional injury prevention Violence and abuse prevention	12 (One recommended revision) 19 (Revisions to 3) 8
Maternal, Infant, and Child Health	Fetal, infant, and child deaths Maternal death and illnesses Prenatal care Obstetrical care Risk factors Developmental disabilities and neural tube defects Prenatal substance exposure Breastfeeding, newborn screening and service systems	3 2 (One recommended revision) 2 (One recommended revision) 2 4 3 (One recommended revision) 2 (One recommended revision) 5 (Revisions to all 5)
Medical Product Safety	—	6 (Recommended deletion of 17-3 and revisions to 3)
Mental Health and Mental Disorders	Mental health status improvement Treatment expansion State activities	5 (Revisions to 4) 6 (Revisions to all 6) 3 (One recommended revision)
Nutrition and Overweight	Weight status and growth Food and nutrient consumption Iron deficiency and anemia Schools, worksite, and nutrition counseling Food security	4 7 3 3 (Recommended deletion of 19-15) 1
Occupational Safety and Health	—	11 (Revisions to 2)
Oral Health	—	17 (Revisions to 3)
Physical Activity and Fitness	Physical activity in adults Muscular strength/endurance and flexibility Physical activity in children and adolescents Access	3 2 6 (One recommended revision) 4 (One recommended revision)

(Table continues on page 297)

Table 16.2

Healthy People 2010: Focus Areas with Midcourse Review (continued)

Focus Area	Care Components	Objectives*
Public Health Infrastructure	Data and information systems	7 (Recommended deletion of 23-1 & 5 and revisions to 2)
	Workforce	3 (Revisions to all 3)
	Public health organizations	5 (Revisions to all 5)
	Resources	1 (Recommended deletion of 23-16)
	Prevention research	1 (One recommended revision)
Respiratory Diseases	Asthma	8 (Revisions to 3)
	COPD	2
	Obstructive sleep apnea	2 (Recommended deletion of 24-12)
Sexually Transmitted Diseases	Bacterial STD illness/disability	3 (Revisions to 2)
	Viral STD illness & disability	2 (One recommended revision)
	STD complications (females)	3 (25-8 moved to HIV focus area)
	STD complications (fetus & newborn)	2 (Recommended deletion of 25-10)
	Personal behaviors	2 (Recommended deletion of 25-12 and revisions to 1)
	Community protection infrastructure	3 (Recommended deletion of 25-14 & 15)
	Personal health services	4 (Recommended deletion of 25-17, 18 & 19 and revisions to 1)
Substance Abuse	Adverse consequences of substance use and abuse	8 (Revisions to 2)
	Substance use and abuse	7 (Revisions to 4)
	Risk of substance use and abuse	2 (One recommended revision)
	Treatment for substance abuse	4 (Revisions to 3)
	State and local efforts	4 (One recommended revision)
Tobacco Use	Tobacco use in population groups	4 (Revisions to 3)
	Cessation and treatment	4 (One recommended revision)
	Exposure to secondhand smoke	5 (Revisions to 2)
	Social and environmental changes	8 (Revisions to 4)
Vision and Hearing	Vision	10 (Revisions to 9)
	Hearing	8 (Recommended deletion of 28-15 and revisions to 6)

Key: COPD, chronic obstructive pulmonary disease; STD, sexually transmitted disease.
* Midcourse Review recommendations are included in parentheses in column 3.
Sources:
U.S. Department of Health and Human Services. (2000c). Tracking Healthy People 2010. Washington, DC: U.S. Government Printing Office. Retrieved August 22, 2006, from http://www.healthypeople.gov/Document/tableofcontents.htm#acking
U.S. Department of Health and Human Services. (2006c). Healthy People Midcourse Review. Retrieved August 22, 2006, from http://www.healthypeople.gov/data/midcourse/

remaining five objectives were developmental in nature, because data was only to be collected and baseline data did not yet exist. Availability of data and interagency collaboration were essential components of this aggressive project to address the health of the nation. This national initiative was an evidence-based approach to addressing the two major goals for a healthier nation.

Midcourse Review Healthy People 2010

The Midcourse Review of Healthy People 2010 was conducted in 2005 on the status of the objectives and was based on public comments and expert evaluation of the data, apparent trends. and emerging knowledge.

Box 16.1 *Healthy People 2010* Focus Area: Health Communications

Goal: Use communication strategically to improve health.
Lead Agency: Office of Disease Prevention and Health Promotion.
- Increase the proportion of households with access to the Internet at home.
- Improve the health literacy of persons with inadequate or marginal literacy skills.
- Increase the proportion of health communication activities that include research and evaluation.
- Increase the proportion of health-related World Wide Web sites that disclose information that can be used to assess the quality of the site.
- Increase the number of centers for excellence that seek to advance the research and practice of health communication.
- Increase the proportion of persons who report that their health-care providers have satisfactory communication skills.

Source: U.S. Department of Health and Human Services. (2000a). Healthy People 2010: Volume I (2nd ed.). Retrieved August 15, 2006, from *http://www.healthypeople.gov/Document/HTML/Volume1/11HealthCom.htm*

As illustrated in Table 16–2, objectives were revised, clarified, and some recommended for deletion if there was not a valid data source. For some developmental objectives, researchers established targets because data were now available for baselines and the objectives could now be measured and tracked. For example, the developmental objective 24–5 on reducing the number of school or work days missed by persons with asthma due to asthma now had an established baseline of about six days for persons aged 5 to 64 years, with a target set to reduce the days to two by 2010 (USDHHS, 2006a).

Other developmental objectives were dropped when no data source could be established, as with the objective to increase the number of state prison systems that provide comprehensive education on sexually transmitted diseases. Some developmental objectives were retained if the data source was identified and the objective clarified with the potential for measurement prior to 2010, as with the objective for reducing the proportion of females with human papillomavirus (HPV) infection (USDHHS, 2006b). Other objectives and subobjectives were retained and were being measured or had revisions in language, baselines, or targets in order to ensure that *Healthy People 2010* remained current and relevant for improving the health of the nation (USDHHS, 2006c).

Reducing health disparities involves addressing the needs of individuals or groups at risk. The needs of these at-risk populations are identifiable in the focus areas and objectives to be addressed. The demographic characteristics identified and targeted for action included: gender, age, race and ethnicity, income and educational level, disability, geographic location, and sexual orientation.

Leading Health Indicators

A component of the *Healthy People 2010* document was the identification of **leading health indicators**

(Box 16–2). "The leading health indicators reflect the major public health concerns in the United States and were chosen based on their ability to motivate action, the availability of data to measure their progress, and their relevance as broad public health issues" (USDHHS, 2000a, p. 24). These 10 indicators, linked to the *Healthy People 2010* objectives, have the ability to provide a "snapshot" at a point in time by which to view the health of the nation. These indicators were intended to "illuminate individual behaviors, physical and social environmental factors, and important health-system issues that greatly affect the health of individuals and communities [and] underlying each of these indicators is the significant influence of income and education" (USDHHS, 2000a, p. 24).

Physical Activity

Although the benefits of physical activity have been demonstrated, sedentary lifestyles are common in the United States, which is a major public health concern. This health indicator targeted perceived barriers to regular, moderate physical activity and sought to prevent

Box 16.2 *Healthy People 2010*: Leading Health Indicators

- Physical activity
- Overweight and obesity
- Tobacco use
- Substance abuse
- Responsible sexual behavior
- Mental health
- Injury and violence
- Environmental quality
- Immunization
- Access to health care

conditions associated with lack of activity. Disparities have been identified with gender, age, race, educational level, geography, and socioeconomic status. At-risk groups are females, the elderly, African Americans, Hispanics, low-income individuals, the disabled, and individuals in the southern and northeastern states (USDHHS, 2000b).

Overweight and Obesity

Increasing trends and associated conditions like heart disease, diabetes, and other chronic illnesses can be directly attributed to overweight and obesity. The interaction with physical activity is evident. The "balance between energy intake and output is influenced by metabolic and genetic factors as well as behaviors affecting dietary intake and physical activity; environmental, cultural, and socioeconomic components also play a role" (USDHHS, 2000b, p. 19–4). Disparities have been reported both within and among population groups related to gender, race, ethnicity, and socioeconomic status. Obesity and overweight have become more and more of a concern in children and adolescents. Objectives in both this area and under physical activity are directed at these population groups.

Tobacco Use

The use of tobacco, whether by smoking, chewing, or exposure to secondary smoke in the physical environment or in utero, has long been associated with serious complications and consequences. Objectives addressed use of specific products in selected groups, cessation efforts, secondhand exposure, and needed social and environmental changes for limitations or cessation in select populations. Disparities exist by age, gender, race and ethnicity, socioeconomic status, educational level, and geography. Several refinements to the objectives, subobjectives, and baseline data were made for this indicator at the Midcourse Review, as with revisions of data sources or elimination of subobjectives due to unreliable sources for data.

Substance Abuse

As a leading health indicator, substance abuse is also an influence on many of the other health indicators and focus areas. Substance abuse represents more than the use of illicit drugs; it includes adverse drug consequences like motor-vehicle and other accidents, domestic violence, intentional or unintentional overdoses, experimentation with other substances, bingeing, lost productivity, and associated conditions. Substance abuse crosses all ages, genders, racial and ethnic groups, regions, educational levels, and socioeconomic groups. In *Healthy People 2010*, it was reported that "alcohol is the most

commonly used substance, regardless of race or ethnicity" (USDHHS, 2000b, p. 26–6). Revised baselines and targets for adolescents were made at the Midcourse Review, reflecting measurability and relevance of this indicator.

Responsible Sexual Behavior

In *Healthy People 2010*, sexually transmitted diseases (STDs) were described as "common, costly, and preventable" (USDHHS, 2000b, p. 25–7). Although they exist in all gender, racial, ethnic, and socioeconomic groups, differences in responsible sexual behaviors have been identified within and among groups that can be used as targets for intervention activities in the stated objectives. An increase in responsible sexual behaviors is the marker to reduce the incidence and complications of STDs. Several developmental objectives were deleted for this indicator at the Midcourse Review and refinements in others have been based on data and current trends. For example, the objective for a reduction in the proportion of cases of human papillomavirus (HPV) infection was made specific to *females* rather than *humans,* as more became known about data sources and the infection.

Mental Health

"Mental health is a state of successful performance of mental function, resulting in productive activities, fulfilling relationships with other people, and the ability to adapt to change and to cope with adversity" (USDHHS, 2000b, p. 18–3). Although differences have been identified within and among groups, "mental disorders occur across the lifespan, affecting persons of all racial and ethnic groups, both genders, and all educational and socioeconomic groups" (USDHHS, 2000b, p. 18–3). Comorbidities and secondary problems are vital considerations for this indicator, as are treatment opportunities. The Midcourse Review resulted in revised data, objectives, and targets for this indicator, including a focus on the homeless. New targets aimed at treatment rather than merely the identification of the proportion of the homeless who are identified with serious mental health problems.

Injury and Violence

Objectives related to this leading health indicator call for the reduction in injuries, disabilities, and deaths related to injury and violence. *Healthy People 2010* noted that "although the greatest impact in injury is human suffering and loss of life, the financial cost is staggering [including costs of] . . . direct medical care and rehabilitation as well as lost income and productivity" (USDHHS, 2000b, p. 15–4). In addition, disparities in rates of injuries by age, racial and ethnic group, and economic status have been noted. The four developmental objectives for this indicator were now measurable and provided with baseline data and targets at the Midcourse Review, as with bicycle helmet use and protective equipment in school sports activities.

Environmental Quality

The environmental quality indicator addresses air and water quality and toxic influences in homes, at worksites, and in the community to promote public health and protection. "Potential risks include indoor air pollution; inadequate heating, cooling, and sanitation; structural problems; electrical and fire hazards; and lead-based paint hazards" (USDHHS, 2000a, p. 8–7). Individuals of certain races and socioeconomic status have been identified as being at greater risk. The Midcourse Review provided data enhancement and refinement, as with the measurability that became available for fish contamination in the nation's lakes and rivers, providing baseline and target data.

Immunization

Infectious diseases increased over the last decade. Strategies in this area include vaccination recommendations and programs, both universal and targeted, as well as concentrating on selected infectious processes and antimicrobial resistance. Particular at-risk populations were identified related to age, ethnicity and race, and geography. Updated information on tuberculosis, hospital-acquired infections, and immunization recommendations arose at the Midcourse Review.

Access to Quality Health-Care Services

Consider the implications of this leading health indicator and its target of 100% health insurance coverage by 2010. The objectives for this indicator address clinical preventive care, primary care, emergency services, and long-term care and rehabilitative services. Disparities have been monitored during the data collection process, with initiatives in place to address the target goals. At the June 2002 progress review, lower levels of insurance were noted in the Latino, Native American, and Alaskan Native populations. Lower levels of health insurance and ongoing sources of care were also noted in populations with lower levels of family income and education. Racial and ethnic representation in the health professions is also under study with this objective, as a component of cultural competence. Little change has been demonstrated, with minority underrepresentation persistent in the health professions. In *Healthy People 2010* (USDHHS, 2000a), access to quality health-care services is viewed through selected indicators that are considered "predictors" of availability and acceptability of quality services. These indicators or predictors include having health insurance, having a regular provider of ongoing care, and the use of prenatal care as a preventive service (USDHHS, 2000a).

A Work in Progress

At the local levels, *Healthy Communities 2010* is involved with initiatives and data collection. States have initiated *Healthy People 2010* plans specific to their population and geography. For example, Alaska has implemented a Talking Circle; Arizona has 12 Focus Areas; Michigan is concentrating on 25 specific Focused Indicators; and Vermont has come up with specific Goals of Healthy Vermonters.

At the national level, ongoing collaboratives to address the public's health continued. For example, preventing medication errors is an issue related to prevention of injury and is included in the focus area of medical product safety. Consider the objectives in Box 16–3 relative to client safety. Following an act of the United States Congress, the Centers for Medicare and Medicaid Services (CMS) sponsored a study by the IOM that was released in July 2006 with the aim of developing a national agenda for reducing medication errors in hospitals, long-term care and ambulatory-care facilities, and in community and home settings (Aspden, Wolcott, Bootman, & Cronenwett, 2006). Activities to address error reduction and adverse drug events address the *Healthy People 2010* goals to eliminate health disparities and increase the quality and years of healthy life. These activities are especially important in light of our aging population and attendant health challenges.

OUR AGING POPULATION

The term *healthy life* applies not only to longevity but also to functional independence and the perception of healthy days. The three major causes of death in people 65 years and older are heart disease, cancer, and stroke. Consider the life expectancy trends reported in Table 16–3. Although life expectancies for both men and women have increased, the 10 to 13 years of functional health and independence after age 65 are less than the 15 to 19 actual remaining years of life. In addition, disparities exist by gender and race. On the other hand, trends in limitation of activities of daily living have declined a little, especially for those **aging adults** 65 years and older living in the community (NCHS, 2006).

The difference between healthy life and unhealthy life is the loss of independence in activities of daily life and increasing dependence on others.

Goal: Ensure the safe and effective use of medical products.

17–1. Increase the proportion of health-care organizations that are monitoring and analyzing adverse events associated with medical therapies within their systems.

17–2. Increase the proportion of health-care providers and organizations that are using information technology.

17–4. Increase the proportion of patients receiving information that meets guidelines for usefulness when their new prescriptions are dispensed.

17–5. Increase the proportion of patients who receive verbal counseling from prescribers and pharmacists on the appropriate use and potential risks of medications.

Note: Objective 17–3 was proposed for deletion due to lack of data source and 17–6 was related to blood donations.

Source: U.S. Department of Health and Human Services. (2006c). Healthy People Midcourse Review. Retrieved August 22, 2006, from *http://www.healthypeople.gov/data/midcourse/*

Table 16.3

Life Expectancy (in Years) at Birth, 65, and 85 Years of Age, by Decade

	1900	1950	1970	1990	2000	2002
At birth	47.3	68.2	70.8	75.4	76.9	77.3
At 65 years	11.9	14.1	15.0	17.3	17.9	18.2
At 85 years	—	—	5.3	6.2	6.3	6.5

Source: National Center for Health Statistics. (2006). Data Warehouse on Trends in Health and Aging. Retrieved August 23, 2006, from *http://www.cdc.gov/nchs/agingact.htm*

The percentage of the population aged 65 years and older has been steadily increasing. Proportional changes have been dramatic. In fact, the population 85 years and older grew more than 500% from 1950 to 1990. According to the 2000 U.S. Census, there were 35 million Americans aged 65 and older, and the projections are that this number will grow to 71.5 million in 2030, with the number of people aged 85 and older expected to rise from 4.2 million in 2000 to almost 21 million in 2030 (Federal Interagency Forum on Aging-Related Statistics, 2006). Despite Medicare coverage, this population of aging Americans is experiencing differences in health-care purchasing power and socioeconomic status. The affordability of health care and medications is a serious concern to our aging population. Consider the following information reported by the Administration on Aging (AOA) (2005):

About 3.6 million elderly persons (10.2%) were below the poverty level in 2003. . . . Another 2.3 million or 6.7% of the elderly were classified as "near-poor" (income between the poverty level and 125% of this level). One of every 12 (8.8%) elderly Whites was poor in 2003, compared to 23.7% of elderly African Americans, 14.3% of

Asians, and 19.5% of elderly Hispanics. Higher than average poverty rates for older persons were found among those who lived in central cities (13.1%), outside metropolitan areas (i.e., rural areas) (11.0%), and in the South (11.9%). (p. 1)

The difference between healthy life and unhealthy life is the loss of independence in activities of daily life and increasing dependence on others for health and routine care. We now see chronic illness rather than acute illness as the major morbidity factor in aging adults. Prevention of disability and promotion of independent functioning are essential and can be aided by healthy behaviors such as smoking cessation, good nutrition, reduction of sodium intake and body weight, reduction in social isolation, regular physical activity, and availability of primary health-care services.

Approximately one-third of people hospitalized are older than 65 years. In the acute-care setting, the average length of stay for individuals over 65 years was 5.8 days compared with 4.8 days for individuals of all ages (AOA, 2005, p. 12). Even though the average length of hospital stays has shortened, those older than 65 years require a great proportion of our health-care resources, both in and out of the acute-care setting. With projections for a dramatic increase in the older population and the associated health-care costs, several national projects have been initiated to promote healthy lifestyles and lifestyle changes for seniors (Box 16–4). As noted by the director of the Centers for Disease Control and Prevention (CDC) (2006b), "the prevention of disease and injury is one of the few tools available to reduce the expected growth of health-care and long-term care costs" (p. 1). For example, think about safety with medications (availability, administration, and interactions) and in the prevention of falls and the associated cost factors.

Theories on and Types of Aging

With the focus on health promotion and quality of life for the growing aging population and the entry of "baby boomers" into this category, research has evolved in several disciplines, all proposing different theories on aging. No agreement on a specific theory has emerged. Research continues, and our knowledge of the aging process grows with biologic, sociologic, psychological, longevity, medical, and nursing theories on aging. For example, *medical theories* highlight disease-related influences on physiologic functioning of the person, while nursing theories propose functional consequences in which age-related changes and age-related factors are the risk factors.

Interestingly, aging has also been classified as successful, usual, or pathologic (Rowe & Kahn, 1987). In *successful aging*, there is a positive interaction between the individual's genes and the environment. Such an interaction results in no serious detriment in functioning from the middle 20s until the early 70s. Minimal measurable changes in functioning are seen, with these individuals as the energetic and functional "survivors" in aging. Successful agers represent only about 5% to 10% of the population. These individuals are the aging "stars" we aspire to be—those active, energetic, and involved elders we revere, admire, or respect.

Usual aging occurs in the vast majority of individuals. With usual aging we observe an interaction between the person's genetic endowment and their environment. A neutral or negative environment has positive or neutral

genes. Think about diet, cholesterol, and heredity, and individual differences for the person as affected by heredity and the unique environment. This raises concern for the reversible risk factors that occur with aging. The gene-environment interaction leads to obvious functional limitations, but the limitations are not serious enough to affect activities of daily living (ADLs) as long as the person makes compromises and adaptations. An example is the person whose mobility is limited but who adjusts to the limitation and is still able to live independently without assistance in daily life. With usual aging, we may also see genetic diseases, but again, adaptations are made that do not significantly interfere with independent daily functioning. This is the quality of life focus for the increasing numbers of aging adults.

At the opposite extreme is *pathologic aging*. Here we see a negative interaction between genetic and environmental factors. Some combination of negative or neutral influences arises from both the individual's genes and the environment. We often see clinical evidence of genetic diseases in these aging individuals. This gene-environment interaction leads to serious functional limitations for the individual, such as being unable to take care of personal needs, inability to perform ADLs, and sometimes the ability to sustain life. These functional limitations require substantial intervention. Prevention of disabilities and quality of life issues in this population are the focus of healthy initiatives.

Characterizing Aging Americans

We have acknowledged that aging adults represent a growing segment of our population, especially those 85 years and older and those who are members of minority groups. As these population proportions increase even more, we will need to consider individual differences, needs of age groups, cultural and ethnic trends, and changing family patterns. Intergenerational issues will involve more than children, parents, grandparents, and great-grandparents. Consider the complexity of a family with two or three older adult groups, those in their middle to late 60s, 80s, and 100s, as well as the family members younger than age 60. The concern also arises as to who will be the caregiver for the frail older adult. Will the 80-year-old be caring for a frail spouse as well as a 99-year-old mother, or will the 60-year-old be caring for both the 80-year-old parents and the 99-year-old grandmother and perhaps be the head of the household also caring for grandchildren? Older women are expected to continue to outnumber men by at least three to two, according to life expectancy projections.

Residential Changes

Living arrangements are an important factor for aging adults. Most aging adults live in the community, usually

---

Box 16.4　Strategies For Health Promotion of Older Adults

- Healthy lifestyles
- Early detection of disease
- Immunization
- Self-management techniques for chronic diseases

Source: Centers for Disease Control and Prevention. (2006b). Healthy aging: Preventing disease and improving quality of life among older Americans—at a glance 2006. Retrieved August 15, 2006, from *http://www.cdc.gov/nccdphp/aag/aag_aging.htm*

with a spouse, alone, or with adult offspring. The proportion of people older than 65 who are living in nursing homes is less than 5%. And approximately 30%, or 9.7 million aging adults, live alone in the community (AOA, 2006, p.1). Decisions about living arrangements should include considerations for optimal promotion of functional independence and health. Opportunities for social interactions and access to resources and caregivers, when needed, are vital considerations.

Various housing options are considered by aging adults. In our more mobile society, being tied to a homestead may no longer be preferable, especially for urban and younger aging adults. Retirement planning may include relocating to a more temperate climate or closer to grandchildren. Instead of the large family home, smaller detached homes, condominiums, town homes, gated retirement communities, continuing care communities, assisted-living apartments, senior homes, and group homes are options, depending on needs, affordability, and accessibility. In addition, a frail elder may relocate again to live with a child or other relative after the death of the spouse, sale of the retirement home, or growing loss of functional independence.

Physical Changes

Characteristics of aging adults continue to be as varied as the individuals themselves. Aging adults come with years of unique experiences that have molded their psychosocial profile. Physically and physiologically, aging adults also differ in development and progression of age-related changes. Aging is progressive and irreversible, but the manner in which these changes occur is variable. Appearance changes and motor activities slow down. But things do not stop without some disease process. Aging adults are more susceptible to disease and environmental factors. Maintaining homeostasis is more difficult.

Age-related changes occur in biologic systems. Skin becomes less elastic. Sweat glands, temperature receptors, pigment, and subcutaneous fat decrease. This makes the aging adults more susceptible to temperature extremes (cold and hot), sunlight, and injury. Other senses are affected by aging as well. Visual and hearing acuity diminish. Adaptation of the lens and ocular muscles decreases, with a decrease in depth perception. Glare and driving at night become stressful, especially if the aging person looks at oncoming headlights. The home environment must be well illuminated, but with nonglare lights. For example, reducing the glare with fluorescent lights can also lower the chance of accidents, especially falls. Print may need to be larger and bolder. Eye examinations are important. The loss of the driver's license may be devastating to an aging person, even if his driving is limited.

Moreover, muscle mass and strength decrease, and joints may be stiff with arthritis. Muscle mass may be replaced with connective tissue. Osteoporosis occurs with calcium losses and hormonal changes, and worsens with inactivity. Low-impact, isometric, and routine exercises can prevent further immobility and loss of function. Digestion and slower motility are improved with small meals. Food may taste and smell bland. Herbs and seasoning can be used, but one must beware of hidden sodium content.

Changes in level of consciousness and delirium are not normal signs of aging. Neurologic changes do occur but may indicate an underlying pathology or drug interaction. As noted in *Healthy People 2010* (USDHHS, 2000b), "in later life, the majority of people aged 65 years and older cope constructively with the changes associated with aging and maintain mental health, yet an estimated 25% of older people (8.6 million) experience specific mental disorders, such as depression, anxiety, substance abuse, and dementia, that are not part of normal aging" (USDHHS, 2000b, pp. 18–3, 18–4). These possibilities should always be investigated further with referrals. Time rather than loss should be the first thought with the delays that may happen; it may take a little more time to remember something, but that does not mean that the memory is lost.

Sexuality and sexual intercourse continue, but adaptation may be needed as well, such as more time for arousal, excitement, and foreplay, or lubrication for vaginal dryness. Impotence should be evaluated for pathology or possible drug side effects. Counseling, erectile aids, reduction in alcohol consumption, and changes in medications all are possible treatments. Sexual activity need not stop because of advancing age, although partner availability may become an issue.

Major Health Problems of Aging Adults

Chronic illness and frailty are primary concerns of aging adults and their health-care professionals. Diseases common to aging include:

- Osteoporosis
- Diabetes
- Stroke
- Depression
- Arthritis
- Alzheimer's disease
- Cancer
- Cardiovascular disease

In 2004, 22.4% of older persons between 65–74 assessed their health as fair to poor, but this number rose for those between 75–84 years (30.4%) and those 85 years and older (35.2%) in the overall population, with little difference between men and women over

65 years (NCHS, 2006). But definite differences among minority older persons were noted in their self-report for these same age groups. Consider the fair-to-poor perceptions of those individuals aged 75–84 years who were African Americans (42.9%) or Hispanic (44.8%) (NCHS, 2006). In addition, older individuals living in the community increasingly report limitations of daily activities as a result of at least one chronic illness—with 18.2% of those 85 and older needing assistance with personal-care needs (NCHS, 2006).

Consider the difference between chronicity and disability. **Disability** is the inability to do something because of a physical or mental impairment. **Chronicity** is related to duration or recurrence of a condition. The individual may have a chronic condition but with healthy behaviors can limit, delay, or prevent disability. Hence, health-promotion behaviors and empowerment of the individual are essential for taking charge of one's own life. Unlike the irreversible normal changes of aging, risk factors can be reduced and in some cases eliminated.

Risks in aging adults include physical, environmental, psychosocial, and chemical factors. *Physical risks* affect the biologic system and related physiologic function. Examples of physical risks are limitations in flexibility leading to falls and vision changes, resulting in automobile accidents. *Environmental risks* can be natural or artificial. Natural environmental risks include ultraviolet radiation and weather extremes. Examples of artificial or human-made environmental risks are air quality, hazards in housing, and poor maintenance of equipment or the environment. *Psychosocial risks* are a part of everyday life, whether the aging person is isolated or active. Stress levels from illness of self, family members, or friends take an increasing toll on the individual. An inward focus on problems may make the aging person more egocentric and, as a result, more isolated. To address these risks, the special needs of aging adults should be considered.

Needs of Aging Adults

The major needs of aging adults roughly parallel the leading health indicators in *Healthy People 2010*. Longevity factors that have been supported by research include genetics, gender, environment, physical activity, alcohol consumption, sexual activity, nutrition, and social factors (such as economics, marital status, and family), religious beliefs, purpose in life, and laughter. Positive behaviors must be directed at promoting and maintaining health and functional independence and at reducing risk factors. The aging adult also requires access to affordable health care, including transportation and acceptability of the provider to the person.

Family needs and issues are another consideration. Given the proportion of aging adults living in the community and projections for population increases, especially in the group 85 years and older, family needs are a major issue in health-promotion and care activities. Much can be found in the literature about family decisions for nursing home placement and the "sandwich generation" of caregivers. But recall that only a small proportion of older adults live in institutional settings, the great majority being cared for in the community. In addition, consider the projected increase in number of aging adults in minority groups and the importance of the extended family in some groups. Likewise, the growing older population stretches available health-care resources, placing a strain on society as a whole.

Lay Caregivers

The fact is that caring for a frail older adult takes a major toll on the caregiver and the family. The number of informal and family caregivers exceeds 23 million nationwide, most of them women caring for relatives, adult children with disabilities, or their grandchildren. The physical and emotional toll on the caregiver can be enormous while the caregiver continues maintaining other family, social, work, and personal obligations. The physical and emotional strains on the caregiver often compromise her health. Financial and economic difficulties can compound the strain on the caregiver.

The concept of respite care, to give the caregiver a break, is ideal but is not always perceived as available, affordable, or even emotionally acceptable. Regardless, the caregiver will need some form of respite, and this must be determined, sought, and used regularly. The reauthorization of the Older Americans Act in 2000 supported demonstration projects on caregiving and authorized the National Family Caregiver Support Program. This program provides support and resources at the state and local levels for informal caregivers providing care for their older relatives or adults with disabilities. A user-friendly Web site is available to provide information on resources and demonstration projects and support for both caregivers and professionals. Note the 10 caregiver survival tips identified by the Support Program listed in Box 16–5. Legislation has been proposed offering tax

ⓞNLINE ⒸONSULT

National Family Caregiver Support Program at
http://www.aoa.gov/prof/aoaprog/caregiver/caregiver.asp

FMLA 29CFR825, The Family and Medical Leave Act of 1993 at
http://www.dol.gov/esa/regs/statutes/whd/fmla.htm

Box 16.5 Caregiver Survival Tips

- Plan ahead.
- Learn about available resources.
- Take one day at a time.
- Develop contingency plans.
- Accept help.
- Make YOUR health a priority.
- Get enough rest and eat properly.
- Make time for leisure.
- Be good to yourself!
- Share your feelings with others.

Administration on Aging. (2004). National family caregivers support program resource room. Retrieved on August 14, 2006, from *http://www.aoa.gov/prof/aoaprog/caregiver/carefam/taking_care _of_others/survival_tips.asp*

benefits for lay care of elders. In addition, family leave through the Family and Medical Leave Act (FMLA) also addresses the need for care of spouses and parents with serious health conditions.

Societal Needs

Societal needs and issues are another consideration for aging adults. Public policy issues include the availability and allocation of health-care resources for aging adults as well as the use of these resources. Some people contend that aging adults are using the vast majority of the health-care resources with their chronic health problems. Focusing on the prevention of these health problems in the "baby boomers" is critical.

Health-care legislation and financing for aging adults occur mainly through the Social Security amendments and budget reconciliation acts, which include Medicare and Medicaid funding. With Medicaid, the role, legislation, and funding levels fall within the domain of the state of residence. But what about part-time residents who spend half the year in a state in which they do not claim primary residence? What about the issue of reverse migration of frail aging adults who, after years of retirement in a satisfactory condition in one state, lose a spouse and become increasingly frail, move to be cared for by their children? Their affluence was spent somewhere else, but when they move near the children, the new community must absorb the cost of chronic health conditions and increasing frailty. Similar situations can have great impact on society and health-care resources.

Elder Abuse

Another area of concern at the individual, family, and societal levels is elder abuse. This includes physical neglect or violence, verbal abuse, psychological or emotional abuse, financial exploitation, and sexual abuse. It may be intended or unintended in active or passive actions of the abuser. Those aging individuals most at risk are the frail elderly who are functionally impaired and depend on others. In fact, the National Center on Elder Abuse (2005) has reported that elder abuse perpetrators are family members, men and women, most often the victim's adult child or spouse. The elders may be in dysfunctional family situations or even in nursing homes, but they often fear being alone more than the abuse or neglect they are experiencing. Assessment, reporting, education, and counseling are responsibilities of health-care providers and members of society. Elder abuse has also been related to caregiver stress. Special efforts being made to address this growing problem include the Older Americans Act and other national legislation for awareness and outreach.

Elder abuse is only one aspect of the broader domestic violence problem in this country. The frail elder is certainly not the only one affected by abuse or violence in the environment. Spouses, parents, and

Elder Abuse

If you suspect that an older person is being abused or neglected, you must call the adult protective services of the state where the elder is located. Proof is not required and calls made are confidential. Some states have separate reporting lines for domestic versus institutional elder abuse. Access the agency to contact in your state at *http://www.elderabusecenter.org/default.cfm?p= statehotlines.cfm*

ⓞ N L I N E ⓒ O N S U L T

Administration on Aging at
http://www.aoa.gov

National Family Caregiver Support Program at
http://www.aoa.gov/prof/aoaprog/caregiver/ caregiver.asp

National Association of State Units on Aging at
http://www.nasua.org

American Society on Aging at
http://www.asaging.org

National Center on Elder Abuse at
http://www.elderabusecenter.org/default .cfm

National Domestic Violence Hotline at
http://www.ndvh.org

significant others are all considerations in cases of domestic violence. In fact, estimates of domestic abuse in America range from 960,000 incidents of violence against a current or former spouse, boyfriend, or girlfriend per year to 3 million women who are subjects of physical abuse annually (National Domestic Violence Hotline, 2006, p.1).

MINORITY HEALTH

In pursuit of the goal to eliminate health disparities, *Healthy People 2010* identified the following demographic groups within which health disparities occur: gender, race or ethnicity, education or income, disability, geographic location, and sexual orientation. In the area of race or ethnicity, *Healthy People* proposed that the identified disparities were "the result of the complex interaction among genetic variations, environmental factors, and specific health behaviors" (USDHHS, 2000a, p. 12). The following disparities between White and minority populations were documented:

- Higher infant mortality rates for African Americans, Native Americans, and Alaskan Natives
- Higher incidence of cancer and heart disease for African Americans
- Higher mortality from HIV/AIDS for African Americans
- Increased diabetes-related deaths for Hispanic Americans and a higher incidence of diabetes for Native Americans and Alaskan Natives
- A higher incidence of hypertension and obesity in Hispanic Americans
- High death rates from unintentional injuries and suicide for Native Americans and Alaskan Natives
- High rates of tuberculosis in Hispanics, Asians, and Pacific Islanders
- High rates of hepatitis in Asians and Pacific Islanders. (USDHHS, 2000a, p. 12)

Clearly, the reasons for the occurrence of the health disparities among ethnic groups are multifaceted and complex and the focus of many different initiatives to address the national goals. A large focus of **minority health** is on the special needs of groups characterized by race or ethnicity. The Office of Minority Health of the CDC (2007a) classifies racial or ethnic minority populations as follows:

- American Indian and Alaskan Native
- Asian
- Black or African American
- Hispanic or Latino
- Native Hawaiian and other Pacific Islander

In a 2001 study conducted by the Commonwealth Fund, racial and ethnic disparities were documented further in the areas of insurance coverage, health perceptions, incidence of and mortality from chronic conditions, and higher utilization of emergency services and no source of regular care (Collins et al., 2002, p. 39). In a further study on racial and ethnic data-collection processes, however, the researchers concluded, "minority data collection and reporting was inconsistent and sometimes contradictory" (Perot & Youdelman, 2001, p. 24). Stabilization was recommended. And we continue to investigate the issues and differences among population groups and the needs of the members. The Commonwealth Fund has identified that racial and ethnic disparities exist in numerous areas of diagnosis, treatment, and preventive care (even when income, insurance status, and other socioeconomic factors are held constant). California, Florida, and Louisiana have been the most active in dealing with minority health issues through statutes (Gamble et al., 2006, p. 2) to address their large aging populations.

Addressing the Disparities

Plans are ongoing to address current and emerging minority issues in order to achieve the goal of elimination of health-care disparities. Federal, state, and local initiatives are actively focusing on the needs of the nation. In 1999, Congress (Public Law 106–129) directed the Agency for Healthcare Research and Quality (AHRQ) to examine priority populations, including minority groups, low-income groups, women, children, the elderly, individuals with special needs, and rural residents. In their 2005 report, AHRQ (2005) noted four major themes: disparities still exist, some disparities are diminishing, opportunities remain for improvement, and that the information on disparities is improving (p. 3).

In 2000, Congress passed the Minority Health and Health Disparities Research and Education Act (Public Law 106–525) establishing the National Center on Minority Health and Health Disparities under the National Institutes of Health (NIH). The NIH, along with its Specialty Institutes and Centers, has integrated this initiative to eliminate health disparities into the strategic plans for the various agencies, including the National Institute of Nursing Research. Initiatives continue to address not only health habits and access to care but also provider-client interactions in their research support.

In 2003, the Kaiser Family Foundation, the Robert Wood Johnson Foundation, and national heart organizations, in response to a meta-analysis research on disparities in cardiac care in different population groups, led a national initiative entitled *Why the Difference* for physician outreach about racial and ethnic disparities in medical care. This research reviewed prior rigorous studies in the literature and documented evidence of racial or ethnic differences in cardiac care, with African Americans less likely to receive certain procedures and care than their White counterparts despite similar patient characteristics (Lillie-Blanton, Rushing, Ruiz, Mayberry, & Boone, 2002). Mixed findings were reported for Hispanic patients.

Health-care providers and communities must address the documented disparities. Doing so requires an understanding of the evidence and the people. Consider the documented increased infant mortality rate in the African-American population. The CDC's Office of Minority Health has developed a fact sheet to encourage health providers and communities to promote healthy behaviors during the prenatal period in order to address the complications of pregnancy that are more prevalent in minority populations and also to promote the reduction in cases of sudden infant death syndrome (SIDS) (Box 16–6) (Office of Minority Health, 2006c). Other similar fact sheets on areas of health disparities are also available (see Online Consult). Nevertheless, delivery of health-care services to specific minority populations such as the Alaskan Native and Hispanic/Latino groups is influenced by the availability, accessibility, and acceptability of services. Difficulty with communication and other problems may hamper acceptance of early prenatal care or access. Acceptability of services may be limited by the clients' health-care beliefs and practices or other factors. Continuing development in cultural competence is essential for the nurse to address minority health-care disparities. A major resource for health-care professionals can be the faith community specific to the particular minority population.

The projection for an increase in minority populations necessitates immediate action for the health of the nation. Improved data collection has been designed for enhanced practice based on better evidence. Initiatives for cultural

ONLINE **C**ONSULT

Access the following Fact Sheets from the CDC Office of Minority Health on

Cancer
Cardiovascular Disease
Diabetes
HIV/AIDS
Immunizations
Infant Mortality
Mental Health
Tuberculosis
Lupus at
http://www.cdc.gov/omhd/AMH/dbrf.htm

competence in the current health-care system, improved communication, and greater diversity of health-care providers are designed to address existing disparities and perceived quality of care and health status. As the Office of Minority Health (2006b) has stated, "culturally appropriate, community-driven programs are critical for eliminating racial and ethnic disparities in health" (p. 1). Collaborative efforts are growing at the national, state, and local levels. Consult the resources listed in the Online Consult to examine current initiatives and progress on the goal for the elimination of health disparities.

RURAL HEALTH

Geographic location was also identified in *Healthy People 2010* as a demographic characteristic for which definable health disparities exist. Until recently, there

Box 16.6 Fact Sheet on Efforts to Reduce Infant Mortality

- Encourage health behaviors: early and regular prenatal care, good nutrition.
- Advise clients about factors that affect birth outcomes, such as maternal smoking, drug and alcohol abuse, stress, chronic illness, or other medical problems.
- Parents and caregivers should place sleeping infants on their backs and reduce bed sharing.

Adapted from Office of Minority Health, CDC. (2006c). Eliminate disparities in infant mortality. Retrieved August 24, 2006, from *http://www.cdc.gov/omh/AMH/factsheets/infant.htm*

ONLINE **C**ONSULT

The Commonwealth Fund at
http://www.cmwf.org

The Kaiser Family Foundation at
http://www.kff.org/whythedifference/about.htm

CDC Office of Minority Health at
http://www.cdc.gov/omh

Health Resources and Services Administration at
http://www.hrsa.gov

Office of Minority Health at
http://www.omhrc.gov

National Institutes of Health at
http://www.nih.gov

was no predominant definition of *rural*. It has been defined in several ways in the literature and at the federal level. The divergent definitions impeded research and policy-making. Most definitions have been based on population or population density of a specified area. In 2002, new criteria based on the 2000 Census were released, defining an **urbanized area** as a central city with a densely populated surrounding area of 50,000 or more. **Rural areas** are defined as areas with a population of less than 2500.

Certain health problems have been identified as particular to people living in rural areas. In fact, *Healthy People 2010* characterizes **rural health** issues as follows:

> Twenty-five percent of Americans live in rural areas, that is with fewer than 2500 residents. Injury-related death rates are 40 percent higher in rural populations than in urban populations. Heart disease, cancer, and diabetes rates exceed those for urban areas. People living in rural areas are less likely to use preventative screening services, exercise regularly, or wear seat belts. In 1996, 20 percent of the rural population was uninsured compared with 16 percent of the urban population. Timely access to emergency services and the availability of specialty care are other issues for this population group. (USDHHS, 2000a, p. 16)

Further complicating matters is the fact that rural communities may share some features but are not all the same. For example, characteristics and problems of rural residents in south Georgia may be quite different from those of rural residents in Montana or New Mexico. It is important to be aware that the large majority of rural residents are not farmers. But for those who are, agriculture is a dangerous occupation with great risk of injury and illness, even for their children.

The National Advisory Committee on Rural Health and Human Services (2003) has characterized the differences between health care in urban and rural areas in terms of scope and scale as follows:

> The urban setting features a high volume of patients with an emphasis on technology-intensive and inpatient services. The rural setting focuses more on ambulatory care and features a much lower patient volume. Rural health-care systems tend to take care of more elderly patients and patients with more advanced or chronic conditions possibly due to the delays in getting health care. Rural residents, particularly those located in more isolated and sparsely populated communities, have higher risk factors than the general population. Rural areas also face greater shortages of health-care providers . . . [and] reimbursement for

providers who practice in rural areas tends to be less than their urban counterparts. (p. 6)

Health issues are of vital concern to this committee that has been commissioned through 2007. The Committee's 2006 report focused on the rural implications of health-information technology, access to pharmacy and pharmaceutical services, and family caregiver support for the rural elderly. The Committee's 2007 goals are directed at Medicare, Head Start, and substance abuse in rural communities (National Advisory Committee on Rural Communities, 2006a, 2006b).

The rural health literature addresses a variety of problems. Two recurring concerns seem to predominate: chronic illness (particularly in the elderly) and inadequate prenatal care. Just consider the issue of access in rural areas, especially with challenges related to reliable transportation, limitations in activities of daily living secondary to a chronic illness, and cost factors with additional child care or loss of income from time off work. Information from the 2000 Census indicates a growth in minority population in rural areas, particularly Hispanic and Latino. Not surprisingly, rural growth also was higher in the more temperate climate areas of the South and the West. Demographic factors such as age, gender, race and ethnicity, socioeconomic status, and educational level are all considerations when rural geography and health status are investigated.

Delivery of health-care services in rural communities is heavily influenced by the availability, accessibility, and acceptability of services. Rural communities have fewer health-care resources. Distance, lack of communication, and other problems may hamper access. Acceptability of services may be limited by the clients' health-care beliefs and practices or other factors. In addition, the rural community health nurse may well be the only health professional in the community, working with very limited resources. Rural residents tend to be religiously and politically conservative, self-sufficient, and wary of outsiders (especially urbanites). Thus, the community health nurse cannot expect to rush eagerly into a rural community with good intentions and gain immediate acceptance. Building rapport with residents of a rural community takes time, and showing respect for their values and beliefs is imperative. In other words, the nurse must be sensitive and must demonstrate cultural competence. A further challenge is presented when the rural residents are also members of an ethnic group that is different from that of the nurse. The rural community health nurse must beware of assuming that these clients (and their problems) are the same as those of their urban counterparts. Their ruralism may be as significant as their ethnic identity.

RURAL HEALTH CLINICS

Under Public Law 95–210, Rural Health Clinics (RHCs) were established to provide primary-care services for residents of medically underserved areas. These clinics are located as permanent facilities or mobile units throughout the nation, with many staffed with advanced practice nurses (APRNs). The clinics are certified by the Centers for Medicare and Medicaid (CMS) and have required staffing and specified reimbursement components. Federal legislation has also created the Federally Qualified Health Center (FQHC) program, which includes the Migrant Health Center (MHC) and Community Health Center (CHC) programs funded under the Public Health Service Act to provide primary care for medically underserved rural populations. Agencies receiving funding under the FQHC program must provide primary health-care services for all age groups including diagnostic and lab, pharmacy, preventive health and dental, transportation, case management after hours care, hospital/specialty care, and emergency medical services either onsite or through provider arrangements. The MHC program is limited to migrant farm workers and their families. The RHC Program requires similar primary health-care services, but pharmacy, preventive health and dental, transportation, case management, and after hours care are not requirements of the program.

In 2000, reimbursement for care under Medicaid was changed from cost-based to a prospective payment system (PPS) developed exclusively for RHCs and FQHCs. This gave states greater flexibility to create new payment mechanisms (USDHHS, HRSA, 2006, p. 5). Further information on payment systems is provided in Chapter 19. In addition, in 2002 RHCs and FQHCs could be designated as health professional shortage area (HPSA) facilities with the opportunity for additional resources.

Reimbursement

Reimbursement policy is a major issue for providers of rural health care. Although some improvements have occurred, especially in designated health professional shortage areas, urban health-care providers are reimbursed by Medicare at a higher rate than rural providers. And states direct Medicaid reimbursements, so these vary. An important consideration is economy of scale, in that certain key services must be available despite the low volume of service in rural health-care agencies compared with their urban counterparts. Home health care is also more costly in the rural area because of low volume and longer travel distances.

Telecommunication

The use of telecommunications technology in health care (*telemedicine* or *telehealth*) has greatly increased in recent years. It is being used extensively in some areas to enhance care of rural residents, as with a specialist at an urban medical center consulting on a patient in a remote rural area via telecommunications. This is also occurring globally, providing consultations, preparation of imaging, or interpretation of findings. There is a tremendous potential for greater access with telemedicine, but it is not without problems. Issues such as reimbursement, liability, and credentials and licensure must be addressed.

The *Rural Healthy People 2010 Project* was developed as a research effort to identify disadvantages and disparities in rural communities and to address the priority health concerns of rural America with featured practice models (Gamm, Hutchinson, Dabney, & Dorsey, 2003a, 2003b). As with the national *Healthy People 2010* initiative, data collected through this project will provide a better understanding of the rural population and its risk factors and will facilitate movement toward the national goals.

COMMUNITY NURSING IN THE CONTEXT OF HEALTHY PEOPLE

The nature of nursing practice in the community is different, dynamic, and responsive. Community health

ONLINE CONSULT

National Rural Health Association at
http://www.nrharural.org

Rural Health Research Gateway database at
http://www.ruralhealthresearch.org/

Rural Healthy People 2010 at
http://www.srph.tamhsc.edu/centers/ rhp2010/publications.htm

National Advisory Committee on Rural Health and Human Services at
http://ruralcommittee.hrsa.gov/ nacpubs.htm

Migrant Health Care Program at
http://bhpr.hrsa.gov/kidscareers/ migrant_program.htm

Economic Research Service, USDA at
http://ers.usda.gov/emphases/rural/

nursing crosses age, demographic, and specialty groups. The client for the community health nurse may be the person, the family, or even the entire community. **Community health nursing** is built upon the principles of nursing and public health, with the broader focus on the client in the context of his environment for health promotion and illness treatment and prevention. Community health nursing crosses many traditional boundaries, is holistic, and is not limited to a particular age group, diagnostic category, or narrow set of specialized skills. Although clients include individuals and families, community health nursing may have a group or even an entire community as a client. Clients may be well or ill. Their health risks or needs may be either physical or mental in nature. In addition, spiritual needs are also a consideration, especially with parish or faith-based nursing care.

Several factors determine the roles, activities, and intervention strategies of an individual community health nurse, working in the context of *Healthy People*:

- Mission, philosophy, and priorities of the employing agency
- Level of prevention at which intervention is aimed
- Definition of client

The mission, philosophy, and priorities of a private agency or a faith-based organization can be quite different from those of an official government agency. The level of funding influences how well the agency is able to implement its priorities, which should be based on identified health needs in the community.

Another factor that influences the functions for the community health nurse is the agency's level of prevention focus. Community health nurses are involved in all three levels of prevention. Historically, however, these nurses have played a key role in primary prevention efforts. For more than 100 years they have been involved in health promotion and disease prevention. Over the past years, and despite initiatives like *Healthy People*, these traditional services have suffered under-

reimbursement, with health departments compelled to provide more direct clinical services. Consequently, many public health nurses have taken on a role that is more illness-oriented. Nevertheless, *Healthy People* priorities clearly reflect a need for community health nurses, especially those in public health agencies, to renew and strengthen their role in primary prevention.

Community health nursing is frequently described in the literature as a synthesis of nursing and public health. Public health is unique because it broadens concerns to the "public" with a population and collaborative focus. The mission of the Public Health Nursing Section of the APHA is "to enhance the health of population groups through the application of nursing knowledge to the community" (American Public Health Association, 2006, p. 1). In published standards of public health, the American Nurses Association (1999), in collaboration with several other public health nursing organizations, identified eight tenets of public health nursing and defined the practice as "promoting and protecting the health of populations using knowledge from nursing, social, and public health sciences" (p. 1). Clearly, an interdisciplinary focus is necessary to address the health of the community and the people who make up that community. One important consideration, as mentioned in *Healthy People*, is the environmental concerns that affect the health of the community.

Challenges exist in many areas for professional nursing practice as we address the health needs of at-risk populations. Whether talking about the aging member of a minority population, the well elder in the community, the rural child with asthma, or the individual with diabetes, health professionals focus on increasing years of healthy life and the elimination of health disparities.

INTERACTIVE EXERCISES

Go to the Intranet site and complete the interactive exercises provided for this Chapter.

EVIDENCED-BASED PRACTICE: CONSIDER THIS . . .

*E*zenwa, Ameringer, Ward, and Serlin (2006) examined the research literature on racial and ethnic disparities in pain management. As a professional you realize that pain, as the fifth vital sign, requires effective pain assessment and management for positive client outcomes. Although these researchers found limitations in the published studies of ethnicity and pain management, they did document that disparities persist in pain management and that non-white individuals in the United States are "short-changed in the advances that have been made in pain management" (p. 232).

Question: How will you use this information as a nurse or nurse-manager to eliminate health disparities?

Source: Ezenwa, M. O., Ameringer, S., Ward, S. E., & Serlin, R. C. (2006). Racial and ethnic disparities in pain management in the United States. *Journal of Nursing Scholarship, 38,* 225–233.

KEY POINTS

■ *Healthy People 2000* addressed three general goals as national health promotion and disease prevention objectives, with a focus on specific age groups and special populations in 22 priority areas.

■ *Healthy People 2010* built upon the information from the prior decade but was developed with the two major goals of increasing the quality and years of healthy life and eliminating health disparities. It uses a framework of 28 focus areas, 467 objectives, and 10 leading health indicators.

■ Leading health indicators reflect the major public health concerns in the nation: physical activity, overweight and obesity, tobacco use, substance abuse, responsible sexual behavior, mental health, injury and violence, environmental quality, immunization, and access to care.

■ Proportional increases in the population of aging adults are predicted, with the greatest increase in those 85 years and older. Women currently account for a large proportion of this group. Predictions include an increase in minority groups represented in our aging population.

■ Chronic illnesses and increasing frailty are the major causes of morbidity in aging adults. Disability is the inability to do something because of a physical or mental impairment. Chronicity is related to duration or recurrence of a condition.

■ Aging adults face physical, environmental, psychosocial, and chemical risk factors. The risks commonly affect many aging adults, creating conditions that interfere with activity. Health-promotion activities are vital in this area to maintain functional ability and reduce the incidence of frailty and disability.

■ Evidence that health disparities exist among ethnic groups of all ages has been documented; however, reasons for their occurrence are multifaceted and complex. Minority health is an important initiative for the health of the nation.

■ The CDC's Office of Minority Health (2007a) classifies racial or ethnic minority populations as: American Indian and Alaskan Native, Asian, Black or African American, Hispanic or Latino, and Native Hawaiian and other Pacific Islander.

■ In 2002, new criteria based on the 2000 Census were released, defining an urbanized area as a central city with a densely populated surrounding area of 50,000 or more. Rural areas are generally defined as areas with a population of less than 2500.

■ Rural health clinics (RHCs) have been established to provide primary care services for residents of underserved areas. Federal legislation has also created the Community Health Center (CHC) and Migrant Health Center (MHC) programs to provide primary care for medically underserved rural populations. In 2002, reimbursement for care was changed to a PPS specific to these clinics and the services provided.

■ Community health nursing is frequently described in the literature as a synthesis of nursing and public health. The mission of the Public Health Nursing Section of the APHA has as its mission "to enhance the health of population groups through the application of nursing knowledge to the community" (American Public Health Association, 2007, p. 1).

Thought and Discussion Questions

1. Consider a goal of *Healthy People 2010, which is* "to increase the quality and years of healthy life." Be prepared to share your impressions on achievement of this national goal in a discussion to be scheduled by your instructor.

2. The second goal set for *Healthy People 2010* was for the elimination of health disparities. Be prepared to participate in a discussion to be scheduled by your instructor to share your impression on achievement of this goal in the area of minority health care.

3. Review the Chapter Thought located on the first page of the chapter, and discuss it in the context of this chapter.

☐ REFERENCES

Adams, P. F., & Barnes, P. M. (2006). Summary health statistics for the U.S. population: National health interview survey, 2004. National Center for Health Statistics. Vital Health Statistics 10(229). Retrieved December 11, 2006, from *http://www.cdc.gov/nchs/data/series/sr_10/sr10_229.pdf*

Administration on Aging (AOA). (2004). Caregiver survival tips. National Family Caregivers Support Program Resource Room. Retrieved on August 14, 2006, from *http://www.aoa.gov/prof/aoaprog/caregiver/carefam/taking_care_of_others/survival_tips.asp*

Administration on Aging (AOA). (2005). A profile of older Americans: 2005. Retrieved August 24, 2006, from *http://www.aoa.gov/PROF/Statistics/profile/2005/profiles2005.asp*

Administration on Aging (AOA). (2006). A statistical profile of older Americans 65+. Retrieved August 24, 2006, from *http://www.aoa.gov/PRESS/fact/pdf/Attachment_1304.pdf*

Agency for Healthcare Research and Qualitty (AHRQ). (2005). National healthcare disparities report. Retrieved August 24, 2006, from http://www.ahrq.gov/qual/Nhdr05/fullreport/Index.htm

American Nurses Association. (1999). *Scope and standards of public health nursing practice* (Publication No. 9910PH). Washington, DC: American Nurses Publishing.

American Public Health Association (APHA). (1991). *Healthy communities 2000: Model standards: Guidelines for community attainment of the year 2000 objectives.* Washington, DC: American Public Health Association.

American Public Health Association (APHA). (2007). Public health nursing section. Retrieved on October 4, 2007, from *http://www.apha.org/membergroups/sections/aphasections/phn/about/*

Aspden, P., Wolcott, J., Bootman, J. L., & Cronenwett, L. R. (Eds.). (2006). *Preventing medication errors.* Washington, DC: National Academies Press.

Centers for Disease Control and Prevention (CDC). (2006a). Healthy aging: Preventing disease and improving the quality of life among older Americans 2006. Retrieved August 24, 2006, from *http://www.cdc.gov/nccdphp/publications/aag/pdf/aag_aging2006.pdf*

Centers for Disease Control and Prevention (CDC). (2006b). Healthy aging: Preventing disease and improving quality of life among older Americans—at a glance 2006. Retrieved August 15, 2006, from *http://www.cdc.gov/nccdphp/aag/aag_aging.htm*

Collins, K. S., Hughes, D. L., Doty, M. M., Ives, B. L., Edwards, J. N., & Tenney, K. (2002). *Diverse communities, common concerns: Assessing health-care quality for minority Americans.* New York: The Commonwealth Fund.

Federal Interagency Forum on Aging-Related Statistics. (2006). Older Americans update 2006: Key indicators of well-being. Retrieved August 24, 2006, from *http://www.agingstats.gov/agingstatsdotnet/Main_Site/Default.aspx*

Gamble, V. N., Stone, D., Ladenheim, K, Gibbs, B. K., et al. (2006). Special Issue: Comparative perspectives on health disparities. *Journal of Health Politics, Policy and Law, 31*(1). Retrieved August 24, 2006, from *http://www.cmwf.org/publications/publications_show.htm?doc_id=368671*

Gamm, L. D., Hutchinson, L. L., Dabney, B. J., & Dorsey, A. M. (Eds.). (2003a). *Rural Healthy People 2010: A companion document to Healthy People 2010* (Volume 1). College Station, TX: Texas A&M University System Health Science Research Center. Retrieved August 15, 2006, from *http://www.srph.tamhsc.edu/centers/rhp2010/publications.htm*

Gamm, L. D., Hutchinson, L. L., Dabney, B. J., & Dorsey, A. M. (Eds.). (2003b). *Rural Healthy People 2010: A companion document to Healthy People 2010* (Volume 2). College Station, TX: Texas A&M University System Health Science Research Center. Retrieved August 15, 2006, from *http://www.srph.tamhsc.edu/centers/rhp2010/publications.htm*

Lillie-Blanton, M., Rushing, O. E., Ruiz, S., Mayberry, R., & Boone, L. (2002). *Racial/ethnic differences in cardiac care: The weight of the evidence.* Menlo Park, CA: Kaiser Family Foundation. Retrieved August 15, 2006, from *http://www.kff.org/whythedifference/6040fullreport.pdf*

National Advisory Committee on Rural Health and Human Services. (2003). Health care quality: The rural context. Retrieved August 24, 2006, from *http://ruralcommittee.hrsa.gov/QR03.htm*

National Advisory Committee on Rural Health and Human Services. (2006a). News and updates from the national advisory committee. Retrieved August 24, 2006, from *http://ruralcommittee.hrsa.gov/nacupdat.htm*

National Advisory Committee on Rural Health and Human Services. (2006b). *The 2006 report to the secretary: Rural health and human services issues.* Retrieved on August 14, 2006, from *ftp://ftp.hrsa.gov/ruralhealth/NAC06forweb.pdf*

National Center for Health Statistics. (NCHS). (1999a). *Healthy People 2000 review, 1998–99.* Hyattsville, MD: Public Health Service.

National Center for Health Statistics (NCHS). (1999b). Healthy People 2000: Maternal and infant health progress review. Retrieved on August 14, 2006, from *http://www.cdc.gov/nchs/about/otheract/hp2000/childhlt/childhlt.htm*

National Center for Health Statistics (NCHS). (2006). Trends in health and aging. Retrieved on August 23, 2006, from *http://www.cdc.gov/nchs/agingact.htm*

National Center on Elder Abuse. (2005). FAQs about elder abuse. Retrieved on August 24, 2006, from *http://www.elderabusecenter.org/default.cfm?p=faqs.cfm#five*

National Domestic Violence Hotline. (2006). Support the National Domestic Violence Hotline. Retrieved on November 18, 2006, from *http://www.ndvh.org/support/index.html*

Office of Minority Health, CDC. (2007a). About OMHD. Retrieved October 4, 2007 from *http://www.cdc.gov/omhd/About/about.htm*

Office of Minority Health, CDC. (2006b). Disease burden and risk factors. Retrieved on August 14, 2006, from *http://www.cdc.gov/omh/AMH/dbrf.htm*

Office of Minority Health, CDC. (2006c). Eliminate disparities in infant mortality. Retrieved August 15, 2006, from *http://www.cdc.gov/omh/AMH/factsheets/infant.htm*

Perot, R. T., & Youdelman, M. (2001). *Racial, ethnic, and primary language data collection in the health care system: An assessment of federal policies and practices.* New York: The Commonwealth Fund.

The President's Advisory Commission on Consumer Protection and Quality in the Health Care Industry. (1998). *Quality first: Better health care for all Americans* (Final report to the President of the United States). Columbia, MD: Consumer Bill of Rights.

Rowe, J. W., & Kahn, R. L. (1987). Human aging: Usual and successful. *Science, 237,* 143–149.

U.S. Department of Health and Human Services (USDHHS). (1995). Healthy people 2000: Midcourse review and 1995 revisions. Retrieved August 15, 2006, from *http://odphp.osophs.dhhs.gov/pubs/hp2000/midcrs1.htm*

U.S. Department of Health and Human Services (USDHHS). (2000a). Healthy People 2010: Volume 1 (2nd ed.). Retrieved August 15, 2006, from *http://www.healthypeople.gov/Document/tableofcontents.htm#volume1*

U.S. Department of Health and Human Services (USDHHS). (2000b). Healthy People 2010: Volume 2 (2nd ed.). Retrieved August 15, 2006, from *http://www.healthypeople.gov/Document/tableofcontents.htm#Volume2*

U.S. Department of Health and Human Services (USDHHS). (2000c). Tracking healthy people. Retrieved August 15, 2006, from *http://www.healthypeople.gov/Document/tableofcontents.htm#tracking*

U.S. Department of Health and Human Services (USDHHS). (2006a). Objective 24–5 school or work days lost, asthma. Healthy People Midcourse Review. Retrieved August 22, 2006, from *http://www.healthypeople.gov/data/midcourse/comments/faobjective.asp?id=24&subid=5*

U.S. Department of Health and Human Services (USDHHS). (2006b). Objective 25–5 human papillomavirus infection, viral STD illness and disability. Healthy People Midcourse Review. Retrieved August 22, 2006, from *http://www.healthypeople.gov/data/midcourse/comments/faobjective.asp?id=25&subid=5*

U.S. Department of Health and Human Services (USDHHS). (2006c). Healthy People Midcourse Review. Retrieved August 22, 2006, from *http://www.healthypeople.gov/data/midcourse/*

U.S. Department of Health and Human Services, Health Resources and Services Administration (USDHHS, HRSA). (2006). Comparison of the rural health clinic and federally qualified health center programs. Retrieved August 25, 2006, from *http://www.cms.hhs.gov/mlnproducts/downloads/fqhc_rhccomparison.pdf*

U.S. Department of Health and Human Services, Public Health Service (USDHHS, PHS). (1992). *Healthy people 2000: Summary report.* Boston: Jones and Bartlett.

☐ BIBLIOGRAPHY

Administration on Aging. (2006). A statistical profile of black older Americans Aged 65+. Retrieved August 24, 2006, from *http://www.aoa.gov/PRESS/fact/pdf/Attachment_1302.pdf*

Administration on Aging. (2006). A statistical profile of Hispanic older Americans Aged 65+. Retrieved August 24, 2006, from *http://www.aoa.gov/PRESS/fact/pdf/Attachment_1303.pdf*

Anderson, N. B., Bulatao, R. A., & Cohen, B. (Eds.). (2004). *Critical perspectives on racial and ethnic differences in health in later life.* Washington, DC: National Academies Press.

Arizona Department of Health Services, Bureau of Community and Family Health Services. (2005). Healthy Arizona 2010. Retrieved August 15, 2006, from *http://www.hs.state.az.us/phs/healthyaz2010*

Centers for Disease Control and Prevention. (2000). *Measuring healthy days: Population assessment of health-related quality of life.* Atlanta, GA: Author. Retrieved on August 14, 2006, from *http://www.cdc.gov/hrqol/pdfs/mhd.pdf*

Doty, M. M. & Holmgren, A. L. (2006, August). Health-care disconnect: Gaps in coverage and care for minority adults. New York: The Commonwealth Fund. Retrieved August 24, 2006, from *http://www.cmwf.org/publications/publications_show.htm?doc_id=386220*

Economic Research Service. (2005). An enhanced quality of life for rural Americans: Rural gallery. Retrieved August 15, 2006, from *http://ers.usda.gov/emphases/ rural/gallery/*

Federal Interagency Forum on Child and Family Statistics. (2006). *America's children in brief: Key national indicators of well-being, 2006*. Washington, DC: U.S. Government Printing Office. Retrieved August 15, 2006, from *http://www.childstats.gov/americaschildren/*

Gamm, L. D., & Hutchison, L .L. (Eds.). (2004). *Rural Healthy People 2010: A Companion Document to Healthy People 2010* (Volume 3). College Station, TX: The Texas A&M University System Health Science Center, School of Rural Public Health, Southwest Rural Health Research Center. Retrieved August 15, 2006, from *http://www.srph.tamhsc.edu/centers/rhp2010/ publications.htm*

Gorina, Y., Hoyert, D., Lentzner, H., & Goulding, M. (2006). Trends in causes of death among older persons in the United States. Aging Trends, No 6. Hyattsville, MD: National Center for Health Statistics. 2006. Retrieved August 24, 2006, from *http://www.cdc.gov/nchs/data/ ahcd/agingtrends/06olderpersons.pdf*

Goulding, M. R. (2005). Trends in prescribed medicine use and spending by older Americans, 1992–2001. Aging Trends, No. 5. Hyattsville, MD: National Center for Health Statistics. 2005. Retrieved August 24, 2006, from *http://www.cdc.gov/nchs/data/ahcd/agingtrends/ 05medicine.pdf*

Hamrick, K. (Ed.). (2002). Rural America at a glance. (ERS Rural Development Research Report No. RDRR94-1). Retrieved on August 14, 2006, from *http://www .ers.usda.gov/publications/rdrr94-1/rdrr94-1.pdf*

Hamrick, K. (Ed.). (2005). Rural Hispanics at a glance. (ERS Economic Information Bulletin No. EIB8). Retrieved on August 14, 2006, from *http://www.ers.usda.gov/ Publications/EIB8/*

Health Resources & Services Administration (HRSA). (2006). Promoting rural health. Retrieved August 15, 2006, from *http://www.hrsa.gov/*

Institute of Medicine. (2003). *Unequal treatment: Understanding racial and ethnic disparities in health care*. Washington, DC: National Academies Press. http://books.nap.edu/catalog.php?record_id=10260

Lillie-Blanton, M., Rushing, O. E., & Ruiz, S. (2003). Key facts: Race, ethnicity and medical care (Report #6069). Menlo Park, CA: The Henry J. Kaiser Family Foundation. Retrieved on August 14, 2006, from *http://www.kff.org/minorityhealth/upload/ Key-Facts-Race-Ethnicity-Medical-Care-Chartbook.pdf*

Maine Rural Health Research Center. (2005). Database for rural health research in progress. Retrieved August 15, 2006, from *http://www.rural-health.org/database.htm*

National Advisory Committee on Rural Health. (2002). A targeted look at the rural health care safety net. Retrieved August 15, 2006, from *ftp://ftp.hrsa.gov/ruralhealth/ NACReportbb.pdf*

National Center for Health Statistics (NCHS). (2005). NCHS data on racial and ethnic disparities. Retrieved August 24, 2006, from *http://www.cdc.gov/nchs/data/factsheets/ racialandethnic.pdf*

Office of Disease Prevention and Health Promotion (ODPHP). (2001). Healthy People in Healthy Communities: A Community Planning Guide Using Healthy People 2010. Retrieved on August 14, 2006, from *http://www.healthypeople.gov/Publications/ HealthyCommunities2001/default.htm*

Pearson, K. B. (Ed.). (2006) Rural health research in progress in the rural health research centers program (10th ed.). Retrieved on August 14, 2006, from *http://muskie.usm.maine.edu/Publications/rural/ ResearchInProgress2006.pdf*

State of Alaska, Health and Social Services. (2006). Healthy Alaskans 2010. Retrieved August 15, 2006, from *http://www.hss.state.ak.us/dph/targets/ha2010/default.htm*

State of Michigan, Department of Community Health. (2007). Critical health indicators. Retrieved October 4, 2007,from *http://www.michigan.gov/mdch/0,1607 ,7-132—17501—,00.html*

Title 42, Chapter 35. (2004). Programs for Older Americans. Retrieved October 4, 2007, from *http://www4.law .cornell.edu/uscode/html/uscode42/usc_sup_01_42_10_35 .html*

U.S. Department of Health and Human Services. (2000). Healthy People 2010: Understanding and improving health. Retrieved August 21, 2006, from *http://www .healthypeople.gov/Document/tableofcontents.htm#uih*

U.S. Department of Health and Human Services, Office of Public Health and Science, Office of Disease Prevention and Health Promotion (USDHHS, OPHS). (2001). *Healthy people in healthy communities: A community planning guide using Healthy People 2010.* Washington, DC: U.S. Government Printing Office.

Ver Ploeg, M., & Perrin, E. (Eds.). (2004). Eliminating health disparities: Measurement and data needs. Retrieved August 15, 2006, from *http://newton.nap.edu/ catalog/10979.html*

■ *Francoise* **Dunefsky**

Quality Health Care

17

> **"***Quality is everyone's responsibility.***"**

The United States continues to examine the definition of quality and its relationship to health-care costs. This effort has been stimulated by a number of factors: the necessity to compete in a global marketplace, where production costs are often significantly lower; the ongoing explosion in technologic advances; exponential expenditures for health-care services; individual and corporate consumer pressures to improve value, safety, and portability of health information; and potential reduction of the fragmentation of care.

Health-care institutions are attempting to understand and apply principles and techniques previously reserved for the business world. In their codes of ethics and standards of practice, professional groups, including nurses and physicians, have historically expressed the intent of ensuring that individual patients receive optimal care. The impact of structures and processes on these individual and aggregate outcomes was previously neither documented nor necessarily understood.

In addition, societal forces are shifting the health-care paradigm from a paternalistic model of delivering care and services to one that responds to customer demands. Making providers accountable for evaluating the quality of care they deliver, and for communicating that quality effectively to the public, is an emerging task influenced by corporate buyers of services, who want to know what they can expect to receive for their money. Much progress has been made in the last decade to create an infrastructure that can be used to improve the entire system of care for all stakeholders.

With its professional commitment to clients, responsibility for coordinating care, and roots in the psychosocial and physical sciences, nursing is poised to play an important role in the ongoing development and implementation of care-delivery models that are effective and efficient, meet customer expectations, and ensure excellent clinical outcomes. The dictionary defines **quality** as "character with respect to fineness or grade of excellence" (Merriam-Webster's Collegiate Dictionary, 1997). In health care, we previously defined it as being "free of mistakes" or perfect relative to process. The standard of perfection or 100% compliance was focused within. The current quality movement is evolving a definition of quality that includes "meeting customer needs" and focusing on outcome. The Institute of Medicine uses the following definition: "The degree to which health services for individuals and populations increase the likelihood of desired health outcomes and are consistent with current professional knowledge" (Institute of Medicine [IOM], 2006, p. 1). A new paradigm for clinical practice across disciplines is contributing to nursing's body of knowledge, current standards of practice, and nursing care outcomes. Commonly referred to as evidence-based practice, quality is defined as "the integration of the best research evidence with our

clinical expertise and our patient's unique values and circumstances" (Strauss, Richardson, Glasziou, & Hayes, 2005).

Health-care providers have consistently looked at clinical care as the measure for quality. Traditionally, the qualifications of clinicians, state-of-the-art technology, and episodic interventions that cure illness or "do no harm" were considered indices of quality. But asking customers how they perceive "quality" has enabled a more complex picture to emerge. The consumer expects expert clinical care. But equally important are timely, courteous, and respectful treatment, easy access to caregivers and information, unfragmented care delivery, reasonable costs, and the ability to maneuver through the system without too many obstacles. Understanding the convergence of the consumer's perspective of quality and use of evidence-based nursing practice, together with an ongoing focus on continuous improvement, are an integral part of meeting our professional commitment.

HISTORICAL PERSPECTIVES

Human societies have always strived for excellence. Reliance on professional associations such as guilds, and inspection by consumers, are century-old methods of judging quality. Societal values, however, are changing the context in which quality is evaluated.

Pre–World War II health-care delivery in the United States was mostly a cottage industry. This time is referred to as the "charitable era of health care." The wealthy and fortunate rural populations relied on services delivered in the home. The poor and urban working classes were sent to hospitals in critical circumstances or died at home. A sudden growth in technology and treatment modalities and the building of hospitals stimulated by the Hospital Survey and Construction Act of 1946, also known as the Hill-Burton Act, began the corporatization of health-care delivery. This "technologic era" lasted for more than 30 years. Extensive development of policies, procedures, standards of practice, and professional disciplines ensued. It took 20 years before the industrial model of reliance on departmental inspection and supervisory audits became part of the fabric of health care. The role of Medicare and federal and state government accelerated this growth.

The early 1970s saw the beginning of formalized measurement of clinical performance and outcomes. Organizations such as the Joint Commission on Accreditation of Healthcare Organizations (JCAHO), professional review organizations (PROs), and some state health departments played a major role in the initial movement. Retrospective audits, investigation of problems, and indicator measurements were all attempts to discover less than acceptable performance by an individual, discipline, or department. The objective was to discover the "bad apples," implement a corrective action plan, and monitor its effectiveness through ongoing measurement. It was assumed that quality was a result of the performance of individuals or groups of individuals. The tools of the corrective action plans were education, disciplinary action, and increased resources such as technology and staffing.

A gradual quality paradigm shift began in the second half of the 1980s. The "economic era" of health care was emerging. Other industries purchasing health care for their employees at rapidly rising costs challenged the health-care sector to provide "more" and "better" for "less." The Japanese were successfully invading the American marketplace as a result of quality methodologies developed by Deming, Juran, and others. Deming had persuaded the Japanese government and industry that they should focus on quality rather than price and costs. Knowing that this focus would take time and commitment, they infused their businesses with the belief that work is performed by interdependent teams, that individuals want to do a good job, that those who do the work itself know its processes better than anyone else, and that mass inspection and fear do not automatically result in quality.

Juran proposed the notion that by planning for quality, one avoids multiple trial-and-error situations and costly rework, often referred to as "the cost of poor quality." Quality could be cost-effective. Improvement required even higher goals for quality. Reliance on systems analysis and statistical methods and techniques produced better-quality products than did supervision and inspection of individual human behaviors.

During the next 10 years, companies began to recognize that care is delivered by individuals who function as members of crossfunctional and interdisciplinary teams,

and that individuals and teams are tools for, rather than objects of, improvement. Currently a body of scientific research is emerging that tests the new theories that care is supported by environmental, managerial, support, and governance structures, and that ensuring accepted clinical outcomes is not enough to meet customer needs.

Many individuals and organizations have contributed to the quality journey over the past 30 years. The Agenda for Change at JCAHO and Donald Berwick and his group at the Institute for Healthcare Improvement are but a few who deserve recognition for being driving forces in the implementation of the new quality-care models. In 1996, the Institute of Medicine (IOM), a member of The National Academies, began a multiple-phase Quality Initiative; its landmark reports include *To Err Is Human: Building a Safer Health System* (2000), *Crossing the Quality Chasm: A New Health System for the 21st Century* (2001), and the study sponsored by the U.S. Department of Health and Human Services Agency for Healthcare Research and Quality, *Keeping Patients Safe: Transforming the Work Environment of Nurses* (2004). These and other IOM reports focus on the quality problems and on the multiple levels of system reform needed. Currently the IOM Quality Initiative focuses on operationalizing the vision described in "The Quality Chasm," including how to keep patients safe and prevent medication errors.

Largely as a result of the IOM's activities and reports, the JCAHO in 2004 approved National Patient Safety Goals. The requirements to meet these goals are surveyed in all health-care organizations seeking their accreditation.

In 2000, the JCAHO began the journey towards the standardization of **core measures** with the ultimate goal by 2010 of performance measures that will be the natural derivative of the care delivery process. During the first half of the decade the focus has been on metrics through the identification and implementation of core performance measures. From 2005 on, the work targets their expansion and enhancement across the national system so there is demonstrable improvement in health-care quality and patient safety. Of note is the collaborative work throughout this endeavor among JCAHO, the Centers for Medicare and Medicaid Services (CMS), and the National Quality Forum (NQF), as well as other partners. Separate systems can now be compared by using core measures in a standardized fashion. By using specific performance measures for conditions such as acute myocardial infarction, pregnancy, surgical infection, and their management, hospitals can be compared, regardless of size or geographical location. In addition, the aim is to minimize redundancy in data collection. Initially, the work has been hospital-based. It is planned to expand the measures to provide a greater scope of selection options in long-term care, home care, behavioral health care and

ONLINE CONSULT

For more information on accreditation initiatives visit:

The Joint Commission for Accreditation of Healthcare Organizations at
http://www.joint commission.org

The Joint Commission's Quality Report at
http://www.QualityCheck.org

The Institute for Healthcare Improvement at
http://www.ihi.org

The Institute of Medicine at
http://www.iom.edu/

ambulatory care, so standardized performance improvement is implemented throughout the entire continuum of care.

The role nursing plays in all of the quality and safety work has been pushed to the forefront. The American Nurses Association, through its National Database of Nursing Quality Indicators (NDNQI), has identified acute-care patient outcomes that are dependent primarily on nursing care, commonly referred to as "nurse sensitive." On the basis of evidence-based practice, targets are being set for nurse-sensitive outcomes, such as urinary tract infections, pneumonia, and cardiac arrest (Pierre, 2006).

THEORETICAL MODELS FOR QUALITY

The models used for quality improvement have come from industry. Some have been adapted for health care, but all share the common theme of using the scientific process.

Deming's Principles for Transformation

W. Edwards Deming was the first to challenge seriously the managerial notion that quality and increased productivity are incompatible. In doing his research and developing the 14 Points for Management, he assumed the new radical approach of listening to those who actually did the work (Deming, 1982, 1986) (Box 17–1). Deming contends that the model can be applied anywhere, including service industries. Nursing leaders at all levels of the organization can apply the principles in their quest to implement quality care. The more pervasive the quality culture in the organization, the easier the model application becomes. The stronger and more visible leadership is in its support for quality, the more rapidly a quality culture can be implemented.

The 14 Points for Management

Following is a brief description of each of Deming's 14 Points of Management.

1. *Create constancy of purpose for improvement of product and service.* Innovation is the foundation for the future. It requires a belief that there is a future and an unshakable commitment to quality

Box 17.1 Deming's 14 Points

1. Create constancy of purpose for improvement of product and service.
2. Adopt the new philosophy.
3. Cease dependence on mass inspection.
4. End the practice of awarding business on the basis of price tag alone.
5. Improve constantly and forever the system of production and service.
6. Institute training.
7. Adopt and institute leadership.
8. Drive out fear.
9. Break down barriers between staff areas.
10. Eliminate slogans and targets in the workplace that urge increased productivity.
11. Eliminate numerical quotas for the workplace and management.
12. Remove barriers that rob people of pride in workmanship.
13. Encourage education and self-improvement for everyone.
14. Take action to accomplish the transformation.

Reprinted from *Out of the Crisis* by W. Edwards Deming by permission of the W. Edwards Deming Institute®. Copyright 1986 by The W. Edwards Deming Institute®.

and productivity. Resources must be put into education and research so we can constantly improve. The aim is to meet our mission and serve our customers, because otherwise we will not stay in business. We must address day-to-day problems without getting stuck in them. Many nurse managers fail to plan their resources, energy, and time to deal with the future. Work better, not harder, to plan new services. Meeting our customers' needs and training and retraining personnel help deal with required change.

2. *Adopt the new philosophy.* Do not accept existing levels of mistakes or staff members who are not adequately prepared to perform. Become the change agent who meets the challenge. Propose, develop, and implement improvements in systems and services.

3. *Cease dependence on mass inspection.* The inspection stage is too late to improve quality. Quality comes from improvement in production processes. Tools, such as 100% case review, will not improve care, are time-consuming, and require resources that could be spent better in improving design or systems. Measuring incomplete records, medication errors, or service delays in and of themselves will not improve the delivery of care.

4. *End the practice of awarding business on the basis of price tags alone.* The nurse manager has a responsibility to include total cost when recommending the purchase of goods or services. This includes not only the "up-front" price but also the cost of disposables and maintenance, amount of vendor support provided, ease of training in use, labor costs, and cross-functional use. It is a managerial responsibility to make well-prepared, comprehensive recommendations to the executive team. Deming believes that limiting the suppliers we deal with and establishing long-term relationships with vendors creates interdependency, which assists in the achievement of quality.

5. *Improve constantly and forever the system of production and service.* Quality must be built and incorporated during the design phase in order to avoid costly rework. Teamwork is essential in this process, especially in service industries such as health care, in which we rely on interdependent, cross-disciplinary teams to deliver the care that is our product. As our customers' needs and available resources change, we are obliged to improve existing systems. Reductions in length of stay, shifts in delivery of care along the continuum, and changing demographics all require us to seek opportunities to "do it better." It is no longer acceptable to think "we always did it this way and it worked."

6. *Institute training.* Learning must be lifelong and pervasive. The principles of adult learning, and an appreciation for the fact that different people learn by different methods, apply at all layers of the organization, regardless of length of employment. All must understand the institution's mission, values, customer needs, and expectations. What the assignment is, what is acceptable work, and how we prepare people all must be defined. For the manager, this includes knowing which processes are assigned and understanding variation in these processes. We must become learning organizations.

7. *Adopt and institute leadership.* The job of management is leadership, namely, vision and communication of that vision, not supervision. The assignment is to work on quality of service, designing for quality, and delivering an actual product. The leader must understand the work supervised and must remove barriers that prevent the staff members from doing their work.

8. *Drive out fear.* Fear of reprisal, fear to admit mistakes, fear of not having the needed new knowledge, and fear of not meeting the deadlines or quotas interfere with seeing opportunities for improvement. Errors, complaints, and areas that appear out of control must be studied and analyzed for opportunities to improve.

9. *Break down barriers between staff areas.* This point has proved especially difficult in health care, where the struggle to establish distinct professional domains fostered accountability, review, and disciplinary actions within professions. The emergence of matrix organizations, patient-care departments, use of product or service line teams, cross-training, and decentralization of services will assist in the implementation of patient-care teams focused on the patient rather than on the professional. Simultaneously, this will create a new challenge to ensure that no one can hide behind or dominate the team. All professional groups must be held accountable for their professional practice and for quality in service delivery.

10. *Eliminate slogans and targets in the workplace that urge increased productivity.* The assumption that one can improve quality and productivity by trying harder does not take into account that most problems come from systems rather than individuals. The role of management is to improve the system with results of sound statistical methods.

11. *Eliminate numerical quotas for the workforce and management.* Quotas assume that the target is correct, not too high or too low, and that all can attain them. They have a negative effect on pride in workmanship. Productivity should be studied, analyzed, and understood. Everyone should know what to do and how to do it. A sustained requirement for all to participate in setting goals and figuring out how to reach them is needed.

12. *Remove barriers that rob people of pride in workmanship.* Make clear what the job is and what the expectations are. Improving the system to make it easier for people to work well will help them invest in the organization, reducing turnover and absenteeism.

13. *Encourage education and self-improvement for everyone.* Study and development should not only focus on the immediate needs of the organization or department. Develop the organization and its members for the future as well as for the present.

14. *Take action to accomplish the* **transformation**. The leaders must adopt the new philosophy with pride. It must be explained often and well to a critical number of individuals. Everyone in the organization must be asked to participate. This requires substantial and sustained commitment and energy.

Obstacles to Quality Transformation

Deming (1982, 1986) also recognized obstacles to the transformation, which are:

- Desire to achieve instant results by hiring a consultant
- Supposition that solving problems creates transformation
- Belief that one can simply transfer systems from another organization
- Belief that the quality department takes care of quality
- Belief that your problems are different
- Poor understanding of statistical methods

More serious blocks, referred to by Deming (1982, 1986) as "deadly diseases" because of their severity and resistance to eradication, include:

- Lack of constancy of purpose
- Emphasis on short-term profits
- Evaluation of performance without long-term improvement in mind
- Mobility of management
- Management by numbers only

When considering the application of Deming's principles for transformation, the nurse has to acknowledge realities in the organization. It may be necessary to maintain annual performance review, existing merit systems, strict organizational and professional hierarchies, and a focus on monthly budget fluctuations. Nevertheless, the general principles of constancy of purpose, focus on improvement, creating a learning environment, reducing fear, and removing barriers to pride in workmanship can be adopted by anyone in any setting.

Juran Trilogy

Deming offers us a framework for how to transform any organization by incorporating quality, but the Juran Trilogy focuses on the tools that organizations can use while doing the work. The two models are complementary and are often used together.

Dr. Joseph Juran (1989) defines *quality* as "fitness for use." This definition assumes both freedom from defects and presence of the multiple elements required to meet the total needs of a customer. The freedom from defect does not guarantee that this is the product the customer wants. The client assumes we can deliver care without errors. Waiting time, ease of access, and cleanliness may be crucial factors in determining whether a client chooses us, for example. Patients may opt to seek urgent-care services in freestanding facilities with shorter wait times, or diagnostic mammograms in Zen-like women's health centers.

The Juran Trilogy utilizes three managerial processes: planning, control, and improvement (Box 17–2). The trilogy's proposed procedural steps and tools are unique.

Quality Planning

Planning for programs or services requires that quality is built into them. This stage of **quality planning** follows five distinct steps:

1. *Determine who the customers of the program or service are.* They can be external customers, internal customers, or both. In health care, clients, families, and payers are all external customers. Departments and providers are internal customers of one another. Nursing receives services from dietary or medical records, and those departments in turn are customers of nursing. Independent medical staff members are often considered both internal and external customers because of their ability to choose the institution and their influence and provision of services within the institution.
2. *Determine the customers' needs.* Surveys, focus groups, individual client interviews, complaint reviews, and market analysis can be used to determine what our customers want.
3. *Develop product features that respond to the customer's needs.* Consider offering services outside traditional business hours. Weekend day surgery, diagnostic procedures early and late in the day, and respite care are but a few examples.
4. *Develop processes that are able to produce those product features.*
5. *Transfer the resulting plans to the implementation team.*

For example, while teaching breast self-examination at a customer-friendly breast clinic, a nurse hears clients express concerns about the time it takes to receive mammography results. In response to complaints, the nurse, working with the department and a local women's group, initiates a formal survey of women who currently use the center and women who do not. The survey reveals that women want to receive test results within 24 hours and to be able to refer themselves for mammography. As a result, the services at the center are redesigned to incorporate these features. The clinic applies for and obtains an expanded license for self-referral. It institutes policies, procedures, and standards to ensure that the improved services are implemented and monitored.

Quality Control

The three steps of **quality control** involve:

1. *Evaluating actual quality performance.* This requires knowledge of statistical methods of measurement and analysis.
2. *Comparing actual performance with quality goals.*
3. *Acting on the difference.* This assumes understanding of common and special cause variation.

BOX 17.2 Juran Trilogy

A. Quality Planning

  1. Determine who the customers are.
  2. Determine the needs of the customer.
  3. Develop product features that respond to the customer's needs.
  4. Develop processes that are able to produce these product features.
  5. Transfer the resulting plans to the operating forces.

B. Quality Control

  1. Evaluate actual quality performance.
  2. Compare actual performance to quality goals.
  3. Act on the difference.

C. Quality Improvement

  1. Establish an infrastructure.
  2. Identify needs for improvement.
  3. Establish project teams for each project.
  4. Provide the teams with resources, motivation, and training.

Variation is part of any process. Constant reaction to it may destabilize an otherwise stable process.

Example: First, measure the number of women who underwent mammography and received their results within 24 hours. Then, compare the number to the agreed upon benchmark. Finally, analyze the discrepancies for special cause variation and develop an improvement plan.

Quality Improvement

Raising performance to unprecedented levels of **quality improvement** requires four steps:

1. *Establishing the infrastructure needed to secure ongoing quality improvement.* The infrastructure, which may comprise a quality council, departmental teams, and assigned roles, ensures that quality improvement is part of the way business is done.
2. *Identifying specific needs for improvement.* Data from quality control, feedback from customers, and goals of the organization help determine what needs to be improved and what needs to be prioritized.
3. *Establishing a project team for each project.* Responsibility must be defined clearly. This includes the objective for improvement and measures of success.
4. *Providing resources, motivation, and training*, so that the teams can diagnose causes of lesser quality, stimulate a remedy, and establish controls to hold the gains in improvements. Example: The special cause variation for the delay in result reporting of the mammograms appears to be linked to the day of the week (Friday) and the shift (evening). The

radiology nursing staff is drastically reduced on Saturdays with only interventional radiology nursing staff covering for the mammography service. After training this staff on the necessary skills to report results adequately, you resume measuring and see a marked improvement.

Juran's work has shown that most of the potential for eliminating errors and improving the system does not lie in changing workers. The 85/15 rule, as it is now commonly referred to, states that 85% of problems can be corrected only by changing systems.

Both Deming and Juran have provided the foundation for today's quality movement in industry and in health care. The *JCAHO Agenda for Change* helped in the transition from quality assurance to quality improvement.

The 10-Step Model for Monitoring and Evaluation

Dr. O'Leary at the JCAHO took the position that improvement requires effective monitoring and that effective monitoring requires good indicators. Quality assurance evolved into quality improvement largely as a result of this position. The monitoring and evaluation process has been revised over time, but the 10 steps remain part of the foundation on which many of quality activities are based. The process requires identifying the most important aspects of care for a particular organization or division, selecting indicators that reflect these aspects, taking opportunities to improve care, taking action, and evaluating the effectiveness of that action. Elements of performance include what is done and how well it is done (Joint Commission on

Accreditation of Healthcare Organizations [JCAHO], 2005). Doing the right thing includes efficacy and appropriateness. Doing it well involves availability, timeliness, effectiveness, continuity, safety, efficiency, and providing services with respect and caring.

Step 1: Assign Responsibility

The leaders in the organization are responsible for fostering quality improvement and setting priorities for assessment and improvement. Leaders are defined as the leadership of the board, the executive team, including the nurse executive, the leaders of the medical staff, and department directors. This step has implications for nurse managers and other leaders in the nursing staff, because they have direct responsibility for quality.

Step 2: Delineate Scope of Care and Service

The scope of care of the organization or service must be defined in order to go on to the next step. We are not all things to all people, and we need to focus our energies on the mission and vision. We have to be clear about who our clients are and what we need to do for them.

Step 3: Identify Important Aspects of Care and Service

What are the key functions that warrant ongoing monitoring? Which functions need prioritization? The key function in outpatient areas are often very different from those in bedded units, as are the ones from services focusing on prevention, action, or chronic illness. Timeliness as an aspect of care may vary based on the scope of service and aspects of care of a particular service.

Step 4: Identify Indicators

Interdisciplinary teams develop and select indicators for those aspects of care that have been prioritized. As an example, turnaround time for laboratory results could be an indicator selected to reflect timeliness in an emergency department.

Step 5: Establish a Means to Trigger Evaluation

The team determines at what level and time evaluations will be triggered. Identifying thresholds that are not met after quarterly reviews is an example of how to implement evaluation. The review of every unexpected return of a patient to the surgical suite within 24 hours after surgery may be another.

Step 6: Collect and Organize Data

Defining data sources and methodology for collection, the actual data collection, and organization all are parts of this process. More often than not, too much peripheral information is collected, which actually hampers meaningful organization of data, is labor-intensive, and interferes with the next step.

Step 7: Initiate Evaluation

Once it is determined that further evaluation is needed, other feedback may be taken into consideration. Intensive evaluation should be performed by teams.

Step 8: Take Action to Improve

Actions include changes in the system, education, designation of clear authority and accountability, and development of standards.

Step 9: Assess the Effectiveness of the Actions

Whether the action improved the care or service and whether it sustained improvement are questions to be answered by evaluation of effectiveness.

Step 10: Communicate Results to Relevant Individuals and Groups

Dissemination of conclusions, actions, and results to those affected and to the leaders is necessary. This may be accomplished through team presentations, committee structures, and department or division meetings.

> Doing the right thing includes efficacy and appropriateness. Doing it well involves availability, timeliness, effectiveness, continuity, safety, efficiency, and providing services with respect and caring.

The 10-Step Model has been used successfully both in the traditional scope of quality assurance and in the context of quality improvement. The steps have remained the same, but the focus from within departments to processes, the level of accountability, the understanding and application of statistical methodologies, and the role of leadership have evolved significantly. Organizational leaders can no longer delegate responsibility to the quality department. Hiding behind professional or departmental boundaries is not acceptable. Leaders of boards, executive and management teams, and the medical staff are all being held accountable for delivery of quality care and for participation in the transformation of the health-care system.

CONTINUOUS QUALITY IMPROVEMENT IN HEALTH CARE

Health-care organizations strive to embed quality in every service they provide. Their success lies in their ability to incorporate quality as a key component of their strategic mission and to implement a model by which they continually evaluate and improve quality.

Quality as Strategy

The guiding members of any organization are responsible for developing the mission, vision, and core strategies chosen to achieve the vision. Not every business will choose quality as a strategy. Competitive pricing, a customer service focus, promoting access to the product, and creating a niche market are all examples of different strategies. It is not accidental that JCAHO-accredited agencies are required to include a quality plan in their strategic plan. To survive and thrive requires a formal, well-thought-out approach with a focus on the communities we serve.

"Doing the right things right" means that we have identified what the "right things" are. They will vary according to the needs of the particular community and the mission and vision of the organization. Not every hospital can or should serve all the health-care needs of its community. Such needs may be met better by other community agencies or tertiary care centers. Once the health-care agency defines what the "right things" are, or what the scope of its services is, it must design quality into the structures and processes, monitor and analyze performance, and identify opportunities for improvement in order to ensure that the right things are "done right" and desired outcomes result.

A successful strategic plan also requires identification of needed core competencies and methods to address existing gaps. **Core competencies** define the organizational capabilities as well as the subsequent employee competencies needed to achieve the vision through utilization of the strategic plan. Core competencies are not stagnant; they change with the organization's strategies. The recruitment, retention, development, and performance management of everyone working in or for the organization play a key role. Creating a **learning organization**, in which skill development is dynamic, is strategic in and of itself. Understanding how to build quality into structures and processes, knowing the tools and measures to be utilized, knowing how to monitor and analyze performance, and understanding team process, group dynamics, and improvement methods require learning, which must be included in the organizational development strategies.

Quality is everyone's responsibility. It is a business strategy, or centralized philosophy, with accountability at every service level. Because quality is everyone's job, everyone must be educated and must demonstrate competence about quality—the leadership, the providers, and the customers.

Total Quality Management and Continuous Quality Improvement

The terms **total quality management** (TQM) and **continuous quality improvement (CQI)** have been used interchangeably. TQM is mostly linked with industrial models, whereas CQI has received wide acceptance in health care. Because the underpinnings of the two terms are the same, CQI is used through the remainder of the chapter.

The basic concepts of CQI are that quality improvement is an ongoing process that utilizes proactive and reactive strategies. The process goes beyond meeting preestablished goals or catching up to the competition; rather, it involves exceeding expectations and creating new opportunities.

Improvements can be large scale or incremental. Quality is defined as satisfying the needs of external and internal customers, including anticipating developing needs and introducing new services. Teamwork is the underlying framework. Improvement activities and measurement are always linked, because without measurement we cannot be sure that improvement has occurred. Additionally, measurement keeps teams focused on concrete opportunities and provides feedback regarding which core strategies helped achieve the vision and mission of the organization. **Benchmarking**, the process of comparing with the best of the industry, requires understanding of statistical methods, including the validity and reliability of the tools and measures used in both organizations, understanding systems variation, and sampling methods.

Transition from Quality Assurance to Continuous Quality Improvement

The traditional model of **quality assurance**—relying on inspection to catch problems and correcting individual performances—has already evolved in many segments of the health-care industry. To assume that the journey through quality assurance was wasted fails to recognize that many of the tools used in quality assurance are still used in quality improvement, and the journey helped define what constitutes quality care. There are many differences, however. CQI is widely recognized as being broader in scope, involving the leadership and many more people, and blurring boundaries. The expectation of perfection is gone, but the search for excellence is essential.

It is important to understand that the evaluation of individual performance must continue. Standards for hiring competent members of the team are more important than ever. Results of individual performance should be looked at for trends across shifts, units, and departments. Findings can be used for staff and leadership development. Individual competence remains a professional obligation. The shift in focus from individual to team does not change our standards or our accountability to those we serve.

Department- or unit-based quality programs remain valuable and should not be demolished. They are an important vehicle for teaching the concepts of CQI and provide needed mechanisms for ongoing measurement and application of standards. They also recognize that much improvement does not require large teams but can occur at the unit level.

Risk management evaluates the legal standards and their application to the delivery of care, the environment of care, and other services and functions. As with quality assurance, it relies on inspection; however, the focus is on how to protect the assets of the organization against liability. Table 17–1 highlights the differences and similarities between quality improvement, quality assurance, and risk management.

An example of how the same problem may be approached differently with the three approaches is in dealing with a medication error. In the environment of quality improvement, the investigation will search for what system weaknesses may have contributed to the

error: is the dispensing system weak, are high-risk medications kept separate, and so on. At the unit level, quality assurance may investigate the individual nurse's competencies and performance. In the risk management arena, the focus may be on documentation problems that could be discoverable in court in a malpractice claim.

Putting a Continuous Quality Improvement Structure in Place

It is now widely accepted that quality journeys are lengthy and costly. They require a well-developed structure and plan to connect the vision with the implementation. Because CQI is, first and foremost, a management philosophy, the leaders must be competent in its principles and methodologies.

The actual mechanisms of setting up the program are beyond the scope of this chapter. Creating a structure usually involves a quality council and designation of a CQI coach. The coach functions as the facilitator, educator, and expert in tools and techniques. For organizations seeking JCAHO accreditation, well-established guidelines and widely used tools are readily available.

The function of the council is to create integration, prioritize efforts, allocate resources, develop a learning organization, and charter cross-functional teams. The journey is usually expected to take between three and five years, depending on the resources available and the readiness for change.

Table 17.1

Comparing Quality Improvement, Quality Assurance, and Risk Management

Quality Improvement	Quality Assurance	Risk Management
Broad in scope	Based at unit or departmental level	Often its own, separate department
Organizational leadership designs and sets priorities	Often uses separate department or committee to design and set priorities	Looks at legally acceptable level of care or service
Purpose is improvement	Compares against standards	Purpose is risk reduction
Focus is on customers	Focus is on the organization	Focus is on preventing loss
Uses problems as opportunities for improvement	Continuous ongoing monitoring identifies problems (inspection)	Continuous ongoing monitoring (inspection)
Focus is on the system as a whole	Focus is on individual performance	Focus is on protecting organization's assets

Leaders and followers alike need to internalize the new beliefs and learn to use the new techniques and tools. Many organizations fail in the quest to implement the new quality organization because the efforts are all focused on the beginning of the journey. **Just-in-time learning**, the process of acquiring knowledge and skills as they are needed and used, tends to eliminate the feeling that CQI may be another managerial gimmick gone awry.

Another common mistake is the failure to prioritize efforts. Improvement activities require resources and should be linked to strategic objectives, serious quality concerns, or identified needs. Quality costs money, especially in the time and effort of human resources, and few organizations can afford to attempt to improve on all fronts at once.

TOOLS AND TECHNIQUES COMMONLY USED IN QUALITY IMPROVEMENT

An entire body of knowledge has been created in the area of valid techniques to be used for improving quality. Innovation requires team techniques such as brainstorming, boarding, decision matrices, multivoting, management of conflict, and quality communication.

Process Teams

Not all improvement projects require a process team. If the project or problem crosses functions and disciplines and cannot be resolved in the day-to-day operations, a process team is usually necessary. These "project" teams focus on improving or developing specific processes, come together to achieve a specific goal, such as analyzing variation, and have a beginning and an end.

Process teams must be chosen carefully to represent those involved in or affected by the process. If the team is very large, the project chosen may be too big and may have to be broken into steps.

How, then, does one choose an improvement project? Listen to your customers. Repeated complaints or requests for a particular service may require action. Suppose the evening charge nurse in a nonsectarian hospital receives ongoing requests for pastoral services from clients and their families. Each request requires multiple telephone calls and often results in delays. The nurse recognizes that the nursing department cannot address this problem alone. It involves not only the hospital but also the community. The nurse develops a proposal for a process team. Other methods for selecting or recognizing processes to be improved include asking the people in the process, reviewing existing reports, and recognizing excess complexity or long delays.

Process teams require resources. Because resource allocation is a leadership function, many organizations require the development of a proposal and subsequent approval by the quality council. All teams should develop an opportunity statement (what is wrong or needs improving), define the expected output of the project, and include measures of success. Members of the team are, at a minimum, a team leader who is invested in the process, a facilitator who brings CQI skills, and a recorder or minute taker. Depending on the skills and information systems available, analytical and statistical support may be necessary.

Because process teams are groups, they will need to go through the stages of group development—forming, storming, norming, performing, adjourning. (Refer to Chapter 8 on Working with Groups.) All teams must mature to perform. It is important to recognize that anxiety, testing of boundaries, competition for control, and minimal completion of work are part of the early stages. Early cohesiveness and work do not start until the norming stage. Real performance and "team" feeling belong to the performing step. Many teams also struggle with the adjourning phase—namely, meeting the final deadlines and dissolving the group.

The process team must adopt a model or method for doing its work. This model is usually organization-wide. There is value in choosing one model, because it minimizes relearning and allows different teams to communicate easily. Some common models are the Juran (1989) quality improvement project model, and Deming's (1982, 1986) PDCA cycle (Plan-Do-Check-Act).

Quality Improvement Tools

Quality improvement (QI) tools can usually be divided into four categories, those used for:

- Process description
- Data collection
- Data analysis
- Process improvement

Many excellent texts provide further assistance in this area. The ultimate purpose of all the **QI tools** is to have data that can be used and translated into information. The novice in quality improvement tools and techniques may need assistance from the CQI coach or further study of these techniques.

⒪ N L I N E Ⓒ O N S U L T

For more information on the PDCA cycle, visit **http://hci.com.au/hcisite2/toolkit/pdcacycl. htm**

Process Description Tools

One tool for process description is the **flowchart**, which describes the process in detail, from beginning to end, as accurately as possible. It is a picture of the movement of information, people, or materials. The top-down flowchart (Fig. 17–1) takes the major steps in the process, writes them in a horizontal sequence, and illustrates the substeps to be taken under each step. Flowcharts show the rework that gets done, the number of substeps or complexity in each area, the number of hand-offs between individuals and departments, and when subteams need to be formed from a particular process team. A flowchart that is too detailed makes it difficult to focus and impedes progress or action.

The **cause-and-effect diagram** (Fig. 17–2), also called the fishbone or Ishikawa diagram, helps identify the root causes of a problem. Typical categories are equipment, personnel, method, materials, and environment. The main arrow points toward the problem or desired result. It is important to remember that cause-and-effect diagrams point only toward possible causes; more data have be collected to identify the root causes. Cause-and-effect diagrams are most effective after the process has been described, because flowcharts help identify what must be included in the diagram.

Tools for Data Collection

Tools for data collection include asking the right questions, and using, among other things, data sheets, check sheets, surveys, focus groups, and interviews. Often, data are collected that turn out to be useless because the question asked was wrong, too broad, or poorly formulated. Data sheets and check sheets are both used to record data (Fig. 17–3). They differ in that **data sheets** need further analysis. Ordinarily, a data sheet is completed for each occurrence or event in the study. The data are subsequently aggregated and then sorted according to categories of interest.

Check sheets are used to record multiple events by simply putting a mark in the appropriate box. The best check sheets are those that are easy to use, do not require much interpretation, and visually display the data. An example in which either tool could be used is the study of the delivery time of medications to a patient care unit. With data sheets, every time a medication is taken from the pharmacy, the runner uses a new data sheet. At the end of the study all the sheets are gathered and analyzed. With the check sheet, the runner could calculate the time it took to deliver the drug and check the appropriate time box.

There are obvious advantages and disadvantages to both tools. Data sheets tend to be more accurate

■ **Figure !7.1** Top-down flowchart.

■ **Figure 17.2** Cause-and-effect diagram.

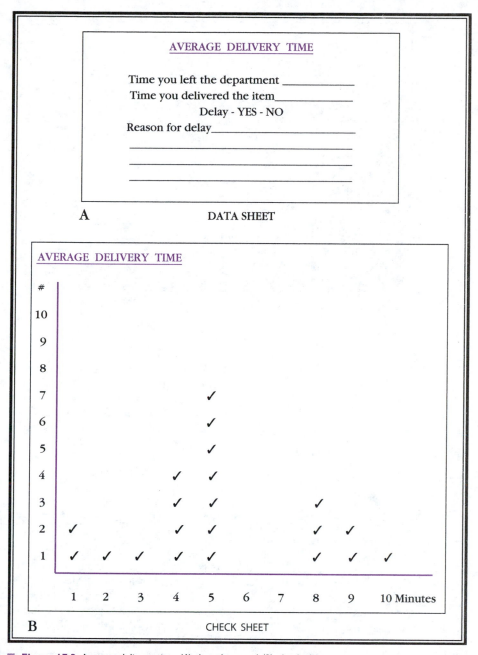

AVERAGE DELIVERY TIME

Time you left the department _____
Time you delivered the item_____
Delay - YES - NO
Reason for delay_____
_____
_____
_____

A   DATA SHEET

AVERAGE DELIVERY TIME

B   CHECK SHEET

■ **Figure 17.3** Average delivery time (A) data sheet and (B) check sheet.

because only one event is recorded on each. Check sheets quickly display trends as they occur without requiring a sometimes lengthy analysis. Data sheets and check sheets should be tested before project-wide work is undertaken, so that improvements can be made in them and only useful data are collected.

Surveys are a tool for obtaining input from large groups. The response rate and the specificity of the questions affect the usefulness and quality of the information obtained. Focus groups and individual interviews are time-consuming and expensive and may require the use of experienced interviewers, but they enable one to ask open-ended questions and probe deeper, if necessary.

Data Analysis Tools

Tools for data analysis include those that compare categories. Bar and pie charts and the Pareto diagram (Fig. 17-4), for example, analyze data within a category, such as numerical and graphic summaries. The

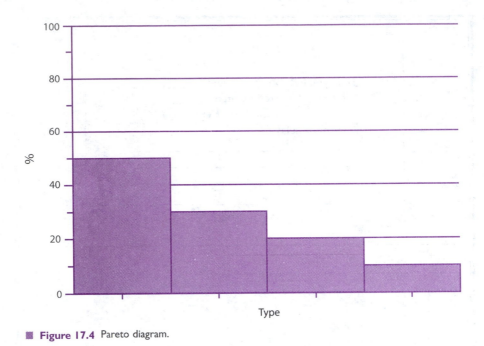

■ **Figure 17.4** Pareto diagram.

Pareto principle, sometimes called the 80/20 rule, was applied to management by Juran. It identifies the few sources of problems that contribute most to the outcome. By ranking problems on a bar graph in descending order, from left to right, Pareto diagrams focus attention on the most common problems and often build consensus about where to concentrate attention and effort.

Analysis of a particular category can include numerical summaries such as average, median, mode, and standard deviation. Graphic summaries—line graphs, histograms, scatter diagrams, and control charts—are especially valuable for working in diverse groups. They provide pictorial display of data, possible analysis and interpretation of patterns, relationships between variables, and the ability to distinguish between common and special cause variation.

Improvement Activities

Criteria-based information and tools are essential in evidence-based practice, performance improvement, and patient safety initiatives. The Agency for Healthcare Research and Quality (AHRQ) launched its website in

More information on the Agency for Healthcare Research and Quality (AHRQ) and "Quality Tools" at
http://www.qualitytools.ahrq.gov

2003 as a repository of practical, ready-to-use tools for assessing, measuring, and improving the quality of health care. Tools have been updated continually throughout 2006 and 2007. They come from clinical practice guidelines, tools for addressing patient and medication safety, benchmarking and comparative data, tools addressing specific diseases, and tools for maintaining a patient's health.

DEVELOPING A MEASUREMENT PROGRAM

As previously mentioned, improvement and measurement or evaluation are linked. Measurement of the capability of the organization, or its competence, determines the organization's ability to provide, and competence in providing, quality care. Measurement of outcome determines whether the process yielded favorable results. For example, the Breast Care Clinic used as an earlier example will not only focus its review on the ability to report examination results within 24 hours and on whether there is a system in place allowing women to self-refer for mammography; it will also measure whether these outcomes actually occur.

Selecting Indicators for Measurement

Indicators are events that are measured. They are categorized by type. They can be structure, process, or outcome indicators chosen in the functions of patient

EVIDENCED-BASED PRACTICE: CONSIDER THIS . . .

*T*he Agency for Healthcare Research and Quality (AHRQ, 2004) presented evidence from the scientific literature on the effects of health care working conditions on patient safety. Part of their findings reported that systems to improve information exchange, transfer of responsibility, and continuity of care between hospital and nonhospital settings ("hand offs") decrease medication errors and, in some settings, hospital readmissions.

Question: How will you use this information as part of a quality initiative at your agency?

Source: The Agency for Healthcare Research and Quality (AHRQ). (2004). The effect of health care working conditions on patient safety. Retrieved October 8, 2006, from *http://www.ahrq.gov/clinic/epcsums/worksum.htm*

care, services that support the delivery of patient care, practices, and leadership/governance. *Structure* encompasses the policies or standards regarding how service is delivered and resources made available. *Process* refers to the activities, and *outcome* is the result of activities based on policies, standards, and resources. An example could be as follows: according to policy, patients receiving conscious sedation shall be monitored by a professional nurse certified in advanced life support (structure). Professional nurses competent in advanced life support are hired and credentialed for that service (process); all patients receiving conscious sedation are monitored according to policy (outcome).

Practice indicators measure professional standards used in the delivery of patient care. Examples of practice indicators include measurement of documentation frequency and content, and utilization of aseptic technique as required. Leadership indicators measure organizational function, namely how the system affects the delivery of care and services.

When standards are clearly written and defined, are valid, and can be measured, indicators are more easily selected and usable. Meaningful indicators are specific, relevant, reliable, valid, and measurable. They use a numerator and denominator, have a target (internal or external benchmark), relate to specific standards, and define where the data or information can be found. An example would be as follows: the number of individuals monitored by an advanced life support credentialed nurse (numerator) of all patients receiving conscious sedation (denominator) based on the standard, as documented in the outpatient record. One hundred outpatient records of

individuals who received conscious sedation during a month are reviewed. Ninety-five of those patient records reflect that the patients were monitored by the ACL credentialed nurse. The standard requires 100% monitoring.

Many national organizations are currently working on indicators that can be used as external benchmarks. The Maryland Indicator Project, JCAHO, the Healthcare Effectiveness Data and Information Set (HEDIS) measures from the National Council for Quality Assurance, and other professional groups continue to refine and expand the available indicators. Utilizing external performance measures exclusively is not sufficient. Internal performance indicators based on the scope of service, mission, vision, strategic plans, core competencies, organizational culture, and values ensure that overall organizational effectiveness is measured. In turn, external benchmarks compare that performance with the best in the industry.

As previously stated, the JCAHO work started around the identification, implementation, and use of standardized tools for measuring and improving patient care. By 2004, the implementation of core measures in all acute-care hospitals was implemented. The goal is to expand further and rotate these measures. In addition, it is planned to replace noncore measures in nonhospital areas by 2010. The selection process will be driven by CMS and NQF as appropriate for long-term care, home care, behavioral health care, and ambulatory care. The JCAHO also plans to develop an approach to allow for access to aggregate data by third parties through mechanisms such as comparisons and control charts.

Understanding Variation

Variation is part of any process. People, equipment, supplies, procedures, techniques, and inaccuracies in the data all contribute to variation in data from an otherwise stable process. *Common-cause variation* is the ongoing, minute variations that are part of nature. *Special-cause variation* is much larger and can be attributed more easily to contributors through statistical methods such as run charts and control charts. These

O N L I N E C O N S U L T

To learn more about indicators and benchmarks, visit the National Council for Quality Assurance at
oryxcore@jointcommission.org
http://www.jointcommission.org/
PerformanceMeasurement/

charts can monitor processes because, even though individual data points may be unpredictable, a fluctuating pattern will emerge over time. The normal pattern is bell-shaped, meaning that most points are near the center.

The manager of a process must know when to react to particular data or situations and when it is necessary to improve the entire process. For example, suppose you have monitored medication errors on your unit for many months. When you calculate the number of errors over the number of doses administered, a percentage ranging between 0.01% and 0.02% emerges. This is probably the common-cause type of variation. You may want to compare that figure against those of other institutions, of similar type or size in your region, to evaluate whether this is an acceptable error rate. If, for the first time ever, you see a rise to 0.03%, it would be wise to analyze the data further before taking action or deciding to wait. Are all the errors of the same type attributable to a few individuals, or have new systems been introduced? Constant tinkering with systems, without understanding what the causes of the variation are, destabilizes the process. Understanding variation is important. Common-cause variation requires an answer to the question "Is this level acceptable when looked at over time?" Special-cause variation needs careful evaluation to identify the cause and to make an appropriate, focused intervention.

CONTINUOUS QUALITY IMPROVEMENT IN CONTEXT

CQI in practice requires a number of cost and implementation considerations and varies significantly with the context of the health-care organization.

Relationship of Continuous Quality Improvement to Delivery Redesign

The rapid changes in health care previously discussed have also required redesign of its delivery. We have a professional obligation to ensure that the way we deliver care is evaluated along the continuum. Despite our frustration with cost containment efforts, we must prudently manage resources to enable us to provide the greatest benefit to the largest number of clients possible. We may need to develop new delivery models that optimize the role of the professional nurse, delegate tasks, and meet the needs of our customers.

Case management and work redesign are currently being used across the country for delivery redesign. The medical, nursing, and other clinical diagnoses, and their required treatment are addressed through collaboration among disciplines. Their outcomes are usually tracked for clinical outcomes, timeliness, and cost effectiveness by a case manager or case management team. The outcomes are monitored on both an individual patient and aggregate basis. Critical pathways are tools commonly used in this process. Brainstorming, data-driven decision-making, consensus seeking, process flowcharting, evaluation of costs, and satisfaction are all tools used in case management as well as in the new quality model.

Work redesign—the process of analyzing how work is done and what system changes need to be implemented to achieve effective and efficient care delivery—also requires quality to be built in up front. Professionals need to participate actively in this evolving course. Reliance on inspection and control will not ensure delivery of quality care. Simultaneously, we cannot insist on doing it the old way. The parameters set by the Robert Wood Johnson University Hospital ProACT model for work redesign include reaching comprehensive patient outcomes (including patient satisfaction) and contributing to staff satisfaction, retention, and productivity as well as to the financial integrity of the organization (Tonges, 1989). Review of studies on the implementation of redesign activities demonstrate that many focused largely on increasing efficiency and that the changes may not have been managed effectively, resulting in loss of trust in the administration and reduction of clinical nursing leadership (IOM, 2004).

Brainstorming, data-driven decision-making, consensus seeking, process flowcharting, evaluation of costs, and satisfaction are all tools used in case management as well as in the new quality model.

Continuous Quality Improvement in the Managed-Care World

Managed care has received some favor as a methodology for controlling escalating health-care costs. Buyers of managed care, such as employers and state and federal governments, have something to say about quality, access, choice, and satisfaction with services. The more competitive the environment becomes, the more important demonstrated quality will become to differentiate between one contract or provider and another. The managed-care industry is already developing nationally accepted outcomes and indicators. Report cards on customer satisfaction with individual providers and organizations have gained popularity. Nursing must take an aggressive professional role in ensuring that the data on care delivery reflect direct nursing care delivery, coordination provided by nursing, client and family teaching, and nursing management along the continuum of care delivery. Recommendations regarding the need to develop reliable and valid methods to measure nursing care requirements and minimum staffing levels in acute-care and long-term care are considered essential (IOM, 2004).

Ongoing Role for Regulatory Agencies

Agencies such as JCAHO, the PROs, and state and federal governments will continue to have a significant role in the assurance that quality, safe health care is delivered. Many of the organizations have already begun to assist in collecting benchmarking information. JCAHO, in particular, is acting as an external change agent with regard to guaranteeing that all providers accept and implement the new paradigm. The hospital associations are helping their members deal with uniform responses to the report cards required by many managed-care contracts. Regulators and providers alike are struggling with the implementation of significant change in the delivery of quality health care.

INTERACTIVE EXERCISES

Go to the Intranet site and complete the interactive exercises provided for this Chapter.

K E Y   P O I N T S

■ Rapid changes in health care have prompted a new way of business.

■ Purchasers require "more" and "better" for "less."

■ Reliance on inspection and control against preestablished standards (the traditional quality assurance model), although of ongoing value, is no longer sufficient.

■ Quality models, such as Deming's Principles for Transformation, the Juran Trilogy, and JCAHO's 10-Step Model, provide an excellent foundation for improving quality of care.

■ Quality improvement does not just entail correcting problems but also requires ongoing improvement.

■ Quality journeys require a vision, a plan to turn that vision into reality, and a well-developed structure to ensure implementation.

■ Most problems are within systems, not individuals.

■ To improve quality, you must improve the system.

■ Specific knowledge, tools, and techniques are required to create a new quality. They include crossfunctional teamwork, lifelong learning, and process improvement.

■ Process teams are required for those improvement activities that cross functions and disciplines and cannot be dealt with in day-to-day operations.

■ Variation is part of all processes. It requires statistical analysis before actions that may destabilize the process are taken.

■ Benchmarking is the process of comparison with the best practices in the industry.

■ Tools for improvement can be divided into four categories: those used for process description, such as flowcharts and cause-and-effect diagrams; those used for data collection, such as data sheets and check sheets; those used for data analysis, such as bar and pie charts and the Pareto diagram; and those used for process improvement.

■ Continuous quality improvement is not a separate management tool. It is a way of doing business.

Thought and Discussion Questions

1. You are the nurse manager of an ambulatory surgery unit. Recently, you have seen a sudden rise in the number of surgical clients coming through the unit. Simultaneously, clients, physicians, and other providers have started to complain about long delays during pretesting.

   - Would you attempt to fix this problem by addressing it during a staff meeting? Why or why not?
   - Compare how to address this problem using a process-team versus using a staff-meeting approach.
   - Describe how you would analyze the process.
   - Explain which tools are appropriate to use for the analysis.

2. Discuss the Chapter Thought located on the first page of the chapter and discuss it (online or in class) in the context of this chapter.

☐ REFERENCES

Deming, W. E. (1982). *Out of the crisis.* Cambridge, MA: Massachusetts Institute of Technology.

Deming, W. E. (1986). *Out of the crisis.* Cambridge, MA: Massachusetts Institute of Technology.

Institute of Medicine (IOM). (2000). *To err is human: Building a safer health system.* Washington, DC: National Academy Press.

Institute of Medicine (IOM). (2001). *Crossing the quality chasm: A new health system for the 21st century.* Washington, DC: National Academy Press.

Institute of Medicine (IOM). (2004). *Keeping patients safe: Transforming the work environment of nurses.* Washington, DC: National Academy Press.

Institute of Medicine (IOM). (2006). *Crossing the quality chasm: The IOM health care quality initiative.* Retrieved on September 14, 2005, from *http://www.iom.edu/CMS/8089.aspx*

Joint Commission on Accreditation of Healthcare Organizations. (2005). *2006 comprehensive accreditation manual for hospitals.* Oakbrook Terrace, IL: Author.

Joint Commission on Accreditation of Healthcare Organizations. (1991). *An introduction to quality improvement in health care.* Oakbrook Terrace, IL: Author.

Juran, J. M. (1989). *Juran on leadership for quality: An executive handbook.* New York: Free Press.

Merriam-Webster's collegiate dictionary (10th ed.). (1997). Springfield, MA: Merriam-Webster.

St. Pierre, J. (2006). Staff nurses' use of report card data for quality improvement: first steps. *Journal of Nursing Care Quality, 21*(1), 8–15.

Strauss, S. E., Richardson, W. S., Glasziou, P., & Hayes, R. B. (2005). *Evidence-based medicine: How to practice and teach EBM* (3rd ed.). Edinburgh; New York: Elsevier/Churchill Livingston.

Tonges, M. C. (1989). Redesigning hospital nursing practice: The professionally advanced care team (ProACT) model: Part 2. *Journal of Nursing Administration, 19*(8), 19–22.

☐ BIBLIOGRAPHY

Berwick, D. M., Godfrey, A. B., & Roessner, J. (1990). *Curing health care: New strategies for quality improvement.* San Francisco: Jossey-Bass.

Bossidy, L., & Charan, R. (2002). *Execution: The discipline of getting things done.* New York: Crown Business.

The Ernst and Young Quality Improvement Consulting Group. (1990). *Total quality: An executive guide for the nineties.* Homewood, IL: Business One Irwin.

Flarey, D. L. (1995). *Redesigning nursing care delivery: Transforming our future.* Philadelphia: J. B. Lippincott.

Gale, F. (Ed.). (1994). *Tales of pursuit of quality in health care.* Tampa, FL: American College of Physician Executives.

Goodstein, L., Nolan, T., & Pfeifer, W. (1993). *Applied strategic planning: How to develop a plan that really works.* New York: McGraw-Hill.

Hamel, G., & Heene, A. (Eds.). (1994). *Competence-based competition.* New York: John Wiley & Sons.

Juran, J. M. (1988). *Juran on planning for quality.* New York: Free Press.

Katz, J. M., & Green, E. (1997). *Managing quality: A guide to system-wide performance management* (2nd ed.). St. Louis, MO: Mosby-Year Book.

Nix, M. P., Coopey, M., & Clancy, C. M. (2006). *Quality tools to improve care and prevent errors.* (Agency for Healthcare Research and Quality). *Journal of Nursing Care Quality, 21*(1), 1–5.

Provance, L., Alvis, D., & Silfen, E. (1994). Quality improvement and public health—tetanus immunization in the emergency department. *American Journal of Medical Quality, 9*(4), 165–71.

Satinsky, M. A. (1995). *An executive guide to case management strategies.* Chicago: American Hospital Publishing.

Schroeder, P. (1994). *Improving quality and performance: Concepts, programs, and techniques.* St. Louis, MO: Mosby-Year Book.

Senge, P. M. (1990). *The fifth discipline.* New York: Doubleday.

Spears, L. (Ed.). (1995). *Reflections on leadership.* New York: Wiley & Sons.

☐ ONLINE RESOURCES

The Institute for Healthcare Improvement (IHI)
http://www.ihi.org/IHI/

The Institute of Medicine
http://www.iom.edu

The Joint Commission for Accreditation of Healthcare Organizations
http://www.joint commission.org
http://www.QualityCheck.org
http://www.jointcommission.org/ PerformanceMeasurent/

To ask questions regarding JCAHO measures, go to:
oryxcore@jointcommission.org

PDCA Cycle
http://hci.com.au/hcisite2/toolkit/pdcacycl.htm

The American Nurses Association's National Database of Nursing Quality Indicators (NDNQI)
http://www.NursingQuality.org

■ *Julia W.* **Aucoin**

Informatics and Computer Use

18

> ❝ *Telecommunications technology,*
> *like the printing press and stethoscope,*
> *are tools or instruments that*
> *can extend the skills of health professionals.* ❞
>
> Myrna Armstrong (Armstrong & Frueh, 2003)

Chapter Objectives

On completion of this chapter, the reader will be able to:

1. Describe computer and informatics applications used in nursing practice, education, and research.
2. Define the basic terminology used in nursing informatics.
3. Describe the relationship between health-care provision and health management information systems.
4. Define the specialty practice of nursing informatics and the integration of that role into the nursing services of a health-care institution.
5. Identify opportunities for interdisciplinary collaboration from an informatics perspective.
6. Explain telehealth applications and their effect on patients and providers.
7. Describe nursing career opportunities in informatics.

Key Terms

Nursing Informatics

Learning Content Management System (LCMS)

Health Management Information Systems

Health Level 7 (HL7)

Electronic Patient Record

Computerized Physician Order Entry (CPOE)

Office Applications

Personal Digital Assistants

Handheld PCs

Evidence-Based Practice

Minimum Data Set (MDS)

"**N**ursing informatics** is a specialty that integrates nursing science, computer science, and information science to manage and communicate data, information, and knowledge in nursing practice" (American Nurses Association [ANA], 2001, p. vii). This specialty was first described by Graves and Corcoran in 1989, was quickly supported by several nursing graduate programs of study, was recognized as a specialty for registered nurses by the American Nurses Association in 1992, and earned credibility through the offering of a certification examination by the American Nurses Credentialing Center. Nursing informatics (NI) as a specialty grows and changes as quickly as the computer industry itself. This chapter reviews nursing informatics and addresses computer applications (software uses) that support nursing activities.

OVERVIEW OF NURSING INFORMATICS

The primary interest of nursing informatics is to expand how data, information, and knowledge are used within nursing practice. Those conducting research on informatics issues are seeking to identify and explain relationships between health-care data and nursing care. Experts in nursing informatics focus their efforts on the science of information and knowledge acquisition and on the design and evaluation of the systems that process and provide data and information (Graves & Corcoran, 1989). The actual work of informatics specialists varies with settings, according to organizational needs, individual practice interests, and specific research questions. The common element in all functions within the informatics practice is the transformation of data to information and, ultimately, to knowledge that supports and advances nursing practice.

The common element in all functions within the informatics practice is the transformation of data to information and, ultimately, to knowledge that supports and advances nursing practice.

Within care delivery institutions such as hospitals, long-term care facilities, and home-health agencies, the NI specialist could be involved with both the tasks of nursing and improvement of the quality of care. Turley (1996) described Nursing Informatics as the intersection between nursing, cognitive, computer, and information sciences. Task-related NI activities include staffing and scheduling systems, standardization and automation of care plans, documentation systems, real-time retrieval of diagnostic results, response to physician order entry, telehealth applications, and interpretation of nursing needs for the interdisciplinary informatics team.

Clinical performance measures initiatives (such as core measures for congestive heart failure, myocardial infarction, and so on), certification programs, as promoted by the Joint Commission on Accreditation of Healthcare Organizations (JCAHO, 2006) and the Centers for Medicare and Medicaid Services (CMS), require the input and retrieval of data demonstrating use of evidence-based practice guidelines. These guidelines are available electronically as well (Box 18–1). The NI specialist is instrumental in creating communication standards and pathways to provide ease in accessing necessary information for reporting to these and other organizations. Several national benchmarking databases accept and return information in only electronic format.

Nursing informatics applications in academic settings have grown to include both the use of technology in the teaching process and the teaching of an informatics-focused curriculum. Many schools of nursing use a **learning content management system (LCMS),** such as BlackBoard or eCollege, to provide Web-enhanced or totally Web-based courses, including discussion boards, chats, interactive exercises, and online testing as part of the teaching modalities (Pittinsky, 2003). The National League for Nursing (NLN) Human Simulator Project, funded in 2003, provided eight simulators to schools of nursing to be used under research-focused leadership (National League for Nursing [NLN], 2003). These simulators are programmed to present a variety of case scenarios and respond to the students' interventions in planned ways. Information can be downloaded from the simulators to provide feedback on time management, decision-making, and nursing competence.

In addition to technology projects conducted within schools of nursing, electronic journals have made articles available online. These publications have gone through the peer-review process of their print counterparts but are more accessible for readers. The *Online Journal of Nursing Informatics* and the *Online Journal*

Box 18.1 Evidence-Based Practice Electronic Resources

National Guideline Clearinghouse at
   http://www.guidelines.gov/
Centers for Disease Control at
   http://www.cdc.gov
Nursing Knowledge International at
   http://www.nursingknowledge.org
The Cochrane Collaboration at
   http://www.cochrane.org/
Agency for Healthcare Research and Quality at
   http://www.ahrq.gov

of Issues in Nursing were the first for nursing professionals. Because they are exclusively online, these journals differ from the electronically accessible versions of printed journals that may be accessed through major publishers, association Web sites, and subscribers to health science libraries. Online journals can give nurses an electronic format to share findings, experience, perceptions, knowledge, and wisdom with nursing colleagues involved in all facets of their specialties. The intent is to exercise the power of cyberspace in order to create an electronic nursing community that provides both virtually accessible and timely information about nursing globally. Online journals also purport to enhance the speed of cybercommunications through an expedited editorial process that provides rapid turnaround and publication times. Downloading one copy of these electronically accessible articles is permitted for scholarly work. Other titles are listed in Box 18–2.

E-books, electronic versions of printed books, are also available. Although they are convenient ways to access reference material, their intent is not to enable you to read an entire book electronically. Libraries generally limit the window for the checkout period to hours or days. "Living books" are a newer entity similar to online journals; chapters of such books are added to the Web site as they are completed (National League for Nursing, 2006). Many textbooks come with electronic support in the form of a Web site (for access to appendices or bonus chapters) or a CD-ROM and DVDs to supplement the materials. Because CD-ROMs are less expensive to duplicate, they are more efficient for distribution.

Given these advances in informatics, one might think that nursing is well evolved in the specialty. The Institute of Medicine (IOM) has formally identified utilizing informatics as a competency for all health professions education. This is one of the five competencies listed (Greiner & Kneibel, 2003); the other four include applying quality improvement, providing patient-centered care, working in interdisciplinary teams, and employing evidence-based practice. "Utilizing informatics" encompasses the responsibility to communicate, manage knowledge, mitigate error, and support decision-making through the use of information technology. It is the only one of the five competencies to which all the Rules for Healthcare in the 21st century apply (Box 18–3). The applications of informatics discussed in this chapter are derived from the specific informatics competencies further described in the IOM report. The least developed of the five health professions education competencies is informatics, as it is not yet completely understood as a discipline. A weakness in nursing is that a number of students continue to be educated in colleges with underfunded computer technology. One recommendation is to have informatics courses developed by discipline, by specialty, and by stage of career progression.

Informatics tools are changing how nurses teach, communicate, and deliver nursing care. Students and practitioners are able to learn more from home, creating new opportunities for nurse educators in all settings. Updating professional skills for those residing in isolated areas and accessing expert consultation for clinicians in distant geographic areas are two more reasons to embrace technology in nursing and health care.

TRANSFORMATION OF DATA TO INFORMATION AND KNOWLEDGE

The transformation of data into information and knowledge is an important informatics concept. A *datum* is a value placed on a variable. It exists without meaning or explanation. An example is the blood pressure (BP)

Box 18.2 Online Journals

The Internet Journal of Advanced Nursing Practice at
http://www.ispub.com/ostia/index.php?xmlFilePath=journals/ijanp/front.xml
Online Journal of Issues in Nursing at
http://www.nursingworld.org/ojin/
Online Journal of Nursing Informatics at
http://www.eaa-knowledge.com/ojni/
Online Journal of Rural Nursing and Health Care at
http://www.rno.org/journal/
Online Brazilian Journal of Nursing at
http://www.uff.br/nepae/objnursing.htm
Health Informatics Europe at
http://www.hi-europe.info/index.html

Box 18.3 Rules for Health Care in the 21st Century

- Care is based on continuous healing relationships.
- Care is customized according to patient needs and values.
- The patient is the source of control.
- Knowledge is shared and information flows freely.
- Decision-making is evidence-based.
- Safety is a system property.
- Transparency is necessary.
- Needs are anticipated.
- Waste is continuously decreased.
- Cooperation among clinicians is a priority.

Source: From Greiner & Kneibel. (2003).

measurement. The value of the BP, such as 90/54, is the datum for the BP. This value has little meaning until it is put into some context along with other data. For instance, if this were a 35-year-old adult, the BP might have one interpretation, but for a 10-year-old child, 90/54 would mean something very different. Age and BP may not be enough data to offer much information. You may also want to know the person's pulse and weight, which would allow you to understand the BP's significance better. Data viewed in association with one another provide meaning. Knowledge arises from using information, often from combined sources, to determine new meanings, make new discoveries, or expand understandings. For example, patient diagnoses arise through the transformation of combined laboratory data, radiology data, symptomatology, and other information into a whole, the outcome of which is knowledge.

An informatics nurse is someone who has a specialty practice in nursing, not simply a computer expert who happens to be working on a nursing-related problem.

Informatics nurses seek to create new knowledge by working first with data and then with information. Informatics specialists work as an integral part of an interdisciplinary team to support, promote, and advance the delivery of nursing care. Indeed, an informatics nurse is someone who has a specialty practice in nursing, not simply a computer expert who happens to be working on a nursing-related problem.

Some elements of nursing informatics are important for all nurses to understand. The data that are used arise from the processes involved in care delivery. To use a clinical analogy: It is important for all nurses who provide direct care to have some understanding of diabetes, yet we still use nurse specialists in diabetes to support and promote the care of diabetic patients. Nursing does not function in the exclusion of the other clinical, administrative, and managerial health professionals. Nor does nursing informatics exist independent of the larger health information management systems that hospitals, clinics, home-health agencies, nursing homes, and health maintenance organizations depend on to manage their various functions (Fig. 18–1). Although

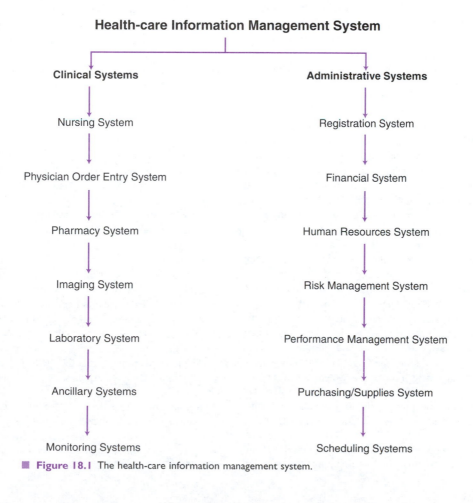

Health-care Information Management System

Clinical Systems

Nursing System

Physician Order Entry System

Pharmacy System

Imaging System

Laboratory System

Ancillary Systems

Monitoring Systems

Administrative Systems

Registration System

Financial System

Human Resources System

Risk Management System

Performance Management System

Purchasing/Supplies System

Scheduling Systems

■ **Figure 18.1** The health-care information management system.

these systems need to be integrated, they sometimes work as separate, noncommunicating units, creating some frustrations in the workplace. In time, these systems will operate seamlessly as we move toward full implementation of a totally computerized patient record. It is becoming more important for nurses to recognize that they are contributing data every time they carry out a nursing function. These data have the potential of providing powerful information when they are well understood within the environment of health-care delivery (Hebda, Czar, & Mascara, 2005).

HEALTH MANAGEMENT INFORMATION SYSTEMS

Because few systems can address every component of health care, there is generally an overriding information system with both clinical and administrative components. Clinical systems include those functions that directly support client care—documentation, order entry, and diagnostic reporting. Administrative systems address the financial, personnel, and managerial functions of the facility. Together, these **health management information systems** provide all the hardware and software needed to process data into information for multiple uses.

The planning for a comprehensive information system requires an organizational strategy based on goals for efficiency, growth, utilization of resources, and technologic leadership. The system design should create workflow so that fewer people can accomplish more work. The system must be able to expand to serve new clinical facilities. Financial and human resources must be considered, as should the amount of technology the organization can support or tolerate. It is important to maintain alignment with the organization's mission and goals in all strategic planning for the information system.

The specific management information needs of health-care institutions differ according to their mode of health-care delivery, third-party payer requirements, accrediting or licensing organizations, and internal reporting protocols. An acute-care facility that manages an inpatient facility, an emergency room, operating suites, extensive clinical laboratories, and a large pharmacy will have different data and information needs from those of a visiting nurse agency. Currently, no one health management information system fits all organizations. This is a significant barrier to the development of a uniform patient record, merging of patient information across institutions, and function in a managed-care environment.

The nursing information system should accomplish two goals. First, it should support the way that nurses operate, giving them flexibility and permitting appropriate documentation. Second, the system should support and improve nursing practice through access to information and tools (Hebda et al., 2005). It is common now for workstations to include Internet access for searches on the World Wide Web or through a literature database such as the Cumulative Index of Nursing and Allied Health Literature (CINAHL) or the National Institute of Health's MedLine (www.pubmed.gov). It is reasonable in an evidence-based practice environment to expect access to health-care databases through the computers at the nurses' station. Consultation with the hospital librarian often results in increased access to appropriate search engines and resources. Additionally, Intranet service often includes access to drug guides, policy and procedures, and patient teaching information. Box 18–4 describes how the integration of systems can help reduce medication errors.

Health Level 7 (HL7) (2006) is an international health-care informatics community collaborating to create a standard for the exchange, management, and integration of health-care information. HL7 serves to define the data, time the interchange, and communicate errors in transmission. The standards support security checks, patient identification, and data exchange structures. The goal is to create seamless systems that exchange information with each other to increase accessibility and safety for patients.

Box 18.4 System Integration to Reduce Medication Errors

1. The provider enters a medication order into the order entry system, eliminating confusion from handwriting.
2. This information is transmitted to the pharmacy.
3. The pharmacy system checks for dosage, allergies, and potential interactions. Alerts are generated.
4. The medication order is filled by the pharmacy, using a bar code or robotic system.
5. The nurse checks the order against the electronic medication administration record and is alerted to administration times as well as any special considerations.
6. The nurse documents that the medication has been administered and notes the patient's response.
7. Reminders for reorders and 24-hour chart checks are generated automatically.

Source: From Cohen, M. R. (2000). *Medication errors: Causes, prevention, and risk management.* Boston: Jones and Bartlett.

Electronic Health Record

A major national effort to develop an **electronic patient (or health) record (EHR)** has been under way for a number of years, and select institutions have had particular success in this area. The EHR is an electronic version of the patient record. The purpose of creating EHRs is to improve the ability to share client-specific information, create permanent lifelong health records, and have ready access to additional information that will improve client care. Advances in the development of large data repositories held within hospitals and other health-care institutions allow linkages between an electronic patient record and administrative, bibliographic, clinical expertise, and research databases.

The IOM produced an extensive report on the importance of developing a computer-based patient record (CPR) system or EHR built on a set of standards shared by all involved parties in both the private and public sectors (Dick & Steen, 1991). More than a decade later, the industry still faces an interesting challenge in the development and implementation of health management information systems and the greater need for client-related information to be communicated and shared by organizations. As it turns out, the simple telephone is still one of the best tools in telehealth. Audio and video systems support transmission of data using home-based monitoring equipment (Burgiss & Dimmick, 2003). Until integration of multiple systems is successful, there still may be faxed referral forms to the home-care agency and photocopied records for interagency patient transfers. The influx of managed care organizations has contributed greatly to the demand for the electronic transmission of health-care data. Many insurers now offer care management and provide regular telephone contact with their clients to help keep their health on track and the insurers' costs low. Consistent contact with a registered nurse who has access to a health history can help patients to partner with the health-care system to improve their health status.

Creating an EHR record is far more difficult than may at first be apparent. Standardized language, data collection, record format, access, confidentiality, and other ethical issues are but a few of the barriers still impeding the widespread development and use of the EHR. To build an EHR that can be shared among institutions, data must be collected and coded in a similar fashion (HL7 is helping). One issue regarding the EHR that has been and will continue to be addressed is client confidentiality. Fortunately, the Health Insurance Portability and Accountability Act (HIPAA) was implemented in 2003 in an effort to eliminate unnecessary, unwarranted, and inappropriate sharing of individual and personal health information. There are now clear guidelines for when information can and cannot be shared and how to handle electronic communication

(CMS, 2006). Password protection for facility and personal computers is recommended if any client identifiers—name, age, gender, social security number—will be stored in the computer. There remain concerns by consumers, however, that their records are not going to be protected and their other information will be accessed. Encryption, passwords, access logs, and firewalls all serve to preserve the integrity of the EHR.

The Center for Nursing Classification and Clinical Effectiveness (CNCCE), housed at the University of Iowa, has taken on the challenge of developing standardized nursing language and has published nursing interventions and outcomes with definitions to be used in documentation systems. (See Appendix B.) The Center also has collaborated with the North American Nursing Diagnosis Association (NANDA) to integrate these interventions and outcomes with nursing diagnosis language. The International Council of Nurses is also working on a language and taxonomy to improve communication of nursing activities across the globe (University of Iowa College of Nursing Centers, 2006).

Computerized Physician Order Entry

Nursing personnel have found both positive and negative attributes of **Computerized Physician Order Entry (CPOE)**. Positive factors include the fact that the provider must take responsibility for the patient-care order and does not rely upon the nurse for interpretation, assistance, or completion. The system cues the provider with correct spellings, dosages, and evidence-based guidelines and alerts the provider to potential and known contraindications and interactions. The provider can view the patient's diagnostic results and initiate appropriate orders from home, office, or other Web-based settings. Until nurses are comfortable with the new flow of

ONLINE CONSULT

See more about the International Council of Nurses International Classification for Nursing Practice, a standardized language, at
http://www.icn.ch/icnp.htm

See information on submitting a nursing diagnosis to the North American Nursing Diagnosis Association (NANDA) at
http://www.nanda.org/html/diagnoses.html

Center for Nursing Classification & Clinical Effectiveness - About Us - The University of Iowa College of Nursing at
http://www.nursing.uiowa.edu/about_us/ nursing_knowledge/clinical_effectiveness/ index.htm

orders, there is often a cognitive processing delay between the provider-entered order and the nurse's recognition of the order, since no chart is flagged and left with the unit secretary for initial transcription. An electronic flag will appear in the patient's record, which indicates that a new electronic order has been entered for this patient; it has simultaneously been sent to the diagnostic or therapeutic department for processing. If a nurse does not acknowledge this electronic flag in a timely manner, the patient may have labs drawn before the nurse has time to inform the patient. The intent is to provide timely communication and intervention for the patient through direct entry of orders and to eliminate careless errors. Providers who engage in this system generally become reliant upon it for real-time modifications to the patient's plan of care.

Computer Applications

Common **office applications**—word processing, spreadsheet, database, and graphics presentations—are also useful in nursing practice, education, and research. Most nursing programs now expect papers to be submitted using word processing and presentations to be made with graphics as a background. Spreadsheet and database management become increasingly important as nurses share in decision-making and must understand the performance improvement data in order to contribute ideas to improve practice. Specialized applications have been created to improve management and dissemination of nursing information. In practice, nurses most commonly use computers to document care and access client data. Documentation often involves selection of interventions and outcomes from a prepared list of appropriate terms, with little need for lengthy narrative comments.

Personal Digital Assistants

Increasingly, reference materials accessible through the computer have become a necessary adjunct to effective care. Handheld computer devices in the form of **personal digital assistants** (PDA) and **handheld PCs** (personal computers) are quite popular with direct care providers since textbook publishers now provide many common nursing references in this electronic format. Although looking up a medication in the drug guide is useful at the nurses' station, it is quite convenient to be able to scroll through an electronic guide on a PDA or handheld PC in the client's presence and answer her questions with confidence and competence. Hunt (2002) suggests that the PDA applications—calculator, drug reference, laboratory reference, blood gas interpretation, note-taking, task lists, calendar, phone lists, e-mail, and quick search—are appropriate for today's busy nurse. Password protection helps the nurse maintain confidentiality and compliance with HIPAA regulations.

Independent Learning Activities

Computers became a quite popular way for nursing programs to provide independent learning activities; computer-assisted instruction (CAI) replaced the video, which replaced the audio-film strip. CAI consists of text, graphics, vignettes, and self-assessment quizzes. These can be loaded onto computers or played from a CD-ROM. Although distance learning has been available since the first continuing education was provided by radio in the 1920s, it has become a convenient way to complete continuing education requirements and degrees (Armstrong, Gessner, & Cooper, 2000). With the advent of the Internet, classes can be delivered from a server on a campus or from a business through a LCMS. Courses can be completed at the student's convenience, with access to numerous resources linked to the course and real-time results through online assessments. A paperless system is created for the submission of journals and assignments, and group discussion can be conducted in a synchronous (live) or asynchronous (everyone at a different time) format. Searching for information on new medications and treatments, current information on obscure conditions, and national standards and guidelines using the search engines is available. Registration for courses, records of educational compliance, and transcripts are managed by learning management systems (Healthstream and NetLearning). Many B.S.N. completion students are likely using a learning content management system to access information for the course supported by this textbook.

A project known as the Simulated E-hEalth Delivery System (SEEDS) represents a successful collaboration between education and practice. Nursing students simulate the management of client cases using the live clinical system that practicing nurses are using to care for clients. The University of Kansas and Cerner Corporation have partnered to permit faculty to prepare clients using the nursing information system; students then respond to changes in client status, plan client care, and document additional findings in a controlled setting (Connors, Weaver, Warren, & Miller, 2002). This creative educational application of a clinical technology has already improved client care for graduates and new employees. Students tend to be satisfied with technology-enhanced learning when faculty demonstrate expertise and creativity (Bloom & Hough, 2003).

Evidence-Based Practice

Evidence-based practice implies that nursing care is delivered on the basis of knowledge generated from research. Practicing nurses have access to this knowledge—and can enhance their practice using this knowledge—by simply searching for it. The National Guideline Clearinghouse is a product of the

U.S. Department of Health and Human Services; nurses can search directly at its Web site or through their professional association Web sites to find the latest guidelines on topics such as pain management, continence care, and teaching protocols for congestive heart failure. The Sigma Theta Tau product Nursing Knowledge International serves as a repository for clinical, research, career, and continuing education resources. This is a huge managed database with links to published, proprietary, and government resources. Using the speed and power of computer search engines, this database places accurate and current information in the hands of practitioners. Many evidence-based practice resources are listed in Box 18–1.

Database Management

In addition to e-commerce, online auctions, live chats, listservs, and other computer-based services, database management and access is a growing application for computers. An agreement between major retailers and the Centers for Disease Control and Prevention (CDC) allows for the organization and reporting of information about geographic purchasing patterns related to disease management and health promotion. When the purchase of flu-related products, for instance, increases in one region, the CDC can respond with investigations and warnings for this area. Often, consumers begin purchasing over-the-counter remedies before seeking medical attention; monitoring of this activity provides information about communicable diseases before formal reporting occurs.

The National Database for Nursing Quality Indicators is an example of an analysis and storage unit for nursing quality information. Members get reports comparing performance of their units to their facility, to other similar facilities and can use the data about falls, skin breakdown, and nurse satisfaction to make decisions about organizational improvements (National Database for Nursing Quality Indicators [NDNQI], 2006).

Telehealth

Telehealth ranges from patient education television in a hospital room to analysis of urine in a smart toilet and transmission of the finding to a monitoring organization. In this age of health-care provider shortages, the time it takes to travel to remote locations suggests that specialists such as mental health providers might better serve groups by hosting a net meeting where all participants can view each other on camera and engage in the therapeutic discussion. One of the oldest telehealth applications is the transmission of pacemaker function via the telephone. By definition telehealth is the use of electronic information and telecommunications technologies to support long-distance clinical health care, patient and professional health-related education, public health, and health administration. Technologies used include: videoconferencing, the Internet, store-and-forward imaging, streaming media, and terrestrial and wireless communications (Health Resources and Services Administration [HRSA], 2006).

HRSA wants to provide access to the underserved populations through telehealth by:

- Fostering partnerships within HRSA, and with other federal agencies, states, and private sector groups to create telehealth projects
- Administering telehealth grant programs
- Providing technical assistance
- Evaluating the use of telehealth technologies and programs
- Developing telehealth policy initiatives to improve access to quality health services
- Promoting knowledge exchange about best telehealth practices

The National Council of State Boards of Nursing has recognized the challenges that practicing across state lines present and embarked upon a multistate regulation initiative called The Mutual Recognition Compact. In order to support telehealth and other interstate nursing practices, 23 states have joined the Compact allowing these nurses to practice in all the listed states and thus provide long-distance services to patients (National Council of State Boards of Nursing, 2006).

Knowing that the American people have many needs that could be addressed electronically and recognizing that private sector, educational institutions, and government together could make a difference, the Office of Technology Policy of the U.S. Department of Commerce (2004) engaged a team of experts to direct the future of telehealth. One factor to explain telehealth's slower than expected development is the consideration that telehealth is a technique and a technical aspect of traditional health care rather than an intervention itself. Many health-care providers have been reluctant to lose *touch* with their patients through electronic means. Nevertheless, homeland security, impending pandemics, and the growing numbers of underserved demand innovation and growth in telehealth. The team's report suggests that:

- Innovation has been impeded by regulatory and legal barriers.
- Creative reimbursement strategies should be explored.
- Stakeholders need to embrace telehealth.
- Inventors need protection for their intellectual property.
- Policy should consider research and development issues.

- Existing programs of the Department of Defense and Veterans Administration have more universal applicability than is currently considered.
- Research must be conducted to demonstrate clinical efficiency and cost-benefit.
- Global considerations will stimulate innovation.

Technologies currently in use include home monitoring with otoscopes, stethoscopes, and ECG monitors, which can transmit data to a home-health agency. A digital image of radiograph or ultrasound image can be conveyed to a radiologist or disease specialist in another location. Robotics can be used to perform skilled procedures when the skilled surgeon is in another location. The electronic ICU allows for experienced critical care nurses to monitor patients in partnership with remotely located critical care nurses. It is interesting to think about the monitoring that is provided by Homeland Security through satellite and heat-sensing surveillance and the possibilities of knowing that an older adult has fallen or has not gotten out of bed for several days through modes previously used only in the national security efforts.

NURSING INFORMATICS: THE SPECIALTY

The goal of nursing informatics is to improve the health of populations, communities, families, and individuals by optimizing information management and communication (ANA, 2001). Although computers have become ubiquitous in homes and businesses, it is not unusual to see implementation of new applications in the health-care setting nearly every day. Without the aid of NI specialists, these applications might offer little improvement in client care and create inefficiencies and errors. NI specialists can guide the collection, documentation, analysis, and aggregation of data with the intent of improving client care, eliminating errors, and developing a body of knowledge based on evidence. Educators skilled in teaching informatics or NI specialists skilled in nursing applications are the best people to teach nurses how to use computer applications. NI specialists possess the characteristics of a specialty (Box 18–5). The activities of the NI specialist include:

- Employment of the information systems life cycle and other tools and processes to analyze data, information, and information system requirements
- Design, development, selection, and evaluation of information technology, data structures, and decision-support mechanisms into an integrated information system
- Facilitation of the creation of nursing knowledge

Box 18.5 Attributes of a Specialty in Nursing

- A differentiated practice
- A defined research program
- Organizational representation
- Educational programs
- A credentialing mechanism

Source: From Panniers, T. L., & Gassert, C. A. (1996). Standards of practice and preparation for certification. In M. E. Mills, C. A. Romano, & B. R. Heller (Eds.), *Information management in nursing and health care*. Philadelphia: Springhouse.

Nursing informatics is interested in the nursing phenomena of client, health, environment, and nurse. It focuses on the structure of the data, information, and knowledge used by nurses in their practice and ensures that nursing's data are represented and included in the electronic processing of health information (Lange, 1997). Nurses in clinical specialties tend to focus on the content of data and information. Currently, NI specialists are working to refine nursing's language, implement efficient telehealth systems, propagate NI educational programs, and expand the use of NI in research. The National Center for Nursing Research (2006) has identified the following priorities for nursing research:

- Investigating effective use of biotechnologies and bioinformatics to enhance adjustment to these new advances and to improve self-management, healthy behaviors, and caregiver activities
- Managing the incorporation of telehealth into nursing interventions, such as enabling long-distance links between clients and clinicians for information exchange and measuring benefits, costs, and client/clinician satisfaction
- Developing and testing creative ways to use the Internet and determining the effectiveness of this method in providing client education and linkages with other clients and health-care providers to maintain and improve health
- Including skills training for interventions that use devices to maintain physiologic function, to ensure that clients and caregivers use these technologies to the best effect

The NI specialty is represented by several professional associations, such as the American Nursing Informatics Association, a working group of the American Medical Informatics Association (AMIA), a group of the International Medical Informatics Association, and other international, regional, and local organizations. Although baccalaureate programs may have a requirement for competency in computers, many offer an elective in computers in nursing. Specialization, however, is at the graduate level, with a master's degree in NI being

ONLINE **C**ONSULT

Read the themes for nursing research at
http://ninr.nih.gov

Learn more about the nursing informatics
specialty at
http://www.ania.org
http://www.imia.org/ni

Explore nursing informatics further by reading the
Online Journal of Nursing Informatics at
www.eaa-knowledge.com/ojni

offered first at the Universities of Maryland and Colorado, and now by others, such as the University of Michigan, University of Iowa, and Excelsior University. A 2006 Internet search yielded approximately 30 master's degree and certificate programs in the specialty of NI, a 100% increase in three years.

The American Nurses Credentialing Center (ANCC) offers certification as a generalist in NI, with a baccalaureate in nursing or a related field. The designation reads RN-BC once awarded. When more candidates have been prepared at the specialty level of master's, an advanced practice test may be developed. Experience and education are required for this examination, which covers systems, ergonomics, technologies, information management and generation, roles, and theories. The examination is based on, and the specialty operates from, the following overarching standards:

- Incorporate theories, principles, and concepts from appropriate sciences into informatics practice
- Integrate ergonomics and human-computer interaction (HCI) principles into informatics solution design, development, selection, implementation, and evaluation
- Systematically determine the social, legal, and ethical impact of an informatics solution within nursing and health care. (ANA, 2001)

CAREERS IN NURSING INFORMATICS

The diversity of informatics projects and programs has led to tremendous professional career opportunities. Managers in the rapidly changing health-care environment demand more and more information; clients receive care in many settings, and organizations have redesigned their services and care models. These changes mean continued growth for nursing and general health information systems and the creation of new positions in nursing informatics.

Many of the future informatics jobs are yet to be defined. As the technology changes, so too will the work necessary to maintain and further the acquisition of information and knowledge. Currently, informatics nurses are working in health-care organizations, for software and hardware vendors, in educational settings, and for insurance companies, to name only a few. In any position, the informatics specialist works closely with professionals from all other health-care disciplines.

Positions in Health-Care Organizations

A variety of roles exist for the specialist in nursing informatics within hospitals, home-health agencies, long-term care facilities, and other health-care facilities. As organizations implement information systems, informatics nurses serve an important function in assessing the institution's information needs, evaluating available products and vendors, and assisting with product installations. As communicator and interpreter, the NI specialist serves as a liaison between the nursing staff and the information systems people. When a system is ready for use (to "go live"), the NI specialist remains on site; later, the specialist is on call to provide expert assistance to staff. Once the system has been installed, modifications are made on the basis of user feedback, and the NI specialist is on to the next project. Informatics is a specialty that changes rapidly.

Long-term care facilities are required to make electronic reports to CMS of the **Minimum Data Set (MDS),** an assessment tool for residents of long-term care facilities. Therefore, nurses must both assess residents on an ongoing basis and report this information using the electronic tools and standardized language. The more than 16,000 long-term care facilities required to comply with this reporting create many job opportunities for registered nurses. Performance improvement functions need NI competencies to navigate through the myriad of systems, reports, and guidelines that direct improvement activities. Compliance offices require access to all the systems in a facility. The annual National Patient Safety Goals (NPSG) (JCAHO, 2006) have created renewing requirements for training staff to better patient safety by improving, in part, data retrieval, management, and reporting. Performance improvement is concerned with NPSG, clinical indicators of quality, and evidence-based practice guidelines. Informatics supports the achievement of these safety goals by providing information retrieval to support medication reconciliation, safe patient handoff, prevention of recording sound-alike look-alike drugs, and accurately recording patient identifiers. From safety reporting to reimbursement opportunities, informatics skills are necessary.

EVIDENCED-BASED PRACTICE: CONSIDER THIS . . .

*Y*our agency just announced that they will be implementing bar-coding technology as one of their safety initiatives. You have just read about this new instrument to measure nurses' satisfaction with and proper use of the technology and to prevent "work-arounds" and errors (Hurley et al., 2006).

Question: How will you use this information to promote effective integration of this new technology and compare rates of adverse drug events?

Source: Hurley, A. C., Lancaster, D., Hayes, J., Wilson-Chase, C., Bane, A., Griffin, M., Warder, V., Duffy, M. E., Poon, E. G., & Gandhi, T. K. (2006). The medication administration system—nurses assessment of satisfaction (MAS-NAS) scale. *Journal of Nursing Scholarship, 38,* 298–300.

Positions with Systems and Software Vendors

Many of the producers of software and information systems seek to hire NI specialists. Nurses work to develop new products, market products and services, and install systems. Experience with documentation and standardized nursing language is helpful. Clinicians with enough patient-care experience to predict barriers to implementation are most useful. NI experts serve as liaisons between the vendor and the health-care organization, because they are able to comprehend and articulate the issues for both parties. Increasingly, nurses with expertise are sought for these positions.

Positions in Educational Settings

With the expectation that beginning and experienced nurses possess informatics competencies (Box 18–6), the responsibilities of educators has grown. Whether it is expertise in instructional design to create a new Web-based course or CD-ROM, or the vision required to implement the SEEDS project, this area presents many opportunities. While these are areas for the experienced nurse educator with a specialty in instructional design, the NI specialist is often consulted. Success in grasping these opportunities is recognized and rewarded—for instance, when Sigma Theta Tau International presents biennial awards for

BOX 18.6 Informatics Competencies for Nurses

Beginning nurses:

- Computer literacy skills
- Information literacy skills
- Identifying, collecting, and recording data relevant to the nursing care of patients
- Analyzing and interpreting patient and nursing information as part of the planning for the provision of nursing services
- Using informatics applications designed for the practice of nursing
- Implementing public and institutional policies related to privacy, confidentiality, and security of information

Experienced nurses:

- Use system applications to manage data, information, and knowledge within their specialty
- Participate as content experts to evaluate information and assist others in developing information structures and systems to support their specialty
- Promote the integrity of and access to information, including confidentiality, legal, ethical, and security issues
- Be actively involved in efforts to improve information management and communication
- Act as advocates or leaders for incorporating innovations and informatics concepts into their specialty

Informatics nurse specialists:

- All the competencies of beginning and experienced nurses
- Operates within Standards of Practice and Professional Performance of Informatics Nurse Specialist

Source: Adapted from American Nurses Association. (2001). *Scope and standards of nursing informatics practice.* (Publication No. NIP21 3M 05/02). Washington, DC: Author.

creativity in the use of technology in both nursing and public education. Nurse-owned companies—such as Health Soft and Professional Development Software, both educational design firms; and NursingCEU.com, a continuing education company—demonstrate the opportunities for entrepreneurship in informatics. Affiliation with any professional association, such as the National League for Nursing, or a commercial venture, such as Assessment Technologies Institute (ATI), will provide opportunities in test development and delivery.

Positions in Managed Care Organizations and Insurance Companies

As forms of managed care continue to develop, the demand for data and information will grow, as will the opportunities for informatics specialists. Informatics nurses are now working directly with care delivery institutions in developing data and information systems as well as with the mechanisms involved in the internal reporting processes. New roles are emerging continuously, many of which have been designed and articulated by NI specialists as this burgeoning new specialty evolves.

For more information, search the various informatics association Web sites and read the *Online Journal of Nursing Informatics*. As with many nursing specialties, nurses should look for opportunities and then create the position that will best serve the organization.

ONLINE CONSULT

Educational design firms at
http://www.healthsoftonline.com
http://www.softwarefornurses.com

Achievement test companies at
http://www.nln.org/testprods/index.htm
http://www.atitesting.com

INTERACTIVE EXERCISES

Go to the Intranet site and complete the interactive exercises provided for this Chapter.

KEY POINTS

■ Nursing informatics is a specialty that integrates nursing science, computer science, and information science to manage and communicate data, information, and knowledge in nursing practice (ANA, 2001, p. vii).

■ Nursing informatics as a specialty grows and changes as quickly as the computer industry itself.

■ The goal of nursing informatics is to improve the health of populations, communities, families, and individuals by optimizing the management and communication of information (ANA, 2001).

■ The NI specialty is represented by several professional associations, is supported by advanced education, and is credentialed through certification.

■ The primary interest of nursing informatics is to expand how data, information, and knowledge are used within nursing practice.

■ Few systems can address every component of health care, so there is generally an overriding information system with both clinical and administrative components.

■ Telehealth has only begun to explore the possible applications and innovations that could advance the provision of health care.

■ In practice, nurses most commonly use computers to document care and to access client data. Yet, there are many applications for education and research.

■ The diversity of informatics projects and programs has led to tremendous professional career and interdisciplinary opportunities.

Thought and Discussion Questions

1. Since the implementation of HIPAA, what challenges have you observed regarding access to patient information?

2. What would happen in your agency if the computer system "went down"? How would the failure affect patient care?

3. What is the representation of nursing informatics in your facility?

4. How can handheld technology improve patient care?

5. What telehealth application would you like to invent to improve access to health care?

6. Review the Chapter Thought on the first page of the chapter, and be prepared to discuss it online or in class.

☐ REFERENCES

American Nurses Association. (2001). *Scope and standards of nursing informatics practice.* (Publication No. NIP21 3M 05/02). Washington, DC: Author.

Armstrong, M., & Frueh, S. (2003). *Telecommunications for nurses: Providing successful distance education and telehealth.* New York: Springer.

Armstrong, M., Gessner, B., & Cooper, S. S. (2000). POTS, PANS, and PEARLs: The nursing profession's rich history with distance education for a new century of nursing. *The Journal of Continuing Education in Nursing, 31*(2), 63–70, 94–95.

Bloom, K., & Hough, M. C. (2003). Student satisfaction with technology-enhanced learning. *CIN: Computers, Informatics, Nursing, 21*(5), 241–246.

Burgiss, S., & Dimmick S. L. (2003). Telehealth in home health care. In M. Armstrong & S. Frueh, *Telecommunications for nurses: Providing successful distance education and telehealth.* New York: Springer.

Centers for Medicare and Medicaid Services (CMS). (2006). HIPAA—general information. Retrieved October 22, 2006, from *http://www.cms.hhs.gov/HIPAAGenInfo/*

Connors, H. R., Weaver, C., Warren, J., & Miller, K. L. (2002, September/October). An academic-business partnership for advancing clinical informatics. *Nursing Education Perspectives, 23*(5), 228–233.

Dick, R. S., & Steen, E. B. (1991). *The computer-based patient record: An essential technology for health care.* Washington, DC: National Academy Press.

Graves, J. R., & Corcoran, S. (1989). The study of nursing informatics. *Image, 21*(4), 227–231.

Greiner, A. C., & Knebel, E. (Eds.). (2003). Health professions education: A bridge to quality. Washington, DC: Institute of Medicine.

Health Level 7 (2006). What is health level 7? Retrieved October 22, 2006, from *http://www.hl7.org/*

Health Resources and Services Administration (2006). Telehealth. Retrieved October 22, 2006, from *http://www.hrsa.gov/telehealth/*

Hebda, T., Czar, P., & Mascara, C. (2005). *Handbook of informatics for nurses and health care professionals.* 3rd ed. Upper Saddle River, NJ: Prentice-Hall.

Hunt, E. C. (2002). The value of a PDA to a nurse. *Tar Heel Nurse, 64*(3), 18–19.

Joint Commission on Accreditation of Healthcare Organizations [JCAHO] (2006). Performance measures initiatives. Retrieved October 22, 2006, from *http://www.jointcommission.org/PerformanceMeasurement/*

Lange, L. L. (1997). Informatics nurse specialist: Roles in health care organizations. *Nursing Administration Quarterly, 21*(3), 1–10.

National Center for Nursing Research (2006). Future themes of nursing research. Retrieved October 22, 2006, from *http://ninr.nih.gov/*

National Council of State Boards of Nursing (2006). Retrieved October 22, 2006, from *https://www.ncsbn.org/158.htm*

National Database of Nursing Quality Indicators (NDNQI) (2006). Retrieved October 22, 2006, from *http://www.nursingquality.org/*

National League for Nursing (2003). Grants. *Nursing Education Perspectives, 24*(6), 326.

National League for Nursing (2006). About living books. Retrieved October 22, 2006, from *http://www.nln.org/ProfDev/onlinecourses/aboutbooks.htm*

Pittinsky, M. S. (2003). *The wired tower.* Upper Saddle River, NJ: Pearson Education.

Turley, J. (1996, Winter). Toward a model for nursing informatics. *Image: Journal of Nursing Scholarship, 28*(4), 309–313.

University of Iowa College of Nursing Centers (2006). Center for Nursing Classification and Clinical Effectiveness. Retrieved October 22, 2006, from *http://www.nursing.uiowa.edu/centers/cncce/*

U.S. Department of Commerce, Office of Technology Policy (2004). *Innovation, demand, and investment in telehealth.* Washington, DC: U.S. Department of Commerce.

☐ BIBLIOGRAPHY

Cohen, M. R. (2000). *Medication errors: Causes, prevention, and risk management.* Boston: Jones and Bartlett.

Mascara, C., Czar, P., & Hebda, T. (1999). *Internet resource guide for nurses & health care professionals.* Menlo Park, CA: Addison-Wesley.

Nicoll, L. (2000). *Computers in nursing's nurses' guide to the internet.* Philadelphia: Lippincott.

Nicoll, L. (2003). Education and networking in nursing informatics. *CIN: Computers, Informatics, and Nursing, 21*(5), 275–286.

Montgomery, K., & Fitzpatrick, J. (2002). *Essentials of internet use in nursing.* New York: Springer.

Panniers, T. L. & Gassert, C. A. (1996). Standards of practice and preparation for certification. In M. E. Mills, C. A. Romano, & B. R. Heller (Eds.), *Information management in nursing and health care.* Philadelphia: Springhouse.

Thede, L. (2003). *Informatics and nursing.* Philadelphia: Lippincott.

☐ ONLINE RESOURCES

American Medical Informatics Association
http://www.amia.org/

American Nursing Informatics Association
http://www.ania.org

British Computer Society—Health Informatics (Nursing) Specialty Group
http://www.bcs.org/server.php?show=conWebDoc.1220

Canadian Nursing Informatics Association
http://www.cnia.ca/

Informatics Nurse Certification
http://www.nursingworld.org/ancc

International Medical Informatics Association, Nursing Group
http://www.imia.org/ni/

NLN Living Books
http://www.nln.org/profdev/onlinecourses/livingbooks.htm

PDA Software
http://www.rnpalm.com
http://www.collectivemed.com

■ *Cyril F.* **Chang** ■ *Susan K.* **Pfoutz**

Health-Care Economics

> " *Health care is different,*
> *and the free market system needs*
> *to be modified appropriately to fit*
> *the special characteristics of health care.* "

Chapter Objectives

On completion of this chapter, the reader will be able to:

1. Understand and apply the basic economic concepts of supply, demand, and market to health care.
2. Describe the structure of the American system of health-care financing and delivery.
3. Describe the roles played by the major participants of the health-care system.
4. Explore health-care issues from the perspective of economics.
5. Examine the varied health-care payment systems.
6. Explain the concept of managed care and the different forms of managed care organizations.
7. Analyze current health-care reforms, such as consumer-driven health plans and the Medicare prescription drug program.

Key Terms

Economics

Health-Care Economics

Demand

Supply

Provider-Driven System

Market-Driven System

Third-Party Payers

Fee-for-Service Payment System

Prospective Payment System

Diagnosis-Related Groups

Managed Care

Capitation

Health Maintenance Organization

Independent Practice Association

Preferred Provider Organization

Point-of-Service Plan

Health Report Card

Effectiveness

Cost-Effectiveness

Evidence-Based Practice Guidelines

I n the past, economic and management issues were not pivotal to nursing practice. In today's health-care market, however, a variety of economic factors are affecting nursing practice and the outcomes of nursing care. This chapter presents a broad survey of current health-care issues from an economic perspective. It prepares nurses to examine relevant economic concepts and integrate them, along with clinical, environmental, and behavioral knowledge, into nursing practice.

Significant changes in the health-care system—specifically, the transformation from a provider-driven system to a market-driven system—require that nurses learn the language and concepts of economics to function effectively. As the single largest group of health-care providers and stewards of health-care resources, nurses are increasingly challenged to defend the value of nursing care. To do so, nurses in a variety of practice settings are examining and analyzing such operational factors as cost, efficiency, and productivity. These economic activities, designed to link clinical outcomes to desirable economic goals, enable nurses to demonstrate the effectiveness and cost-effectiveness of nursing care.

Economics focuses on how consumers, business firms, government entities, and other organizations make choices in an environment of scarce resources. **Health-care economics**, a specialty area of economics, analyzes how the different parts of a health-care system work together to deliver service that meets the needs of patients. Nurses are critical participants in this delivery process. They must learn the basic language of economics and the financial realities in order to deliver high-quality nursing care and contribute meaningfully to the common goals of efficient resource utilization and cost containment.

Obtaining economic knowledge and applying it to nursing practice can be both personally and professionally rewarding. In personal terms, nurses who approach health care from a broader, economic perspective can compete effectively in today's health-care marketplace. In professional terms, having this additional knowledge and related skills enables nurses to participate more fully in the design and delivery of health-care services and to achieve the best possible outcomes at the lowest possible cost. A good beginning point for this learning process is to review the American system of health-care delivery and explore the roles played by the system's major participants.

THE AMERICAN SYSTEM OF HEALTH-CARE DELIVERY: AN OVERVIEW

The health-care system in the United States is composed of three major groups of participants (Box 19–1).

Box 19.1 The Three Groups of Health-Care Participants

Consumers are the millions of individuals who use health care and pay for the services either out of pocket or through an insurance policy bought individually, received through employment, or offered by a government agency.
Providers are doctors, nurses, pharmacists, and other health-care professionals who work in hospitals, nursing homes, and a wide range of other health-care settings to provide services for consumers and who receive payments from consumers directly or through a third-party payer.
Third-party payers are insurance companies, health plans, and government agencies that arrange for the services to be delivered and the necessary payments for these services.

The first group is clients, who are the consumers of health-care services. Only a small percentage of consumers pay for their health care out of pocket. For example, the total amount paid out of pocket by consumers accounted for approximately 15.1% of total national health-care expenditures in the year 2004 (Center for Medicare and Medicaid Service [CMS]). Most consumers are insured by private insurance companies through their employers or by a government-sponsored insurance program.

The second group of participants consists of health-care providers, such as hospitals, nurses, physicians, and other health-care workers, who participate directly and indirectly in the production and delivery of health care. The third group, called third-party payers, includes insurance companies and government health-care agencies that provide health insurance coverage to specific groups of individuals, such as employees of businesses, union members, the elderly, and low-income individuals.

In this vast and largely decentralized market for health-care services, consumers demand services to meet their health needs. Meanwhile, providers deliver the demanded services and bill the third-party payers for payment. The third-party payers collect insurance premiums or taxes to pool financial resources from a large number of individuals and businesses to raise the necessary funds to pay for the anticipated expenses. The roles played by each of the three major parties of the health-care system, along with the critical economic and health-care delivery issues, are examined later in this chapter.

Demand for Health Care

The **demand** for health care refers to the varying amount of health care that a consumer is willing and able to purchase at each of the possible prices. A number of key factors, called the *determinants of demand*, affect the demand for health care:

- Consumer needs and expectations for illness cure, supportive care, preventive care, and health-promotion services
- Individual values derived from the conceptualization of health, culture, ethnicity, religious beliefs, education, and gender
- Access to health care and a set of economic variables that affect access, including price of care, income, employment status, wealth, and adequacy of insurance coverage

Consumer Need

The total demand for health care by all consumers in a country is fundamentally related to the size and health status of the general population. As the population grows larger and older, the demand for health care naturally rises. The demand for health care is also influenced by the incidence of illnesses and injuries. A large natural disaster or a sudden outbreak of influenza, Bird Flu, or severe acute respiratory syndrome (SARS) undoubtedly places greater demands on health care. Still another factor that affects the demand for health services is consumers' expectations from the utilization of various health-care services. The consumers who expect a full recovery from a particular treatment demand a greater amount of the service than those otherwise identical consumers who expect less from the same treatment.

Consumer Conceptualization

The demand for health care is also influenced by consumers' conceptualization of health care. Although good

ONLINE CONSULT

AcademyHealth at
http://www.academyhealth.org

The Economics of Health Care at
http://www.oheschools.org/index.html

The Kaiser Family Foundation at
http://kff.org/

The Center for Studying Health System Change at
http://www.hschange.com/

The Robert Wood Johnson Foundation at
http://rwjf.org

The Commonwealth Fund at
http://www.cmwf.org/

health is desired universally, it is not the only goal in one's life. Individuals routinely make tradeoffs between health and nonhealth goals (rent, food, personal desires) when they conflict with one another. There is no universally held conceptualization of what health means to consumers (Fuchs, 1993). Conceptualizations of health vary widely with such individual characteristics as life expectancy, capacity for work, need for health care, and ability to perform a variety of personal and social functions. The wide variation in conceptualizations of health impedes the potential for the establishment of a public policy that can be consistently implemented and financed. In fact, the wide variations are reflected in the continuing inability of health-care reform efforts to develop a consensus on whether or not to finance a national health plan.

Consumer Access

The demand for health care is also influenced by consumer access to health-care services. Consumer access to health-care services is the ability of the individual physically to reach and to use health-care facilities and services. Geographic proximity influences access to health-care services, as do eligibility for insurance benefits, income level, prices of health services, and individual values and preferences. Urban medical centers tend to concentrate technology and providers within a small geographic area, whereas rural areas often have a scarcity of specialty health-care providers and limited technologic support. Income level influences both the ability to pay for health insurance and health-care services. Some individuals cannot afford private insurance, yet their income exceeds the level that would qualify them for state-funded coverage.

Prices of health care are far more complicated than the prices of ordinary consumer goods and services like a hamburger or a haircut. Health-care consumers know very little about the prices of the various health-care services and products that they buy. They know even less about the relationship between the prices paid and the quality of care purchased. This uneven distribution of knowledge between the buyer and seller is referred to in economics as the phenomenon of "information asymmetry." Providing more information on health-care quality and prices to consumers and the various other factors that influence access to health care has been a central focus of discussion in recent national health-care reform debates (Federal Trade Commission and the Department of Justice, 2004).

The Influence of Delivery System Characteristics on Demand

In addition to the demand-determining factors just discussed, the amount and quality of health care actually delivered to consumers are also influenced by the characteristics of the delivery system. In a provider-driven health-care system, for example, providers dominate health-care demand. In such a system, providers not only prescribe services that they consider necessary and appropriate but also furnish them for a fee. Providers have the control over which and how many health-care services consumers use. This approach is intended to meet the needs of consumers as determined by providers on the basis of their best professional judgment. Such a system does not address the preferences and perceived demand of consumers, as is the case with most other consumer goods and services that are bought and sold every day.

In contrast, a market-driven system responds directly to the demands of the purchaser, whether those demands relate to type of product, quality, or price. The purchaser in this system is not necessarily the consumer who ultimately uses the service or product. In most cases, the purchaser is the health plan or an employer that provides insurance coverage. A market-driven system supports the emergence of competitive delivery plans that seek to attract purchasers by offering more of what consumers want—amenities as well as services and competitive prices. A good example is the attention given to quality improvement by hospitals and physician groups in response to the demand of purchaser alliances that have grown popular across the country.

It is important to note that these days, employers who purchase health insurance and individual consumers are becoming more educated and informed. They freely voice their preferences concerning health-care issues and seek a more active role in the management of their

care. It is useful to examine how different factors affect the health-care services demanded by consumers in the American system (Box 19–2).

Supply of Health Care

Health-care supply is as complex as health-care demand. The **supply** of health-care services refers to the ability and willingness of providers to deliver health care. The supply of health care is affected by the geographic location of both providers and consumers, availability of health-care facilities and technology, consumer and provider cultural values, and, again, the characteristics of the delivery system.

In a **provider-driven system**, the dominant providers, such as physicians and hospitals, make major decisions on the location of services, types of providers, and technology available. The types of services offered, the location of services, as well as provider educational support are determined primarily by the dominant providers and secondarily by market factors. Two secondary market factors, for example, are state licensing laws and available reimbursement. Each type of provider category (e.g., physician, advanced practice nurse, physician assistant, registered nurse, unlicensed assistant) must comply with such laws in order to practice. Providers must also be willing to provide their services for the amount of reimbursement available.

By contrast, in a **market-driven system**, the number of providers at each level of education and the locations and types of services provided are determined by the needs and locations of consumers, rather than by the needs and location of providers. Technology is funded

BOX 19.2 Factors Affecting Health Services Demanded

1. Consumer needs and expectations for cure, care, prevention, and health promotion services
2. Individual values derived from the conceptualization of health, culture, ethnicity, religious beliefs, education, and gender
3. Access to health care is affected by many variables: geographic location, times of service, transportation, price of care, income and wealth, and adequacy of insurance coverage:

   - **Availability** of health care includes characteristics that allow a consumer to reach health care and feel accepted: geographic location, times of service, transportation, and feeling of being personally and culturally welcomed.
   - **Price** of health care is broadly defined as a wide range of sacrifices consumers must make in order to obtain the desired health-care service. It includes both the amounts of deductible, copayments, and other out-of-pocket payments and noncash costs such as travel time and other inconveniences involved in accessing the needed care.
   - **Income** and wealth significantly influence whether or not an individual can afford health insurance, which in turn affects the amount of services demanded.
   - **Insurance coverage** significantly influences the quality of health care demanded by consumers. An insured consumer demands a much greater amount of service than an otherwise identical consumer who has no insurance.

and provided on the basis of consumer need rather than the availability of a skilled provider. For instance, approximately 34% of consumers are using nontraditional health-care therapies to meet their health-care needs in addition to treatment for the same condition from a medical doctor (Eisenberg et al., 1993). As a result, many nurses and other traditional health-care organizations are supplying a growing variety of alternative services that are reimbursed by third-party payers.

A Hybrid System of Supply and Demand

The current health-care delivery system in the United States is a hybrid of the provider-dominant and market-driven systems. In general, the market forces of supply and demand are allowed to function in health care to provide the efficiency and cost savings that are customarily associated with a market-driven system. In other words, competition on the supply side is generally perceived to be healthy and appropriate for health care. Nevertheless, the free-for-all type of rampant competition that often characterizes the highly competitive and sometimes volatile private sector of the U.S. economy is uniformly considered to be excessive and wasteful for health care. Hence the market-driven American health-care system is heavily tempered by rules and regulations driven by dominant providers and sanctioned by the government. The government recognizes that health care is different and that the free market system needs to be modified appropriately to fit the special characteristics of health care (Federal Trade Commission and the Department of Justice, 2004).

Financing Our Health Care System

Health care is expensive and must be paid for. How we pay for health care is important because it affects both the quantity and quality of services accessible to consumers and is a critical factor in determining the cost of health care.

Role of Third-Party Payers

In health insurance terms, insurance companies and government agencies that provide insurance coverage are called **third-party payers**. The consumers and providers of health care are, respectively, the first and second parties to a health-care transaction. Most business transactions outside of health care involve only two parties—a buyer and a seller. But very few people can afford to pay large medical bills out of their own pockets. Health care in the United States is financed primarily by employers in the private sector or by the government in the public sector. Some large employers choose to be self-insured; that is, they have

elected to pay for the medical costs of their employees themselves without buying health insurance from an insurance company. Most employers, especially medium-sized and small ones, buy health coverage from insurance companies and share the costs of premiums with their employees.

The major function of third-party payers is to serve as a financial intermediary. In this role, third-party payers define the services to be provided, estimate the costs of insuring a given population, and collect premiums to cover the anticipated costs of services and administration. Third-party payers play another important role—that of a health-plan administrator. This role is a complex process of determining the range of services to be covered and the amounts of co-payments and deductibles that enrollees must pay for each service delivered. It also involves processing the claims submitted by providers and paying providers for the services delivered. Finally, health-plan administrators also monitor outcomes of services, including consumer satisfaction, clinical outcomes, quality and appropriateness of the services provided, and the cost of services.

Unlike Canada or the United Kingdom, where a single payer provides insurance coverage for the entire country (Box 19–3), a large number of health plans are evident in the American health insurance landscape. Private employers are free to choose among many private for-profit and nonprofit insurance companies, with each offering a variety of health plans to suit the needs and preferences of purchasers. In the United States, government is also involved in the provision of insurance coverage. At the federal level, for example, Medicare provides insurance coverage for elderly and disabled individuals and families. Medicaid is a government insurance program for low-income individuals that is financed jointly by the federal and state governments and is administered by the states.

The main advantages of a multiple-payer system are that it offers greater competition, choice of health plans and services, and incentives to increase efficiency and reduce health-care costs. The disadvantages, however, include multiple layers of administration and higher administrative costs, such as those imposed on providers who must deal with multiple payers and their unique administrative structures. Another disadvantage of a multiple-payer system is that many individuals may fall through the cracks and become uninsured because they do not work for an employer that offers insurance and/or cannot afford to pay the premium. Employers must also consider the impact of cost of health care on their business when deciding whether to offer health insurance.

Payment Systems

There are two broad categories of payment for services in the American system of health-care delivery: the

BOX 19.3 The Health-Care Systems in the UK and Canada

The British National Health Service (NHS) is the largest national health-care system in Europe. It was set up in 1948 to provide health care for all British citizens on the basis of need, not the ability to pay. The NHS is funded by the taxpayer. This means it is accountable to Parliament. It is managed by the Department of Health, which is directly responsible to the secretary of state for health. The department sets overall health policy in England, is the headquarters for the NHS, and is responsible for putting policy into practice. It also sets targets for the NHS and monitors performance through its four directors of health and social care. About one million people work for the NHS in England, and it cost more than £50 billion a year to run in 2002.

Canada's "single-payer" health-care system has long been a source of national pride. Unlike the UK's NHS, the Canadian system is characterized by local control, doctor autonomy, and consumer choice. It is a taxpayer-supported national health-care system that covers everyone living in Canada. It is called a single-payer system because government is the only source of payment for services provided. The service is free at the point of delivery, and the 10 provinces have the authority and responsibility for planning, financing, and evaluating the services for residents in each province.

fee-for-service system and the prospective payment system. The fee-for-service system dominated health care for many years, but the prospective payment system has had a strong presence since the early 1980s.

Fee-for-Service Payment

The **fee-for-service (FFS) payment** system, also known as the retrospective system, gives providers maximum control of services provided to the consumer. Preapproval by third-party payers for services is usually not required in this model. In this provider-driven system, it is the health-care providers who determine the need for and type of services. Few limits are placed on the length of hospital stay, the location of the services, or the amount and type of diagnostic procedures, pharmaceuticals, or treatment procedures. Services are typically considered separately or unbundled; that is, the different services that are required for a procedure or an episode of care are billed separately, with a fee generated by each service or procedure provided. Payments to hospitals and other providers are based on providers' costs in providing the services plus an acceptable markup. Under the FFS system, all costs related to care delivery, including the costs of products, services, salaries, construction, uncompensated care, and capital equipment, are passed on to consumers and their third-party payers.

Prospective Payment System

The **prospective payment system (PPS)** has emerged in response to concerns about access to care, and spiraling health-care costs. It is a pricing model that sets payment rates for hospital services before treatment begins. The Medicare program is an example of a prospective pricing model. In 1982, Medicare transitioned to a PPS based on a diagnostic classification system called **diagnosis-related groups** (DRGs). Under the DRG system, inpatient services are grouped together, or bundled, by DRG into a package of care with a predetermined price allowed for each DRG. If the

hospital can provide the service package for less than the DRG price, it can keep the difference. Conversely, if the care costs the hospital more than the allowable price, the hospital has to absorb the loss. More than 450 DRGs have been identified on the basis of the principal diagnosis, use of the operating room, age of patient, comorbidity, and complications (Table 19–1).

The DRG system used by Medicare in the public sector of health care is the most widespread example of prospective pricing. Originally, DRGs applied only to hospital inpatient services. Most physician services and all outpatient services were excluded. In the early 2000s, different versions of DRGs were introduced in hospital outpatient care, skilled nursing-home care, and home health care. Private sector PPSs are gaining popularity, and varieties of models have been implemented. These models include capitated managed care programs, health maintenance organizations, preferred provider organizations, independent physician associations, and physician hospital organizations.

Managing Risk Related to the Cost of Health Care

The different systems of paying for health care result in different burdens or risks to the various parties in the health-care transaction. There are financial risks and incentives associated with each type of payment system as described below.

Fee-for-Service System

In a traditional FFS system, the health-care provider bills the insurance company for each procedure or service delivered. As long as that service is covered by the insurance policy, the provider can expect to be paid the agreed-upon amount. Because the provider has a fairly good idea about the potential income, he or she bears little risk for the total amount of cost for

Table 19.1

Leading Diagnosis-Related Groups (DRGs) in 2001

DRG Code	Description	Average Days of Care	Average Cost per Discharge
005	Extracranial vascular procedures	5.9	$18,572
012	Degenerative nervous system disorders	6.1	$18,226
014	Specific cerebrovascular disorders	3.3	$17,344
015	Transient ischemic attack and pre-cerebral occlusions	8.3	$13,464
024	Seizure and headache, age >17 yr with complications and comorbidities	5.8	$15,217

Source: From The 2003 Medicare and Medicaid Statistical Supplement to Healthcare Financing Review at http://www.cms.hhs.gov/apps/review/supp/2003/table29.pdf

services. The health-care provider increases income by increasing the number of services delivered. The incentive is for the health-care provider to provide more services. For a patient with coronary artery disease, for example, the provider would encourage diagnostic tests, invasive procedures, and prolonged rehabilitation services.

Prospective Payment System

In a prospective payment system, the health-care provider is paid one fee for an episode of care—a term used to measure the various health-care services and encounters rendered in connection with an identified injury or period of illness. With this payment arrangement, the provider shares some financial risk, because the payment remains the same regardless of how many diagnostic tests, equipment, supplies, and institutional facilities are required. Although the amount for each episode is limited, providers could increase income by increasing the volume of episodes of care or decreasing the number of expensive services provided. With this system, treatment of a patient with coronary artery disease now would consist of only needed testing, discharge from the hospital as soon as possible, and limited rehabilitation services. To increase income, the health-care provider would seek to increase the number of patients with coronary artery disease.

Capitated System

In a capitated system, providers bear much more financial risk. The provider is paid a specified amount per patient per month regardless of what services the

patients use. The incentive here is to keep persons in good health by encouraging healthy lifestyles and aggressively treating early signs of cardiovascular risk. Critics of this system are concerned that managed care organizations (MCOs) and providers may deny some needed services in order to maintain the income of the health-care providers. To maintain income, the health-care insurer and provider will seek to enroll healthy people rather than ones who already have coronary artery disease.

Financial Risks for the Consumer of Health-Care Services

There are financial risks for the consumer with all payment systems. As described previously in the chapter, consumers of health-care services have little knowledge of the cost of health care and are not really the purchasers of the services. Therefore, the incentive for the consumer is to use as many health services as he desires. To encourage consumers to use only needed health services, the portion of the cost of health services paid by the consumer is important. This *copayment*, the portion of the cost of health-care services paid by consumer out-of-pocket, has been rising. In theory, this will encourage consumers to use services more wisely. There is a risk that people may not receive health-promotion services, early screening of high blood pressure, or early treatment. This can result in coronary artery disease, for example, being more advanced by the time they seek health care. They may also not be able to afford their portion of the cost of prescriptions or other treatments.

MANAGED CARE

No single definition can adequately describe managed care because it encompasses a complex range of organizational forms that are still evolving. Defined broadly, however, **managed care** is a health-care system willing to be held accountable for both the clinical and financial outcomes of an enrolled population. The charge for managed care services is based upon a capitated (fixed) payment per month per person that is determined by the covered services and enrollment size (Folland, Goodman, & Stano, 2001).

More Americans are enrolled in managed care health plans (including health maintenance organizations, preferred provider organizations, and point-of-service plans) than ever before. According to the Henry J. Kaiser Family Foundation (2006a), enrollment in all forms of managed care plans increased from 27% of workers covered by employer plans in 1988 to 97% in 2005. Preferred provider organization (PPO) enrollment increased from 11% to 61% of covered workers from 1988 to 2005; HMO enrollment increased from 16% in 1988 to 31% in 1996, but has since declined to 21% in 2005. In contrast, enrollment in the traditional fee-for-service plans has declined from 73% of total enrollment in 1988 to 3% in 2005. Among Medicare enrollees, managed care enrollment rose from 1.3 million or 4% of total in 1990 to 4.7 million or 11% in 2004. Managed care enrollment grew even faster among Medicaid enrollees, rising from 9% in 1990 to 61% in 2004 (Henry J. Kaiser Family Foundation, 2006a).

Compared with the traditional FFS health plans, managed care has two distinctive characteristics. First, it integrates the financing and delivery functions of health care into a single organized system. Second, it emphasizes the delivery of a coordinated continuum of services, from wellness care to acute care, with incentives to achieve cost efficiency. Typically, enrollees must choose a primary health-care provider who will coordinate all of their health-care services. This health-care provider must be a participant in the managed care organization. This primary-care provider serves as a *gatekeeper* by limiting access to specialty care.

> [M]anaged care is a health-care system willing to be held accountable for both the clinical and financial outcomes of an enrolled population.

Under FFS systems, insurance companies reimburse hospitals and physicians after the needed services are delivered. Providers earn more if they provide more. By contrast, under managed care, keeping patients healthy means more profit for the managed care organization. Managers of managed care plans are therefore motivated, at least theoretically, to emphasize communication and coordination of care among physicians, nurses, and other health-care providers across different delivery settings. The essence of this delivery concept is that specific patient outcomes are achieved by economizing use of resources within a fixed budget. Managed care can be defined most practically by reviewing the major participants, the concept of capitation, and the managed care models.

Major Participants of Managed Care

There are four main participants in any managed care system: managed care organizations, purchasers, enrollees, and providers. Each participant will be covered in turn.

Managed Care Organizations

Managed care organizations (MCOs) are the health-care entities that arrange for the provision of services for a group of individuals who are enrolled in the health plan. Purchasers of health plans pay MCOs a fixed monthly payment called a capitation rate for each enrollee. This rate is based on the covered services and the size of enrollment. MCOs then arrange for the delivery of services through a variety of organizations: an HMO, a PPO, a point-of-service (POS) plan, or a combination of these plans.

Purchasers

Purchasers are employers, groups of employers, trade unions, professional associations, governmental agencies, and other legal entities that buy health insurance coverage for their participating members or employees. The purchasers arrange for the necessary legal agreements to contract with MCOs for health services. They also collect the premiums, pay the MCOs, and ensure that the MCOs fulfill their financial and clinical obligations.

Enrollees

The members or enrollees of an MCO are the employees or association members who are insured. They receive the health services and, together with their employers or associations, pay for the covered services. It is very expensive for people to purchase health insurance individually so it is very rare. Enrollees are the final consumers of health services but are not necessarily the purchasers or buyers of health care. The self-insured employers and insurance companies are the buyers of health services. In recent years, enrollees have become more educated and vocal about their preferences and more willing to take action when they are denied care or are dissatisfied with service quality. In response, Congress and many state legislatures have debated a variety of patients' rights bills designed to

A growing number of large purchasers have in recent years chosen to insure themselves (National Center for Health Statistics, 1997; Park, 2000). They no longer buy insurance products from an insurance company; instead, they have become their own insurers. Because the health-care costs of a large group of people can be predicted, self-insured entities save money by not paying for the expenses and profits of an outside insurance company. Many of these self-insured purchasers still contract with an insurance company or MCO to manage the different health plans offered to their employees. However, the MCO in this instance is no longer an insurer; it has become a management service organization that processes insurance claims and provides case management for a fee.

safeguard patients' rights to health care and to provide avenues of recourse for denied services or unfavorable outcomes result.

Providers

The last group of participants within a managed care system includes the institutional and individual providers, such as hospitals, physicians, nurses, and other health-care professionals. They are usually organized into provider networks that deliver services to members of an MCO for specified payments. The mechanisms for payment are determined by the managed care model. In many cities, providers are organized and represented by management services organizations (MSOs). MSOs are paid to provide contracting and administrative services for provider organizations. They specialize in the management of all business aspects of medical practices for the providers.

Models of Managed Care

MCOs can be for-profit or nonprofit. They may be owned by a variety of entities, including for-profit insurance companies, nonprofit companies such as Blue

○NLINE ○ONSULT

The Managed Care Information Center at
http://www.themcic.com/

Wikipedia: The Free Encyclopedia at
http://en.wikipedia.org/wiki/Managed_care

American Association of Retired Persons (AARP) at
http://www.aarp.org/health/insurance/managed_care/

Cross and Blue Shield associations, physician groups, hospitals, and health management firms. MCOs can be organized in a variety of ways and are customarily classified into three major types: (1) health maintenance organizations (HMOs), (2) preferred provider organizations (PPOs), and (3) point-of-service (POS) plans.

Health Maintenance Organization

A **health maintenance organization** is a managed health plan that either administers or arranges for health care to be provided to its members for a capitated monthly fee (Fox, 2001). The philosophy of an HMO is to emphasize preventive health services, such as routine physical examinations, prenatal care, and proactive management of chronic conditions, in order to avert more costly treatments related to progression and complications. In the United States, the number of people enrolled in HMOs jumped from 38.8 million in 1992 to 78.9 million in 2000, but declined to 66.1 million in 2004 (Henry J. Kaiser Family Foundation, 2006a).

Health services provided to patients must be procured from hospitals, physicians, nurse practitioners, nurses, and other health-care providers who participate in the plan. Therefore, the relationship that an HMO maintains with its providers is paramount to its success. Without providers' cooperation, HMO enrollees will not receive cost-effective health services. It is therefore critical to develop a thorough understanding of the different ways that HMOs maintain relationships with their providers (Box 19–4).

Depending on the financial arrangement and organizational relationships with providers, HMOs can be organized in a number of ways. The major HMO models are the staff model, the group model, the independent practice association model, and the network model.

Staff Model
The staff model of HMO employs its own salaried physicians, advanced practice nurses, and ambulatory care nurses. These providers deliver health services only to plan members and usually practice at clinics owned and operated by the HMO. A major advantage of this model is that it exercises tight control over the providers' practice, thereby making it easier for the HMO to monitor utilization and costs. A major drawback is that the physicians in a staff model, who earn a fixed income and work for a fixed number of hours to satisfy mandated encounter times, may give patients less attention than physicians working elsewhere.

Group Model
Unlike the staff model, which hires its own physicians and nurse practitioners and operates at specific practice sites, the group model involves contracting exclusively with a group of physicians and, separately, with hospitals to provide services to its enrollees. The HMO

BOX 19.4 Examples of HMO Relationships with Providers

- **Selecting, recruiting, and credentialing providers**: A successful HMO must develop an effective provider network by recruiting and selecting providers of different specialties who have the appropriate credentials and are willing to work in a managed care environment.
- **Primary care physician**: Sometimes referred to as a "gatekeeper," the primary care physician (PCP) in an HMO promotes the health of specified members. The PCP is responsible for organizing the medical care process, either by referring a patient on for specialized diagnosis and treatment or by caring for that patient then and there. Primary care physicians often participate in teams made up of specialists and other health professionals to study and improve how care is provided, particularly for patients at highest medical risk.
- **Practice guidelines**: Practice guidelines are systematically developed statements on medical practices that help a practitioner make decisions about appropriate health care for specific medical conditions. Managed care organizations commonly use these guidelines to evaluate appropriateness and medical necessity of care. Practice guidelines are developed with the "long view" of health in mind. This approach is fundamental to managed care organizations that want to keep the customers they have. Physicians in managed care environments, therefore, have the incentive to provide high-quality medicine.

usually pays the group practice a monthly capitation fee per enrollee for the provision of health-care services. The major difference between a staff model and a group model is that the staff model HMO pays physicians directly, whereas physicians in a group model are paid by the physician group that contracts with an HMO.

Physicians in a group model can maintain greater autonomy and may experience less direct pressure from the HMO to cut costs than in a staff model because they are paid by the practice group and not by the HMO directly. The practice group bears the financial consequences of practice patterns of individual physicians that may be outside the HMO norms, however. For example, the cost of specialty referral services may come out of the per member per month (PMPM) fees, reducing the practice group's income.

Independent Practice Association Model

In an **independent practice association** (IPA), the fastest-growing HMO model, the HMO enters into a contractual relationship with solo or group practitioners to provide physician and nurse practitioner services (Chang, Price, & Pfoutz, 2001, p. 307). Unlike the group model in which the HMO enters into an exclusive contract with a physician group for physician services, the IPA involves contracting with individual solo practitioners, solo practitioners in practice groups, or both, for services. In general, the IPA receives a PMPM capitation fee under a risk contract with the health plan purchaser to take full responsibility for the health-care needs of the covered enrollees. The IPA then reimburses physicians for their services through either a subcapitation or a discounted FFS subcontract.

A *subcapitation* is a secondary capitation arrangement between the IPA and a group of physicians. This payment arrangement shifts the financial responsibilities of providing services for all or part of the enrollees of an HMO to the contracted physicians or physician

group. A discounted FFS system, on the other hand, is a payment arrangement whereby the physicians are still paid according to the services delivered—hence the term fee-for-service—but the fees are negotiated at a discount to ensure a steady flow of patients from an HMO. The arrangement for payment of specialty services is legally identified in the contract between the IPA and its providers.

Network Model

Like the IPA model, the network model HMO contracts with more than one physician group practice to provide services. Some HMOs contract with many small primary care practices (e.g., family practice, internal medicine, and pediatrics) under a subcapitation agreement that pays the physicians a fixed monthly fee for each patient under the physician's care. These physician groups can make referrals to specialists but are themselves financially responsible for reimbursing these referrals. Some network model HMOs contract with broad-based multispecialty groups that can provide a wide range of services from primary care to highly specialized services. The network model allows referrals to a wider range of physicians than either the staff model or group model.

Preferred Provider Organization

A PPO comprises networks of hospitals, private practice physicians, and other health-care practitioners that provide comprehensive health services to an enrolled population for a negotiated fee. There are more than 1000 PPOs in the United States that serve more than 20% of the insured population and account for half of the total enrollment in managed care plans (Fox, 2001).

A variety of entities, including insurance companies, professional organizations, hospitals, and physician groups, may sponsor PPOs. It is also common for a PPO to be jointly sponsored by a hospital and physicians. Unlike HMOs, PPOs do not assume the financial risk of arranging and providing health services; the sponsoring organizations do. In other words, it is the responsibility of the insurance companies or the professional organizations that sponsor the PPOs to bear the financial risk for the enrolled population. PPOs also do not perform many of the functions customarily assumed by HMOs, such as utilization review and insurance underwriting. Put simply, PPOs are merely networks of physicians that agree to accept discounted FFS for a steady flow of patients.

For example, participating providers such as physicians and advanced practice nurses in a PPO are usually reimbursed 15% to 20% less than the local prevailing reimbursement rates. In return for lower fees, enrollees of a PPO agree to use health-care providers and facilities with whom the PPO has established a contractual relationship.

One disadvantage of a PPO is the limitation of choice of providers. Consumers prefer health-care providers with whom they are familiar. They are often very reluctant to change health plans when their personal health-care provider is not included.

Point-of-Service Plan

A point-of-service (POS) plan combines the classic HMO characteristics, such as capitation and coordination of service delivery, with characteristics of a PPO, such as enrollee choice of providers. Patients in a POS plan are required to select a primary care provider to manage and coordinate the health-care needs of patients under his care. Patients may choose a nonparticipating, out-of-plan provider but must receive a referral from the primary care provider, who, in addition to providing primary care, serves as a "gatekeeper." They must also pay a higher deductible or copayment for this privilege, because the out-of-plan providers are usually paid at an FFS rate. The POS plan appeals to enrollees who prefer the option of choosing providers outside the plan and are willing to pay extra for it.

The options within managed care are continually evolving to include new forms designed to appeal to purchasers and enrollees. The main goal remains the same—to reduce costs by integrating the delivery and payment of services. The managed care formats that develop to achieve this goal are responsive to health-care markets.

THE COST-QUALITY TRADEOFF

Cost issues have dominated recent public debates on health-care reform. Central to the ongoing debates is the issue of whether costs can be managed without

sacrificing quality. Decision makers at managed care organizations, health-care providers including nurses, and consumers of health care often disagree about the proper role of cost containment, choice, and quality in the delivery of health-care services. In the midst of these emotion-laden debates, it is easy to lose sight of the fact that quality of care is the key to success for individual and institutional providers. Health care is different from ordinary consumer goods in that consumers not only demand but also are willing to pay for high-quality services as long as the benefits outweigh the costs. It is critical that individual providers recognize that the winning strategy in an increasingly competitive environment is to compete in terms of quality while keeping costs at a reasonable level. The concepts of efficiency, clinical effectiveness, and cost-effectiveness play an important role in managing the relationship between quality and cost.

Recent health-care reform efforts have heightened the need for objective measures of health-care quality (Box 19–5). To this end, federal agencies, such as the Center for Medicare and Medicaid Services (CMS) and the Agency for Healthcare Research and Quality (AHRQ), and many state governments have made progress in increasing public disclosure of morbidity and mortality rates as well as data from facility inspections and physician malpractice and licensure actions. Private nonprofit and for-profit organizations such as the National Center for Quality Assurance (NCQA), the Joint Commission on Accreditation of Healthcare Organizations (JCAHO), and HealthGrades.Com have also made health-care quality data more readily available to both providers and consumers.

Health Report Card

Current efforts to develop comparative quality indicators that can be shared across institutions and with consumers have resulted in the "report card" phenomenon. A health report card is a summary of information about doctor and hospital performance and consumer satisfaction designed for consumers/patients and health-care buyers. Health plan providers, employer groups, and care providers have initiated several collaborative efforts to formulate report cards that identify and measure the quality of patient care. Examples of report cards are the ANA Nursing Report Card for Acute Care (American Nurses Association [ANA], 1995b), the Health Plan Employer Data and Information Set (HEDIS), the Leapfrog Group's Hospital Survey, and the *U.S. News and World Report's* "America's Best Hospitals" exclusive rankings. These reports include cost benchmarks as well as selected quality indicators, but the results have been hampered by serious gaps in information and lack of standard indicators and uniform means for data collection and analysis.

BOX 19.5 Public and Private Entities that Monitor and Report on Quality of Health Care

National Center for Quality Assurance (NCQA) is an independent, 501(c)(3) nonprofit organization whose mission is to improve health-care quality. NCQA evaluates health care in three different ways: through accreditation (a rigorous on-site review of key clinical and administrative processes); through the Health Plan Employer Data and Information Set (HEDIS, a tool used to measure performance in key areas, such as immunization and mammography screening rates); and through a comprehensive member satisfaction survey. Although participation in the accreditation and certification programs is voluntary, more than half the nation's HMOs currently participate. And almost 90% of all health plans measure their performance using HEDIS (http://www.ncqa.org/).

The Joint Commission on Accreditation of Healthcare Organizations (JCAHO) evaluates and accredits more than 16,000 health-care organizations and programs in the United States. An independent, not-for-profit organization, JCAHO is the nation's predominant standards-setting and accrediting body in health care. Since 1951, JCAHO has developed state-of-the-art, professionally based standards and has evaluated the compliance of health-care organizations against these benchmarks (http://www.jointcommittee.org/).

The Leapfrog Group is an initiative driven by over 170 major health-care purchasers who are committed to initiating breakthrough improvements in the safety, quality, and affordability of health care for Americans. It is a voluntary program aimed at mobilizing employer purchasing power to alert America's health industry that big leaps in health-care safety, quality, and customer value will be recognized and rewarded. Leapfrog gathers and reports information on hospital quality and patient safety efforts to help patients make informed decisions about where to receive hospital care (http://www.leapfroggroup.org/home).

HealthGrades.Com is a private, for-profit, health-care quality ratings and services company. Its mission is to improve the quality of health care nationwide. With its proprietary, objective provider ratings and expert advisory services, HealthGrades gives clients targeted solutions that enable them to measure, assess, enhance, and market health care (http://www.healthgrades.com).

Health Resources and Service Administration (HRSA) Center for Quality (CQ) was established in the HRSA with the mission to strengthen and improve the quality of health care, especially as it relates to HRSA programs and service populations. The CQ operates jointly with the Office of the Chief Medical Officer (CMO) (http://www.ask.hrsa.gov/Quality.cfm).

The **Institute of Medicine (IOM)** was chartered in 1970 as a component of the National Academy of Sciences. The Institute provides a vital service by working outside the framework of government to ensure scientifically informed analysis and independent guidance. The IOM's mission is to serve as advisor to the nation to improve health. The Institute provides unbiased, evidence-based, and authoritative information and advice concerning health and science policy to policymakers, professionals, leaders in every sector of society, and the public at large (http://www.iom.edu/).

The ANA has been active in the identification of nursing-sensitive outcomes—those that respond to nursing interventions. The currently identified nursing-sensitive outcomes are nosocomial infections, medication errors, pressure ulcer, falls, patient and family complaints, and mortality (Aiken, Smith, & Lake, 1994; ANA, 1995a and 1995b; Blegen, Goode, & Reed, 1998; Whitman, Kim, Davidson, Wolf, & Wang, 2002). Use of indicators from such a report card and incorporation of a nursing minimum data set (NMDS) in retrievable format can facilitate the identification of the contribution of nursing care within the larger health-care episode.

In addition to documenting quality, historical measures of treatment outcomes and costs must be translated into new indicators for capitated delivery models. Ongoing programs to assess patient satisfaction need to identify appropriate indicators of satisfaction and how they relate to continuing use of facility services. Traditional patient care issues, such as functional status, physiologic status, symptom management, and safety, continue to be applicable, but they should now be specifically related to patient outcomes. New quality indicators for providers and health-plan managers also must be developed. These efforts assist in the development of meaningful and reportable measures of not only the effectiveness but also the cost-effectiveness of the services delivered.

Effectiveness, Cost-Effectiveness, and Financial Performance

Effectiveness measures how well a prescribed treatment has accomplished the anticipated outcome. Cost-effectiveness measures whether the prescribed treatment has accomplished the desired outcome at a lower cost than any other available treatment alternatives. The delivery of effective and cost-effective services enables providers to maintain quality while keeping cost at an affordable level. Many medical services are beneficial to patients, but not all of them are cost-effective. The delivery of a noncost-effective service may benefit a few patients but will drain scarce resources away from other patients whose needs have not been met. An emphasis on cost-effectiveness helps providers deliver the greatest possible health outcome while remaining mindful of today's financial constraints and limited resources. The attention paid to cost-effectiveness will pay dividends to providers, health plans, and, most importantly, patients.

Traditionally, financial performance in health care was evaluated on the basis of a variety of financial indicators measuring profitability, cash flows, liquidity, capital structure, asset efficiency, and other aspects of the financial health of a business entity. These indicators, both individually and taken as a whole, could provide a comprehensive picture of the financial position of a health-care institution such as a hospital. The *Almanac of Hospital Financial and Operating Indicators*, published annually by the Healthcare Financial Management Association in association with the Ingenix, Inc., includes more than 150 indicators related to these categories collected from audited financial statements, strategic operating indicator data submitted by hospitals, and Medicare cost reports (Healthcare Financial Management Association [HFMA], 2006). New measures of financial performance for prospective capitated payments must be developed. The growing trend toward allocating resources on the basis of the number of enrolled members per month and the number of days per 1000 member-days requires new systems and processes to identify, allocate, and measure costs.

Policies to Improve Quality

Quality has always been an important issue in health care. Historically, government involvement in quality improvement focused on the regulation of the professions in terms of licensing, educational requirements, and other issues related to the quality of providers. The quality of care was mostly left to the purview of private professional groups. For example, many hospitals historically have been monitored by the Joint Commission of Accreditation of Healthcare Organizations (JCAHO), with impressive results.

A major event in government involvement in outcome regulation occurred in 1972 with the creation of professional standards review organizations (PSROs). Part of the 1972 Medicare amendment to monitor the quality of federally funded care for Medicare beneficiaries, PSROs were to ensure that beneficiaries receive the most efficient and most appropriate services. In 1983, PSROs were replaced by peer review organizations (PROs). These were private, nonprofit organizations under contract with the Healthcare Financing Administration (HCFA, now CMS) for utilization review and quality of care assessments of hospitals, HMOs, and some office practices.

After the backlash in the early 1990s against managed care and media reports of managed care mistreatment of patients and other related quality issues, President Bill Clinton signed an executive order in September 1996, creating the Presidential Advisory Commission on Consumer Protection and Quality in the Healthcare Industry. The President appointed a 32-person commission to make recommendations on how to improve quality of health-service delivery and reduce medical errors. In 1999, the reputable and influential Institute of Medicine (IOM) issued a controversial report, *To Err Is Human: Building a Safer Health System* (Institute of Medicine [IOM], 1999), which revealed, for the first time to the American public, that between 44,000 and 98,000 people a year die unnecessarily as a result of medical errors in hospitals. In spring 2001, the IOM released another damning report, *Crossing the Quality Chasm: A New Health System for the 21st Century* (IOM, 2001), which made recommendations for achieving threshold quality improvement in health-care delivery. In November 2003, the IOM released *Keeping Patients Safe: Transforming the Work Environment of Nurses* (IOM, 2003) as a companion to the IOM's earlier patient safety report, *To Err Is Human*. The 2003 report identifies solutions for problems in hospital, nursing home, and other organization work environments that threaten patient safety through their effect on nursing care.

Nurses, as the largest number of health-care professionals, can participate in the evolution of the nation's health-care system to ensure long-term effectiveness.

Encouraged by the release of a series of government reports and taking advantage of the advancement in the World Wide Web, many private health information providers have begun to offer online quality data on hospitals, nursing homes, and individual physicians. Today, anyone with access to a computer and the Internet can instantly obtain information on health-care quality. An example is the HealthGrade.Com Web site (*http://www.healthgrades.com*), which offers online quality information on hospitals, nursing homes, and physicians. Another example is the Web site of the Leapfrog Group (*http://www.leapfroggroup.org/*), a nonprofit quality improvement organization committed to mobilizing employer purchasing power to advance the idea that big leaps in health-care safety, quality, and customer value should be recognized and rewarded.

Pay-for-Performance (P4P) Programs

Pay for performance is emerging health care quality-improvement movement in the United States. Unlike the traditional fee-for-service payment system that pays providers according to the number of services delivered, providers are rewarded for quality of health-care services under the pay-for-performance arrangement.

According to Integrated Healthcare Association, a California-based leader in the P4P movement, Pay-for-Performance is based on two fundamental principles. The first principle is a common set of performance measures for physician groups, developed collaboratively by health plan and physician group medical directors, researchers, and other industry experts. The second is the practice of significant health plan financial payments based on that performance, with each plan independently deciding the source, amount, and payment method for its incentive program *(http://www.iha.org/)*. Across the country, many private health plans as well as government insurance programs including Medicare *(http://www.cms.hhs.gov/apps/media/press/release.asp?Counter=1343)* are experimenting with various forms of the P4P programs.

Evidence-Based Practice Guidelines in Disease Management

Incorporation of research and other available evidence to guide practice is another strategy to improve the quality of care. According to Huffman (2005), **evidence-based practice guidelines** are specific procedures or protocols that are developed based on empirical evidence, health research, and professional clinical expertise to provide clinicians with treatment routines that demonstrate the best patient outcomes. One example of evidence-based guidelines is using standard clinical pathways for decreasing the congestive heart failure (CHF) hospitalization rate (Peterson, 2004).

Evidence-based practice is also a part of the concept of disease management (Huffman, 2005). According to the Disease Management Association of America (DMAA, 2007), *disease management* is an approach to delivering health care to persons with chronic illness that aims to improve patient outcomes while containing health-care costs. For full programs of disease management, six components are required:

- Identification of specific population (usually related to chronic conditions such as CHF and diabetes)
- Use of evidence-based practice guidelines
- Collaboration among physicians, formal and informal home health care (HHC) providers
- Patient/family self-management education
- Outcome measurement, evaluation, and management
- Feedback and reporting loop

In addition, disease management occasionally includes various technologies to enhance favorable outcomes and financial savings for clients and HHC agencies (Huffman, 2005). Several authors have identified the use of evidence-based practice guidelines *and disease management* as key to improving health outcomes (Peterson, 2004; Institute of Medicine, 2001 and Hunt et al., 2001).

The small size and limited resources of some health-care agencies hinder their widespread implementation of these principles, however (Peterson, 2004; Institute of Medicine, 2001).

HEALTH-CARE REFORM

The preceding discussions of performance measures and quality improvement are useful for individual and institutional providers in their quest for quality improvement and cost control. But the United States as a country faces a host of health-system problems that require effective national health reform, such as persistent cost inflation and racial and ethnic disparities in access to quality health care.

With breakthrough advances in medical science such as the mapping of the human genome and better understanding of the basic disease processes, health care in the 21st century offers an array of promising technologic solutions to diseases and medical conditions. Health-care providers in the United States continue to have success in applying advanced medical technologies to previously untreatable diseases and illnesses. The need for these high technology services increases as the population ages. The United States, however, ranks behind developed countries, such as England, Canada, and many Scandinavian countries—which spend a smaller percentage of their GDPs (gross domestic products, or total value of all goods and services produced within their borders) on health care—in basic system performance standards such as infant mortality and life expectancy (Anderson, Reinhardt, Hussey, & Petrosyan, 2003).

Numerous reform measures have been attempted in the last 30 years to improve the functioning of the American system of health-care delivery. Historically, the demand for health-care reform has come from three different sources:

- Businesses, whose employee health-care costs rise every year
- The middle class, who represent a majority of the workforce and the voting public
- Advocacy groups that lobby for the poor and the economically disadvantaged

On the supply side of the reform movement, the key players have been health policy experts, politicians, and public officials who work in key health-care agencies that are charged with the responsibilities of administering public policies. In recent years, many reform measures have been pushed and implemented in three major areas of public concerns: access, cost, and quality.

Policies to Improve Access

The United States spent about 16% of its GDP on health care in 2004 (Smith, Cowan, Heffler, Catlin, & National Health Accounts Team, 2006), and yet 45.8 million of its citizens or about 15.7% of the total population remain uninsured (DeNavas-Walt, Proctor, & Lee, 2005). Even among the insured populations, many people have inadequate insurance coverage or limited coverage that leaves many medical expenses uncovered. Concurrent reform efforts by federal, state, and local governments have been under way to plug the holes in the insurance system and to bring health insurance to the near-universal level. These efforts include the following programs.

The Federal SCHIP Program

The State Children's Health Insurance Plan (SCHIP) was created under the Balanced Budget Act of 1997 as a new children's health insurance program under Title XXI of the Social Security Act. The purpose was to encourage states to initiate and expand health insurance coverage for uninsured children. Many of these children are in families with too large of an income to be eligible for Medicaid but with an income too low to pay for coverage themselves. In 1999, Congress allocated $24 million over five years to help the states expand their insurance coverage for uninsured children. The funds cover the costs of insurance, as well as outreach services to enroll children, and reasonable costs for administration. Funds must be used to cover previously uninsured children and not to replace existing public or private coverage.

The statute set the broad outlines of the program's structure and established a partnership between federal and state governments. States were given great flexibility in tailoring the programs to meet their own needs. States could create or expand their own separate insurance programs, expand Medicaid, or combine the two approaches. States could choose among several benchmark benefit packages, develop a benefit package that is actuarially equivalent to or better than one of the benchmark plans, or use the Medicaid benefit. States also had the opportunity to set eligibility criteria regarding age, income, resources, residency, and duration of coverage within broad federal guidelines. The federal role is to provide technical assistance to the states and to ensure that programs meet statutory requirements designed to ensure meaningful coverage under the program.

To date, all 50 states plus the U.S. Virgin Islands have established their SCHIP programs. The rapid expansion of this federally assisted health insurance program has recently been credited by the U.S. Bureau of the Census for reducing the number of uninsured children in this country (DeNavas-Walt et al., 2006).

Individual State Initiatives

Rather than waiting for Congress and the federal government to solve their problems, many states have engaged in a variety of reforms to expand insurance coverage for their residents. These programs have been developed along two major paths: health insurance mandates and expansion of Medicaid coverage.

Insurance mandates are government laws and regulations that require the provision of certain benefits to ensure consumer access to services deemed to be desirable and necessary. State governments have issued hundreds of mandates on a wide range of health issues, including patient safety, coverage of preventive services, staffing requirements in hospitals and nursing homes, and parities of mental health care with regular health care. These state initiatives reflect the states' impatience with federal health reform, the widespread dissatisfaction with a range of health-care issues at the grass-roots level, and a genuine desire for improvement in access to and quality of health care.

In addition to benefit mandates, many states have chosen to expand insurance coverage through a variety of mechanisms. One of these has been the application of the federal Section 1115 waivers to expand insurance coverage to the previously uninsured and underinsured populations. Tennessee, for example, initiated an experimental managed care program called TennCare in 1994 to add half a million previously uninsured and uninsurable individuals to its Medicaid population. The program now covers about 1.4 million individuals, or one in every four residents of Tennessee. Since its inception, TennCare has been plagued by an assortment of administrative and cost-control problems. But it has played a major role in reducing the percentage of individuals with no insurance in Tennessee to 12.7%, or 2.8 percentage points below the national average of 15.5% (DeNavas-Walt et al., 2005).

Oregon chose a different approach to Medicaid expansion, opting for an innovative rationing program called the Oregon Health Plan. The goal of the plan was to provide insurance coverage to all residents in the state through a combination of public and private insurance programs. Central to the Oregon Health Plan is the establishment of a "prioritized list of health services," a list created by the Oregon Health Services Commission to rank more than 700 individual medical services from most to least important. Each year, the state legislature sets the funding level to cover a certain number of services on the list, but it cannot rearrange the list. Thus, in Oregon, the legislative branch of the state government determines the spending level and the predetermined priority list ensures that the most critical services are provided.

In April 2006, Massachusetts implemented a groundbreaking private, market-based reform that would make health insurance available to every resident of Massachusetts by 2009. The reform requires everyone in the state to purchase health insurance by July 1, 2007, and all businesses with more than 10 employees to pay a contribution of up to $295 per year for each worker if they do not provide insurance. Of the approximately 500,000 uninsured, about a fifth are estimated to be eligible for Medicaid. Others will either receive premium assistance on an income-based sliding scale for policies with no deductibles if their income is below 300% of the federal poverty level or purchase lower-cost policies in the private market if their income is above 300% of the federal poverty level. Premium assistance will be financed by redirecting a portion of the one billion dollars currently spent by state government on the uninsured.

Medicare Reform and Prescription Drug Benefits

The Medicare program has been the nation's major health insurance program for the elderly and disabled since 1965. Despite rapid and continued increases in budget allocation for this federally funded insurance program, many critical services—such as prescription drug coverage, and long-term care services, including home health care—remain uncovered or insufficiently covered. In recent years, the proposal to offer prescription drug benefits under Medicare received strong bipartisan support in Congress.

During the 2000 presidential election, candidates from both political parties championed the passage of prescription drug benefits for seniors. Since capturing the White House, President George W. Bush has made the provision of prescription drug benefits a legislative priority. Throughout 2003, various versions of the prescription drug plans were proposed in both the Senate and the House of Representatives. The two houses passed separate versions of prescription drug plans in the fall of 2003, and the final legislation was passed by both the House and the Senate in late November 2003 (Table 19–2).

The new Medicare drug benefit became available to all 43 million elderly and disabled beneficiaries in January 2006. As of April 2006, CMS reported that 35.8 million beneficiaries have prescription drug benefits, including 19.7 million enrolled in the Part D plans, 10.3 million with private retiree plans, and another 5.8 million with drug benefit coverage through the VA health system or other sources (The Henry J. Kaiser Family Foundation, 2006b). Controversy emerged related to the large number of plans and the confusing nature of

Table 19.2

What Do You Gain Under the Medicare Prescription Benefit?*

If Annual Medications Costs are ($):	You Pay ($)[†]	You Save ($)	Change in Out-of-Pocket Spending
500	32.50	0	47% more[‡]
1000	857.50	142.50	14% less
1500	982.50	517.50	35% less
2000	1107.50	892.50	45% less
2500	1420.00	1080.00	43% less
3000	1920.00	1080.00	36% less
5000	3920.00	1080.00	22% less
10,000	4265.00	5735.00	57% less

*How the voluntary drug benefit, which started in January 2006, would have affected individual enrollees with no other drug insurance or low-income subsidies.
[†]Includes $250 annual deductible, estimated $35 monthly premium, and different levels of copayments.
[‡]Individual enrollees with drug costs of under $810 a year would pay more out of pocket than they would get back in subsidies.
Source: Adapted from AARP Public Policy Institute.

the benefits. Ongoing evaluation will determine the positive and negative outcomes of this program.

Policies to Contain Cost

During the last three decades, federal and state governments have tried a variety of cost-containment policies to restrain the cost of health care. Some of them were designed to regulate specific targets, such as the amount of capital investment in the hospital industry and the numbers of medical and nursing school graduates. Still others regulated the prices of specific services, such as physician fees and hospital reimbursement rates. A summary of these programs follows.

Certificate-of-Need (CON) Regulation

The Certificate-of-Need (CON) program was initiated in the early 1970s to control hospital costs. It was designed to regulate hospital expenditures for new beds, equipment purchases, and facility constructions. CON requires that individuals or health-care facilities seeking to initiate or expand capacity or services submit applications to a state agency. Approval must be obtained before initiation of projects that require capital expenditures above certain dollar thresholds, introduction of new services, or expansion of bed numbers or services. The rationale is that excessive hospital growth—and the resulting need to maintain underutilized facilities—is the root cause of hospital cost inflation. Further, excess supply of hospital beds presents temptations for hospital administrators and physicians to increase hospital admissions so as to raise occupancy rates for hospitals and income for physicians. The CON approach to hospital cost control has had a modest effect on hospital costs, according to many health economists who studied the program (Salkever & Bice, 1979; Conover & Sloan, 1998). It is a very conservative approach to cost control, focusing on the hospitals and large medical practices only, and it provides no new incentives to change patient or physician behavior.

The Medicare PPS Program with DRGs

As mentioned earlier, the federal government changed its method of paying hospitals for treating Medicare patients in 1983, creating an incentive for hospitals to economize. The Medicare PPS pays hospitals a fixed, predetermined sum of money for a particular admission. If a hospital can provide the service at a cost below the fixed amount, it pockets the difference. If more resources and money are used than the predetermined amount, the hospital incurs a loss. Under this payment system, whereby reimbursements are determined before treatment begins, hospitals are encouraged to shorten hospital stays and reduce use of unnecessary resources in order to keep costs below the predetermined reimbursement amounts. This program initially limited the growth in spending, but this benefit did not continue.

Diagnostic-Related Groups

The reimbursement rates under PPS are determined by DRGs. Medicare patients who need hospitalization are admitted according to their initial diagnosis, one of 495 DRGs. Each DRG defines a medical condition and the related processes of care. Each DRG is assigned a flat payment rate based on the national average costs for that DRG.

The DRG rates vary according to several factors. For example, they are modified somewhat for different regions of the country to reflect differences in local wage rates. Rates are also higher for teaching hospitals, in recognition that their teaching and training functions necessitate higher costs. Finally, the DRG rates are adjusted annually by Medicare, subject to approval by Congress, to reflect changes in the health-care environment and the resulting increases in national norms of hospital costs.

Managed Care

As already discussed, managed care was designed to help control costs by combining the financing and delivery of health services into one entity. Managed care was credited for playing a key role in slowing down the health inflation rates in the middle and late 1990s (Staines, 1993; Levit et al., 2000). Studies published since 2000 have revealed, however, that the cost-constraining effect of managed care was mostly "one time" in nature and did not last as long as expected (Gabel et al., 2001; Levit et al., 2003, 2004).

ONLINE CONSULT

Summaries of the Institute of Medicine books can be accessed online as follows:

To Err Is Human: Building a Safer Health System at
http://www.iom.edu/report.asp?id=5575

Crossing the Quality Chasm: A New Health System for the 21stCentury at
http://www.iom.edu/report.asp?id=5432

Keeping Patients Safe: Transforming the Work Environment of Nurses at
http://www.iom.edu/report.asp?id=16173

Evidence-based practice guidelines at
http://www.guideline.gov/

KEY POINTS

■ Economics focuses on how consumers, business firms, government entities, and other organizations make choices in an environment of scarce resources.

■ Health-care economics, a specialty area of economics, analyzes how the different parts of a health-care system work together to deliver service that meets the needs of patients.

■ Demand in health care refers to the varying amount of health care that a consumer is willing and able to purchase at each of the possible prices.

■ The supply of health-care service refers to the ability of providers to deliver health care.

■ In a provider-driven system, the location of services, types of providers, and technology available are controlled by the dominant providers, such as physicians and hospitals.

■ In a market-driven system, the providers' level of education and the locations and types of services provided are determined by the needs and location of consumers rather than the needs and location of providers.

■ Third-party payers are insurance companies and government agencies that provide insurance coverage.

■ The fee-for-service payment system gives providers maximum control over services provided to the consumer. Preapproval for services is usually not required in this system.

■ The prospective payment system has emerged in response to concerns about access to health care and spiraling health-care costs. The federal Medicare program is an example of this system.

■ A diagnosis-related group is a prospective pricing system based on a diagnostic classification system.

■ Managed care, broadly defined, is a health-care system willing to be held accountable for both clinical and financial outcomes of an enrolled population.

■ Managed care organizations (MCOs) are the entities that arrange for the provision of services for a group of individuals who are enrolled in the health plan.

■ Capitation is a system in which MCOs are prospectively paid a per-member-per-month amount for a specified range of health services for enrolled individuals.

■ A health maintenance organization (HMO) is a managed health plan that either administers or arranges for health care to be provided to its members for a capitated monthly fee.

■ An independent practice association (IPA) is a type of HMO that enters into a contractual relationship with solo or group practitioners to provide physician and nurse practitioner services. IPAs are the fastest-growing type of HMO.

■ A preferred provider organization (PPO) consists of networks of hospitals, private practice physicians, and other health-care practitioners that provide comprehensive health services to employers and their employees for a negotiated fee.

■ A point-of-service plan combines HMO features such as capitation and coordination of service delivery with the PPO feature, allowing enrollee choice of providers.

■ A health report card is a summary of information of doctor and hospital performance and consumer satisfaction designed for consumers/patients and health-care buyers.

■ Effectiveness measures how well a prescribed treatment has accomplished the anticipated outcomes.

■ Cost-effectiveness measures whether the prescribed treatment has accomplished the desired outcome at the lowest possible cost.

(Key points continue on page 366)

KEY POINTS   (continued)

■ The American health-care system is far from ideal, and it suffers from a number of health system problems, including access, health-cost, and quality disparities.

■ Both the government and the private sector have experimented with a wide range of reform measures to improve access, contain cost, and improve health-care quality.

EVIDENCED-BASED PRACTICE: CONSIDER THIS . . .

*H*ealth-care providers, economists, payors, and consumers are carefully evaluating the costs related to efficacy, especially in the case of diagnostic procedures. In one NGC guideline provided by the University of Michigan Health System, diagnosis, treatment, and follow-up recommendations were provided for women with a diagnosis of a urinary tract infection (UTI). For example, phone triage and urinalysis were recommended, whereas a urine culture is not indicated in the vast majority of UTIs and only in the case of recurrent UTI or in the presence of complicating factors (NGC, 2005, p. 1).

Question: Consider this information from the perspectives of the various groups: providers, economists, payors, and consumers. What are your thoughts?

Source: National Guideline Clearinghouse (NGC). (2005). Urinary tract infection. Retrieved October 9, 2006, from *http://ngc.gov/summary/summary.aspx?doc_id=7407&nbr=004377&string=Cost+AND+effective#top*

Thought and Discussion Questions

1. Discuss the values and demands for health care from the perspectives of:
   - An employer who is trying to choose a health plan
   - An employee who will be using the services of the health plan

2. Describe how you would evaluate the clinical effectiveness and cost-effectiveness of strategies designed to limit costs. Provide examples of nursing-sensitive patient outcomes.

3. Discuss how the movement to share with health-care providers the financial risk of providing care is changing patterns of practice in your community for:
   - Ambulatory services
   - Hospital care
   - Preventive services
   - Rehabilitation

4. Review the Chapter Thought at the beginning of the chapter, and be prepared to discuss its meaning in the context of the chapter.

☐ REFERENCES

Aiken, L. H., Smith, H. L., & Lake, E. T. (1994). Lower Medicare mortality among a set of hospitals known for good nursing care. *Medical Care, 32*(8), 771–787.

American Nurses Association. (1995a). *Report and recommendations on Joint Congress Task Force on Quality Indicators.* Congress of Nursing Practice and Congress on Nursing Economics, June 1995.

American Nurses Association. (1995b). *Nursing report card for acute care.* Washington, DC: American Nurses Publishing.

Anderson, F. G., Reinhardt, U. E., Hussey, P. S., & Petrosyan, V. (2003). It's the prices, stupid: Why the United States is so different from other countries. *Health Affairs, 22*(3), 89–105.

Blegen, M. A., Goode, C. J., & Reed, L. (1998). Nurse staffing and patient outcomes. *Nursing Research, 47*(1), 43–50.

Centers for Medicare and Medicaid Services (CMS). Health care system: Facts and figures. Retrieved October 2007 from *www.cms.hhs.gov/TheChartSeries*

Centers for Medicare & Medicaid Services (CMS). The 2003 Medicare and Medicaid statistical supplement to Healthcare Financing Review. Available at http://www .cms.hhs.gov/apps/review/supp/2003/table29.pdf

Chang, C. F., Price, S. A., & Pfoutz, S. K. (2001). *Economics and nursing: Critical professional issues.* Philadelphia: F. A. Davis.

Conover, C. J., & Sloan, F. (1998). Does removing certificate of need regulations lead to a surge in health care spending? *Journal of Health Politics, Policy and Law, 23*, 455–481.

DeNavas-Walt, C., Proctor, B. D., & Lee, C. H. (2005). *Income, poverty, and health insurance coverage in the United States: 2004.* (U.S. Census Bureau, Current Population Reports, P60–229). Washington, DC: U.S. Government Printing Office.

Disease Management Association of America (DMAA). (2007). DMAA definition of disease management. *Available from http://www.dmaa.org/dm_definition.asp*

Eisenberg, D. M., Kessler, R. C., Foster, C., Norlock, F. E., Calkins, D. R., & Delbanco, T. L. (1993). Unconventional medicine in the United States: Prevalence, costs, and patterns of use. *New England Journal of Medicine, 328*(4), 246–252.

Federal Trade Commission and the Department of Justice. (2004, July). *Improving health care: A dose of competi-tion.* Washington, DC: Government Printing Office. Available at *http://www.ftc.gov/opa/2004/07/ healthcarerpt.shtm* and *http://www.usdoj.gov/atr/ public/health_care/204694.htm*

Folland, S., Goodman, A. C., & Stano, M. (2001). *The eco-nomics of health and health care* (3rd ed.). Upper Saddle River, NJ: Prentice-Hall.

Fox, P. D. (2001). An overview of managed health care. In P. R. Kongsvedt (Ed.), *Essentials of managed health care* (4th ed., pp. 3–16). Gaithersburg, MD: Aspen Publishers, Inc.

Fuchs, V. R. (1993). *The future of health policy.* Cambridge, MA: Harvard Press.

Gabel, J., Levitt, L., Pickreign, J., Whitmore, H., Holve, E., Rowland, D., Dhont, K., & Hawkins, S. (2001). Job-based health insurance in 2001: Inflation hits double digits, managed care retreats. *Health Affairs, 20*(5), 180–186.

Healthcare Financial Management Association. (2006). *Almanac of Hospital Financial and Operating Indicators 2003.* Salt Lake City, UT: Ingenix, Inc.

Henry J. Kaiser Family Foundation. (2006a). *Trends and indicators in the changing health care marketplace.* Menlo Park, CA: Author. Online available at: *http://www.kff.org/insurance/7031/index.cfm*

Henry J. Kaiser Family Foundation. (2006b). *The Medicare Prescription Drug Benefit Fact Sheet.* (Publication Number 7031). Menlo Park, CA: Author. Online available at: *http://www.kff.org/medicare/upload/7044-03-2.pdf*

Huffman, M. H. (2005). Disease management: A new and exciting opportunity in home healthcare. *Home Healthcare Nurse, 23*(5), 290–296.

Hunt, S. A., Baker, D. W., Chin, M. H., Cinquegrani, M. P., Feldmanmd, A. M., Francis, G. S., et al. (2001, December).

ACC/AHA guidelines for the evaluation and management of chronic heart failure in the adult. *Circulation, 104*(24), 2996–3007.

Institute of Medicine (IOM). (1999). *To err is human: Building a safer health system.* Washington, DC: National Academy of Science.

Institute of Medicine (IOM). (2001). *Crossing the quality chasm: A new health system for the 21st century.* Washington, DC: National Academy of Science.

Institute of Medicine (IOM). (2003). *Keeping Patients Safe: Transforming the Work Environment of Nurses.* Washington, DC: National Academy of Science.

Levit, K., Cowan, C., Lazenby, H., Sensenig, A., McDonnell, P., Stiller, J., & Martin, A. (2000). Health spending in 1998: Signals of change. *Health Affairs, 19*(1), 124–132.

Levit, K., Smith, C., Cowan, C., Lazenby, H., Sensenig, A., & Catlin, A. (2003). Trends in U.S. health care spending, 2001. *Health Affairs, 22*(1), 154–164.

Levit, K., Smith, C., Cowan, C., Sensenig, A., Catlin, A., & the Health Accounts Team. (2004). Health spending rebound continues in 2002. *Health Affairs, 23*(1), 147–159.

National Center for Health Statistics. (1997). *Employer-sponsored health insurance.* Hyattsville, MD: Author.

Park, C. H. (2000). Prevalence of employer self-insured health benefits. *Medical Care Research and Review, 57*(3), 340–360.

Peterson, L. E. (2004). Strengthening condition-specific evidence-based home healthcare practice. *Journal for Healthcare Quality, 26(3),* 10–18.

Salkever, D. S., & Bice, T. W. (1979). *Hospital certificate-of-need controls: Impact on investment, costs, and use.* Washington, DC: American Enterprise Institute.

Smith, C., Cowan, C., Heffler, S., Catlin, A., & the National Health Accounts Team. (2006). National health spending in 2004: Recent slowdown led by prescription drug spending. *Health Affairs, 25*(1), 186–196.

Staines, V. S. (1993). Potential impact of managed care on national health spending. *Health Affairs 12*(Suppl.), 249–257.

U.S. Bureau of Census (2003). *Health insurance coverage in the United States, 2002.* Washington, DC: Author.

Whitman, G. R., Kim, Y., Davidson, L. J., Wolf, G. A., & Wang, S. L. (2002, December). The impact of staffing on patient outcomes across specialty units. *Journal of Nursing Administration, 32*(12), 633–639.

☐ ONLINE RESOURCES

AARP
http://aarp.org/

Centers for Medicare and Medicaid Services (CMS)
www.cms.hhs.gov/TheChartSeries

The Commonwealth Fund
http://cmwf.org/

The Kaiser Family Foundation
http://kff.org/

The Robert Wood Johnson Foundation
http://rwjf.org/

■ *Robin S.* **Vogt**

Protecting the Populace

20

> ❝*Every nation, in every region,*
> *now has a decision to make.*
> *Either you are with us,*
> *or you are with the terrorists.*❞
>
> George W. Bush, September 20, 2001

Chapter Objectives

On completion of this chapter, the reader will be able to:

1. List the five areas of the Centers for Disease Control and Prevention plan for bioterrorism.
2. List the categories of biologic agents used in bioterrorism and the agents in each category.
3. Define each biologic agent and discuss the symptoms and communicability of the agent.
4. Describe your community's bioterrorism plan.
5. List the categories of chemical agents.
6. Discuss the initial treatment, assessment, and identification of the patient with suspected chemical exposure.

Key Terms

Bioterrorism

Category A Agents

Category B Agents

Category C Agents

Chemical Agents

Smallpox

Anthrax

Plague

Botulism

Tularemia

Filoviruses

Arenaviruses

Q Fever

Brucellosis

Glanders

Alphaviruses

Ricinus Communis

Epsilon Toxin of *Clostridium Perfringens*

Enterotoxin B

Nipah Virus

Hantavirus

Tickborne Hemorrhagic Fever Viruses

Tickborne Encephalitis Viruses

Yellow Fever

Multidrug-Resistant Tuberculosis

Avian Influenza (Bird Flu)

Chemical Weapons

Personal Protective Equipment (PPE)

Historically, there have been numerous attempts at biologic and chemical terrorism. It is documented that as early as the sixth century BC, the Assyrians poisoned the wells of their enemies with rye ergot. In the 15th century, during his conquest of South America, Pizarro improved his chances of victory by presenting to the natives, as gifts, clothing laden with the variola virus. In 1767, during the French and Indian War, the British general Sir Jeffrey Amherst gave blankets laced with smallpox to Indians loyal to the French. The epidemic devastated the tribes, resulting in a successful British attack on Fort Carillon. In 1940, the Japanese released plague bacteria at Chuhsien, resulting in the deaths of 21 people. During the Vietnam War in the 1960s, the Vietcong used feces-contaminated spear traps (Eitzen & Takafuji, 1997).

In 1978, Georgi Markov, a Bulgarian exile living in London, was injected in the leg with a steel ball impregnated with ricin. He died three days later. In 1995, it was reported that on at least 10 occasions, Aum Shinrikyo, a Japanese cult, attempted to disperse anthrax, botulinum toxin, Q fever, and Ebola virus against the mass population and authority figures in Japan; no reported infections occurred. And in 2001, a 38-year-old assistant to NBC anchorman Tom Brokaw handled a letter containing white powder, which turned out to be the cause of the first case of cutaneous anthrax.

Biologic terrorism and chemical terrorism are common terms in today's society. Since September 11, 2001, we have realized that these events can and do truly occur. It is critical for the nursing professional to be aware of current threats of terrorism with biologic and chemical agents. As technology and knowledge progress, so do the threats to society. Being educated and knowledgeable on how to handle and identify situations that arise has become necessary as core knowledge for the nursing professional. Nurses can provide leadership to other health-care professionals in the identification and care of patients exposed to biologic and chemical agents.

BIOLOGIC AND CHEMICAL PREPAREDNESS

Nursing leaders recognize the need for preparedness and identification of diseases. English, Cundiff, Malone, and Pfeifffer (1999) developed a template to help prepare health-care professionals for bioterrorism. After all, health-care clinics and nurses may have the first opportunity to respond to a bioterrorism outbreak. Being informed about the most likely agents used, their symptoms, and immediate treatment will help prepare communities in the fight against terrorism. Being prepared also entails understanding your own community's emergency response system. Such systems vary from

locality to locality, depending on investment in public health. Preparedness provides the best civil defense against bioterrorism (Henderson, 1997).

Federal Mandates

Before September 11, 2001, Congress had passed three major laws aimed at preventing the acquisition and use of chemical or biologic weapons:

- The Biological Weapons Act of 1989 made it a federal crime knowingly to develop, manufacture, transfer, or possess any biologic agent, toxin, or delivery system for use as a weapon (Public Law 101–298).
- The Chemical and Biological Weapons Control Act of 1991 (CBWCA) established a system of economic and export controls preventing the export of goods or technologies used in the development of chemical and biologic weapons to designated nations (Public Law 102–182).
- The Anti-Terrorism and Effective Death Penalty Act of 1996 expanded the government's powers under CBWCA to cover individuals or groups who attempt or even threaten to develop or use a biologic weapon (Public Law 104–132).

The Centers for Disease Control and Prevention (CDC) was charged with establishing regulations to supplement and detail these laws. CDC's regulations, which took effect April 15, 1997, identified 24 microorganisms and 12 toxins. Possession of these microorganisms or toxins requires registration with CDC, and their transfer involves filing out of forms by both shipper and receiver (Centers for Disease Control and Prevention [CDC], 1997).

On June 12, 2002, President George W. Bush signed into law the Public Health Security and Bioterrorism Preparedness and Response Act of 2002 (Public Law 107–188). Building on the USA Patriot Act (Public Law 107–56), the new law was aimed at preventing, preparing for, and responding to a bioterrorist attack against the United States.

Role of the Centers for Disease Control and Prevention

As part of a Congressional initiative started in 1999 to upgrade national public health capabilities for response

ONLINE **C**ONSULT

Bioterrorism Readiness and Response: Levels of Personal Protective Equipment at
http://www.unmc.edu/bioterrorism/ equipment.htm

Military and troop protection has been of greatest concern for risk of bioterrorism. Protecting civilians differs from protecting the military. In the civilian population, there is a wide variation of age groups and health concerns. There may be more vulnerability in foodborne or waterborne terrorism in the civilian population. It is because of these differences that an attack on civilians may have greater consequences than an attack on military personnel. Agencies must work together to plan for public protection in the civilian population.

to acts of biologic terrorism, the CDC was designated the lead agency for overall public health planning. On the basis of the overall criteria and weighting, biologic agents were assigned to one of three priority categories, A through C, for initial public health preparedness efforts.

The CDC has also established a multilevel laboratory response network for bioterrorism that links public health agencies to advanced-capacity facilities for the identification and reporting of critical biologic agents (CDC, 1998). They have established regional chemical terrorism laboratories that will provide diagnostic capacity during terrorist attacks involving chemical agents. And, they have established a rapid-response laboratory within the CDC to provide around-the-clock diagnostic support to bioterrorism response teams and to expedite molecular characterization of critical biologic agents.

The CDC has also created an action plan (1998) focusing on five specific areas:

1. Preparedness and prevention
2. Detection and surveillance
3. Diagnosis and characterization of biologic and chemical agents
4. Response
5. Communication

This chapter concentrates on the third focus by covering the most likely biologic and chemical threats, along with their definitions, symptoms, and communicability.

AGENTS

It is important for nurses to be familiar with the agents—both chemical and biologic—that have the greatest potential to be used in an act of terror.

Biologic Agents

Bioterrorism is defined as the use of microorganisms that cause human disease, or the toxins released from them, to harm people or elicit widespread fear or intimidation of society. Biodefense research is similar to that of other emerging infectious diseases. It entails research to understand the pathogenesis of these microbes, how the host responds to them, and the translation of this knowledge into useful treatments, diagnostics, and vaccines.

Biologic agents used by terrorists are divided into three categories, A, B, and C. They are categorized according to priority (CDC, 1998).

Category A agents are "high-priority" agents. They pose a risk because they:

- Can be easily transmitted from person-to-person
- Cause high mortality and potential for a major public health impact
- May cause public panic and social disruption
- Require special action for public health preparedness

Category B agents, the second-highest-priority agents, pose a risk because they:

- Are moderately easy to disseminate
- Cause moderate morbidity and low mortality
- Require specific enhancements of CDC's diagnostic capacity and enhanced disease surveillance

Category C agents are the third-highest-priority agents and include emerging pathogens that could be engineered for mass dissemination in the future because of:

- Availability
- Ease of production and dissemination
- Potential for high morbidity and mortality and a major health impact

Examples of agents in all three categories are listed in Table 20–1.

Chemical Agents

Chemical agents may range from warfare agents to toxic chemicals commonly used in industry. "Priority" chemical agents include those that:

- Are chemical agents already known to be used as weapons
- Are available to potential terrorists
- Are likely to cause major morbidity or mortality
- Have potential to cause public panic and social disruption
- Require special action for public health preparedness

ONLINE CONSULT

Category A, B, and C biologic agents at
**http://www.bt.cdc.gov/agent/
agentlist-category.asp**

Chemical terrorism agents at
**http://www.bt.cdc.gov/agent/
agentlistchem.asp**

Bioterrorism Readiness and Response: Levels of
Personal Protective Equipment at
**http://www.unmc.edu/bioterrorism/
equipment.htm**

Chemical agents that have the potential to be used by terrorists are listed in Table 20–2.

Hundreds of new chemicals are produced monthly. Varied combinations of chemicals produce new threats each month, making it impossible to keep track of all newly developed chemicals. This situation, as well as the limited capability of antiterrorist groups to detect new chemical weapons, creates an advantage in the use of chemicals for warfare. Treatment of suspected chemical terrorism or exposure should focus on the clinical syndrome rather than the specific agent. Because response plans vary by community, their consideration is beyond the scope of this chapter. One of the most important steps nurses can take to be prepared, however, is to become familiar with biologic and chemical agents. These agents are reviewed in detail below.

Table 20.1

Biologic Agents with Potential as Terrorist Weapons

Category A	Variola major (smallpox)
	Bacillus anthracis (anthrax)
	Yersinia pestis (plague)
	Clostridium botulinum toxin (botulism)
	Francisella tularensis (tularemia)
	Filoviruses:
	■ Ebola hemorrhagic fever
	■ Marburg hemorrhagic fever
	Arenaviruses:
	■ Lassa (Lassa fever)
	■ Junin (Argentine hemorrhagic fever) and related viruses
Category B	*Coxiella burnetii* (Q fever)
	Brucella species (brucellosis)
	Burkholderia mallei (glanders)
	Alphaviruses:
	■ Venezuelan encephalomyelitis
	■ Eastern and western equine encephalomyelitis
	Ricin toxin from *Ricinus communis* (castor beans)
	Epsilon toxin of *Clostridium perfringens*
	Staphylococcus enterotoxin B
	Others in this group include pathogens that are foodborne or waterborne.
Category C	Nipah virus
	Hantaviruses
	Tickborne hemorrhagic fever viruses
	Tickborne encephalitis viruses
	Yellow fever
	Multidrug-resistant tuberculosis

Table 20.2

Chemical Agents with Potential as Terrorist Weapons

Nerve agents	Tabun
	Sarin
	Soman
	GF (cyclohexylmethylphosphonofluoridate)
	VX (o-ethyl-{S}-{2-diisopropylaminoethyl} methylphosphonothiolate)
Blood agents	Hydrogen cyanide
	Cyanogen chloride
Blister agents	Lewisite
	Nitrogen and sulfur mustards
	Phosgene oxime
Heavy metals	Arsenic
	Lead
	Mercury
Volatile toxins	Benzene
	Chloroform
	Trihalomethanes
Pulmonary agents	Phosgene
	Chlorine
	Vinyl chloride
Incapacitating agents	BZ (3-quinuclidinyl benzilate)
Pesticides, persistent and nonpersistent	Tetraethyl pyrophosphate (TEPP)
	Parathion
Dioxins, furans, and polychlorinated biphenyls (PCBs)	Organochlorines (industrial byproducts)
Explosive nitro compounds and oxidizers	Ammonium nitrate combined with fuel oil
Flammable industrial gases and liquids	Gasoline
	Propane
Poison industrial gases, liquids and solids	Cyanides
	Nitriles
Corrosive industrial acids and bases	Nitric acid
	Sulfuric acid

BIOLOGIC TERRORISM

Category A, B, and C biologic agents are described here by definition, symptom, and communicability.

Category A Agents

These agents are considered by the CDC to have the highest priority. The following information has been extracted from the CDC Website on bioterrorism.

Smallpox

Definition

Smallpox is a serious, contagious, and often fatal infectious disease caused by the variola virus (CDC, 2003k). There is no specific treatment, and currently, the only prevention is vaccination. The name smallpox is derived from the Latin word for "spotted" and refers to the raised bumps that appear on the face and body of an infected person. There are two clinical forms of smallpox, variola major and variola minor. Variola major is the more severe (and more common) form with an extensive rash and higher fever. The fatality rate is 30%. Variola minor is a less severe form with only about a 1% fatality rate.

Symptoms

The normal incubation period for smallpox is 12 to 14 days but may range from 7 to 17 days. First symptoms include fever (sometimes high [101°F–104°F]), malaise, head and body aches, and vomiting. The person is usually too sick to engage in normal activities. This "prodrome phase" may last 2 to 4 days.

A rash follows the prodrome phase. It spreads and progresses to raised bumps that crust, scab, and fall off after about 3 weeks, leaving pitted scars. Usually, the greatest concentration of these bumps is on the face and extremities. Most of the lesions are deep-seated, firm, round, and well-defined. The bumps are all in the same stage of development on any part of the body.

Communicability

Generally, direct and fairly prolonged face-to-face contact is required to spread smallpox from one person to another. Smallpox also can be spread through direct contact with infected bodily fluids or contaminated objects, such as bedding and clothing. Rarely, smallpox has been spread through the air in enclosed settings such as buildings, buses, and trains. Humans are the only natural hosts of variola. Smallpox is not known to be transmitted by insects or animals. The person is contagious from the first appearance of the rash until the last scab falls off. If there is an outbreak of smallpox, a person experiencing symptoms of the prodrome should be isolated until the onset of a rash or until smallpox can be ruled out in order to decrease the spread of this disease.

Anthrax

Definition

Bacillus anthracis, the etiologic agent of **anthrax,** is a large, gram-positive, nonmotile, spore-forming bacterial rod. Human anthrax has three major clinical forms: cutaneous, inhalation, and gastrointestinal. If left untreated, anthrax in all forms can lead to septicemia and death (CDC, 2006a).

Symptoms (Divided by Type)

Cutaneous anthrax is the most common naturally occurring type of infection (95%) and usually occurs after skin contact with contaminated meat, wool, hides, or leather from infected animals. The incubation period ranges from 1 to 12 days. The skin infection begins as a small papule, which progresses to a vesicle in 1 to 2 days and is followed by a necrotic ulcer. The lesion is usually painless, but patients may also have fever, malaise, headache, and regional lymphadenopathy. Most anthrax infections (about 95%) occur when the bacterium enters a cut or abrasion on the skin. Skin infection begins as a raised bump that resembles a spider bite, but (within 1 to 2 days) it develops into a vesicle and then a painless ulcer, usually 1 to 3 cm in diameter, with a characteristic black necrotic area in the center. Lymph glands in the adjacent area may swell. About 20% of untreated cases of cutaneous anthrax result in death. Deaths are rare if patients are given appropriate antimicrobial therapy.

Inhalational anthrax is the most lethal form of anthrax. Anthrax spores must be aerosolized in order to cause inhalational anthrax. The number of spores needed to cause human infection is unknown. The incubation period of inhalational anthrax among humans is unclear, but it is reported to range from 1 to 7 days, possibly up to 60 days. Inhalational anthrax resembles a viral respiratory illness, initial symptoms being sore throat, mild fever, muscle aches, and malaise. These symptoms may progress to respiratory failure and shock, frequently with development of meningitis.

Gastrointestinal anthrax, which usually follows the consumption of raw or undercooked contaminated meat, has an incubation period of 1 to 7 days. It is associated with severe abdominal distress followed by fever and signs of septicemia. The disease can take an oropharyngeal or abdominal form. Lesions at the base of the tongue, sore throat, dysphagia, fever, and regional lymphadenopathy usually characterize involvement of the

ONLINE CONSULT

Check the Web site showing vaccine information from the Centers for Disease Control at **http://www.bt.cdc.gov/agent/smallpox/ vaccination/infopacket.asp** pharynx. Lower bowel inflammation usually causes nausea, loss of appetite, vomiting, and fever, followed by abdominal pain, vomiting blood, and bloody diarrhea.

Communicability
Anthrax is not contagious; the illness cannot be transmitted from person to person.

Plague

Definition
Plague is an infectious disease of animals and humans caused by the bacterium *Yersinia pestis.* This bacterium is found in rodents and their fleas and occurs in many areas of the world, including the United States (CDC, 2004).

Symptoms (Divided by Type)
- *Bubonic plague*: Enlarged, tender lymph nodes; fever, chills, and prostration
- *Septicemic plague:* Fever, chills, prostration, abdominal pain, shock, and bleeding into skin and other organs
- *Pneumonic plague:* Fever, chills, cough, and difficulty breathing; rapid shock and death if not treated early

Communicability
Bubonic plague is usually transmitted to humans by the bites of infected rodent fleas. During rodent plague outbreaks, many animals die and their hungry fleas seek other sources of blood to survive. People and animals that visit places where rodents have recently died from plague risk getting the disease from fleabites. Persons also can become directly infected through handling of infected rodents, rabbits, or wild carnivores that prey on these animals when plague bacteria enter through breaks in the skin. House cats are also susceptible to plague. Infected cats become sick and may transmit plague directly to persons who handle or care for them. Also, dogs and cats may bring plague-infected fleas into the home. *Y. pestis* is easily destroyed by sunlight and drying. Even so, when released into air, the bacterium will survive for up to 1 hour, although this period may vary with conditions. Inhaling droplets expelled by the coughing of a plague-infected person or animal (especially a house cat) can result in plague of the lungs (plague pneumonia). Transmission of plague pneumonia from person to person is uncommon but sometimes results in dangerous epidemics that can spread quickly.

Botulism

Definition
Botulism is a muscle-paralyzing disease caused by a toxin made by a bacterium called *Clostridium botulinum.* The three main kinds of botulism are as follows:

- *Foodborne botulism* occurs when a person ingests preformed toxin, which leads to illness within a few hours to days. Foodborne botulism is a public health emergency because the contaminated food may still be available to other persons besides the patient.
- *Infant botulism* occurs in a small number of susceptible infants each year who harbor *C. botulinum* in their intestinal tracts.
- *Wound botulism* occurs when wounds are infected with *C. botulinum* that secretes the toxin (CDC, 2005b).

Symptoms
The classic symptoms of botulism are double vision, blurred vision, drooping eyelids, slurred speech, difficulty swallowing, dry mouth, and muscle weakness. Infants with botulism appear lethargic, feed poorly, are constipated, and have a weak cry and poor muscle tone. These are all symptoms of the muscle paralysis caused by the bacterial toxin. If untreated, these symptoms may progress to cause paralysis of the arms, legs, trunk, and respiratory muscles. In foodborne botulism, symptoms generally begin 18 to 36 hours after consumption of contaminated food, but they can occur as early as 6 hours or as late as 10 days.

Communicability
Botulism is not spread from one person to another. Foodborne botulism follows ingestion of toxin produced in food by *C. botulinum*. The most common source is home-canned food prepared in an unsafe manner. Wound botulism occurs when *C. botulinum* spores germinate within wounds. Intestinal colonization botulism occurs when *C. botulinum* spores germinate and produce toxin in the gastrointestinal tract.

Tularemia

Definition
Tularemia is an infectious disease caused by a hardy bacterium, *Francisella tularensis*, found in animals (especially rodents, rabbits, and hares) (CDC, 2003i).

Symptoms
Symptoms of tularemia include sudden fever, chills, headaches, muscle aches, joint pain, dry cough, progressive weakness, and pneumonia. People with pneumonia may experience chest pain and bloody sputum, and may have trouble breathing or sometimes stop breathing. Other symptoms of tularemia depend on how a person was exposed to the tularemia bacteria. They can include ulcers on the skin or mouth, swollen and painful lymph glands, swollen and painful eyes, and a sore throat. Symptoms usually appear 3 to 5 days after exposure to the bacteria but can take as long as 14 days to manifest.

Communicability

Tularemia is not known to be spread from person to person, so people who have tularemia do not need to be isolated. People who have been exposed to *F. tularensis* should be treated as soon as possible. The disease can be fatal if it is not treated with the appropriate antibiotics. The most common means of contracting the disease is inoculation through the skin or mucous membranes from infected deer flies or ticks or insufficiently cooked rabbit meat.

Viral Hemorrhagic Fevers

Viral hemorrhagic fevers (VHFs) are a group of illnesses caused by several distinct families of viruses. In general, the term viral hemorrhagic fever is used to describe a severe multisystem syndrome. Characteristically, the overall vascular system is damaged, and the body's ability to regulate itself is impaired. These symptoms are often accompanied by hemorrhage; however, the bleeding is rarely life-threatening. Although some types of hemorrhagic fever viruses can cause relatively mild illnesses, many cause severe, life-threatening disease. This latter category includes the filoviruses and arenaviruses.

Filoviruses
Definition

Filoviruses belong to a virus family called *Filoviridae* and can cause severe hemorrhagic fever in humans and nonhuman primates. So far, only two members of this virus family have been identified: Marburg virus and Ebola virus. Four species of Ebola virus have been identified: Ivory Coast, Sudan, Zaire, and Reston. Ebola-Reston virus is the only known filovirus that does not cause severe disease in humans (CDC, 2003e).

Symptoms

People infected with Ebola virus have sudden fever, weakness, muscle pain, headache, and sore throat, followed by vomiting, diarrhea, rash, limited kidney and liver functions, and both internal and external bleeding. Death rates range from 50% to 90%.

Symptoms of Marburg virus occur after an incubation period of 5 to 10 days. The onset of the disease is sudden and is marked by fever, chills, headache, and myalgia. Around the fifth day after the onset of symptoms, a maculopapular rash, most prominent on the trunk, may occur. Nausea, vomiting, chest pain, a sore throat, abdominal pain, and diarrhea then may appear. Symptoms become increasingly severe and may include jaundice, inflammation of the pancreas, severe weight loss, delirium, shock, liver failure, massive hemorrhaging, and multiple-organ dysfunction.

Communicability

Viruses causing hemorrhagic fever are initially transmitted to humans when the activities of infected reservoir hosts or vectors and humans overlap. The viruses carried in rodent reservoirs are transmitted when humans have contact with urine, fecal matter, saliva, or other body excretions from infected rodents. The viruses associated with arthropod vectors are spread most often when the vector mosquito or tick bites a human or a human crushes a tick. Some of these vectors may spread the virus to animals, such as livestock; humans then become infected when they care for or slaughter the animals.

Once a human is infected, person-to-person transmission is the means by which further infections occur. Specifically, transmission involves close personal contact between an infected individual or their body fluids and another person. During recorded outbreaks of hemorrhagic fever due to filovirus infection, people who cared for or worked very closely with infected individuals were especially at risk of becoming infected themselves. Nosocomial transmission, through contact with infected body fluids via reuse of unsterilized syringes, needles, or other medical equipment contaminated with these fluids, has also been an important factor in the spread of disease. When close contact between uninfected and infected persons is minimized, the number of new filovirus infections in humans usually declines. Although in the laboratory the viruses display some capability of infection through small-particle aerosols, airborne spread among humans has not been clearly demonstrated.

Arenaviruses
Definition

The *Arenaviridae* family of viruses (**arenaviruses**) is generally associated with rodent-transmitted disease in humans. Each virus usually is associated with a particular rodent host species in which it is maintained. Arenavirus infections are relatively common in humans in some areas of the world and can cause severe illnesses (CDC, 2003c). Lassa fever is the most common type of Arenavirus.

Symptoms

Signs and symptoms of Lassa fever typically occur 1 to 3 weeks after the patient comes into contact with the virus. These include fever, retrosternal pain (pain behind the chest wall), sore throat, back pain, cough, abdominal pain, vomiting, diarrhea, conjunctivitis, facial swelling, proteinuria, and mucosal bleeding. Neurologic problems have also been described, such as hearing loss, tremors, and encephalitis. The symptoms of Lassa fever are so varied and nonspecific, however, that clinical diagnosis is often difficult.

The incubation period of Lassa fever infection is usually between 8 and 13 days. A characteristic biphasic febrile illness then follows. The initial phase, which may last as long as a week, typically begins with any or all of the following symptoms: fever, malaise, anorexia, muscle aches, headache, nausea, and vomiting. Other, less common symptoms are sore throat, cough, and joint, chest, testicular, and parotid pain. After a few days of remission, the second phase of the disease occurs, consisting of symptoms of meningitis or characteristics of encephalitis.

Communicability. The viruses are shed into the environment in the urine or droppings of their infected hosts. Human infection with arenaviruses is incidental to the natural cycle of the viruses and occurs when an individual comes into contact with the excretions or materials contaminated with the excretions of an infected rodent, such as ingestion of contaminated food, or through direct contact of abraded or broken skin with rodent excrement. Infection can also occur through inhalation of tiny particles soiled with rodent urine or saliva. The types of incidental contact depend on the habits of both humans and rodents.

Some arenaviruses, such as Lassa and Machupo viruses, are associated with secondary person-to-person or nosocomial transmission. This occurs when a person infected by exposure to the virus from the rodent host spreads the virus to other humans, in a variety of ways. Person-to-person transmission is associated with direct contact with the blood or other excretions of infected individuals that contain virus particles. Airborne transmission has also been reported in connection with certain viruses. Contact with objects contaminated with these materials, such as medical equipment, is also associated with transmission.

> According to the World Health Organization (WHO), "143 cases of Ebola virus had been reported, including 128 deaths, in the districts of Mbomo and Kéllé in the Cuvette Ouest Département by May 2003. Thirteen of the cases were confirmed by laboratory tests and 130 were epidemiologically linked." (WHO, 2003)

Category B

Category B agents are the CDC's next level of priority, as illustrated in the following extracts.

Coxiella burnetii (Q Fever)

Definition
Q fever is a zoonotic disease caused by *Coxiella burnetii*, a species of bacteria that is distributed globally. In 1999, Q fever became a notifiable disease in the United States, but reporting cases of Q fever is not required in many other countries. Because the disease is underreported, scientists cannot reliably assess how many cases of Q fever have actually occurred worldwide. Many human infections are not apparent. Cattle, sheep, and goats are the primary reservoirs of *C. burnetii*. Infection has been noted in a wide variety of other animals, including other breeds of livestock and domesticated pets. Humans are often very susceptible to the disease, and very few organisms may be required to cause infection (CDC, 2003l).

Symptoms
Only about half of all people infected with *C. burnetii* show signs of clinical illness. Most acute cases of Q fever begin with sudden onset of one or more of the following: high fevers (up to 104°F to 105°F), severe headache, general malaise, myalgia, confusion, sore throat, chills, sweats, nonproductive cough, nausea, vomiting, diarrhea, abdominal pain, and chest pain. Fever usually lasts for one to two weeks. Weight loss can occur and persist for some time. From 30% to 50% of patients with a symptomatic infection experience pneumonia. Additionally, a majority of patients have abnormal results of liver function tests, and some have hepatitis. Most patients recover to good health within several months without any treatment. Only 1% to 2% of people with acute Q fever die of the disease.

Communicability
In the United States, Q fever outbreaks have resulted mainly from occupational exposure of veterinarians, workers in meat-processing plants, sheep and dairy workers, livestock farmers, and researchers at facilities housing sheep. Prevention and control efforts should be directed primarily toward these groups and environments.

Coxiella burnetii is a highly infectious agent that is rather resistant to heat and drying. It can become airborne and inhaled by humans. A single *C. burnetii* organism may cause disease in a susceptible person.

Brucella Species (Brucellosis)

Definition
Brucellosis is an infectious disease caused by bacteria of the genus *Brucella*. These bacteria are primarily passed among animals, and they cause disease in many different vertebrates. Various *Brucella* species affect sheep, goats, cattle, deer, elk, pigs, dogs, and several other animals. Humans become infected by coming in contact with animals or animal products that are contaminated with the bacteria. In humans, brucellosis can cause a range of symptoms similar to those of the flu—fever, sweats, headaches, back pains, and physical weakness. Severe infections of the central nervous systems or lining of the heart may occur. Brucellosis can also cause long-lasting or chronic symptoms such as recurrent fevers, joint pain, and fatigue (CDC, 2003d).

Symptoms
Symptoms of brucellosis are extremely variable. Symptoms of the acute form (< 8 weeks from illness onset) are nonspecific and "flu-like," including fever, sweats, malaise, anorexia, headache, myalgia, back pain, and, uncommonly, death. In the undulant form

(< 1 year from illness onset), symptoms include undulant fevers, arthritis, and orchiepididymitis. Neurologic symptoms may occur acutely in up to 5% of cases. Symptoms of the chronic form (> 1 year from onset) include chronic fatigue syndrome-like symptoms, depressive episodes, and arthritis.

Communicability

Transmission of brucellosis is zoonotic, commonly through abrasions of the skin from handling infected mammals. In the United States, transmission occurs more frequently through ingestion of contaminated milk and dairy products. The disease is highly infectious in the laboratory via aerosolization. Direct person-to-person spread of brucellosis is extremely rare. Mothers who are breast-feeding may transmit the infection to their infants. Sexual transmission has also been reported.

Burkholderia mallei (Glanders)

Definition

Glanders is an infectious disease caused by the bacterium *Burkholderia mallei*. Primarily a disease affecting horses, it also affects donkeys and mules and can be contracted naturally by goats, dogs, and cats. Human infection, although not seen in the United States since 1945, has occurred rarely and sporadically among laboratory workers and people in direct and prolonged contact with infected domestic animals (CDC, 2003f).

Symptoms

The symptoms of glanders depend on the route of infection with the organism. The types of infection are localized, pus-forming cutaneous infections, pulmonary infections, bloodstream infections, and chronic suppurative infections of the skin. Generalized symptoms of glanders include fever, muscle aches, chest pain, muscle tightness, and headache. Additional symptoms are excessive tearing of the eyes, light sensitivity, and diarrhea.

- *Localized infections:* If there is a cut or scratch in the skin, a localized infection with ulceration will develop within 1 to 5 days at the site where the bacteria entered the body. Swollen lymph nodes may also be apparent. Infections involving the mucous membranes in the eyes, nose, and respiratory tract cause increased mucous production from the affected sites.
- *Pulmonary infections:* In pulmonary infections, pneumonia, pulmonary abscesses, and pleural effusion can occur. Chest x-rays show localized infection in the lobes of the lungs.
- *Bloodstream infections:* Glanders bloodstream infections are usually fatal within 7 to 10 days. Generally, symptoms are respiratory distress, severe headache, fever, diarrhea, development of pus-filled lesions on the skin, muscle tenderness, and disorientation.

- *Chronic infections:* The chronic form of glanders involves multiple abscesses within the muscles of the arms and legs or in the spleen or liver. Mortality has decreased markedly since sulfa drugs were introduced, although it can still be fatal in severe cases.

Communicability

Glanders is transmitted to humans through direct contact with infected animals. The bacteria enter the body through the skin or through mucosal surfaces of the eyes and nose. The sporadic cases have been documented in veterinarians, horse caretakers, and laboratory workers. In addition to animal exposure, cases of human-to-human transmission have been reported, including two suggested cases of sexual transmission and several cases in family members who cared for the patients.

Alphaviruses

The **alphaviruses** include Venezuelan encephalomyelitis (VEE) and Eastern and Western equine encephalomyelitis (EEE and WEE, respectively).

Definition

WEE is a member of the antigenically similar group of viruses known as *Togaviridae*, which encompasses EEE and VEE. These alphaviruses are spherical and have a diameter of 60 to 65 nm (CDC, 2003b).

Symptoms

Diffuse central nervous system involvement characterizes WEE in its more severe stages. The large number of immunologically active cells that enter the brain parenchyma and perivascular areas mediate much of the damage. Focal necrosis is often found in the striatum, globus pallidus, cerebral cortex, thalamus, pons, and meninges. Neutrophils and macrophages may infiltrate the brain parenchyma and cause neuronal destruction, neuronophagia, focal necrosis, and spotty demyelination. Vascular inflammation with endothelial proliferation, small-vessel thrombosis, and perivascular cuffing may also occur. Cell death occurs primarily in the glial and inflammatory cells.

Communicability

The alphaviruses are spread primarily via the vector mosquito *Culex tarsalis*. Other mosquitoes (e.g., *Aedes* species) and, occasionally, small wild mammals also have been known to spread the virus. *C. tarsalis*, a mosquito that is often found on the West Coast of the United States, prefers warm, moist environments. In these locations, cycles of wild bird and mosquito interactions and infectivity allow the virus to remain endemic. No known cases of bird transmission of the disease exist, making mosquitoes the primary vector and birds simply the reservoirs. Epidemic outbreaks in the equine or pheasant population often precede human epidemics of the alphaviruses.

Ricin Toxin

Definition

The seeds from the castor bean plant, **Ricinus communis**, are poisonous to people, animals, and insects. One of the main toxic proteins is "ricin." Now we know that the agglutination observed with ingestion of the seeds is due to another toxin also present, called *Ricinus communis agglutinin* (RCA). Ricin is a potent cytotoxin but a weak hemagglutinin, whereas RCA is a weak cytotoxin and a powerful hemagglutinin. Poisoning by ingestion of the castor bean is due to ricin, not RCA, because RCA does not penetrate the intestinal wall and does not affect red blood cells unless given intravenously. If RCA is injected into the blood, it will cause the red blood cells to agglutinate and burst by hemolysis (CDC, 2003g).

Symptoms

- *Inhalation:* Within a few hours of inhalation of significant amounts of ricin, the likely symptoms would be coughing, tightness in the chest, difficulty breathing, nausea, and aching muscles. In the next few hours, the body's airways would become severely inflamed, excess fluid would build up in the lungs, breathing would become even more difficult, and the skin might turn cyanotic. Excess fluid in the lungs would be diagnosed on x-ray or by listening to the chest with a stethoscope.
- *Ingestion*: Someone who swallowed a significant amount of ricin would have internal bleeding of the stomach and intestines that would lead to vomiting and bloody diarrhea. Eventually, the liver, spleen, and kidneys might stop working, and death could result.
- *Injection*: Injection of a lethal amount of ricin would at first cause the muscles and lymph nodes near the injection site to die. Eventually, the liver, kidneys, and spleen would stop working, and the person would have massive bleeding from the stomach and intestines. The person would die from multiple organ failure.

Death from ricin poisoning could take place within 36 to 48 hours of exposure, whether by injection, ingestion, or inhalation. If the person lives longer than 5 days without complications, she will probably recover. Presentation with the preceding signs and symptoms does not necessarily mean, however, that a person has been exposed to ricin.

Communicability

Contracting ricin could only be the result of a deliberate act to make ricin and use it to poison people. Accidental exposure to ricin is highly unlikely. People can breathe in ricin mist or powder and be poisoned. Ricin can also get into water or food and then be swallowed. Pellets of ricin, or ricin dissolved in a liquid, can be injected into people's bodies. Depending on the route of exposure, as little as 500 micrograms of ricin could be enough to kill an adult. A 500-microgram dose of ricin would be about the size of the head of a pin. A much greater amount would need to be inhaled or swallowed to be fatal. Ricin poisoning is not contagious. It cannot be spread from person to person through casual contact. Some reports have indicated that ricin may have been used in the Iran-Iraq war during the 1980s and that quantities of ricin were found in al-Qaeda caves in Afghanistan. Because of the similarity of the symptoms of many biologic and chemical agents, nasal or throat swabs and induced respiratory secretions may be collected for toxin assay. Blood can be collected for serum and toxin assays as well as measurement of antibody response using serum.

Epsilon Toxin of Clostridium perfringens

Definition

Epsilon toxin is a potent toxin produced by the bacterium *Clostridium perfringens*. Each of the types of *C. perfringens* produces a unique spectrum of toxins. Of the five types known (A through E), only B and D produce toxin. These strains have a limited host range, being isolated mainly from sheep and lambs, occasionally from goats and cattle, and rarely from humans. The two strains, along with strain C, are responsible for producing a very severe and often fatal form of enterotoxemia (Northstar Preparedness Network, n.d.).

Symptoms

Diarrhea is accompanied by severe abdominal cramping and bloating. There seems to be little or no information about the effects of epsilon toxin on humans. Extrapolation from studies with experimentally infected animals indicates that neurologic signs or pulmonary edema may be possible in humans. The toxin increases intestinal permeability, ensuring its absorption into the circulation, where it damages vascular endothelium, leading to fluid loss and edema. Stress responses to cerebral edema trigger catecholamine release, resulting in adenylate cyclase activation, hyperglycemia related to cyclic adenosine monophosphate (cAMP), and glycosuria, a common finding in enterotoxemia. Postmortem autolysis is rapid. Subserous and subendocardial hemorrhages and excess fluid in the body cavities are sometimes seen. Cerebral hemorrhaging and degenerative lesions are common in less acute cases.

Communicability

It is possible for the epsilon toxin to be transmitted in contaminated food and water or by aerosol. Specific information is not available for the epsilon toxin. Toxins are not generally transmitted from animal to animal or from animal to people.

Because of the similarity of the symptoms of many biologic and chemical agents, nasal or throat swabs and induced respiratory secretions may be collected for toxin assay. Blood can be collected for serum and toxin assays as well as measurement of antibody response using serum.

Staphylococcal Enterotoxin B

Definition
Staphylococcal **enterotoxin B** (SEB) is one of several exotoxins produced by *Staphylococcus aureus* (CDC, 2003h).

Symptoms
From 3 to 12 hours after aerosol exposure, high fever (103°F to 106°F), chills, headache, myalgia, and non-productive cough may appear. Some patients may have shortness of breath and retrosternal chest pain. If pulmonary edema or adult respiratory distress syndrome (ARDS) develops, there may be a cough with frothy sputum. Fever may last 2 to 5 days and cough may persist for up to 4 weeks. Ingestion of the toxin leads to acute salivation, nausea, and vomiting followed by abdominal cramps and diarrhea. Fever and respiratory involvement are not seen in foodborne SEB intoxication. Higher exposure can lead to septic shock and death if left untreated.

Physical findings in SEB intoxication are often unremarkable. Postural hypotension may be present, particularly with ingestion of SEB, because of fluid loss. Conjunctivitis or rale may also be found.

Communicability
SEB toxin is heat stable and water-soluble. The incapacitating dose is 30 ng/person by inhalation. SEB, one of several exotoxins produced by *S. aureus*, may be aerosolized or used to sabotage food supplies. Although it would be effective in causing illness that incapacitates victims for up to 2 weeks, it would not be a weapon likely to produce significant mortality rates.

Category C

The agents in Category C are regarded as lower priority by the CDC, as illustrated in the following extracts.

ⓞNLINE CONSULT

The New York Health Department has developed a concise table identifying—on the basis of symptoms—different types of biologic terrorism. It includes the testing to be done, as well as the treatment.
http://www.health.state.ny.us/nysdoh/bt/pdf/rapid_response_card.pdf

Nipah Virus

Definition
Nipah virus and Hendra virus are newly recognized zoonotic viruses. They are typically grouped together and are members of the *Paramyxoviridae* family. It is currently believed that certain species of fruit bats are the natural hosts of both Nipah and Hendra viruses. Although members of this group of viruses have caused only a few focal outbreaks, the biologic ability of these viruses to infect a wide range of hosts and to produce a disease causing significant mortality in humans has made this emerging viral infection a public health concern (World Health Organization [WHO], 2001).

Symptoms
The incubation period for Nipah and Hendra viral infections is between 4 and 18 days. In many cases the infection is mild or not apparent, and diagnosis is determined through assays. Treatment is supportive. In symptomatic cases, the onset is usually with "influenza-like" symptoms, with high fever and myalgia. The disease may progress to encephalitis with drowsiness, disorientation, convulsions, and coma. Of people with clinically apparent infection, 50% die.

Communicability
The mode of transmission from animal to animal, and from animal to human, is uncertain but appears to require close contact with contaminated tissue or body fluids. Nipah antibodies have been detected in pigs as well as other domestic and wild animals. The role of species other than pigs in transmitting infection to other animals has not yet been determined.

It is unlikely that Nipah virus is easily transmitted to humans. Despite frequent contact between fruit bats and humans, there is no serologic evidence of human infection from bat carriers. Pigs were the apparent source of infection in most human cases in the Malaysian outbreak of Nipah virus, but other sources, such as infected dogs and cats, cannot be excluded. Human-to-human transmission of Nipah virus has not been reported.

Hantaviruses

Definition
Hantavirus pulmonary syndrome (HPS) is caused by a hitherto unknown virus, subsequently isolated and named Sin Nombre Virus (SNV). Commonly referred to as

ⓞNLINE CONSULT

Review the number of recent outbreaks of SARS and West Nile virus and find out when was the last reported case of smallpox at
http://www.cdc.gov/

hantavirus disease, HPS is a febrile illness characterized by bilateral interstitial pulmonary infiltrates and respiratory compromise usually requiring supplemental oxygen and clinically resembling acute respiratory disease syndrome (ARDS) (CDC, 2003a).

Symptoms

Early symptoms are fatigue, fever, and muscle aches, especially of the large muscle groups—thighs, hips, back, and sometimes shoulders. These symptoms are universal. There may also be headaches, dizziness, chills, and abdominal problems, such as nausea, vomiting, diarrhea, and abdominal pain. Because there have been so few cases of HPS, the incubation time is not quite clear. On the basis of limited information, however, it appears that symptoms may develop between 1 and 5 weeks after exposure to potentially infected rodents and their droppings. Typical clinical laboratory findings are hemoconcentration, left shift in the white blood cell count, neutrophilic leukocytosis, thrombocytopenia, and circulating immunoblasts. (CDC, 2005d)

Communicability

Some rodents are infected with a type of hantavirus that causes HPS. In the United States, deer mice (as well as cotton rats and rice rats in the southeastern states and the white-footed mouse in the Northeast) are the rodents carrying the hantaviruses that cause HPS. These rodents shed the virus in their urine, droppings, and saliva. The virus is mainly transmitted to people when they breathe in air contaminated with the virus. This happens when fresh rodent urine, droppings, or nesting materials are stirred up and aerosolized. The types of hantavirus that cause HPS in the United States cannot be transmitted from one person to another; these viruses are not known to be transmitted by any types of animals other than certain species of rodents.

Tickborne Hemorrhagic Fever Viruses

Definition

Crimean-Congo hemorrhagic fever (CCHF), one of the **tickborne hemorrhagic fever viruses**, is a viral hemorrhagic fever of the Nairovirus group. Although it is primarily a zoonosis, sporadic cases and outbreaks of CCHF affecting humans do occur (CDC, 2005c).

Symptoms

The length of the incubation period for the illness appears to depend on the mode of acquisition of the virus. After infection via tick bite, for example, the incubation period is usually 1 to 3 days, with a maximum of 9 days. The incubation period after contact with infected blood or tissues is usually 5 to 6 days, with a documented maximum of 13 days.

Onset of symptoms is sudden, with fever, myalgia, dizziness, neck pain and stiffness, backache, headache, sore eyes, and photophobia. There may be

nausea, vomiting, and sore throat early on, which may be accompanied by diarrhea and generalized abdominal pain. Over the next few days, the patient may experience sharp mood swings and may become confused and aggressive. After 2 to 4 days, the agitation may be replaced by sleepiness, depression, and lassitude, and the abdominal pain may localize to the right upper quadrant, with detectable hepatomegaly.

Communicability

The CCHF virus may infect a wide range of domestic and wild animals. Many birds are resistant to infection, but ostriches are susceptible and may show a high prevalence of infection in endemic areas. Animals become infected with CCHF from the bite of infected ticks. The most important source for acquisition of the virus by ticks is believed to be infected small vertebrates on which immature Hyalomma ticks feed. Once infected, the tick remains infected through its developmental stages, and the mature tick may transmit the infection to large vertebrates, such as livestock.

Patients with suspected or confirmed CCHF should be isolated and cared for with the use of barrier nursing techniques. Specimens of blood or tissues obtained for diagnostic purposes should be collected and handled with universal precautions. Sharps and body wastes should be safely disposed through appropriate decontamination procedures. Health-care workers are at risk of acquiring infection from sharps injuries during surgical procedures. In the past, CCHF infection has been transmitted to surgeons operating on patients to determine the cause of the abdominal symptoms in the early stages of disease.

Tickborne Encephalitis Viruses

Definition

Tickborne encephalitis (TBE), also known as spring-summer encephalitis, is a viral infection of the central nervous system transmitted by bites of certain vector ticks. Human infections follow bites of infected *Ixodes ricinus* ticks, usually in people who visit or work in forests, fields, or pastures. Infection with **tickborne encephalitis viruses** also can be acquired by consuming unpasteurized dairy products from infected cows, goats, or sheep (CDC, 2005c).

Symptoms

Symptoms of TBE include sudden fever, headache, vomiting, photophobia, stiff neck, confusion, drowsiness, and

ONLINE CONSULT

Review the universal precautions and determine when it is appropriate to utilize them at **http://www.cdc.gov/ncidod/dhqp/pdf/ guidelines/Isolation2007.pdf** clumsiness. Symptoms requiring emergency treatment include loss of consciousness, stupor, coma, seizures, muscle weakness or paralysis, and sudden severe dementia. TBE is a virus of the central nervous system. Focal epilepsy and flaccid paralysis often characterize this type of encephalitis. Once the virus enters the bloodstream it can make its way into the brain, causing inflammation of the brain cells and the surrounding membranes. White blood cells try to fight off the infection, but in the process, they invade the brain tissue. Cerebral edema occurs and can cause destruction of nerve cells, bleeding in the brain, and brain damage.

Communicability
The TBE virus is transmitted by the bite of an infected tick. Ticks and mammals conjoined appear to be the true reservoir. Sheep, deer, rodents, small mammals, and birds serve as sources of tick infection. Humans become infected through the bite of an infected tick or the consumption of milk from certain infected animals. The virus cannot be transmitted from human to human.

Yellow Fever

Definition
Yellow fever is a mosquito-borne viral disease that occurs in tropical and subtropical areas. Yellow fever is seen only in Africa and South America. Sporadic infections occur almost exclusively in forestry and agricultural workers due to occupational exposure in or near forests (CDC, 2003j).

Symptoms
Initial symptoms may be dengue fever-like and include fever, headache, vomiting, and backache. As the disease progresses, the pulse slows and weakens, and gums start to bleed. Bloody urine and jaundice may also occur. The incubation period is usually 3 to 6 days, after which symptoms of fever, malaise, headache, photophobia, nausea, vomiting, and irritability appear. Physical examination at this time shows a patient who is febrile, is toxic in appearance, and has hyperemic skin, injected conjunctiva, coated tongue, and epigastric or hepatic tenderness. Faget's sign, a relative bradycardia with a fever, may be present. After 3 to 5 days, the patient either recovers or goes onto the next stage, fulminant disease.

Fulminant disease consists of significant hepatic injury with jaundice, yielding the name "yellow fever." Renal failure is not uncommon. A hemorrhagic diathesis, consisting of epistaxis, oozing at the gums, petechiae, ecchymosis, hematemesis, melena, hematuria, thrombocytopenia, and disseminated intravascular coagulation, may occur. Myocarditis, encephalopathy, and shock may also ensue. The case fatality rate is 20% to 50%. Anyone who survives can expect to recover fully.

Communicability
Yellow fever is a viral disease transmitted to humans by a mosquito. The vector is the *Aedes aegypti* or *Haemagogus* mosquito. Vertical transmission occurs when the virus is passed on to the mosquito's ovum. This feature is advantageous for continuation of the life cycle during the dry season, when the eggs may lay dormant. When the rainy season returns, the eggs hatch, allowing the virus to carry on. Horizontal transmission occurs when either an animal (typically monkeys) or humans are infected by the mosquito. The mosquito is the true reservoir of the virus; yellow fever is never transmitted from person to person or animal to person.

Multidrug-Resistant Tuberculosis

Definition
Tuberculosis (TB) is an infectious disease caused by a germ called *Mycobacterium tuberculosis*. **Multidrug-resistant tuberculosis** (MDR TB) is a form of tuberculosis that is resistant to two or more of the primary drugs used for the treatment of tuberculosis. Resistance to one or several forms of treatment occurs when the bacteria develop the ability to withstand antibiotic attack and relay that ability to their progeny (CDC, 2005a).

Symptoms
TB primarily attacks the respiratory system, although it can affect other organs as well. The symptoms of TB include fever, night sweats, weight loss, chest pain, and coughing. TB may be fatal, especially for HIV-infected persons.

Communicability
Tuberculosis is spread through the air when a person sneezes, coughs, or breathes. MDR TB is resistant to at least two of the main drugs used to treat TB—isoniazid (INH) and rifampin. Because that entire strain of bacteria inherits the capacity to resist the effects of the various treatments, resistance can spread from one person to another. On an individual basis, however, inadequate treatment or improper use of the antituberculous medications remains an important cause of drug-resistant and multidrug-resistant tuberculosis.

Other Uncategorized Threats

Avian Influenza

Definition
Avian influenza is an infection caused by avian (bird) influenza (flu) viruses. These influenza viruses occur naturally among birds. Wild birds worldwide carry the viruses in their intestines, but usually do not get sick from them. Avian influenza, however, is very contagious among birds and can make some domesticated birds, including chickens, ducks, and turkeys, very sick to the point of death.

Symptoms

Symptoms in birds and other animals vary, but virulent strains can cause death within a few days. Vaccines to protect humans against H5N1 viruses currently are under development. The reported symptoms of avian influenza in humans have ranged from typical influenza-like symptoms (e.g., fever, cough, sore throat, and muscle aches) to eye infections (conjunctivitis), acute respiratory distress, viral pneumonia, and other severe, life-threatening complications (CDC, 2006b).

Communicability

Wild birds can carry the viruses, but usually do not get sick from them. But some domesticated birds, including chickens, ducks, and turkeys, can become infected, often fatally. One strain of avian influenza, the H5N1 virus, is endemic in much of Asia and has recently spread into Europe. Avian H5N1 infections have recently killed poultry and other birds in a number of countries. Although not certain, some small outbreaks suggest person-to-person transmission may have occurred. To date, however, the vast majority of cases can be linked to poultry exposure as the source, rather than transmission from an infected person.

CHEMICAL TERRORISM

Chemical weapons are defined as chemical substances intended for use in military operations to kill, seriously injure, or incapacitate people through physiologic effects. Such weapons are generally separated according to severity of effects: lethal (choking, nerve, and blood agents), blistering, and incapacitating. Chemical agents are also a direct threat as terrorist agents (CDC, 2000). Because hundreds of new chemicals are produced

There is evidence that a handful of terrorist organizations have been exploring biologic weapons. Producing germs and being able to disseminate them widely among a civilian population requires hundreds of millions of dollars of research. Some groups may have acquired a fundamental biologic weapons capability, and investigation and experimentation with biologic weapons will most likely continue. This does not automatically translate into an ability to conduct a mass-casualty attack with a biologic warfare agent. There are many technical hurdles to developing an effective large-scale chemical or biologic weapons program. This task may be so insurmountable that terrorists would choose to remain reliant on more conventional methods of attack.

ONLINE CONSULT

CDC Bird Flu Facts at
http://www.cdc.gov/flu/avian/gen-info/facts.htm

monthly, treatment should focus on clinical syndrome rather than specific agent.

Patient Arrival in the Emergency Department

Typically, the emergency department (ED) staff members are the first point of contact for patients who have not been decontaminated. When such a patient arrives in the ED, staff should:

- Try to determine the chemical agent's identity on the basis of the symptoms discussed later. Classification into a group of chemicals is helpful. Do not waste time trying to ascertain this information.
- Prepare personal protection equipment (PPE), decontamination supplies, and antidotes.
- Determine whether there is high suspicion of a chemical hazard. If there is, don personal protective equipment and set up a hot line.
- Clear and secure all areas that could become contaminated.
- Secure hospital entrances and grounds.
- Notify local emergency management authorities if needed.
- If a chemical is a military agent, inform the Army.
- If an organophosphate is involved, notify the hospital pharmacy that large amounts of atropine and 2-PAM may be needed.

The term **personal protective equipment** refers to clothing and respiratory apparatus designed to shield an individual from chemical, biologic, and physical hazards. There are different levels of PPE depending on the type of exposure expected.

When the Patient Arrives Without Warning

A contaminated patient may present at an emergency department (ED) or any office or health-care facility without prior warning. In such circumstances, ED staff should:

- Determine whether a chemical hazard exists. If there is no chemical hazard, handle the patient routinely.
- Determine whether there is suspicion or serious risk of a chemical hazard. Look for liquid on the patient's clothes or skin, symptoms in other patients and

emergency medical technicians (EMTs), an odor (H, L, phosgene, chlorine), or positive reaction on M-8 paper.

- Keep the patient outside until preparations are complete, and don personal PPE to assist EMTs as necessary.
- If the patient is grossly contaminated (liquid on skin, positive M-8 paper) or if there is any suspicion of contamination, decontaminate the patient before allowing his entry into the building.

Treatment and Identification of the Chemical Agent

Here are some general treatment suggestions followed by specific ways to treat exposure to particular chemical agents:

- Establish the airway, if necessary.
- Give artificial respiration, if the patient is not breathing.
- Control bleeding, if the patient is hemorrhaging.

For any patient with symptoms of specific agents, as described below, staff should check for other possible chemical exposures, looking for decreased level of consciousness without head trauma, an odor on the clothes or breath, and specific signs or symptoms of other chemical agents.

Nerve Agent Symptoms

If the following symptoms are present or there is a suspicion of cholinesterase poisoning, the problem is considered to be a nerve agent.

- Pinpoint pupils
- Difficulty breathing (wheezing, gasping, and so on)
- Local or generalized sweating
- Fasciculations
- Copious secretions
- Nausea, vomiting, diarrhea
- Convulsions
- Coma
- Sudden headache

Nerve Agent Treatment

Treatment recommendations for contamination with a nerve agent are as follows:

- If there is severe respiratory distress: Intubate and ventilate. Give atropine (Adults: 6 mg IM or IV. Infants/children: 0.05 mg/kg IV) and 2-PAM C1 (Adults: 600–1000 mg IM or slow IV. Infants/children: 15 mg/kg slow IV).
- If there are major secondary symptoms: Give atropine (Adults: 4 mg IM or IV. Infants/children:

0.02–0.05 mg/kg IV) and 2-PAM C1 (Adults: 600–1000 mg IM or slow IV. Infants/children: 15 mg/kg). Open the IV line.
- Repeat the atropine as needed until the secretions decrease and breathing is easier. (Adults: 2 mg IV or IM. Infants/children: 0.02–0.05 mg/kg IV.)
- Repeat 2-PAM C1 as needed. (Adults: 1.0 gm IV over 20–30 minutes; repeat every 1 hour times 3 as needed. Infants/children: 15 mg/kg slow IV.)
- If there are seizures: Give diazepam. (Adults: 10 mg slow IV. Infants/children: 0.2 mg/kg IV.)
- Reevaluate every 3 to 5 minutes. If signs worsen, repeat atropine, 2-PAM C1, and diazepam. *Note:* Warn the hospital pharmacy that unusual amounts of atropine and 2-PAM may be needed.

Chlorine Agent Symptoms

If any of the following symptoms are present, the problem is considered to be a chlorine agent.

- Dyspnea or shortness of breath
- Coughing, chest tightness
- Burning sensation in the nose, throat, and eyes
- Watery eyes, blurred vision
- Nausea and vomiting
- Burning pain, redness and blisters if in contact with skin (similar to frostbite)

Chlorine Agent Treatment

Treatment recommendations for contamination with a chlorine agent are as follows;

- If there is dyspnea, try bronchodilators and give oxygen by mask. A chest x-ray will be needed. Pulmonary edema can occur in 2 to 4 hours. The patient will have to be admitted to the hospital.
- Treat other problems and reevaluate. (Consider phosgene.)
- If phosgene poisoning is a possibility, refer to the phosphene agent section.
- Give supportive therapy; treat other problems and/or discharge.

Lewisite Agent Symptoms

If there were thermal burns, did they begin within minutes of poisoning? If they did, consider the problem a lewisite agent (can be from vapors or liquids).

- Immediate burning and blistering of any part of the body contacted.
- Burns of eyes—immediate edema of lids, conjunctiva, and cornea. Burns can also affect mucous membranes and lungs.
- Skin—immediate burns, erythema within 15 to 30 minutes, and vesication within a few hours.

The most familiar historical use of a chemical agent was by a Japanese cult. In 1995 Aum Shinrikyo released sarin gas, a nerve agent, in the Tokyo subway system, killing 12 people and injuring 5500. The sarin produced by the cult was an impure form and not nearly as lethal as military grade. It is reported that this cult also attempted to develop a biologic agent but was unsuccessful, even with a reported six laboratories and a budget of $300 million.

Blisters start small and expand to cover entire site. Maximum blistering may take up to 4 days. Blisters are less fragile than those due to mustard agents.
- Burns usually less severe than with mustard agents.
- Systemically absorbed lewisite, by any route, can cause "lewisite shock," potentially resulting in death.

Lewisite Agent Treatment

Treatment recommendations for contamination with a lewisite agent are as follows:

- Survey the extent of injury.
- Treat the affected skin with British antilewisite (BAL) ointment (if available).
- Treat affected eyes with BAL ophthalmic ointment (if available).
- Treat any pulmonary or severe effects. (BAL in oil, 0.5 mL/25 lb body wt. deep IM to max of 4.0 mL. Repeat every 4 hours times 3.)
- Give morphine as needed for pain.
- If there is severe poisoning, shorten the interval for BAL injections to every 2 hours.

Mustard Agent Symptoms

If the patient experienced burns or eye irritation beginning 2 to 12 hours after exposure, consider the problem a mustard agent:
- Mild to severe conjunctivitis with recovery in 1 to 2 weeks.
- Mild to severe corneal erosions and necrosis resulting in potential blindness.
- Skin exposure is latent; it may be several hours before lesions are noted. (This is the hallmark of mustard agents.)
- Erythema with slight edema and itching is seen 2 to 48 hours after exposure.
- Blisters are uncomfortable and tense and rupture easily.
- Deep burning (up to full-thickness loss) is possible anywhere but most likely in the genital and axillary areas.
- Rhinorrhea, burning throat pain, and hoarseness start 4 to 6 hours later.
- Bone marrow can be depleted, causing leukopenia and aplastic anemia.

- Nausea, vomiting, and diarrhea occur.
- Systemic absorption can cause central nervous system involvement.

Mustard Agent Treatment

There is no specific treatment for contamination with a mustard agent; the following measures are recommended:

- The goal of therapy is to relieve symptoms, prevent infection, and promote healing.
- If there is airway obstruction, a tracheostomy may be needed.
- If there are large burns, establish an IV line. (Do not push fluids as for thermal burns.)
- Drain vesicles: unroof large blisters and irrigate the area with topical antibiotics.
- Treat other symptoms appropriately.

Phosgene Agent Symptoms

If the patient has immediate eye pain, respiratory symptoms (immediate if inhaled, later if absorbed through the skin), and skin irritation (white with circular erythema), consider the problem a phosgene agent:

- Immediate skin irritation—exposed skin turns white and is surrounded by a circular zone of erythema, giving the appearance of a target. Within 24 hours, there is edema, and severe necrosis can develop.
- Inhalation causes immediate respiratory symptoms leading to pulmonary edema. Severe skin exposure can lead to delayed respiratory symptoms and/or pulmonary edema.

Phosgene Agent Treatment

No specific treatment is available for contamination with a phosgene agent. The following measures are recommended:
- Restrict fluids, perform a chest x-ray, and obtain blood gas measurements.
- If the patient is experiencing dyspnea, oxygen with positive end-expiratory pressure (PEEP) will be needed.
- Observe the patient closely for at least 6 hours. If severe dyspnea develops or x-ray or blood gas findings are consistent with phosgene poisoning, the patient will have to be admitted, with oxygen via PEEP, fluid restriction, and monitoring with chest x-rays and blood gas measurements. The patient will be seriously ill.

INTERACTIVE EXERCISES

Go to the Intranet site and complete the interactive exercises provided for this Chapter.

EVIDENCED-BASED PRACTICE: CONSIDER THIS . . .

*T*hrough the use of historical data sources, "researchers at the National Institutes of Health (NIH) conclude that the regional spread of annual influenza epidemics throughout the United States is more closely connected with rates of movement of people to and from work than with geographical distance or air travels" (U.S. Department of Health and Human Services [USDHHS], 2006, p. 1).

Question: How will you use this information as an occupational health nurse to implement evidence-based practice?

Source: U.S. Department of Health and Human Services (USDHHS). (2006). Interregional spread of influenza through United States described by virus type, size of population, and commuting rates and distance. *NIH News*. Retrieved October 8, 2006, from *http://www.nih.gov/news/pr/apr2006/fic-19.htm*

KEY POINTS

■ Biologic agents used in terrorism are divided into three categories: Category A (high priority), Category B (second-highest priority), and Category C (third-highest priority).

■ Category A agents pose a risk because they (1) are easily transmitted from person to person, (2) cause high mortality and the potential for a major public health impact, (3) can cause public panic and social disruption, and (4) require special action for public health preparedness.

■ Category B agents pose a risk because they (1) are moderately easy to disseminate, (2) cause moderate morbidity and low mortality, and (3) require specific enhancements of CDC's diagnostic capacity and enhanced disease surveillance.

■ Category C agents pose a risk because they (1) are readily available, (2) are easily produced and disseminated, and (3) have a potential for high morbidity and mortality as well as a major health impact.

■ Chemical agents range from warfare agents to common toxic chemicals used in industries today. Hundreds of new chemicals are produced monthly. Identification and treatment of chemical exposure focuses on the clinical syndrome rather than the specific agent.

■ Knowledge of what to do and what not to do is imperative in the treatment of chemical exposure.

■ Don personal protective equipment (PPE) prior to decontaminating the patient. Assess and establish the airway after PPE is in place.

■ Major groups of chemicals used as weapons are: (1) nerve agents, (2) chlorine agents, (3) lewisite agents, (4) mustard agents, and (5) phosgene agents.

Thought and Discussion Questions

1. The CDC has identified five focus areas for terrorism. The emphasis of this chapter has been on the third focus, diagnosis and characterization of biologic and chemical agents. Discuss what your community has done for focus number one, preparedness and prevention. What has your educational institution done to prepare for a terrorist attack if it should occur while you, as a student, are at a clinical site?

2. Be prepared to discuss the chronology of a chemical terrorist attack in your community. Discuss how to triage patients properly and give your views on allowing patients to expire who are determined to be beyond the ability to save.

3. Discuss how this story ends: You are working at a hospital. You have been notified that there are two confirmed cases of smallpox at the local school. The city has become aware. The school is in a panic,

(Thought and Discussion Questions continue on page 386)

Thought and Discussion Questions (continued)

and the next day, 25% of the students are kept at home. You have received eight call-ins for various reasons but realize the underlying fear is exposure. The local supermarket is closed because of staffing issues. What would be your course of action? How would you handle staffing issues? Would you let your children attend school? Would you return to work?

4. Discuss the central nervous system involvement of the Alphaviruses in the severe stages.

5. Discuss how the Nipah virus is transmitted.

6. When a patient arrives with an unknown chemical exposure, how do you know what to treat?

7. Review the Chapter Thought on the first page of the chapter, and discuss your views on how to prevent terrorist attacks and how to deal with countries that launch such attacks.

☐ REFERENCES

Centers for Disease Control and Prevention. (1997). *Additional requirements for facilities transferring or receiving select agents.* (42 CFR Part 72/RIN 0905-AE70.) Atlanta, GA: U.S. Department of Health and Human Services.

Centers for Disease Control and Prevention. (1998). *Preventing emerging infectious diseases: A strategy for the 21st century.* Atlanta, GA: Author.

Centers for Disease Control and Prevention. (2000). *Biological and chemical terrorism: Strategic plan for preparedness and response. Recommendations of the CDC Strategic Planning Workgroup. MMWR, 49*(4).

Centers for Disease Control and Prevention. (2003a). *All about hantavirus.* Retrieved June 21, 2006, from *http://www.cdc.gov/ncidod/diseases/hanta/hps/*

Centers for Disease Control and Prevention. (2003b). Public health and emergency preparedness and response: Facts about alphaviruses. Retrieved June 21, 2006, from *http://www.cdc.gov/ncidod/dvbid/arbor/arbdet.htm*

Centers for Disease Control and Prevention. (2003c). *Arenaviruses.* Retrieved June 21, 2006, from *http://www.cdc.gov/ncidod/dvrd/spb/mnpages/dispages/arena.htm*

Centers for Disease Control and Prevention. (2003d). *Brucellosis: Frequently asked questions.* Retrieved June 21, 2006, from *http://www.cdc.gov/ncidod/dbmd/diseaseinfo/brucellosis_g.htm*

Centers for Disease Control and Prevention. (2003e). *Filoviruses.* Retrieved June 21, 2006, from *http://www.cdc.gov/ncidod/dvrd/spb/mnpages/dispages/filoviruses.htm*

Centers for Disease Control and Prevention. (2003f) *Glanders (Burkholderia mallei): Frequently asked questions.* Retrieved June 21, 2006, from *http://www.cdc.gov/ncidod/dbmd/diseaseinfo/glanders_g.htm*

Centers for Disease Control and Prevention. (2003g). Public health and emergency preparedness and response: Facts about ricin. Retrieved June 21, 2006, from *http://www.bt.cdc.gov/agent/ricin/*

Centers for Disease Control and Prevention. (2003h). Public health and emergency preparedness and response: Facts about staphylococcal enterotoxin B. Retrieved June 21, 2006, from *http://www.cdc.gov/nchs/data/dvs/2a2005a.pdf*

Centers for Disease Control and Prevention. (2003i). Emergency preparedness and response. *Frequently asked questions (FAQ) about tularemia.* Retrieved June 21, 2006, from *http://www.bt.cdc.gov/agent/tularemia/faq.asp*

Centers for Disease Control and Prevention. (2003j). *Yellow fever—disease and vaccine.* Retrieved June 21, 2006, from *http://www.cdc.gov/ncidod/dvbid/yellowfever/*

Centers for Disease Control and Prevention. (2003k). Public health and emergency preparedness and response: Smallpox fact sheet. Retrieved June 21, 2006, from *http://www.bt.cdc.gov/agent/smallpox/overview/disease-facts.asp*

Centers for Disease Control and Prevention. (2003l). Viral and rickettsial zoonoses branch. *Q fever.* Retrieved June 21, 2006, from *http://www.cdc.gov/ncidod/dvrd/qfever/index.htm*

Centers for Disease Control and Prevention. (2004). Emergency preparedness and response. *Facts about pneumonic plague.* Retrieved June 21, 2006, from *http://www.bt.cdc.gov/agent/plague/factsheet.asp*

Centers for Disease Control and Prevention. (2005a). Public health and emergency preparedness and response: Emerging infectious diseases. Retrieved June 21, 2006, from *http://www.cdc.gov/ncidod/eid/index.htm*

Centers for Disease Control and Prevention. (2005b). Emergency preparedness and response. *Facts about botulism.* Retrieved June 21, 2006, from *http://www.bt.cdc.gov/agent/botulism/factsheet.asp*

Centers for Disease Control and Prevention. (2005c). Public health and emergency preparedness and response: Facts about hemorrhagic fever virus. Retrieved June 21, 2006, from *http://www.cdc.gov/ncidod/dvrd/spb/mnpages/dispages/cchf.htm*

Centers for Disease Control and Prevention. (2005d) *Hantavirus.* Retrieved June 21, 2006, from *http://www.cdc.gov/nceh/ehs/Topics/Hantavirus.htm*

Centers for Disease Control and Prevention. (2006a). Emergency preparedness and response. *Fact sheet: Anthrax information for health care providers.* Retrieved June 21, 2006, from *http://www.bt.cdc.gov/agent/anthrax/anthrax-hcp-factsheet.asp*

Centers for Disease Control and Prevention. (2006b). *Key facts about avian influenza (bird flu) and avian influenza A (H5N1) virus.* Retrieved June 21, 2006, from *http://www.cdc.gov/flu/avian/gen-info/facts.htm*

Eitzen, E. M., & Takafuji, E. T. (1997). Historical overview of biological warfare. In F. R. Sidell, E. T. Takafuji, & D. R. Franz (Vol. Eds.), *Medical aspects of chemical and biological warfare* (pp. 415–424). *Textbook of military medicine: Warfare, weaponry, and the casualty.* Washington, DC: Office of the Surgeon General at TMM Publications.

English, J. F., Cundiff, M. Y., Malone, J. D., & Pfeiffer, J. A. (1999). CDC Hospital Infections Program Bioterrorism Working Group. Retrieved June 21, 2006, from *http://www.hospitalsoup.com/public/bioplan.pdf*

Henderson, D. A. (1997). Bioweapons and bioterrorism. *Journal of the American Medical Association, 278,* 351–370, 389–436.

New Jersey State Health Department (2002). What you should know about Q fever. Retrieved June 21, 2006, from *http://www.cdc.gov/ncidod/EID/vol9no2/02-0271.htm*

Northstar Preparedness Network. (n.d.). *Clostridium perfringens toxins.* Retrieved June 21, 2006, from *http://www.preparednessnetwork.org/northstar/warfare/cpt.html*

Osterholm, M., & Schwartz, J. (2001). *Living terrors: What America needs to know to survive the coming bioterrorist catastrophe.* Belmont, CA: Wadsworth.

World Health Organization (WHO). (2001, September). Fact sheet no. 262. *Nipah virus.* Retrieved June 21, 2006, from *http://www.who.int/mediacentre/factsheets/fs262/en/index.html*

World Health Organization (WHO). (2003, May 7). Epidemic and pandemic alert and response (EPR). *Ebola haemorrhagic fever in the Republic of the Congo—Update 12: Disease outbreak reported.* Retrieved June 21, 2006, from *http://www.who.int/csr/don/2003_05_07/en/*

BIBLIOGRAPHY

Department of Defense. (2001). *21st century bioterrorism and germ weapons. U.S. Army field manual for the treatment of biological warfare agent casualties (anthrax, smallpox, plague, viral fevers, toxins, delivery methods, detection, symptoms, treatment, equipment).* Washington, DC: Progressive Management.

Federal Emergency Management Agency. (2003). *Guidelines for public sector hazardous materials training.* Washington, DC: Author.

Henderson, D. A., Inglesby, T. V., & O'Toole, T. (Eds.). (2002). *Bioterrorism: Guidelines for medical and public health management.* Chicago, IL: American Medical Association.

U.S. Government. (2002). 2002 *Bioterrorism after the anthrax attacks: Complete revised guide to biological weapons and germ warfare, anthrax, smallpox, medicines, treatment, preparedness, White House, Homeland Security, CDC, HHS, FDA, NIH, Military manuals.* Washington, DC: Progressive Management.

Venzke, B. (1998). *First responder chem-bio handbook.* Alexandria, VA: Tempest Publishing.

Vorobyov, A. (1994, April). Criterion rating as a measure of probable use of bio agents as biological weapons. In: *Papers presented to the working group on biological weapons control of the committee on international security and arms control. National Academy of Sciences.* Washington, DC.

■ Rose **Kearney-Nunnery** ■ Jimmie E. **Nunnery**

The Politically Active Nurse: An Imperative

> " *There are risks and costs to a program of action, but they are far less than the long-range risks and costs of comfortable inaction.* "
>
> John F. Kennedy, 1917–1963

Chapter Objectives

On completion of this chapter, the reader will be able to:

1. Explain why it is important for nurses to possess political efficacy.
2. Discuss the process for the enactment of laws and associated regulations.
3. Identify the major committees at the federal and state levels, especially those that influence health policy.
4. Identify how nurses can influence the passing of legislation.
5. Analyze statutes and regulations governing nursing practice.
6. Examine the roles and activities of nurses and professional associations in influencing health policy decisions.
7. Demonstrate political involvement on a current health policy issue.

Key Terms

Political Efficacy
Government
Law
Bill
Committee Structure
Conference Committee

Regulations
Precedent
Nurse Practice Acts
Title Protection
Lobbying
Grassroots Effort

Political Action Committees
Workplace Issues
Community or Civic Involvement
Professional Organizations
Voice of Agency

Hillary Rodham Clinton once observed:

> A political life, I've often said, is a continuing
> education in human nature, including one's own . . .
> In each place [of my involvement], I met someone
> or saw something that caused me to open my mind
> and my heart and deepen my understanding of the
> universal concerns that most of humanity share.
> (Clinton, 2003, p. x)

Politics is a process for finding solutions to these universal concerns of humanity, one being the concern for public health and safety. Nurses likewise are engaged in finding solutions to problems of humanity on a daily basis. These problems are not restricted to a location or practice area. The nursing professional advocates for the health of people and policies aimed at health protection and promotion. This imperative for change requires a broader view of what is involved in making changes in public policy at the local, state, and national levels. Nurses have become increasingly interested in public policy, realizing that both their personal and their professional lives are significantly influenced by governmental policy and programs.

Nurses are effective in the political process when they understand the sources of power and are willing to be involved and make a difference. Interestingly, Wilson and DiIulio (1998) have defined **political efficacy** as having two components: internal political efficacy and external political advocacy. Internal political efficacy is personal competence or the "ability to understand and take part in political affairs" (Wilson & DiIulio, 1998, p. 102). External political advocacy is the "ability to make the system respond to the citizenry" (Wilson & DiIulio, 1998, p. 102). Nurses must develop their internal political efficacy by being increasingly able to take part in the political process. This will further the external political advocacy of the nursing profession. These two components are the political imperative of the profession. Political efficacy is possible by virtue of the number of nurses in the profession who are skillful in promoting change. In addition, we see the active involvement of nursing organizations in political initiatives to effect change in health policy. As described by Leininger (2002), "political aspects of nursing are now a dominant and frequent topic in hospitals and schools of nursing in the current era" (p. 189).

Both internal efficacy and external political advocacy are growing with the increasing involvement of nurses. As noted by Mason and colleagues (2006), health care is a political endeavor at all levels of government and is influenced by health-care institutions in the private sector. This is one area of influence for nursing professionals and their political efficacy. The first step in the development of political efficacy is understanding the political process in government.

STRUCTURE AND FUNCTION OF GOVERNMENT

When we think of the term **government**, different images may come to mind. We may be thinking of the federal structure with its three components—executive, legislative, and judicial. Or, at the local level, we may be envisioning the organizational, local, and state influences on the operation of the health-care unit. Government is merely the controlling entity that has the authority to make decisions and regulations for the public good. Milstead (2003) describes government as an "iron triangle" of congresspeople, bureaucratic staff, and interest groups. Nursing has the responsibility to contribute to the decisions by providing the information needed and offering support for wise policy decisions that protect the public and the profession. To participate most effectively in the political process, one must understand the structure of government at each level. Because government structures do vary, it is essential to be familiar with your own local and state governing bodies.

Branches of Government

Each branch of government plays a significant role in the development and implementation of health policy. The federal government and most state governments have three branches: legislative, executive, and judicial. The powers of the three federal branches are vested in accordance with the U.S. Constitution.

Executive Branch

At the federal level, the executive branch consists of the president, the cabinet-level departments, and regulatory agencies. The executive branch is responsible for the administration of government and the laws enacted. The president sets the legislative agenda for Congress and the annual budget for the nation. The president's budget influences the funding available for health-care programs, reimbursement, and education. In addition, the agenda set by the president determines what programs have a high priority for the administration. The president can recommend legislation and can approve or veto legislation passed by Congress. It is also the executive branch that makes appointments to government departments, courts, boards, and committees, as with the appointment of the surgeon general or the secretary of U.S. Department of Health and Human Services. The Constitution mandates that certain executive appointments be confirmed by the legislative branch.

Legislative Branch

The legislative branch comprises the two houses or chambers of Congress, the Senate and the House of

Representatives. Congress is responsible for lawmaking, representation, and administrative oversight, including oversight of the agencies of the executive branch. Congress also provides the operational funding for the administrative agencies. The composition of and qualifications for the U.S. Congress are listed in Table 21–1. Compare these qualifications with those for the president. Also consider the reelection cycle and how the priorities, policies, and laws can be influenced by executive and legislative agendas and majority control.

Judicial Branch

The judicial branch includes the Supreme Court, which interprets laws and, through its judicial review process, can declare an act of Congress or the president unconstitutional. The nine federal Supreme Court justices are appointed for life by the president after their selection has been confirmed by the Senate. The federal system also comprises lower courts and appellate or circuit courts. Federal judges are nominated by the executive branch and confirmed by the Senate. This system of

checks and balances manages to create an equilibrium, vesting limited power in each branch with oversight by another branch.

State and Local Systems

State government structures are similar to those described at the federal level. They also receive their mandates from the U.S. Constitution with which their respective state constitutions must abide. Like the president, the governor can sign legislation into law and use the power of the veto. State legislatures can also override a governor's veto. In some states, members of the state board of nursing, or other important health commissioners, are appointed by the governor. As with the federal government, some legislative branches must confirm selected executive appointments. State supreme courts and lower courts interpret the law and make decisions under their power of judicial review.

County government generally entails a board of supervisors or an elected board of commissioners and a county executive or county manager. Cities, towns, and

Table 21.1

Qualifications for Service in the U.S. Congress or Executive Office

	Senate	House of Representatives	Presidency
Number	■ 100 senators (two from each state) ■ Equal representation ■ Senior senator (elected first) and junior senator	■ 435 members ■ Representation based on state population; minimum of one from each state with reapportionment every 10 years based on the U.S. Census ■ The House also includes delegates from the District of Columbia, Guam, the Virgin Islands, American Samoa, and Puerto Rico, who have voting rights in committees but not in matters before the full House of Representatives	■ One; in the case of the inability of the president to fulfill his or her role, succession of power occurs as follows: vice president as second in line, then speaker of the house, and then president pro tempore of the Senate
Terms	■ Elected for a term of six years, on alternate schedule	■ Elected for a term of two years	■ Elected for a term of four years
Reelection	■ Every two years, one third of senators face reelection	■ Entire membership is up for reelection every two years	■ Eligible for reelection once (two-term limit)
Qualifications	■ At least 30 years of age ■ Citizen of United States for nine years ■ Resident of the state represented when elected	■ At least 25 years of age ■ Citizen of United States for seven years ■ Resident of the state represented when elected	■ At least 35 years of age ■ A natural-born citizen of the United States and a resident for at least 14 years

villages also have a variety of elected officials similar to those of county government. Local health policies and politics must be consistent with state and federal law but can also have a profound influence on the health and welfare of a community, as with public utilities and local programs.

Although nurses are most often involved with the legislative branch of government, the executive branch and the judicial branch can also be of great importance to nursing and health care. It is essential that nurses understand the functions of the different branches of government and how laws and regulations are enacted and implemented.

HOW LAWS ARE MADE

A **law** is a mandate of prescribed conduct, grants certain rights, requires certain responsibilities, or a combination of these attributes. A law can come from a constitution, from the legislature, or from the courts. Administrative agencies promulgate regulations, which supplement and further interpret the laws. Consider the types of laws and regulations identified in Table 21–2.

The idea for a law may originate with an individual, a professional group, a legislator, or the executive branch. *Statutory law* is legislation that has been approved by both legislative houses of Congress and signed by the executive branch. The legislation starts as a **bill** or a proposal for a law authored or sponsored by either a representative or a senator, who introduces it after it has been written in appropriate language by the legislative counsel of either the House or the Senate.

A bill may also be introduced from a legislative committee. A bill proposed in the Senate is designated "S." followed by a number, and a bill introduced in the House of Representatives is designated "H.R." followed by a number.

Congressional Committees

At the federal level, bills are referred to full committee and sometimes to a subcommittee, because of the thousands of bills introduced each year. The U.S. Senate has 16 standing committees, with a variable number of associated subcommittees, depending on the scope and work of the committee, and four select or special committees. The House of Representatives has 19 standing committees and additional special or select committees. There are also four joint committees, staffed by both houses, which focus on common oversight functions for printing, taxation, the Library of Congress, and economics.

It is within the **committee structure** that most of the work of Congress takes place, at both the federal and state level. Committee action is perhaps the most important phase of the congressional process because it is at this phase that proposed measures are given the most intensive consideration and people have an opportunity to provide testimony for consideration and incorporation into the record. The committee or subcommittee level is where nursing can have a powerful impact. The subcommittee studies the issues contained in each bill carefully, holds hearings, and reports back to the full committee with recommendations. Each committee has jurisdiction over certain subjects. Some of the committees identified in Table 21–3 focus specifically on health-related issues.

Table 21.2
Types of Law

Type	Description	Example
Constitutional	▪ Specific guarantees granted by the U.S. Constitution	Freedom of speech
Statutory	▪ Formal laws enacted by federal, state, and local legislative branches of government	Nurse practice acts
Administrative	▪ Regulations created by administrative agencies under the direction of the executive branch of government	Regulations associated with nurse practice acts to assist with implementation
Court, case, or common law	▪ Laws created from judicial decisions ▪ Judgments create a precedent on which future decisions are based	"Miranda Rights" must be read to an arrestee before he or she is taken into custody

Table 21.3

Major Committees of the U.S. Congress

Senate	
Standing committees (16)	Agriculture, Nutrition, and Forestry Appropriations* Armed Services Banking, Housing and Urban Affairs Budget* Commerce, Finance and Transportation Energy and Natural Resources Environment and Public Works Finance* Foreign Relations Governmental Affairs Health, Education, Labor, and Pensions* Judiciary Rules and Administration Small Business and Entrepreneurship Veteran's Affairs*
Select, special, & other committees (4)	Indian Affairs* Aging* Ethics Intelligence
House	
Standing committees (19)	Agriculture Appropriations* Armed Services Budget* Education and The Workforce* Energy & Commerce* Financial Services Government Reform House Administration International Relations Judiciary Resources Rules Science Small Business Standards Of Official Conduct Transportation And Infrastructure Veteran's Affairs* Ways and Means*
Select or special committees	Aging* Children, Youth, and Families* Homeland Security Intelligence

*Frequently address health-related matters.

States operate much like the federal government. In a particular state, there are also specific committees and subcommittees that handle selected topics. For example, in South Carolina, the Medical, Military, Public, and Municipal Affairs Committee for the House and the Medical Committee of the Senate generally handle the topics of concern to nursing and health care. But state structures differ, and it is important to be aware of the differences and to know the committees in which the issues of major concern to nursing arise. Appointment to the committees is often based on Congressional seniority or priority. Members often have special interests in an area. Because these members represent their constituents, it is important to know on which committees your congressperson serves and that he or she has valid information, resources, and background to address your concerns. Testimony, either written or in person, provides valuable information to the committee member, whether information from constituents, special interest groups, experts, or other public officials.

Committee action is perhaps the most important phase of the congressional process, because it is at this phase that proposed measures are given the most intensive consideration.

How a Bill Becomes a Law

Consider a bill, for instance, that has been sponsored by your legislator, a member of the House of Representatives. It has been sent to the applicable subcommittee or committee for review. After consideration by the full committee, several things may happen to this bill:

- It may be reported out of committee favorably and be scheduled for debate by the full House.

- It may be reported out favorably, but with amendments or "markups" to the bill.
- It may be reported out unfavorably or not acted upon at all; thus, it is "killed" or "dies in committee."

Generally, once the bill has been reported favorably out of a House committee, it goes to the Rules Committee, which schedules bills and determines (1) how much time will be spent on debate and (2) whether or not amendments will be allowed. A written report is drafted, including a summary of the bill, along with impact statements. Impact statements are provided to project how the proposed legislation would affect existing laws and present and future resources. Bills are then placed on the calendar and scheduled for action. After a bill is debated under the procedural rules of the House, possibly amended, voted upon, and passed, it is sent to the Senate, where it goes through the same procedure. If the bill also passes the Senate without any changes, it is sent to the president or governor for signature. If minor changes were made in the Senate, it is referred back to the originating chamber (in this case the House of Representatives) for concurrence before submission to the executive branch. If significant changes were made to the bill in the Senate, the bill is sent to a **conference committee,** composed of representatives of both chambers, who reconcile differences and prepare a conference report for approval by both chambers. If it does not get approved, the bill dies. After the conference report, the bill must be accepted or rejected, because no further amendments may be made.

If the bill is approved in both houses, it goes to the executive branch. If the president or governor signs the bill, it becomes law, and the Congress is notified. If the bill is vetoed, it is referred back to the House and Senate. A two-thirds vote by both chambers is required to override the veto. The bill may also become law if the president or governor fails to veto or return the bill to Congress with objections within a specified time.

Once the bill is signed or passed, it becomes an act, and is *enacted* into law. Laws are enforceable if they do not violate the Constitution. Once a law is passed, it is assigned to the appropriate department of the executive branch of government, where the process of developing regulations to interpret the law takes place. The department studies the law and drafts the regulations for implementation. Administrative agencies, governed by the executive branch, promulgate **regulations** or rules, which serve the purpose of detailing and applying the laws. For example, the Health Insurance Portability and Accountability Act (HIPAA) was enacted as Public Law 104–191 in 1996. The Department of Health and Human Services (HHS) published a final Privacy Rule in December 2000 with a general compliance date of

April 14, 2003, and a compliance date of April 14, 2004, for small health plans. All of this activity involved detailing regulations for application of the law.

The legislative process (Fig. 21.1) can seem endless, especially when the bill stays in committee, perhaps during a recess or between legislative sessions. In addition, proposed regulations from the executive branch may require public hearings for input prior to finalization and enforcement. In the United States Congress, a legislative session spans a two-year period, with the 110th Congressional session running from January 1, 2007, through December 31, 2008. Variable legislative sessions occur in the different states; however, special sessions may be called for special circumstances.

Impact of Laws

Laws and regulations govern behavior and relationships with others in society. Consider the impact of laws that have been passed and their effect on nursing. When the federal government implemented diagnosis-related groups (DRGs) for Medicare reimbursement, patients began to be discharged from hospitals "sicker and quicker." Although this law applied only to Medicare clients, it set a precedent that other insurance carriers followed. In law, a **precedent** is a decision or verdict from a prior case that becomes the principle to follow in future cases. A precedent is more than an everyday custom to follow. If the precedent is set in a higher court, like the Supreme Court, it becomes mandatory in lower court decisions.

Awareness of laws and regulations governing health care is essential in professional nursing practice so that nurses can help to influence the making of policy and laws. Nurses can and do play a significant role at several points in the legislative process, whether through lobbying or providing testimony or information to legislators and regulatory bodies (Box 21–1).

REGULATING NURSING PRACTICE

Nursing practice and education are directly regulated by law. **Nurse practice acts** are contained in state statute (laws) and associated regulations that dictate practice parameters. As part of the statute, nursing education programs in different forms are regulated. For example, most states require a new, beginning nursing program to receive approval from the board of nursing according to specified standards before it can open. These standards ensure that the organization, curriculum, faculty, and services are appropriate for preparation of students and protection of the public. Nursing education is further regulated indirectly through the accrediting bodies that are authorized by the Department of Education.

> The state boards of nursing and their associated practice acts define the scope of practice; establish the requirements for licensure, entry into practice, continuing competency, and advanced practice; create and empower a board of nursing; and identify grounds for disciplinary action.

Nurse Practice Acts

Nurse practice acts are developed by each state to protect the public health, safety, and welfare by regulating and overseeing nursing practice. The various state boards of nursing and their associated practice acts define the scope of practice; establish the requirements for licensure, entry into practice, continuing competency and advanced practice; create and empower a board of nursing; and identify grounds for disciplinary action. An important component in many practice acts

1. Concerned party contacts legislator, bill drafted

2. Sponsors obtained, introduced to House and/or Senate

3. To committees for recommendation/amendments

4. Debate on floor

5. Vote and recommendation to other chamber

6. Consideration in a similar manner by the other chamber

7. Passage or to Conference Committee

8. Back to both houses for concurrence

9. If agreement by both chambers, to president or governor for signature

10. If executive veto, back to chambers for potential override with a 2/3 vote of Congress or the legislature

■ **Figure 21.1** The legislative process.

Box 21.1 Nurses' Involvement in the Legislative Process

- Meeting with legislators, their aides, or staff to influence the introduction of a bill as private citizens or as members of a professional organization
- Providing information to assist in drafting the bill and gathering support for legislators or bill sponsors on the proposed legislation
- Providing testimony in committee or subcommittee hearings about their position on the bill
- Contacting legislators to support or not support proposed legislation, both in the home district and the capitol
- Contacting either the president or the governor to sign or veto the proposed legislation
- Responding to requests for comments, either written or verbal testimony, by regulatory agencies or committees
- Submission of an *Amicus Curiae* (friend of the court) brief for consideration by the court

is **title protection**. This is a part of the law that maintains the use of the title *nurse* only for the licensee authorized by the board. The term *nurse* is used in some contexts outside of professional practice, and more states are moving to protect the integrity and identity of this title.

Nurse practice acts can be revised or completely eliminated through a single legislative action, so the prospect of "opening the practice act" in the legislature can cause great anxiety. Although state practice acts (statute and regulations) are specific to the state, there is general content common to many state acts. For example, the National Council of State Boards of Nursing (NCSBN) has a model act and model rules that illustrate standard contents of the legislation and associated regulations for implementation (Box 21.2). In addition, in 1998 a mutual recognition model for interstate practice among the "compact states" was introduced. This mutual recognition model requires further specific language to be incorporated into state law to allow a nurse to have one license (in the state of residency) and to practice in

other states that are members of the compact. The nurse is required to practice in accordance with each state's specific practice law and regulations.

Appointments to a state board of nursing are often made by the governor. The state board should be composed of a variety of members who represent practice throughout all areas of nursing. In four states, there are separate boards for licensed practical nurses/licensed visiting nurses (LPNs/LVNs) and registered nurses (RNs), but the boards are combined in the remaining jurisdictions. RN boards address both professional nursing and advanced practice nurses (APRNs) except in two states that currently have separate APRN boards. APRN regulations may also be addressed in the respective practice acts of other health professions such as the board of medicine. In addition, boards of nursing may have advisory committees or practice committees that research issues for recommendations to the board on practice or policy issues. Review your state's practice act for the composition of members on the board or perhaps seek a seat on the board. In many cases, serving on a board of nursing is both a humbling and an enlightening experience, and allows you to serve your state and your profession.

Because changes proposed by a state board can lead to law and rules that have the same force as law, it is imperative for nurses to remain aware of the activities of the board that regulates practice within their state. The American Nurses Association (ANA) provides recent updates to practice acts and the status of proposed legislation on its Web site. In addition, some states issue advisory opinions; although such opinions do not have the same impact as law, they do guide acceptable standards of practice. Nurses are often unaware that changes are even being proposed. Some states distribute the state nurses association newsletter to all registered nurses, whether or not they hold membership in the ANA or the state association. Many of the newsletter issues (print or online) contain periodic informational alerts concerning changes in or interpretations to the statute or advisory opinions by the board.

State boards and their respective members are concerned about nurses' current understanding of their

Box 21.2 Nurse Practice Acts

General content for both statute and regulations:

- Title and purpose
- Definitions, scope, and standards of practice
- Board of nursing—authority and how it functions
- Application of other state statutes and the state's administrative law act
- Licensure
- Titles and abbreviations
- Approval of nursing education programs
- Violations and penalties
- Discipline and proceedings
- Emergency relief for public protection
- Reporting requirements
- Exemptions
- Revenue and fees
- Implementation of the statute and regulations

respective state law. To encourage and increase nurses' knowledge about their respective practice acts, several states award continuing education credits for specific courses. These courses and the multiple-choice posttests specific to the state are available through the NCSBN at *http://www.ncsbn.org*. It is vital that nurses understand the content of their respective practice acts. This understanding must be ongoing, beyond the point of original licensure or title recognition. Put a bookmark in your computer's Internet browser with the Web site of your nursing board(s) to give yourself quick information and links to related resources.

Additional State and Federal Laws Affecting Nursing Practice

Many states have passed laws, for example, allowing some nurses to be directly reimbursed by clients or insurers. Legislation varies from state to state, but APRNs, particularly nurse anesthetists, nurse practitioners, and nurse midwives, are most commonly covered. Over 240,000 APRNs (over 8% of the total number of RNs) are providing essential health-care services as certified nurse midwives, certified registered nurse anesthetists, nurse practitioners, and clinical nurse specialists, with a demonstrated increase in APRNs from the 2000 survey (American Nurses Association [ANA], 2007a).

State laws that affect practice can be passed with the support of nursing. Some states have passed laws to allow registered nurses to pronounce death. Others are addressing safe practice through staffing requirements, title protection, tort reform, and prohibitions on mandatory overtime. Still others are addressing delegation to assistive personnel. Public protection is a concern at all levels of government. In the area of advanced practice, for example, states differ in level of supervision or collaboration and prescriptive authority for advanced practice nurses. Nurses must be politically astute and must continue to develop their internal political efficacy and the external efficacy of the profession.

INFLUENCING LEGISLATION

As mentioned previously, the idea for a law may originate from a concerned citizen or special interest group, a legislator, a professional group, or the executive branch to address a community problem or a public policy issue. Many laws originate from the legislature itself, which is composed of individuals who are elected by constituents with specific interests, needs, and concerns. Legislators' knowledge and recognition of particular needs and concerns come about through influence. For instance, special interest groups representing large numbers of the voting public can have a lot of influence on legislators.

Special interest groups have become more politically savvy at influencing the creation of public policy, and more controls have emerged, as with campaign financing reforms. Special interest groups influence legislators through lobbying activities, professional lobbyists, professional organizations, political action committees, and grassroots efforts. Each of these groups represents the dollars and votes of a particular special interest group, and each group uses expert communication and interpersonal skills to influence change.

Lobbying

Activities to influence legislators vary from formal to informal and often take the form of lobbying. **Lobbying** may be defined as attempting to persuade a legislator or legislative aide of the merits of your viewpoint in order to influence legislation. Individuals may "lobby" through face-to-face interviews, letter-writing, telephone calls, faxes, e-mails, letters to the editor, and testimony (verbal or written). Valuable clues on and guidelines for letter-writing are provided by professional associations that recognize the value of individual constituents contacting their elected legislators. These professional organizations often provide special alerts or suggestions to the members to assist with lobbying activities. For example, some professional organizations provide an alert when congresspersons are on recess and should be contacted in their home states. Other organizations may include lobbying tips on their Web sites, along with background issues and talking points to assist in lobbying activities.

But there is definitely an art at getting your point across. The bottom line is that numbers mean something to the legislative aide or legislator, especially from constituents. There are other considerations, however, such as time. The impact of a well-composed, factual, meaningful, and succinct letter far outweighs the form letter that has less impact or a letter that

ONLINE CONSULT

Governmental Affairs

ANA at
http://nursingworld.org/gova/

National League for Nursing at
http://www.nln.org/Policy/index.htm

American Association of Colleges of Nursing at
http://www.aacn.nche.edu/Government/index.htm

Also look for governmental affairs on Web sites of some nursing specialty organizations.

rambles on. Another consideration is the form of the correspondence. Postal delays cannot compete with the immediacy of e-mail, for instance. For a personal appointment, be aware of the congressional calendar, and do not be disappointed if you meet with a legislative aide. The aide may be more knowledgeable about your issue and can be persuaded to communicate the information to the legislator.

The professional lobbyist is a person on the staff of a professional association or hired consultant who has outstanding skills in persuasion, in-depth knowledge of the organization, and an acute sense of the intricacies of the political system. These professionals understand the legislators and their political agendas. The professional lobbyist is present at the appropriate time with the correct message, especially in the case of the undecided legislator. The role of the professional lobbyist is to provide the facts and the support base to persuade the legislator. The ANA has several professional lobbyists working at the federal level. A significant number of constituent state associations (CNAs) and specialty professional organizations also hire professional lobbyists.

Lobbying is especially effective when there is an associated strong **grassroots effort** that responds with mobilization of a group to provide additional correspondence and support on the position presented to the legislator or legislative aide. This approach has been used effectively by many professional organizations to influence public policy. Various nursing and other grassroots networks have been established to lobby in support of the legislative goals and objectives of the state nurses associations. There are specific channels of communication for response to a key issue. Key contacts for each legislator or legislative district must be active and ongoing.

ANA creates political action through grassroots efforts and successful lobbying. ANA's N-STAT is an example of this grassroots lobbying system. Established in 1993, N-STAT continues to grow, with more nurses providing a rapid response on legislative and policy issues. Information is provided on current topics as they move through Congress. Then, when the time to speak out on an issue is beneficial, nurses are assisted with electronic contact information and content for contacting their senators and representatives.

Nurses can register online, receive periodic alerts, and take an active step toward political efficacy. Sign up today, or periodically refer to the ANA Web site for particular national and state initiatives and legislative alerts at *http://www.nursingworld.org/MainMenuCategories/ANAPoliticalPower.aspx*.

Professional Organizations

Nurses have always had a great deal of potential power by virtue of numbers, but have now begun to use their power collectively. This is one important reason to join professional organizations. Only through united efforts will nurses be seen as a powerful group and will their voices be recognized in the policy arena. This has been demonstrated continually by many vocal and powerful organizations readily visible on Capitol Hill, on surrounding streets in Washington, DC, or in your state capitol, such as the American Medical Association (AMA) and the American Hospital Association (AHA). In a study conducted in 2003, the ANA was listed along with the AMA and the AHA in the top 20 of groups with most influence on Capitol Hill (Heaney, 2003). And consider the number of professional nursing organizations with headquarters located in the Washington, DC, area (refer to the professional organizations listed on the Intranet site and in Appendix A).

The ANA and its 54 constituent state members are also associated with the Washington, DC, area organizational affiliate members. The legislative or political arm of the ANA is known as its Department of Governmental Affairs. It actively advocates for legislation and works with administrative agencies on regulations for implementation of laws and health policy. ANA regularly monitors the work of more than a dozen federal agencies that affect health-care policy. It monitors agencies like the Centers for Medicare and Medicaid Services (CMS) and the Agency for Health Research and Quality (AHRQ). The ANA (2002), in association with other affiliated nursing organizations, also promoted an *Agenda for the Future: A Call to the Nation*, that identified and demanded action on the following 10 areas of concern:

- Leadership and planning
- Delivery systems/nursing models
- Legislation/regulation/policy
- Nursing/professional culture
- Recruitment/retention
- Economic value
- Work environment
- Public relations/communication
- Education
- Diversity.

To address this agenda in addition to its lobbying activities, ANA establishes legislative and regulatory initiatives for each session of Congress. For example, for the 109th Congress, the ANA specified an advocacy agenda for nurses that focused on the nursing shortage, appropriate staffing, workplace rights, workplace health and safety, and patient safety and advocacy. These are broad-based initiatives with well-developed statements of the issue, background, and the ANA position.

The ANA's Department of Government Affairs also contains the political action unit N-STAT, made up of the grassroots lobbying network that functions through the activities of Congressional district coordinators, Senate coordinators, and the ANA's political action committee (ANA-PAC).

Political Action Committees

As a result of campaign reform in the 1970s, restrictions were placed on contributions made by individuals or organizations to a candidate for a federal office. This campaign financing reform also allowed for the creation of **political action committees (PACs)**, through which organizations could make openly reported contributions. Although any organization can form a PAC, most PACs are sponsored by corporations, labor groups, and special interest groups who want their message heard and promoted. It is a political reality that legislators are more likely to see and listen to a group of people who have contributed money to their campaign.

The ANA (2007b) formed a PAC more than three decades ago to create power and influence for the nursing profession. Contributions to the ANA-PAC support candidates, current legislators, and legislation aligned with the ANA Legislative Agenda. It is bipartisan, supporting candidates of both national parties. The PAC is focused on the public office and the candidate for that office, whether incumbent or opponent. Endorsements and financial contributions are based on the candidates' support for the ANA legislative agenda and stance on health policy. In addition, some state constituents of ANA have separate state-associated PACs working on behalf of nursing issues in their particular states and at the federal level. Other specialty professional nursing organizations have PACs as well, representing issues critical to their respective missions.

GAINING SKILL IN POLITICAL EFFICACY

The initial step in developing political efficacy is understanding the process and having the willingness to be involved. But even more basic is possessing an understanding of people and policy needed for public health and welfare. This understanding of people and their health-care needs is basic to nursing practice. The next prerequisite to political efficacy is an understanding of the issues involved. It is vital that nurses use their voices and individual power to empower nurses and nursing. As Milstead (2003) has observed, "involvement in policy making is not an option for a professional nurse—it is a necessity" (p. 15). This is your imperative for action. Nurses, particularly with their focus on health issues, can influence change in the workplace and health policy in their communities, in professional organizations, and in government.

Workplace Issues

As illustrated with management in the organizational setting, the workplace is a significant area for nurses to promote policy changes, particularly regarding workplace advocacy and client safety and advocacy. Nurses are highly regarded by clients and the public. In addition, they have the five general bases of power identified by Mintzberg (1983): control of resources, control of a technical skill, control of a body of knowledge, exclusive rights or privileges to impose choices (legal prerogatives), and access to people who have and can be relied on for the other four. To be influential, nurses must take an active role in institutional decision-making, either at the unit level or by volunteering to serve on various committees. To contribute to policy decisions, they must remain current on health policy issues and must provide factual information. This involvement with **workplace issues** provides the basis for the improvements needed in the delivery of care and positive outcomes for both clients and the profession.

Community or Civic Involvement

A prime responsibility for all citizens is to be part of the electorate—to be registered and to vote in local, state, and national elections. Nurses have traditionally been involved in the community, whether serving on committees like the local school or hospital board or helping out with a local health fair. These activities constitute **community** or **civic involvement.** In the community, nurses can identify potential health hazards that require the attention of local officials or businesspersons, and can intervene in the case of health risks or hazards. Nurses are adept at understanding community issues, and active involvement of professional nurses in community or civic activities is truly an imperative.

Professional Organizations

Active involvement in **professional organizations** provides both constant development and valuable information. As illustrated with the governmental functions of the ANA, professional organizations offer policy analysis and updates, and they can lead effective campaigns to influence policy change. As already described, Nursing's Agenda for the Future (ANA, 2002) addresses many policy areas that the ANA and the other professional organizations on the steering committee are committed to addressing. Nurses should remain knowledgeable about the positions of the professional organizations on issues that are likely to come before Congress.

This awareness can assist with needed action on health policies and legislation through participation in grassroots efforts of the organization. It can also lead to service in elected and appointed positions or opportunities to provide testimony on behalf of the organization.

Government

Be aware of who your legislators and other elected or appointed officials are at local, state, and national levels. Keep yourself informed on how they support the issues, especially those related to health policy. Communicate with these officials. Nurses have the expertise in the care for clients and they witness the impact of health policy on a daily basis. Legislators want to hear the concerns of their nurse constituents and will appreciate the information you provide to help address the concerns of all their constituents. Often, legislators' only view of the health-care arena is through the care they or family members receive and the views imparted to them by their legislative aides and constituents. At times, this perspective can be narrow and very personal. The issues being confronted by federal, state, and local legislators on health policy can have long-term and wide-ranging effects on both the profession and care of clients. Nurses are serving in growing numbers in important roles to assist with the passage of health policy for the good of both the public and the profession.

At the state level, nurses have successfully lobbied to enact legislation that allows them to bill insurance companies directly for the care they provide. Prescriptive authority, interstate practice, amendments or revisions to practice acts, and safe staffing requirements are current issues in many state legislatures. To have legislation enacted, individual nurses or a nursing organization can seek a sponsor and co-sponsors to introduce it. Once the legislation is introduced, nurses must lobby legislators to provide information on how passage of the bill will benefit the legislator's constituents. Nurses elected to leadership positions and appointed to serve on boards at the state government level are becoming more common, but there is a great need to increase the numbers who are willing and prepared to serve in these roles. Often it is through involvement at the local level that nurses gain experience and the confidence to move on to state positions.

To effectively influence policy, nurses must establish a relationship with legislators and their legislative aides whenever possible. These officials are elected to serve—and are concerned about the needs of their constituents. They expect constituents to inform them of their concerns. Watch the interactions that occur at your next community or state function attended by a legislator. It may not be an election year, but the legislator is present because the particular function is of importance to a group the legislator represents. A nurse's offer to serve as a personal resource is frequently welcomed by the legislator and her staff. This is particularly true at the local and state levels, at which legislators may not have extensive staff to assist with legislation involving health policy. Nurses can also be valuable in providing testimony for regulatory change. Practice and preparation are needed for developing proficiency, effectiveness, and ease in these activities, particularly in dealing with the media. Being knowledgeable and articulate in both subject matter and presentation is essential.

Nurses must be part of the process, whether providing needed facts and background on the issues or serving in an office. Buresh and Gordon (2006) have described this as the **voice of agency,** a strong and authentic voice as talking about what you do as a nurse and being more visible and vocal as individuals and as members of

EVIDENCED-BASED PRACTICE: CONSIDER THIS . . .

*T*he American Association of Critical-Care Nurses (AACN) issued a practice alert on family presence during CPR and invasive procedures in 2004.

You are the nurse manager in an Emergency Department (ED). The VP for Patient Care has come to you with a problem. Last night, a city council member complained that one of his constituents called him because she was not allowed to be with her spouse during CPR in the ED last night. Currently, the patient is in ICU following a myocardial infarction and is in guarded condition. You are aware of the practice alert and have been trying to establish a policy in the ED and ICU. The VP for Patient Care has asked that you meet with the council member and his constituent on this issue.

Question: What is your plan for meeting with the council member and his constituent?

Source: American Association of Critical-Care Nurses. (AACN). (2004). Practice alert: Family presence during CPR and invasive procedures. Retrieved October 8, 2006, from *http://www.aacn.org/AACN/practiceAlert.nsf/Files/FP/$file/Family Presence During CPR 11-2004.pdf/*Source: Coopey, M., Nix, M., & Clancy, C. (2006). Translating research into evidence-based nursing practice and evaluating effectiveness. *Journal of Nursing Care Quality, 21*(3), 195–202.

organizations (p. 25). It is being the "agent" for both nursing and the consumer of nursing services. Nurses must increasingly be involved in advocating beyond the hospital or health-care unit environment. We have unique insights and the knowledge base to effect change and improve health care and health policy. This is the political imperative: be involved, be active, continue to develop interpersonal and political skills, and continue to understand the evolving needs of people and the profession.

INTERACTIVE EXERCISES

Go to the Intranet site and complete the interactive exercises provided for this Chapter.

Box 21.3 Tips for Talking to Legislators

- Before meeting with your legislator, get to know as much as possible about his or her background, special interests or initiatives, voting record, committee assignments, and involvement with health policy issues.
- Prepare your position, including a list of talking points to assist you during the discussion.
- Investigate both sides of the issue but stay focused on the facts.
- Request a meeting of at least 15 to 30 minutes.
- Practice your presentation with a friend or colleague to gain comfort with the content and to anticipate questions that may arise.
- If the legislator is not available, meet with the legislative aide or staff member who has a good knowledge of the issues.
- Be on time, and be professional.
- Introduce yourself and thank the legislator or legislative aide for his or her time and interest.
- Be prepared to explain what you do as a nurse, your philosophy of care, and the impact of pending legislation on health care and care delivery for the legislator's constituents.
- Use concise and explicit examples from your practice to illustrate your position.
- Be prepared to offer additional information or solutions, but stick to the facts.
- If the legislator or legislative aide indicates support for your position, ask what you can do to reach other legislators or sponsors.
- Provide an opportunity to answer any questions and offer any additional assistance on the circumstances of the proposed legislation or regulation.
- Send a follow-up thank you note for the time spent, in which you restate your position. You may even want to follow your interview with a well-worded letter on your position to the editor of the local newspaper—and perhaps gain further support among other constituents.

BOX 21.4 Tips for Presenting Testimony

Be prepared, with:

- A full, well-developed written statement and talking points.
- An understanding of the committee process and regulatory structure.
- An anticipation of any follow-up questions that may be asked of you.
- Be on time.
- Be confident in your abilities and knowledge base, and remain calm.
- Be flexible; you may not have the time for your presentation that you were told you would.
- Recognize the members of the body ("Mr./Madam Chairperson and members of the ___ Committee") and thank them for allowing you the opportunity to address them.
- Introduce yourself and be respectful.
- Do not read your written testimony; ask to have it placed in the record.
- Use the talking points to present your case and focus on the facts.
- Again, try to use concise and explicit examples from your practice to illustrate your position.
- Do not go over your allocated time.
- Leave time at the end of your presentation for any questions from the members.
- Thank the committee for the opportunity to present your testimony at the end.

KEY POINTS

- Internal political efficacy is personal competence or the "ability to understand and take part in political affairs," and external political advocacy is the "ability to make the system respond to the citizenry" (Wilson & Dilulio, 1998, p. 102).

- Laws are mandates based on the Constitution, enacted by federal or state legislatures, and interpreted by the courts. Administrative agencies, governed by the executive branch, promulgate regulations or rules, which serve the purpose of detailing and applying the laws.

- The enactment of a law begins with introduction of the bill by the sponsoring legislator to either the House or the Senate. Then, it is referred to committee for recommendations and amendments.

- Common law is created by judicial decisions that form a precedent upon which future decisions are based.

- Nurse practice acts are statutory law with associated administrative regulations developed by each state to protect the public health, safety, and welfare. They define the scope of practice; establish requirements for licensure, entry into practice, continuing competency and advanced practice; create and empower a board of nursing to oversee licensees; and identify grounds for disciplinary action.

- Title protection is the part of the nursing practice act that protects and restricts the use of the term *nurse* to the licensee authorized to practice by the board.

- Activities to influence legislators vary from formal to informal. Lobbying may be defined as attempting to persuade a legislator or legislative aide of the merits of your viewpoint and to influence legislation.

- Lobbying is especially effective when there is an associated strong grassroots effort that provides additional correspondence and support on the issues.

- Special interest groups have become more politically savvy at influencing the creation of public policy, and more controls have emerged, as with campaign financing reforms. One form of a special interest group is the political action committee (PAC).

- Buresh and Gordon (2006) define a voice of agency as a strong and authentic voice talking about what you do as a nurse and being more visible and vocal as individuals and as members of organizations (p. 25). Nurses can influence change in the workplace, the community, professional organizations, and government.

Thought and Discussion Questions

1. Consider the laws allowing direct reimbursement of nursing services by insurance companies. Discuss the processes that led to passage of these laws.

2. Identify how you will demonstrate both internal political efficacy and external political advocacy. Be prepared to participate in a discussion in class or online to be scheduled by your instructor.

3. Select a current issue of concern and develop an action plan to present your views to a legislator.

4. Review the Chapter Thought located on the first page of the chapter, and discuss it in the context of the chapter.

☐ REFERENCES

American Nurses Association. (2002). *Nursing's agenda for the future.* Retrieved October 16, 2006, from *http://nursingworld.org/MainMenuCategories/ HealthcareandPolicyIssues/Reports/ AgendafortheFuture.aspx*

American Nurses Association. (2007a). *Nursing facts.* Retrieved October 16, 2007, from *http://www.needlestick .org/readroom/fsdemogr.htm*

American Nurses Association. (2007b). American Nurses Association Political Action Committee (ANA-PAC). Legislative Branch. Retrieved October 16, 2007, from *http://nursingworld.org/MainMenuCategories/ ANAPoliticalPower/ANAPAC.aspx*

Buresh, B., & Gordon, S. (2006). *From silence to voice: What nurses know and must communicate to the public* (2nd ed.). Ithaca, NY: Cornell University Press.

Clinton, H. R. (2003). *Living history.* New York: Simon & Schuster.

Heaney, M. T. (2003, October 1). PhRMA tops health groups with most pull on Hill. *The Hill*, Special Section: Health Care.

Leininger, M. (2002). Cultures and tribes of nursing, hospitals, and the medical culture. In M. Leininger & M. R. McFarland, *Transcultural nursing: Concepts, theories, research, and practice* (3rd ed., pp. 181–204). New York: McGraw-Hill.

Mason, D. J., Chaffee, M. W., & Leavitt, J. K. (2006). *Policy and politics in nursing and health care* (4th ed.). Philadelphia: WB Saunders.

Milstead, J. A. (2003). Interweaving policy and diversity. *Online Journal of Issues in Nursing, 8*(1). Retrieved May 28, 2006, from *http://www.nursingworld .org/MainMenuCategories/ANAMarketplace/ ANAPeriodicasl/oinn/TableofContents/Vol82003/ Num1Jan31_2003/InterweavingPolicyandDiversity.aspx*

Mintzberg, H. (1983). *Power in and around organizations.* Englewood Cliffs, NJ: Prentice-Hall.

Wilson, J. Q., & DiIulio, J. J. (1998). *American government: Institutions and policies.* Boston: Houghton Mifflin.

U.S. Constitution. *Preamble.* Retrieved May 28, 2006, from *http://www.usconstitution.net/const.html*

☐ BIBLIOGRAPHY

Federal Election Commission. (2006). *Administering and enforcing federal campaign finance laws.* Retrieved May 28, 2006, from *http://www.fec.gov*

Mason, D. J., Chaffee, M. W., & Leavitt, J. K. (2006). *Policy and politics in nursing and health care* (4th ed.). Philadelphia: WB Saunders.

Milstead, J. A. (2004). *Health policy and politics: A nurse's guide* (2nd ed.). Boston: Jones and Bartlett.

Oleszek, W. J. (2004). *Congressional procedures and the policy process* (6th ed.). Washington, DC: CQ Press.

THOMAS: Legislative information from the Library of Congress. [U.S. Congress on the Internet]. Available from *http://thomas.loc.gov*

U.S. Department of Health and Human Services. (2003). *Summary of the HIPAA privacy rule.* Available from *http://www.hhs.gov/ocr/privacysummary.pdf*

U.S. General Services Administration, Office of Citizen Services and Communications. *USA.gov: government made easy.* [Official government Web portal]. Available from *http://www.firstgov.gov*

☐ ONLINE RESOURCES

American Association of Critical-Care Nurses (AACN) **http://www.aacn.nche.edu**

American Nurses Association (ANA) **http://www.nursingworld.org/gov**

National League for nursing (NLN) **htttp://www.nln.org**

Parliament of Canada **http://parl.gc.ca**

THOMAS **http://thomas.loc.gov**

U.S. Government Portal **http://firstgov.gov**

U.S. House of Representatives **http://www.house.gov**

U.S. Senate **http://www.senate.gov**

■ *Sister Rosemary* **Donley**

Nursing's Health-Care Agenda

> " *Nursing in its broadest sense may be defined as an art and a science which involves the whole patient—body, mind, and spirit; promotes his spiritual, mental, and physical health by teaching and by example; stresses health education and health preservation, as well as ministration to the sick; involves the care of the patients' environment—social and spiritual as well as physical; and gives health service to the family and community as well as to the individual.* "

Sr. M. Olivia Gowan, founding Dean, The Catholic University of America,
School of Nursing, June, 1944

Chapter Objectives

On completion of this chapter, the reader will be able to:

1. Discuss the issues on nursing's health-care agenda.
2. Describe the interaction between issues.
3. Discuss how the nursing shortage influences nursing's ability to influence change and advance its agenda.

Key Terms

Nurse Reinvestment Act of 2002

Community Benefit

Hospitalists

Surgicenters and Urgicenters

Niche Services

Staffing Ratios

Best Practice

Cost-Benefit-Burden Ratios

Evidence-Based Practice

Tiered Payments

Technological Imperative

Health Disparities

Medicare Parts A, B, C, D

The Prescription Drug Act of 2003

Medicaid

SCHIP

The Nursing Shortage

New Education Pathways: Clinical Nurse Leader and Doctor of Nursing Practice

In the past 30 years, nurses have become interested and engaged in health-care policy. Most schools of nursing teach classes or entire courses in health policy. Professional and specialty nursing organizations monitor federal and state legislation, provide information about health and nursing issues, lobby or make financial contributions to candidates, members of Congress or state legislators, or join political action committees (PACs) in support of legislators who embrace nursing's legislative and policy agenda. Many local and global factors contribute to nurses' interest in policy and politics. The nursing shortage, the growing number of uninsured, an increased recognition of the impact of health disparities on health status, and changes in the health-care delivery system and modes of reimbursement have altered the practice of nursing and the nursing care of patients in all health-care settings. Recent events in the world, the tragic events of September 11, 2001, and threats of bioterrorism have made nurses aware of their positions as first- and second-line responders. Nurses realize that many of the problems that affect the health of all Americans can be addressed only at the policy level by informed and collective action. In the 21st century, policy competence is a professional responsibility. This chapter addresses current issues on nursing's policy agenda, specifically:

- Health care as a business
- Health-care costs
- Uninsured persons
- Health disparities
- Medicare, Medicaid, and SCHIP
- Nursing shortage
- Evolving medical and nursing roles

HEALTH CARE AS A BUSINESS

The United States is the only first-world country without a universal program of health insurance sponsored by its government. The United States government becomes engaged with health care in several ways. The federal government encourages biomedical and health-care research. Scientists at the National Institutes of Health (NIH), a division in the Department of Health and Human Services (DHHS), conduct studies within their own clinical center in Bethesda, Maryland. The major research thrust, financed and supported by NIH, is carried out in the medical and nursing schools and academic health centers around the United States. Other federal agencies also sponsor extramural research. The Centers for Disease Control and Prevention (CDC), the Centers for Medicare and Medicaid Services (CMS), the Agency for Healthcare Research and Quality (AHRQ), the Substance Abuse and Mental Health Services Administration (SAMHSA), and the Center for Nursing Research (CNR) are just a few of the federal agencies that support studies to improve the health of the nation.

The federal government and some state governments also provide scholarships and loans to students who study nursing or medicine. In some cases, these loans are forgiven if nurses or physicians work within the state, or in the case of federal grants, in underserved areas after graduation. This is one recent example of federal assistance to nursing. Recognizing the impact of the nursing shortage, **The Nurse Reinvestment Act of 2002** created a loan-forgiveness program to support the education of teachers. Aimed at increasing the number of nurse educators, the program will forgive 85% of student loans if graduates teach in schools of nursing for four years (Donley et al., 2002).

However, the federal government's most significant engagement is in the business of health care through its insurance programs: Medicare, Medicaid, and the State Children's Health Insurance Program (SCHIP). When most people talk about the government and health care, they think of Medicare. However, anyone interested in public policy is interested in Medicaid and SCHIP, as well as Medicare, because these programs pay for the health care of the poor, the disabled, poor children, and the poor elderly.

Public/Private Model of Health Care

In America, health care contributes significantly to the economic well-being of the country. In this way, America provides a model of private and public (government) collaboration around health. For some eligible persons, military personnel on active duty, their dependents, military retirees, especially veterans with service-connected illnesses or disabilities, Native Americans, and prisoners, the federal government operates its own health systems and provides direct care. These delivery systems are significant. For example, the Veterans Administration Nursing Service is the largest nursing service in the United States. Some public hospitals and long-term care facilities are also run by state or local governments. The Cook County Hospital in Illinois is one example of a county-owned public hospital that provides care to underserved people in Chicago.

Most people in this country receive health care in the private sector: physicians' offices, clinics, ambulatory care centers, and for-profit or not-for-profit hospitals. Although both state and federal governments play a role in the private sector by licensing health-care providers, such as doctors and nurses, and establishing and maintaining safety and health standards in institutions, the responsibility of providing preventive, therapeutic, or rehabilitative care is in the hands of doctors and nurses who are not employees of the government. These health professionals participate as an integral part of the private sector economy.

Because this public-private model of health care is unique among first-world nations, it is often cited in discussions of health-care costs and health-care outcomes. The United States spends more than 15% of its gross domestic product (GDP) on health care, ranking above Japan, Great Britain, Canada and the countries of Western Europe in health-care expenditures (USDHHS, 2005). Yet when health outcomes, as measured by public health indicators such as mortality, morbidity, infant mortality, low-birth-weight babies, and immunizations are examined, the United States ranks behind other countries that spend less money on health care (National Center for Health Statistics, 2006; World Health Organization, 2006).

Supporters of private sector involvement in health care note that America's health-care system is the envy of the world. Its technology and expertise are exported to many countries; its medical and nursing schools and hospitals are the training sites for many multinationals; the United States is a major developer of new drugs; and its biomedical researchers contribute to scientific advancement throughout the world. Closer to home, hospitals are often the largest employers in communities, providing jobs to a wide range of workers. Physicians and nurses with graduate degrees are at one end of the employment spectrum. At the other end, hospitals offer jobs and career advancement opportunities to persons who have not completed high school. Hospitals often have desirable benefit packages for full-time employees that include health insurance, retirement plans, on-the-job training and development, and tuition support programs. Health careers are sought after; places in medical school are coveted; and jobs in the health-care sector seem to be stable even in periods of recession. Hospitals fuel local economies by providing jobs. Hospitals are also major purchasers and contribute to the economic and political development of their communities.

For-Profit Versus Not-For-Profit Health Care

The majority of hospitals in America are not-for-profit. Profit, the positive difference between income and expenditures generated by not-for-profit hospitals, is reinvested in the hospitals or in their local communities. **Community benefit** is the term that describes the pro bono services that not-for-profit health-care centers provide in their communities (Catholic Health Association, n.d.). In for-profit institutions, most nursing homes, some hospitals, most clinics, ambulatory care centers, and managed care companies, profit is shared among the investors. In the for-profit health sector, the focus is upon making the business (in this case health care) profitable, competitive, and therefore attractive to investors. Individuals in private or group practices, physicians and some advanced practice nurses, must run

profitable health-care operations to stay in business. This fact of life is most evident in the practice of medicine, in which most physicians are self-employed or share medical partnerships with nurse practitioners or other doctors. These providers' incomes depend on the number of patients on their panels and the nature of their practices. Specialist physicians earn more than primary care physicians; surgeons earn more than internists; and physicians earn more than nurse practitioners. American physicians have adjusted their practices to the financial incentives present in their communities. In fee-for-service medicine, physicians perform more tests and examinations because fee-for-service physicians are paid according to the number and type of services they provide. Malpractice concerns also influence testing and treating protocols in all settings.

When managed care became the dominant form of health insurance in the United States, hospitals and the physicians learned that financial incentives had changed (Relman, 1992). Hospitals accepted that shortening length of stay influenced their profit margin. Hospitals that could provide care within the time frames specified by the insurers were selected for contracts by managed care groups. Managed care companies offered special financial incentives to physicians who used less expensive tests and treatments, made fewer referrals, and were able to keep their patients out of hospitals. Physicians realized that they could make more money by providing fewer tests and referrals. Managed care's control of tests, procedures, and treatments has had some effect on health-care costs and the practice protocols of physicians. However, these practices have distorted the traditional idea that physicians are agents of their patients (Feldstein, 2003). Patients and families are no longer certain whether medical advice benefits them, their insurance programs, or the financial well-being of doctors. This conflict of interest has caused a loss of trust in doctors and the health-care system itself. Changes in practice patterns have intensified the underlying business reality that physicians in managed care systems are working for themselves and the insurance companies as well as their patients. Some critics of this public/private American plan blame rising health-care costs and the failure to achieve good outcomes on business involvement in health care. These critics address the link between employment and health insurance, the for-profit influence on health care, and the placing of efficiency and economic gain above the care of patients. In the United States, health-care providers are encouraged to be entrepreneurs.

Competition in Health-Care and the Hospitalist Movement

American health care operates in competitive markets. Competition exists between physicians and nurses, especially physicians and advanced practice nurses, between physicians and hospitals, among hospitals and health-care systems, and among hospitals, physicians, and insurers. The most complex form of competition occurs between insurance companies and hospitals. In the 1990s, insurance companies bought hospitals and physician practices, and hospitals acquired insurance companies and recruited physicians to refer patients or become employees and practice within the hospital walls. Hospitals had employed physicians to manage radiology, anesthesia, and emergency care. Hospitals then acquired physicians (intensivists) to direct and manage care in intensive care units. As more patients were treated by primary care doctors and fewer medical residency positions were funded by Medicare, a number of hospital-based physicians, **hospitalists**, were employed to manage inpatient care and to advise and support the nursing staffs, particularly on medical-surgical units (Wachter & Goldman, 2002).

In a true marketplace, competition drives down prices and allows the most competent and efficient to survive (Feldstein, 2003). Health care is not the best example of a marketplace economy. Ill patients are often unable to do research or make the judgments that are in their best interests. The health-care industry and providers are regulated; regulation restricts competition. At another level, medical societies influence state legislators. Revision of state practice acts to permit more independence for advance practice nurses, nurse practitioners, nurse anesthetists, clinical specialists, and midwives is often blocked by local medical societies. Although studies have demonstrated the competence and cost-effectiveness of nurse practitioners, the role that advance practice nurses could play in lowering the cost of health care without affecting its quality has never been adequately tested because of the control that medical societies and their lobbyists have on state legislatures.

Physician and physician group relations with hospitals are complex. The simplicity and availability of technology, changes in reimbursement, and the pressure to limit hospital stays and provide care in less expensive settings have encouraged many physicians to join together in freestanding ambulatory care businesses that compete with hospitals. Physicians and nurses in these **surgicenters** and **urgicenters** can safely perform biopsies, cataract surgery, and many orthopedic, gynecologic, and urologic procedures in attractive and convenient settings. Insurance companies recognize that these centers operate without the high overhead of hospitals because they do not provide costly emergency and intensive care services. Ambulatory centers are one type of **niche services** that meet particular needs.

Hospitals also engage in significant competition with one another. Before the changes in Medicare initiated during the early 1980s, hospitals competed by offering amenities such as family-centered maternity care.

However, after diagnostic-related groups (DRGs) became the standard of payment for inpatient care, hospitals began to compete on price. Hospitals that could not compete on price lost managed care contracts and experienced lower occupancy rates. Price competition stimulated hospitals that could provide quality care within the DRG payment structure to compete aggressively for managed care contracts. However, because the payment system based on DRGs encouraged patients to be admitted late and discharged early, all hospitals, even efficient ones, experienced reduced occupancy. Hospitals responded by decreasing in size and reorganizing. This downsizing triggered a reduction in nursing and support staff. Some commentators trace the current nursing shortage to staffing decisions made by hospitals in the mid-1980s (Aiken, Clarke, & Sloane, 2002). The decade of the 1980s saw many hospitals merge or become organized into health systems. Vertical organization became the term in the hospital literature to describe hospital systems that organized along similar service lines. For example, vertical health systems were a collection of hospitals or a collection of nursing homes. As an alternative to vertical organization, some hospitals built integrated service networks to become one organization that offered all the health services that patients might need. These sophisticated horizontal organizations provided acute care, home care, extended care, durable medical equipment, and pharmacy services. Hospitals that joined horizontal organizations hoped that they could compete more successfully for managed care contracts because they could offer patients and insurers a form of one-stop shopping. Other values encouraged hospitals to merge or form horizontal or vertical systems: economies of scale and access to capital for expansion, acquisition of new services including physician practices, and more success in bargaining with insurance companies for higher rates. The idea behind these business arrangements was to control the delivery of health care within communities, and manage the flow of health-care dollars.

Business Influence on Health Care

The relationship of private and public sectors in health care has been expanded in the past 30 years. The influence of business is evident by the health community's adoption of the language and ethics of business. It is not uncommon for patients to be described as "consumers" or "market share" and for health or nursing care to be described as "product lines." Nurses have not been immune to the influence of business on their practices and language. Some have tried to learn or at least adapt to the business model in providing health care. Others have tried to practice what they believe is important to patients. Some have joined unions or advocated for legislation to mandate **staffing ratios** to ensure a sufficient number of nurses to care for patients, especially those who are hospitalized (Buerhaus & Needlemen, 2000).

One positive influence of the business community on health care is its insistence that outcomes are more important than processes. For years, the health-care community relied on structure and process to ensure quality of care. In the new era, the business community wants health-care outcomes that show some demonstrable change or benefit to patients and some positive cost-benefit ratio to society. The professional community, especially physicians and nurses, have responded to these mandates. This response has caused nurses and other health-care professionals to examine the outcomes or results of their interventions and to base their practices on evidence derived from analyses of outcomes. There is also a growing interest in the health community in finding and then using best practices. Simply put, a **best practice** is something that works, accomplishes the goal, and produces the desired outcomes. Discovering and sharing best practices is one mode, research is another, of obtaining evidence for nursing practice. Evidence-based practice is increasingly important to the professional practice of nursing. Health professionals have added another factor to business concerns with the **cost-benefit-burden ratio**. Considerations of burden look at the patients' or societal perceptions and experiences of planned diagnostic or therapeutic interventions. This approach puts the patient or the common good at the center of clinical decision-making. **Evidence-based practice** is based on outcome, cost, and benefit/burden analysis.

The business community wants health-care outcomes that show some demonstrable change or benefit to the patient and some positive cost-benefit ratio to society.

HEALTH-CARE COSTS

Health-care costs appear on nursing's policy agenda, probably because these costs have risen for more than 40 years and directly affect patient care and nurse staffing. As medical technology and drug therapy have become more sophisticated, people live longer, and as the "baby boomer" generation nears retirement, there is renewed concern because no system or method consistently reduces health expenditures in the United States. In the 1990s, policy makers and the Congress of the United States had great hope that managed care would control rising health-care costs. The latest available data (2003) show that the United States spends an average of $5,670 per person for health care per year, approximately twice that spent in European countries. Initially, policy makers were encouraged by managed

care protocols because health costs increased by only 5% to 5.3% from 1996 to 1998. Since then, costs have begun to rise. By 2002 health-care spending had grown by 9.3%, the sixth straight year of reported increases (Brown, 2004). Researchers at the Centers for Medicare and Medicaid Services identified the following explanatory factors for the growth of expenses:

- Technology, especially those technologies delivered in acute care hospitals
- Physician services
- Home health care
- Prescription drugs. (Levit et al., 2004)

Prescription drugs rose 15% in 2002. This increase, notable in itself, is of particular interest because of the new prescription drug benefit enacted as Medicare Part D in 2003.

Rising health-care expenditures confirm that managed care has lost its ability to control health-care costs. Why did this happen? The American public, physicians, and hospitals became tired of the control exerted by managed care officials' second-guessing of clinical decisions. There was a public outcry against practices such as the same-day discharge of new mothers and babies, which some called "drive-by deliveries." People believed that their health providers, not their insurance companies, should make health-care decisions. Managed care companies responded to public and legal pressure and gave patients more choice of primary care providers and greater access to certain specialists. Loss of a rigorous gatekeeping function was a factor in the growth of health-care costs.

Managed care companies and employers have responded to both the increasing cost of health care and the cost of providing health insurance to employees by changing payment and benefit structures. Managed care companies have designed plans with fewer benefits. Employers are sharing or passing on increases in health insurance premiums to employees (Feldstein, 2003). Employees now pay more money to participate in their employer-based plan: higher premiums, higher deductibles (the amount the person must pay before the insurance pays), and more in copayments for any health service: medical visits, tests, visits to the emergency department, therapy, and drugs. Many insurance plans have **tiered payments** so that patients pay one fee to visit their primary care providers and a higher fee to visit specialists. This same pattern of tiered payments applies to prescription drugs included in managed care benefit programs and Medicare's prescription drug benefit program. Generally:

- Generic drugs have a small copayment (tier one).
- Midrange drugs have a higher copayment (tier two).
- New, breakthrough drugs and most drugs protected by patents have the highest copayments (tier three).

The size of the copayments varies with the prescription drug benefit plan.

The belief that the cost of health services will be controlled only if all participants share costs is evident in the new prescription drug plan, Medicare Part D. The introduction of cost-sharing into Medicare Part D represents policy makers' latest effort to manage Medicare expenditures. Currently, Medicare Part D is an optional program. Those who enroll must select a drug benefit program and abide by its costs/benefit/ burden structures. These new prescription benefit packages are another example of public/private partnerships involving the nonprofit and the for-profit private sector. Medicare Part D plans differ in the cost of their participation fees and in the number, type, and cost of drugs in each tier. Seniors are advised to compare their current medication profiles with the benefit packages offered by the prescription drug plans in their states. If they can find, select, and afford a plan where all their drugs are in tier one (the most economical tier) or tier two, they will reduce their out-of-pocket drug costs. Seniors are advised to ask their doctors to change their drug protocols to drugs that are offered in tier one of their drug benefit plans. Some prescription drug plan managers also write to doctors asking them to adjust the drug protocols of patients in their plans. Although this approach to prudent drug management is attractive to those concerned with rising costs, many seniors find that analyzing the drug coverage in the plans available in their states to be burdensome. Some were unwilling, unable, or afraid to ask physicians to change their drugs.

Seniors realized that their drug protocols change with their age and health status. They also realized the companies that offered prescription drug benefits are free to cease participating in the program, change the drugs offered within each tier and, at the end of the contract year, change prices. While the growth of Medicare costs, since its inception in 1965, is impressive and certain to grow as the large cohort of baby boomers becomes eligible for Medicare in 2010, it is interesting that senior citizens were selected to test the impact of cost sharing on health-care costs.

"High-Tech" Acute Care

American-style health care is expensive because it emphasizes acute care rather than prevention or primary care. In other countries, where health-care costs are less, there is more emphasis on primary care. Because Americans have invested in high-technology medicine, they are caught up in technologic revolutions, medical and informational. Hospitals are familiar with the need to upgrade and advance their medical technology. However, because of managed care, Medicare regulations, and the multiple settings of health care, the health-care system has become increasingly dependent on informational

technology, its infrastructure, and its privacy and security systems. Medical and computer-assisted technologies, too numerous to enumerate, explain why America is the leader in health care. However, costs of high-technology medicine must be weighed in light of cost, benefit, and burden. Used wisely, these technologies benefit everyone. Medical technology gives patients more control over their chronic illnesses. Informational technology provides providers and patients rapid access to medical records and reports of diagnostic tests. The Internet offers access to scientific reports and research findings. Many of these technologies:

- Reduce length of stay (e.g., laparoscopic surgery)
- Shorten time in surgery (e.g., lens implants)
- Avoid painful, intrusive, and sometimes dangerous tests (e.g., magnetic resonance imaging)
- Enable patients to monitor their own status at home (blood pressure or glucose readings)
- Permit patients, primary care providers, home-care nurses, and specialists to observe and communicate (telehealth technologies)
- Obtain consultation across state lines (information technologies)

The practice of high-technology medicine does not occur in a vacuum. Americans are pragmatic and want results and innovation. Americans trade up, they choose faster computers, smaller appliances, and more fuel-efficient cars. These cultural factors support America's investment in technologic medicine. At another level, many health providers perceive losing a patient to disease as failure. In the American medical psyche, there is an impetus to treat, to try another intervention, and not to give up. Because technology is so readily available, there is a **technologic imperative**: If the technology is there, it should be used. Some patients undergo more technologic interventions than they want or perhaps need. It is not by chance that the majority of health expenditures for Medicare recipients are incurred in the last 6 months of a patient's life (Hoover, Crystal, Kumar, Sambamoorthi, & Cantor, 2002).

Medical Error

Today, there is a greater sensitivity to the cost of error (Leape, 1992). Several studies by the Institute of Medicine (IOM) have alerted the public and providers about the frequency, seriousness, and cost of medical error. One IOM study, *To Err Is Human: Building a Safer Health System* (Kohn, Corrigan, & Donaldson, 2000), addresses the importance of developing a culture of safety in contemporary health-care systems. A second IOM study, *Crossing the Quality Chasm: A New Health System for the 21st Century* (Committee on Quality Health Care, 2001) presents recommendations to reduce error and enhance the quality of health care. Accreditors and health systems have directed dollars and programs to decrease errors, especially medication errors. Hospitals, nurse practitioners and physicians, especially physicians and nurse practitioners in certain specialties, recognize the cost of malpractice insurance and the effect of malpractice claims on their reputation and practice patterns (Wilensky, 2004).

UNINSURED PERSONS

Many of the issues on nursing's policy agenda are interrelated. There are connections among the role that health care plays in the economy, the cost of health care, and the number of people in the United States who do not have health insurance. As has been stated earlier in this text, health insurance in America is not a right associated with citizenship. Lacking a system of national health insurance, Americans either must qualify for a government program because they fit entitlement categories—military (Veterans, Tricare), age or disability (Medicare), poverty (Medicaid or SCHIP)—participate in their companies' health insurance plans, or insure themselves. However, even eligible people described in these categories are not always insured. Ironically, all persons who meet the government's entitlement criteria are not enrolled in the programs for which they are eligible. Children provide the most compelling illustration of this finding. It is estimated that 80% of the 9 million uninsured children would be eligible for existing programs, Medicaid or SCHIP, if their parents applied (Kaiser Family Foundation, 2004). Before this can happen, cultural, linguistic, informational, and bureaucratic hurdles must be remedied. The United States does not require companies to provide insurance for its workers. Consequently, there exists a large group of uninsured workers: the self-employed; persons employed by firms that do not offer health insurance benefits; or persons who do not enroll in their companies' health-care plans. In summary, the insurance structure in the United States, which connects health-care coverage to employment, does not address the 46.6 million uninsured people. When the uninsured become ill, they delay care or seek care in hospital emergency departments. Uninsured people contribute to the rising cost of health care because their health status is compromised by delaying treatment and their care is usually not paid for. Another IOM panel has estimated that the cost to society of having over 43 million people uninsured (the number of uninsured at the time of study) is between $43 billion and $130 billion a year (Committee on the Consequence of Uninsurance [CCU], 2004). (Current figures place the uninsured rate at 46.6 million.)

The quality of care that uninsured people receive is also worthy of examination. This same IOM panel (CCU, 2004) discussed the health consequences of being an uninsured working adult with a common illness, such as cancer, diabetes, human immunodeficiency virus (HIV) infection and acquired immunodeficiency syndrome (AIDS), heart or kidney disease, mental illness, or trauma. The main findings of the report are that uninsured working age people (roughly 30 million, or 1 in 7 workers):

- Receive too little medical care
- Receive it too late
- Are sicker
- Die sooner
- Receive poorer care, even when hospitalized for trauma. (CCU, 2004)

It is relevant to note that the number of uninsured people continues to rise. This figure increased by 5.7% in 2002, when an estimated 15.2% of the population, or 43.6 million people, were without health insurance for the entire year (U.S. Census Bureau, 2004). The 2002 Census data reveal some interesting information about uninsured Americans:

- Young adults (18 to 24 years old) were less likely to be insured than other age groups.
- Poor workers were less likely to have insurance than nonworkers.
- Hispanics (67.6%) were less likely to have health insurance.
- Although Medicaid insured 14 million people, another 10.5 million poor people (some 30.4% of the poverty population) had no insurance.
- The percentage of people covered by employment-based insurance dropped from 62.2% to 61.3%.
- The number covered by governmental programs, notably Medicaid, rose slightly, from 25.3% to 25.7%.
- The number of uninsured children remained at 11.6% of all uninsured children, or 8.3 million.

In 2006, the Congress passed a law which requires persons to show proof of citizenship or legal residency before they can qualify for the federally financed health programs, Medicare, Medicaid, and SCHIP. This provision is tied to an effort to limit access to services to persons who cannot prove that they are legal or permanent residents in the United States. While the actual impact of this law on cost of health care or care delivery is unknown, it is recognized that immigrants, particularly poor immigrants, have poor health status. Lacking insurance or the ability to benefit from public programs, these persons have no recourse but emergency care. They and their children will find access to preventive services very difficult (Kaiser Commission on Medicaid and the Uninsured, 2006).

The Agency for Healthcare Research and Quality (AHRQ) (n.d.) indicates that from 1998 to 2001, three measures of the uninsured seemed to remain stable: between 21 and 31 million people were uninsured all year; at any point in time, about 40 million people were uninsured; and during some part of the year, 60 million people were uninsured. As is evident from the growth in the number of uninsured people, the problem of the uninsured is not going away.

HEALTH DISPARITIES

The Surgeon General's report, *Healthy People 2010*, established two ambitious goals (U.S. Department of Health and Human Services, 2000):

- Increase quality and years of healthy life
- Eliminate health disparities

In discussing the second goal, the elimination of **health disparities**, the report states that socioeconomic status, race, ethnicity, and access to care must be considered along with disease in understanding and addressing differences in health status among Americans. As was illustrated in Chapter 16, it also identifies a list of leading health indicators that are helpful in assessing the health status of individuals and populations. These factors should be integrated into nursing assessments (USDHHS, 2000, p. 24).

- Physical activity
- Overweight and obesity
- Tobacco use
- Substance abuse
- Responsible sexual behavior
- Mental health
- Injury and violence
- Environmental quality
- Immunization
- Access to health care

The idea that factors other than biology or genetics contribute to health status, severity of disease, response to treatment, morbidity, and even death is not new. Representations of the significance and the interplay of factors that explain health, like the one presented in

ONLINE CONSULT

For information about the 28 focus areas where health disparities exist and tool kits to help nurses and other health professionals address the gaps in health care and health status in this country, go to the Healthy People Web site at
www.healthypeople.gov

Figure 22–1, are well documented in the community-health and public-health literature. What is new and exciting is that the surgeon general's report highlights the importance of assessing the person's lifestyle and environment.

> The idea that factors other than biology or genetics contribute to health status, severity of disease, response to treatment, and even death is not new.

It is also significant that the message of *Healthy People 2010* reminds nurses of the 1948 World Health Organization's definition of health as more than the absence of disease. An interesting source of information on health disparities can be found in the IOM's study, *Unequal Treatment: Confronting Racial and Ethnic Disparities in Health Care* (Smedley, Stith, & Nelson, 2003).

MEDICARE, MEDICAID, AND SCHIP

Because uninsured people have limited access to care and suffer greater health disparities than people who do have health insurance, the contemporary practice of professional nursing requires that nurses understand how care is financed. This section addresses three governmental health-care financing programs: Medicare, Medicaid, and SCHIP.

Medicare

Until 2003, **Medicare**, a federal health insurance program that since 1965 primarily served (1) the elderly and (2) disabled people younger than 65 years who receive Social Security cash payments and have fulfilled the 2-year waiting period, changed little (Feldstein, 2003). Most of the amendments made to Medicare reduced health-care costs, limited utilization of health services, and adjusted methods of payment. There are some exceptions to this pattern. In 1972, persons with end-stage renal disease were made eligible for Medicare regardless of age. In 1982, the mode of Medicare payment changed from reimbursement after care had been delivered to prospective payment based on diagnostic-related categories. In 1983, Congress added a hospice benefit (Longest, 2006).

However, in late 2003, President George W. Bush signed the Medicare Prescription Drug Improvement and Modernization Act of 2003 (**Prescription Drug Act of 2003**), which significantly changed the structure of Medicare because it was based on cost sharing. There is every indication that Medicare will change again by the end of the decade. In 2010, a demonstration project in six

Source: U.S. Dept. Of Health and Human Services, 2000, p. 7.

■ **Figure 22.1** Determinants of health. (From U.S. Dept. of Health and Human Services. [2000]. *Healthy People 2010* [p. 7]. Washington, DC: U.S. Government Printing Office.).

metropolitan areas will put Medicare in competition with private health insurance plans. The theory is that because Medicare serves an older, sicker, and more expensive population, the costs of traditional Medicare will force more people into private plans and Medicare will be privatized (Understanding the New Medicare, 2003).

Because the cost of prescription drugs became an issue early in the 2004 presidential campaign, the press has focused its reporting on the prescription drug benefit component of the new law. This benefit, which became effective in 2006, adds a costly and complex program to Medicare. Its payment structure is particularly confusing. Initially, after the beneficiary has paid a premium and an annual deductible of $250, **Medicare part D** will pay 75% of the drug bill. The beneficiary will pay the remaining 25% until expenses reach $2,250. At this point, the coverage stops and the beneficiary is responsible for all drug costs until the total expenditure reaches $5100. By this time, when the beneficiary has spent $3600 out-of-pocket, catastrophic coverage begins. For the rest of the year, beneficiaries pay a flat copayment of $2 for each generic and $5 for each brand-name drug. At the end of the year, the person begins the cycle anew. There is no policy rationale for what is described as the "doughnut hole," the start-stop-start again prescription drug benefit. The payment scheme was an attempt to reduce the cost of the benefit and keep it within the $400 billion ceiling set by President Bush. Most beneficiaries do not understand the complexities of the Prescription Drug Act. Some commentators believe that the real beneficiaries of this legation are the drug companies and the managed care

industry (Understanding the new prescription drug benefit, 2003).

The contemporary **Medicare** program has four parts, each offering different benefits. **Part A** provides hospital insurance (HI). **Part B** provides supplemental medical insurance (SMI) and pays for outpatient and physician services. **Part C** offers Medicare beneficiaries a choice of managed health plans or traditional Medicare. In 2003, Medicare Part C was named Medicare Advantage. People enrolled in Medicare Part C have prescription drug benefits. The new Prescription Drug Act is **Part D**.

Medicaid, a means-tested health insurance program for the poor, pays for medical and long-term care to almost 14% of the population (Insurance Coverage, 2001). The Medicaid population consists of five groups: pregnant women, adults in families with dependent children, poor children, persons with disabilities, and the poor elderly (Centers for Medicare and Medicaid Services, 2004). Administered by each state, the policy-making is shared with the federal government, which pays between 50% and 76% in matching funds on the basis of each state's financial capacity (per capita income) (Feldstein, 2003). The influx of federal dollars into the states makes Medicaid a less expensive approach to expanding access to medical care to persons of low income. The states may expand eligibility beyond the five federally mandated population groups, but to qualify for federal matching funds, they must offer the following benefits to these groups: inpatient care, outpatient care, laboratory services, early and periodic screening, diagnosis, and treatment (EPSDT) for children, and other services such as prescriptions and home health care. Some persons because of their age, disability, and poverty are eligible for both Medicare and Medicaid. The care of many persons in long-term care settings is supported by both of these programs.

The State Children's Health Insurance Program (SCHIP) is a newcomer to federal investment in health care. This program, Title XXI of the Social Security Act, was originally passed as part of the Balanced Budget Act of 1997. In many ways, **SCHIP** has a policy structure similar to that of Medicaid, but it is targeted to less-poor children. It is designed to help states expand health coverage to uninsured children, especially those whose family income is above the federal poverty line or too high to qualify them for Medicaid. The federal poverty level is the standard used to determine whether people qualify for programs like Medicaid and SCHIP. Most Medicaid programs cover people whose income is at 100% to 150% of the federal poverty level. The latest federal poverty level (FPL) for a family of four, living in the 48 contiguous states is $20,000 (USDHHS, 2006). SCHIP covers children who live in families with higher incomes, usually at 200% of the FPL (for example, $40,000 for a family of four).

NURSING SHORTAGE

The **nursing shortage** represents a paradox in both recruitment and retention (Donley et al., 2002). Nursing has failed to project a contemporary image of professional practice and career opportunities to school counselors, other health professionals, and the public (Nurses for a Healthier Tomorrow, n.d.). Consequently, stereotypes and myths about nursing are passed on. Some young people do not see nursing as an attractive career option (Steinbrook, 2002). It is perceived as too demanding, too dangerous, and too undervalued. For others, nursing is an exciting, meaningful, and socially relevant profession. Although the inability to project an attractive image of contemporary professional nursing to the public is not the only cause of the shortage, a documented 6-year decline in enrollment in all levels of nursing education—diploma, associate, and baccalaureate degrees—which began in the 1990s, has contributed to the shortage (American Association of Colleges of Nursing [AACN], 2002). Concern about enrollment is intensified by a shortage of teachers and by the age of the nurse faculty (Spratley, Johnson, Sochalski, Fritz, & Spencer, 2001). Some observers note that the nursing shortage will not be addressed until more teachers are prepared. Faculty shortage continues to limit enrollment in schools around the country (AACN, 2006).

Even the most optimistic do not expect that the number of nursing students will increase to meet the needs of the baby-boomer generation. The population cohort is smaller, and the current career opportunities for women (who account for about 90% of registered nurses) are much more numerous than they were for women born in the mid-1940s. The positive side of the nursing shortage is that new graduates have a wide choice of jobs, the opportunity to enter specialty practice after graduation, higher salaries, and an enhanced ability to move up the career ladder. It is a good time to be a nursing student (Johnson & Johnson Health Care Systems, 2002).

Although shortages are not new to the profession, the contemporary shortage has been troublesome. It has called attention to the practice of nursing and the level of dissatisfaction within the nursing workforce, especially in hospital nursing (Steinbrook, 2002; Norrish & Randall, 2001):

- Poor staffing ratios that affect patient safety and quality of care
- Mandatory overtime
- A workplace culture that is not respectful of the nurses' knowledge or experience
- Poor communication with administrators and physicians
- Overreliance on agency or travel nurses, especially in specialty areas
- Lack of opportunities for professional development or job advancement
- Lack of involvement in decisions that affect nurses and their patients

The public, the federal government, physicians, the hospital industry, health-workers unions, and nurses themselves have made strides in responding to the crisis in nursing (AHA Commission, 2002; Joint Commission on Accreditation of Healthcare Organizations [JCAHO], 2002; AACN, 2001; SEIU, 1993) by developing white papers, commissioning studies, and presenting testimony to Congress advocating for:

- More scholarships for students of nursing
- Demonstration projects to address retention and nurse satisfaction
- Involvement of professional nurses in governance structures in their places of work
- Loan forgiveness programs for nurses who study to be teachers

In 2002, President Bush signed the Nurse Reinvestment Act, Public Law 107–205. This visionary piece of legislation addresses the nursing shortage from the viewpoint of recruitment: public image programs; scholarships and loan forgiveness programs; and support for the advanced nursing education of clinical specialists, teachers, administrators, and practitioners. It also addresses the nursing shortage from the retention side: demonstration funds to support innovation in practice and career development. As the title of the public law indicates, the country has reinvested in nurses as a national resource.

There is also a renewed impetus within nursing to promote and accredit magnet hospitals, workplaces that attract and retain qualified nurses (McClure & Hinshaw, 2002). The American Nurse Credentialing Center (ANCC) (2004) describes magnet hospitals as institutions that demonstrate certain attributes:

- Professional nursing practice
- Support for nursing excellence in the delivery of patient care
- Dissemination of successful nursing practices and strategies
- Positive patient outcomes

EVOLVING MEDICAL AND NURSING ROLES

The American Association of Collegiate Schools of Nursing (AACN) has also moved to advance nurses' career development by proposing two new educational programs: Clinical Nurse Leader and the Doctor of Nursing Practice. The **Clinical Nurse Leader (CNL)**, prepared at the masters' level, is educated to assume clinical, managerial, and leadership roles, particularly in hospitals. Students are not educated to assume advanced practice roles as clinical specialists, practitioners, midwives, or nurse anesthetists. The **Doctor of Nursing Practice (DNP)** prepares advance practice nurses who do not seek a research-oriented degree, a PhD. Supporters of practice doctorates argue that nurses are disenfranchised because they lack the credentials enjoyed by other health-team members, physicians, pharmacists, physical therapists, and social workers. The AACN envisions that the Doctor of Nursing Practice will be the standard preparation for anyone who prepares for advanced practice. Opponents

argue that this new degree will contribute to an already confusing pattern of nursing education and weaken traditional, research-oriented doctorates (PhDs) (Meleis & Dracup, 2005). Initially, the Doctor of Nursing Practice was described as a curriculum to prepare nurses for advanced practice. As the thinking about the Doctorate of Nursing Practice developed, it was conceptualized as preparation for advanced practice, management of patients and systems, policy development, and clinical teaching. This conceptualization flows from the AACN's (2004) definition of practice:

> . . . any form of nursing intervention that influences health-care outcomes for individuals or populations, including the direct care of individual patients, management of care for individuals and populations, administration of nursing and health-care organizations, and the development and implementation of health policy. Preparation at the practice doctorate level includes advanced preparation in nursing, based on nursing science, and is at the highest level of nursing practice. (AACN, 2004, p.3)

The American Medical Association (AMA)(2006) has been a vocal opponent of the practice doctorate, a position expressed in 2006 by AMA's resolution 211. Organized medicine has argued that patients will confuse the doctor of nursing practice with the doctor of medicine.

Nurses are needed at policy tables. The issues on the nursing agenda, outlined in this chapter, address many of the domestic issues in the country. They affect the health of the public and the future of professional nursing. By becoming competent in policy, you can play a role in advocating for the nursing agenda as students and as practitioners. Keep informed and get involved.

INTERACTIVE EXERCISES

Complete the Interactive exercises provided for this Chapter on the Intranet site.

EVIDENCED-BASED PRACTICE: CONSIDER THIS . . .

*Y*ou have now considered the SCHIP Program and the increases to address uninsured children as a health-promotion strategy. When considering the national enrollments in this program, you recognize the dramatic increase from over 660,000 children enrolled in 1998 to the 2006 enrollment figure of over 6.6 million children.

Question: What is the SCHIP enrollment in your state and what policy improvements would lead to more participation and a decline in the rate of uninsured children?

Source: Centers for Medicare and Medicaid Services. (CMS) (2008). National SCHIP policy overview: SCHIP ever enrolled in years. Retrieved January 11, 2008, from *http://www.cms.hhs.gov/NationalSCHIPPolicy/downloads/SCHIPEverEnrolledYearGraph.pdf*

KEY POINTS

■ Health care in the United States is a business partnership between the public sector and the private sector and is a model of collaboration around health.

■ Some critics of the public/private American plan blame rising health-care costs and the failures to achieve good outcomes on business involvement in health care and the link between employment and health insurance, the for-profit nature of health care, and the placing of efficiency and economic gain above the care of patients.

■ The influence of business is also evident in the adoption of the language and ethics of business. Two recent influences from the business community are its insistence that outcomes are more important than processes and the use of best practices.

■ The simplicity and availability of technology, changes in reimbursement for hospitals and physicians, and the pressure to limit hospital admissions and provide care in less expensive settings have encouraged the development of surgicenters and urgicenters as freestanding ambulatory care niche businesses that compete with hospitals and force hospitals to lower their costs.

■ Values that encouraged hospitals to merge or form systems include: economies of scale and access to capital for expansion, acquisition of new services including physician practices, the enlargement of the system itself, and the concept of one-stop shopping for patients.

■ Most companies have responded to rises in both the cost of health care and the cost of providing health insurance to employees by changing payment and benefit structures.

■ American-style health care is expensive because it emphasizes acute care rather than prevention or primary care and supports the technologic imperative.

■ Uninsured Americans have limited access to care and suffer greater health disparities than people who do have health insurance.

■ Medicare, a federal health-insurance program that primarily serves the elderly and disabled people younger than 65 years who receive Social Security, has four Parts (A, B, C, and D), each offering different benefits and using different financing mechanisms. In 2003, Public Law 108-173 became a new section, Medicare Part D. It was added to provide outpatient drug coverage for beneficiaries who have not enrolled in Medicare Part C.

■ Medicaid is a means-tested health program that pays for medical and long-term care for five indigent groups: pregnant women, adults in families with dependent children, children, persons with disabilities, and the poor elderly.

■ SCHIP is a federal health-insurance program designed to help states expand health coverage to uninsured children who live in families that are slightly above the federal poverty level, usually 200% above the poverty level.

■ The current nursing shortage represents a failure in both recruitment and retention. The Nurse Reinvestment Act, Public Law 107–205, is designed to address nurses as a national resource by promoting both recruitment and retention and encouraging the education of teachers.

■ Legislation to mandate staffing ratios has been introduced in an effort to ensure a sufficient number of nurses to care for patients.

■ The AACN has promoted new educational pathways, the Clinical Nurse Leader (CNL) and the Doctor of Nursing Practice (DNP).

■ Competence in health policy is within the reach of each nurse and student of nursing.

Thought and Discussion Questions

1. A student, not a nursing student, asks you whether she should buy health insurance. She is a 29-year-old single mother with two preschool-age children. Everyone in the family is healthy.

   - How would you advise your fellow student?
   - Give reasons for your advice, using the cost-benefit-burden equation.
   - What governmental programs may be helpful to this woman and her children?

2. What populations are most at risk for health disparities?

3. Explain how you can integrate the leading health indicators into your assessments of patients.

4. Identify three factors associated with recruitment and retention in nursing.

5. Discuss the advantages and disadvantages of new educational pathways for nurses.

6. Review the Chapter Thought located on the first page of the chapter, and discuss it in the context of the chapter.

☐ REFERENCES

Agency for Healthcare Research and Quality (n.d.). The uninsured in America—1996–2002, MEPS Statistical Brief No. 24. Retrieved December 24, 2006, from *http://www.ahrq.gov*

AHA Commission on Workforce for Hospitals and Health Systems (2002, April). *In our hands now: How hospital leaders can build a thriving workforce.* Chicago: American Hospital Association.

Aiken, L., Clarke, S., & Sloane, D. (2002). Hospital restructuring: Does it adversely affect care and outcomes? *Journal of Nursing Administration, 30*(10), 457–465.

American Association of Colleges of Nursing (AACN). (2001). *Tri-council for nursing: Strategies to reverse the new nursing shortage.* Retrieved December 24, 2006, from *http://www.aacn.nche.edu/Publications/positions/tricshortage.htm*

American Association of Colleges of Nursing (AACN) (2002). *Nursing faculty shortage fact sheet.* Retrieved December 24, 2006, from *http://www.aacn.nche.edu/media/backgrounders/facultyshortage.htm*

American Association of Colleges of Nursing (AACN) (2004). Position statement on the practice doctorate in nursing. Retrieved December 24, 2006, from *http://www.aacn.nche.edu/DNP/DNP/PositionStatement.htm*

American Association of Colleges of Nursing (AACN) (2006). Nursing faculty shortage fact sheet. Retrieved December 24, 2006, from *http://www.aacn.nche.edu/Media/FactSheets/FacultyShortage.htm*

American Medical Association (2006). Need to expose and counter nurse doctoral programs (NDP) misrepresentation. Resolution 211(A-06). Retrieved December 24, 2006, from *http://www.ama-assn.org/ama1/pub/upload/mm/471/211a06.doc*

American Nurses Credentialing Center. (2004). ANCC magnet program. Retrieved November 1, 2007, from *http://nursecredentialing.org/magnet/*

Brown, D. (2004, January 9). Health care spending increases for sixth year. *Washington Post,* Health section, A3.

Buerhaus, P., & Needleman, J. (2000). Policy implications of research on nurse staffing and quality of patient care. *Policy, Politics, & Nursing Practice, 1*(1), 5–15.

Catholic Health Association. (n.d.) *Community benefit.* Retrieved December 24, 2006, from *http://www.chausa.org/Pub/MainNav/ourcommitments/CommunityBenefits/*

Centers for Medicare and Medicaid Services. (2004). State Children's Health Insurance Program (SCHIP). Retrieved December 24, 2006, from *http://www.cms.hhs.gov/home/schip.asp*

Committee on the Consequences of Uninsurance (CCU). (2004). *Insuring America's health: Principles and recommendations.* Washington, DC: The National Academy Press.

Committee on Quality Health Care. (2001). *Crossing the quality chasm: A new health system for the 21st century.* Washington, DC: The National Academy Press.

Donley, R., Flaherty, M. J., Sarsfield, E., Taylor, L., Maloni, H., & Flanagan, E. (2002, December 12). What does the nurse reinvestment act mean to you? *Online Journal of Issues in Nursing, 8*(1), Manuscript 5. Retrieved December 24, 2006, from *http://www.nursingworld.org/MainMenuCategories/ANAMarketplace/ANAPeriodicals/OJIN/TableofContents/Volume62001/Number1January2001/NurseReinvestmentAct.aspx*

Feldstein, P. (2003). *Health policy issues.* Chicago: Health Administration Press.

Hoover, D., Crystal, S., Kumar, R., Sambamoorthi, U., & Cantor, J. (2002). Medical expenditures during the last year of life: Findings from the 1992–1996 Medicare beneficiary survey. *Health Services Research, 37*(6), 1625–1642.

Insurance Coverage 2001 (2001). *Almanac of Policy Issues.* Retrieved December 24, 2006, from *http://www.policyalmanac.org/health/archivehealth_insurance_coverage.shtml*

Johnson & Johnson Health Care Systems, Inc. (2002). Discover nursing. Retrieved December 24, 2006, from *http://www.discovernursing.com*

Joint Commission on Accreditation of Healthcare Organizations (JCAHO). (2002). *Health care at the crossroads: Strategies for addressing the evolving nursing crisis.* Chicago: Author.

Kaiser Commission on Medicaid and the Uninsured. (2006). *Health coverage for low-income populations: A comparison of Medicaid and SCHIP (Report number 7495).* Washington, DC: Author

Kaiser Family Foundation. (2004, September). *Health coverage for low-income children.* Retrieved December 24, 2006, from *http://www.kff.org/uninsured/214403:cfm*

Kohn, L., Corrigan, J., & Donaldson, M. (Eds.) (2000). *To err is human: Building a safer health system.* Washington, DC: National Academy Press.

Leape, L. (1992). Unnecessary surgery. *Annual Review of Public Health, 13,* 363–383.

Levit, J., Smithe, C., Cowan, C., Sensenig, A., Cathlin, A., & the Health Accounts Team. (2004). Health spending rebound continues in 2002. *Health Affairs, 23*(1),147–159.

Longest, B. B. (2006). *Health policymaking in the United States.* Washington, DC: AUPH Press.

McClure, M. L., & Hinshaw, A. S. (Eds.) (2002). *Magnet hospitals revisited: Attraction and retention of professional nurses.* Washington, DC: American Nurses Association.

Meleis, A., & Dracup, K. (2005). *The case against the DNP: History, timing, substance, and marginalization.* Retrieved December 24, 2006, from *http://www.nursingworld.org/MainMenuCategories/ANAMarketplace/ANAPeriodicals/OJIN/TableofContents/Volume102005/Number3/tpc28_216026.aspx*

National Center for Health Statistics (2006). *Health, United States 2006.* Retrieved December 24, 2006, from *http://www.cdc.gov/nchs/hus.htm*

Norrish, B. R., & Randall, T. G. (2001, March). Hospital restructuring and the work of registered nurses. *The Milbank Quarterly, 79*(1), 55–79.

Nurses for a Healthier Tomorrow. (n.d.). Campaign news. Retrieved December 24, 2006, from *http://www.nursesource.org/campaign_news.html*

Relman, A. S. (1992). What market values are doing to medicine. *The Atlantic Monthly, 269,* 99–106.

Service Employees International Union (SEIU). (1993). *The national nurse survey: 10,000 dedicated healthcare professionals report on staffing, stress. and patient care in U.S. hospitals and nursing homes.* Washington, DC: SEIU, AFL-CIO.

Smedley, B. D., Stith, A. Y., & Nelson, A. R. (Eds.). (2003). *Unequal treatment: Confronting racial and ethnic disparities in health care.* Washington, DC: The National Academies Press.

Spratley, E., Johnson, A., Sochalski, J., Fritz, M., & Spencer, W. (2001, September). *The registered nurse population, March 2000, Chart 17.* Rockville, MD: Health Resources and Service Administration, Bureau of Health Professions, Division of Nursing.

Steinbrook, R. (2002, May 30). Nursing in the crossfire. *New England Journal of Medicine, 346*(22), 1757–1766.

Understanding the new prescription drug benefit (2003, November 25). Retrieved December 24, 2006, from *http://209.85.165.104/search?q=cache:IRVVBARoDbkJ:www.familiesusa.org/assets/docs/11-25_Q_A42bf.doc+Understanding+the+new+prescription+drug+benefit+Familiesusa.org&hl=en&ct=clnk&cd=1&gl=us*

U.S. Census Bureau. (2004). Retrieved December 24, 2006, from *http://www.census.gov*

U.S. Department of Health and Human Services (USDHHS). (2000). *Healthy people 2010.* Retrieved December 24, 2006, from *http://www.healthypeople.gov*

U.S. Department of Health and Human Services (USDHHS). (2005). *Effects of health care spending on the U.S. economy.* Retrieved December 24, 2006, from *http://aspe.hhs.gov/health/costgrowth*

U.S. Department of Health and Human Services (USDHHS). (2006). *The HHS poverty guidelines.* Retrieved December 24, 2006, from *http://aspe.hhs.gov/poverty/06poverty.shtml*

Wachter, R. M., & Goldman, L. (2002, January). The hospitalist movement 5 years later. *Journal of the American Medical Association, 287*(4), 487–494.

Wilensky, G. (2004, January 28). Health cost drivers and the uninsured. [Testimony presented to Committee on Health, Education, Labor, and Pensions.] Retrieved December 24, 2006, from *http://help.senate.gov/Hearings/2004_01_28/2004_01_28.html*

World Health Organization (2006). *The world health report 2006—working together for health.* Retrieved December 24, 2006, from *www.who.int/whr/2006/en/*

ONLINE RESOURCES

American Association of Colleges of Nursing (AACN)
http://www.aacn.nche.edu

Healthy People 2010
http://www.healthypeople.gov

Expanding the Vision

> **❝***There is no security on this earth; there is only opportunity.***❞**
>
> General Douglas MacArthur, 1880–1964

Chapter Objectives

On completion of this chapter, the reader will be able to:

1. Evaluate trends in professional practice.
2. Continue to evaluate your personal philosophy.
3. Envision personal competencies in professional nursing practice.
4. Develop personal strategic initiatives for future contributions to professional nursing practice.

Key Terms

Competencies
Collaboration
Collegiality
Continued Competence

Continued Professional
Nursing Competence
Involvement

We have seen nursing and health care change radically in recent years. With restructuring of health care, nursing professionals have responded with refinements, advancements, and innovations. Nursing has moved from the functional service mode of the mid-1900s to a cost-, community-, quality-, research-, and consumer-focused orientation. It is no longer the nursing care plan for the patient, but is now the collaborative care plan of the client. And this care must be framed in the context of safety and client involvement in an environment with shortages of health-care providers, especially nursing professionals.

To address the health of people, all health professions are now faced with the challenges of transformation, innovation, and collaboration. We have options and challenges ahead. Collegiality and collaboration extend beyond the structural walls of a single institution or the boundaries of a community. In a global society, we can reach out to colleagues and clients physically or electronically. Critical components of professional practice continue to expand and be enhanced through technology. And we continually strive to envision the challenges ahead. It is now time to expand the vision and address the challenges ahead.

HEALTH-CARE PROFESSIONALS OF THE 21ST CENTURY

Several initiatives have led to the changes in practice and the profession during the last decade.

The Pew Health Professions Commission

The Pew Charitable Trust Foundation established the Pew Health Professions Commission, which worked from 1989 to 1999 to address issues of health-care reform and health policy across the professions. At that time, the health-care industry was in the midst of redesigning services and roles and containing costs with declining resources. The Commission identified 21 specific competencies for health professionals for the year 2005. These competencies addressed ethics, critical thinking and evidence-based practice, primary and preventive health care, access, diversity and health disparities, consumer empowerment and outcomes, the use of informatics and interdisciplinary practice, quality and continuous improvement, leadership and public policy, and continued learning. **Competencies** are those qualities that illustrate effectiveness and appropriateness in our respective professional roles. In 1995, reports from the commission produced strong reactions and responses throughout the professional communities, with predictions for redesign needed in education

and health care and for a rapid transformation in the health professions workforce. The four "Rs" were redesign, reregulate, right size, and restructure. The view of the health-care system presented by the Commission was market-driven and integrated with more managed and primary care. In addition, this health-care system and its professionals would be more accountable to the public and responsive to consumers; would be more efficient, effective, and innovative; and would focus primarily on education, prevention, and care management rather than treatment (Finocchio, Dower, McMahon, Gragnola, & Taskforce on Health Care Workforce Regulation, 1995).

The work of the Pew Commission continued, concentrating on the assets and needs of each of the health professions to address the nation's health. The commission proposed five strategies to prepare nurses with the professional competencies that would be essential in the year 2005. Further, the Commission made 10 recommendations aimed at state regulation for protecting and promoting the public's health concerning the following areas:

- Standardization of terms and regulations
- Entry-to-practice requirements
- Scopes of practice
- Assessment of continuing competence and disciplinary processes
- Professional boards
- Providing information and public accountability
- Data collection
- Evaluation processes
- Development of partnerships to streamline regulation

The recommendations directed at the profession of nursing involved public accountability, recognition of our assets, the need for clarity in our roles and functions, and the need to meet the demands of the marketplace.

The final major report of the Commission detailed professional characteristics of nursing, stating that "over the past 50 years, nursing has changed substantially from a largely supportive role in health care to one with many independent and complex responsibilities in care delivery" (O'Neil & Pew Health Professions Commission, 1998, p. 61). Recommendations presented for nursing professionals included: the need to develop a more diverse and younger workforce; specific competencies through educational mobility and advancement; educational curricula addressing differentiated practice, learning experiences, advanced education and skills; and faculty experience in clinical practice and research (O'Neil, 1998a).

As a result of the findings of the commission and the associated reactions from different professional groups, O'Neil (1998b) identified strategic directions for nursing that included addressing differentiated practice, curricula changes, core competencies, a commitment to research, the creation of strategic partnerships, and enhanced leadership. Later that year, however, the focus changed from the future competencies of health professionals to a call for immediate attention to client safety.

The Institute of Medicine Quality Chasm

The health professions came under fire with the release of two reports from the Institute of Medicine (IOM) of the National Academies on the high incidence of medical errors, changing the focus from the future of health care to the current need to improve safety to clients. The IOM is a nonprofit organization designed to provide science-based advice as a public service. Its quality initiative is described as "the degree to which health services for individuals and populations increase the likelihood of desired health outcomes and are consistent with current professional knowledge" (Institute of Medicine [IOM], 2006, p. 1). The 2001 report from the IOM, *Crossing the Quality Chasm*, proposed 10 rules for the health system in the 21st century for quality health care (see Chapter 1, Box 1.4). The six overall aims—that care should be safe, effective, patient-centered, timely, efficient, and equitable—underlie the 10 rules (IOM, 2006, p. 1). A further report after a Health Professions Education Summit led to the identification of the five core competencies for all health professionals:

- Provide patient-centered care.
- Work in interdisciplinary teams.
- Employ evidence-based practice.
- Apply quality improvement.
- Utilize informatics. (Greiner & Knebel, 2003)

Client safety and effectiveness of outcomes became major national objectives and directed additional attention to nursing. Research by the Agency for Healthcare Research and Quality (AHRQ) (2002) focused on expanding the knowledge base on how the quality of the health-care workplace affects the quality of health care provided, especially in the areas of workload and

working conditions, effects of stress and fatigue, reducing adverse events, and the organizational climate and culture. Client outcomes were now being investigated, along with nursing-sensitive indicators and factors that promote safe and effective practice.

In late 2003, the IOM focused on nursing itself in its report, *Keeping Patients Safe: Transforming the Work Environment of Nurses.* The IOM's Committee on the Work Environment and Patient Safety provided specific recommendations to both acute-care and long-term care organizations on issues of management practices, workforce capability, work design, and the organizational safety culture (Page, 2004, p. 3). The following risk factors were identified for patient safety in nursing work environments:

- More acutely ill patients
- Shorter hospital stays
- Redesigned work
- Frequent patient turnover
- High staff turnover
- Long work hours
- Rapid increases in new knowledge and technology
- Increased interruptions and demands on nurses' time. (Page, 2004, pp. 37–45).

Although these facts were no surprise, their identification as risk factors to clients was significant. Nurses have been reporting these factors but now they were included in a major national report. This committee also documented the national shortages of both nurses and nursing assistants. Recommendations to nursing leadership and management on how to address the deficiencies in the documented work environments called attention to the following areas:

- Leadership, communication skills, collaborative decision-making, and resources
- Emphasis on safety goals *along with* productivity and financial goals
- Management practices promoting safety, trust, change, engagement, and learning collaboratives
- External support for evidence-based management practices

In addition, at the staff level, the committee found "strong evidence that nurse staffing levels, the knowledge and skills level of nursing staff, and the extent to which workers collaborate in sharing their knowledge and skills affect patient outcomes and safety" (Page, 2004, p. 161). This finding provides further support for the need to incorporate the five core competencies into professional nursing practice on a consistent basis. In addition to client-centered care, evolving technologies, evidence-based collaborative practice, and continued competence are essential components for quality improvement in the delivery of health care to consumers.

In subsequent years, the IOM investigated health disparities, the role of the government including Medicare, rural health, health-care reimbursement practices, and mental health conditions, among still other quality improvement initiatives. Of particular note were two studies mandated by the United States Congress, on insurance and reimbursements and preventing medication errors. In July 2006, the IOM report released on *Preventing Medication Errors* presented information available on the incidence of medication errors in acute-care settings, long-term care, and in ambulatory care—including errors in the homes of consumers—in an effort to develop an agenda for the nation to reduce preventable errors and adverse drug events and enhance medication safety. Although the incidence rates were approximated based on the data, the report did emphasize that these rates were most likely underestimates, based on available and reportable data and the incidence of adverse events. It was reported, however, that at least 25% of all harmful adverse drug events are *preventable* (Aspden, Wolcott, Bootman, & Cronenwett, 2006, p. 4).

Based on the 10 rules from the earlier *Quality Chasm Report* in 2001, the IOM (Aspden et al., 2006) recommended the transformation of the entire system to a patient-centered, integrated-use system with specific action agendas to support the consumer-provider partnership:

- For health-care organizations
- For the pharmaceutical, medical device, and health information technology industries
- For applied research on safe medication use
- For oversight, regulation, and payment

The seven recommendations provided by the IOM (Aspden et al., 2006) focused further on:

- Consumer empowerment for self-medication management
- Improvement and standardization of resources by governmental agencies
- Implementation of patient-information and decision-support technologies nationwide
- Improved labeling, packaging, and distribution, including studies on use of samples
- Establishment of standards for drug information technologies, including design and alert systems
- Broad, federally-funded research on safe and appropriate medication use across settings, focused on error prevention
- Use of legislation, regulation, accreditation, payment mechanisms, and the media for adoption of practices, technologies, and professional behaviors focused on safety and error reduction.

Concerted efforts must now be collaborative among professionals, governmental agencies, suppliers, educators,

ONLINE CONSULT

Agency for Healthcare Research and Quality (AHRQ) at
http://www.ahrq.gov

Institute of Medicine (IOM) at
http://www.iom.edu

and regulators with the consumer involved in the process. Evidence-based practice is the standard with a focus on safety, positive client outcomes, and the use of known and evolving technologies.

The Professional Nursing Practice Environment

Changes in the practice environment have received serious attention with the focus on safety and client outcomes. The IOM Committee on the Work Environment and Patient Safety (Page, 2004) identified necessary client safeguards in the environment (Box 23-1). These recommendations call for leadership, collaboration, and action.

Leadership in the practice environment is essential for client safety but also for the satisfaction, involvement, and commitment of dedicated health-care professionals. One area that is receiving serious consideration at the national and state levels is adequacy of staffing. In addition, the American Nurses Association (ANA) has been actively looking at the roles of both the employer and the nurse to promote healthy work hours and consider the effect of fatigue on safety for both clients and nurses. The focus on productivity and appropriate staffing has led to a renewed emphasis on quality outcomes. Indicators that are nursing sensitive, like infection rates, client satisfaction, and nursing hours per patient day, are being studied in relation to staffing. As noted by Clark et al. (2005), we cannot simply tell staff to do more, "rather, we need to create systems that support staff in their efforts and set them up for success" (p. 8).

The American Association of Colleges of Nursing has identified selected characteristics of work environments that support professional nursing practice (American Association of Colleges of Nursing [AACN], 2002):

- Magnet status
- Preceptorships and residencies
- Differentiated practice
- Interdisciplinary collaboration

Recognition as a magnet hospital requires that applicant health-care organizations meet specific eligibility

Box 23.1 Necessary Client Safeguards in the Work Environment

- Governing boards that focus on safety
- Leadership and evidence-based management structures and processes
- Effective nursing leadership
- Adequate staffing
- Organizational support for ongoing learning and decision support
- Mechanisms that promote interdisciplinary collaboration
- Work design that promotes safety
- Organizational culture that continually strengthens patient safety

From Page, A. (Ed.). (2004). *Keeping patients safe: Transforming the work environment of nurses.* Washington, DC: National Academies Press.

criteria, including strong nursing leadership in line with national standards of practice. The self-assessment requirement for the institution applying for magnet recognition is described as revealing and "creating opportunities for organizational advancement, team building, and enhancement of individuals' professional self esteem" (American Nurses Credentialing Center [ANCC], 2006, p. 1). Retention and appropriate staffing are characteristics of magnet organizations. Further, the Joint Commission on Accreditation of Healthcare Organizations (JCAHO) (2005) has released a position paper on the nursing shortage, acknowledging the successes of magnet hospitals with retention and calls for redesigned processes, effective staffing, use of information and ergonomic technologies, but, "most importantly, workplace cultures that empower, value, and reward nurses" (p. 37).

Retention is enhanced when professionals have had an opportunity to expand their knowledge base and skills with a rapidly changing practice environment through preceptorships for students and residencies for graduates. Joel (2002) correlates this to the student teacher, resident, or law clerk engaging in hands-on experiences that are intended "to socialize the neophyte into the field and provide a transition to professional accountability" (p. 6). Mentorship is an important component to advance the skills of the neophyte and of the seasoned clinician. Matching the knowledge and skills of the professional with the requirements of the position is an ongoing consideration. This can be promoted through mentorship programs and activities for continuing education, competency, and differentiated practice.

Differentiated nursing practice (see Chapter 15), the third characteristic identified by AACN in the supportive practice environment, is illustrated through

advancement structures in the organization based on experience, additional education, certification, or other identified indicators of excellence (AACN, 2002, pp. 6–7). Implementation of differentiated practice has historically been difficult; the combination of skills matched to the position requirements must be delineated. As Nelson (2002) has proposed, it is not feasible to try to differentiate practice along current educational points of entry when the roles have not been translated into the practice setting (p. 7).

Interdisciplinary collaboration, illustrated through teamwork, trust, shared responsibility, and respect, also enhances client outcomes. The AACN (2002) proposed eight hallmarks of excellence in the professional nursing practice environment. Consider how these hallmarks for the practice environment (Table 23–1) also address the core competencies for all health professionals identified by the IOM. Note the focus on quality care for clients, collaboration, competency, and leadership throughout. As documented by Gordon (2005), however, collaboration and collegiality in practice place inevitable challenges to nursing and can undermine the care of clients.

COLLABORATION AND COLLEGIALITY

Essential activities of contemporary practice include strategic partnerships, leadership, and collaboration. This collaboration and collegiality must occur within the profession and be interdisciplinary. Collaboration is especially critical with the end of the moratorium on the development of single-focus specialty hospitals in 2006. See Box 23–2. The initial step in collaboration and collegiality is valuing our colleagues who provide clinical nursing care, medical care, specialty care, advanced clinical practice, education, or administrative functions. Collaboration and collegiality are both intradisciplinary within the discipline of nursing, and interdisciplinary among other health-care professionals.

ONLINE CONSULT

American Association of Colleges of Nursing (AACN) at
http://www.aacn.nche.edu

American Nurses Credentialing Center (ANCC) at
http://nursecredentialing.org/magnet/index.html

Joint Commission on Accreditation of Healthcare Organizations (JCAHO) at
http://www.jointcommission.org

Table 23.1

Hallmarks of Professional Practice and Core Competencies

Hallmarks of the Professional Nursing Practice Environment*	Core Competencies for Health Professionals [†]			
	Provide Patient-Centered Care	Work in Interdisciplinary Teams	Employ Evidence-Based Practice	Apply Quality Improvement
Manifest a philosophy of clinical care emphasizing quality, safety, interdisciplinary collaboration, continuity of care, and professional accountability.	☑	☑	☑	☑
Recognize contributions of nurses' knowledge and expertise to clinical care quality and patient outcomes.	☑	☑	☑	☑
Empower nurses' participation in clinical decision-making and organization of clinical care systems.	☑	☑	☑	☑
Promote executive-level nursing leadership.	☑	☑	☑	☑
Maintain clinical advancement programs based on education, certification, and advanced preparation.	☑	☑	☑	☑
Demonstrate professional development support for nurses.	☑	☑	☑	☑
Create collaborative relationships among members of the health-care provider team.	☑	☑	☑	☑

*From American Association of Colleges of Nursing (AACN). (2002). *Hallmarks of the professional nursing practice environment.* Washington, DC: Author.
[†]From Greiner, A. C., & Knebel, E. (Eds.). (2003). *Health professions education: A bridge to quality.* Washington, DC: Institute of Medicine.

Collaboration

The health-care team should be an ideal example of collaboration. See also Chapter 7. **Collaboration** involves actively working together to meet some identified goal, such as the client's treatment goals. Within the discipline, nurses from each area of nursing would contribute to that goal—the admission nurse or discharge planner, the student in a clinical rotation, the operative nurse, the acute-care nurse practitioner, and other professional nurses providing care to raise the client's level of well-being. As noted by Weston (2006), however, this sense of teamwork may be particularly challenging for the four different generations of nurses in practice—veterans, baby boomers, generation Xers, and millennials—with their different characteristics and perspectives that can either enhance or traumatize the practice environment. In times of limited staffing and growing responsibilities, seeing the broader picture with collaboration is necessary to ensure effective client outcomes.

Box 23.2 Single-Focus Specialty Hospitals

"As defined by Congress, specialty hospitals are hospitals exclusively or primarily engaged in caring for one of the following categories of patients: patients with a cardiac condition or an orthopedic condition; or patients receiving a surgical procedure" (Centers for Medicare and Medicaid Services [CMS], 2006, p. 1).

A moratorium on the development of these specialty hospitals expired in 2006. The issues involved payment and transparency in the case of physicians referring patients to these single-focus care settings in which they had some ownership. But with the development of these physician-owned hospitals, there is a consumer focus as customer service and specialty care.

Consider the interdisciplinary and collaborative opportunities and challenges.
Find "Specialty Hospital Issues" at the CMS site at *http://www.cms.hhs.gov/PhysicianSelfReferral/ 06_specialty_hospital_issues.asp*

A cooperative spirit with collaboration will bring more efficient achievement of goals and greater personal reward for both colleagues and clients. Questions of authority and responsibility arise with this cooperative or collaborative spirit, such as who is the leader of the team and who is responsible for ensuring quality client outcomes. This ownership of responsibility must be shared in a true collaborative relationship rather than create "turf" issues in a more competitive environment. The goal is the effectiveness of the client outcomes with collaboration as the means to reach the goal. Effective communication and clinical skills, along with trust, leadership, and collegiality, are important attributes of the health-care professional collaborating with other health-care professionals. Consider the lessons for collaboration described by Gardner (2005) that are listed in Box 23–3.

One morning, suppose that you were on an acute-care unit and see the pulmonologist arrive to see his patient with COPD. You know that the respiratory therapist is currently working with the client on a treatment. You know all parties involved, the client's wife is present but concerned about at-home compliance, and there is a need for good follow-up and discharge teaching. How will you capitalize on this opportunity for interdisciplinary collaboration for home care? How can you get all parties involved and create a win-win situation for all, focused on the efficacy of treatment for this client? These skills are critical for the efficient use of scarce human and physical resources in a consumer environment that must be focused on effectiveness of client outcomes and overall safety.

Collegiality

Collegiality is sharing responsibility and authority to achieve a goal or prescribed outcome. Power and responsibility for outcomes related to clients' health and well-being are invested in more than one person. Mutual respect and collaboration are important components of a collegial relationship. All colleagues contribute to the intended goals and are accountable for the outcomes.

Collaboration and Collegiality in Practice

Both collaboration and collegiality are specified by the American Nurses Association as standards of professional performance in its document *Nursing: Scope and Standards of Practice.* As identified in Chapter 1, the document contains six standards of practice and nine standards of professional performance, with objectives and measurement criteria (ANA, 2004, pp. 21–45). The standards of practice reflect the steps of the nursing process, whereas the standards of performance are those behaviors expected of the professional. Collaboration is measured by virtue of communication, consultation, documentation, and referrals within and outside the nursing discipline. Measures of collegiality include sharing knowledge and skills, providing constructive

Box 23.3 Characteristics for Collaboration

- Knowing yourself—your biases, values, and goals
- Valuing and managing diversity
- Developing constructive conflict-resolution skills
- Creating win-win situations
- Demonstrating clinical competence, cooperation, and flexibility
- Making time for practicing collaboration skills
- Using all multidisciplinary opportunities for building partnerships
- Appreciating that collaboration can occur spontaneously
- Being reflective, seeking feedback, and admitting mistakes for autonomy and unity
- Understanding that collaboration is not required in all situations

Adapted from Gardner, D. B. (2005, January 31). Ten lessons in collaboration. *Online Journal of Issues in Nursing, (10)*1. Retrieved August 28, 2006, from *http://www.nursingworld.org/MainMenuCategories/ ANAMarketplace/ANAPeriodicals/OJIN/TableofContents/ Volume102005/No1January31/tpc26_116008.aspx* feedback, enhancement of practice, and creating and supporting a learning and work environment. In the revised standards, additional measurement criteria have been added for the advanced practice nurse and specialty nurse to accommodate the additional expectations in interdisciplinary practice.

Nursing professionals also are responsible for promoting collaboration and collegiality among the professions. As described throughout this text, health-care delivery systems are becoming more and more integrated and interdisciplinary. In our present multidisciplinary health-care system, collaboration must be effective among all members of the various health professions and care disciplines. Collegiality between professionals is also critical for the team to function effectively.

In 1998, the President's Advisory Commission on Consumer Protection and Quality in the Healthcare Industry reported that "the challenge for industry leaders is to harness the tremendous talent, energy, and commitment of the 10 million people who have been drawn to work in the health-care industry because of its strong sense of mission" (President's Advisory Commission, 1998, p. 197). Since then, the IOM report *Keeping Patients Safe* has recommended that healthcare organizations "should take action to support interdisciplinary collaboration by adopting such interdisciplinary practice mechanisms as interdisciplinary rounds, and by providing ongoing formal education and training in interdisciplinary collaboration for all health-care professionals on a regularly scheduled, continuous basis . . ." (Page, 2004, p. 216). The IOM also identified two necessary precursors to collaboration—individual clinical competence and mutual trust and respect—and the following four characteristics of collaboration:

- Shared understanding of goals and roles
- Effective communication
- Shared decision-making
- Conflict management. (Page, 2004, pp. 212–213)

An additional characteristic is also necessary—continued competence to maintain safety and quality care for the client and effective interdisciplinary practice.

COMPETENCE

The issue of competence is vital to all professionals. Although not restricted to nursing, professional competence has received greater attention after the reports from both the Pew Health Professions Commission and the IOM. Professional competence is of great concern to health professionals, their regulatory bodies, and consumers. It is an issue of definition, ownership, policy

development, and demonstration. Regulatory bodies are required to assure the public of safe and competent professional practice by the professionals they regulate. But definitions vary by statute, and measurement issues are complex. Consider two different ways in which competence can be measured: by continuing practice and through continuing education. But then the following question arises: Is the continuing practice safe and effective in meeting appropriate client outcomes using evidence-based practice? Or, in the case of continuing education, are the programs or sessions selected directed at the area of practice to improve and enhance practice or merely counting hours toward license renewal without a focus on clients and responsible professional practice? In fact, measurement issues are further complicated by the different levels of practice that must be regulated—new graduate, continued practice, and advanced practice.

Entry into practice occurs through licensure on the basis of performance on a psychometrically sound instrument, the National Council Licensure Exam NCLEX®. Advanced practice is regulated differently in the various jurisdictions but often through advanced education and the certification process. But, how should the regulators monitor continued professional competence for the clinician not governed by specialty practice certification and what about variable requirements for recertification? And consider the role of both the nurse and the employer in monitoring continued professional competence.

The issue of **continued competence** is not restricted to state and federal regulatory bodies. As described in *Nursing's Social Policy Statement* (ANA, 2003), regulation of practice also includes the following:

- Self-regulation, through personal accountability and peer review
- Professional regulation, with education requirements and a defined scope of practice
- Legal regulation, through statutory and regulatory requirements

Glaser (1999) has stated that "the primary goal of continued competence is to assure safe, *quality,* nursing care/practice to clients/the public" (p. 1). In 1996, the National Council of State Boards of Nursing (NCSBN) illustrated a collaborative model for continued competence that included the individual nurse, the employer, the regulatory body, the educator, and the consumer of nursing care (NCSBN, 2005a). But further work and understanding of best practices continues. In some Canadian provinces and in other countries, nurses are required to use a portfolio system to document their continued competence. This system requires critical reflection and assessment of continued competence by the nurse with documentation of evidence in a portfolio, often including some form of peer review in the process. The International Council of Nurses has pointed out that the development of systems to identify continued competence is relatively new but that employers, nurses, providers of continuing education, and regulatory bodies all have a stake in both the definition and the process (Bryant, 2005, p. 21).

Although continued competence is ultimately the professional responsibility of the individual clinician, the professional education level must be appropriate to the defined scope of practice and professional standards, the health-care employer must ensure the competence in the practice setting, and the client must be assured (and should assure himself) of safe and effective practice. As noted by the NCSBN (2005b), however, "responsibility for interpreting and enforcing nursing scopes of practice, including the determination of the appropriate education, training and experience necessary to support a given scope of practice, rests solely with the boards of nursing" (p. 1).

The professional performance standard of education of the *Scope and Standards of Practice* states that for continued competence, "the nurse attains knowledge and competency that reflects current nursing practice" (ANA, 2004, p. 35). In addition, nurses are required to be "lifelong learners," taking advantage of appropriate, adequate, and innovative learning opportunities and solutions (ANA, 2004, p. 20). Ongoing educational activities occur through continuing education—formal, noncredit (CE), and on-the-job. In research conducted by the NCSBN, respondents "rated contributions of work experience, initial professional education, and mentors above the contributions of CE in assisting them to their current levels of ability" (Smith, 2003, p. 25). Concerning continued learning in the work environment, the IOM report *Keeping Patients Safe* recommended that health-care organizations should "dedicate budgetary resources equal to a defined percentage of the nursing payroll to support nursing staff in their ongoing acquisition and maintenance of knowledge and skills" (Page, 2004, p. 210). Further, the concept of a learning environment is extended beyond its start in an educational setting to one encouraged in the practice setting. But budgetary considerations have resulted in associated cuts in funding education departments and programs in some agencies. A learning environment in the practice setting supports the core competencies and ongoing professional competence. The individual professional must determine, seek, request, and utilize resources to maintain his continued competence in the safe and effective performance of nursing practice activities.

> Although continued competence is ultimately the professional responsibility of the individual clinician, the professional education level must be appropriate to the defined scope of practice and professional standards, the health-care employer must ensure the competence in the practice setting, and the client must be assured of safe and effective practice.

After the report of a special panel, the ANA defined **continuing professional nursing competence** as the:

> . . . ongoing professional nursing competence according to level of expertise, responsibility, and domains of practice as evidenced by behavior based on beliefs, attitudes, and knowledge matched to and in the context of a set of expected outcomes as defined by nursing scope of practice, policy, Code of Ethics, standards, guidelines, and benchmarks that assure safe performance of professional activities. (Whittaker, Carson, & Smolenski, 2000, p. 1)

This definition of competence requires demonstration of skillful, effective, and evidence-based practice both in nursing and interdisciplinary endeavors, with a view of the core competencies and the challenges ahead.

Both professional and personal contributions are the ingredients of your professional career. Skills, which are the ingredients of professional nursing practice, require ongoing refinement. The International Leadership Institute of Sigma Theta Tau, International Honor Society of Nursing (2006), has proposed eight skills (Box 23–4) to be used as guideposts by the nurse navigating a "healthy career," from before entry into nursing education and nursing to obtaining further credentials, demonstrating career growth, and moving into an active retirement. Notice that these skills include those in the practice setting as well as personal life. These skills are also not restricted to nursing or health care. Your own demonstration of these skills is defined by your views on practice, human beings, the environment, health, and nursing.

ONLINE CONSULT

American Nurses Association (ANA) at
http://www.nursingworld.org

American Nurses Credentialing Center (ANCC) at
http://www.nursecredentialing.org

National Council of State Boards of Nursing (NCSBN) at
https://www.ncsbn.org/172.htm

CHALLENGING PRACTICE

The recommendations and changes in the health-care environment present all nurses with additional career opportunities and responsibilities, whether they are in acute, ambulatory, home, or long-term care settings or in a nontraditional setting as a clinician, case manager, researcher, administrator, consultant, educator, advanced practice nurse, or nurse entrepreneur. These challenges in your future are dynamic and evolve daily as we address the themes of safety, quality client outcomes, evolving technology, and interdisciplinary practice. Consider the implications of the following challenges in the workforce or in a specific delivery setting:

- A culture supportive of safe and quality client outcomes
- Appropriate staffing patterns and skill mixes
- Appropriate delegation activities
- Training and supervision of unlicensed assistive personnel
- Competencies and continued knowledge development of professionals
- Differentiated practice
- Coordination of care across practice settings
- Changes in populations and health-care needs
- Strategies to improve health and eliminate health disparities
- Cost containment
- Evidence-based interdisciplinary practice
- Consumer satisfaction
- Using information technologies and quality-based indicators

The challenges in your future truly depend on you, your practice environment, colleagues, and future initiatives. Consider how the Michigan Nurses Association (MNA) challenged nurses to improve the nursing culture in their practice environment with 101 ways in the 10 areas of communication, respect,

support, education, conflict management, collegiality, leadership, diversity, development of others, and professionalism (Ervin, 2006). This initiative promoted by the MNA Congress on Practice was designed to encourage nurses to be proactive in the work environment and to take positive steps toward improvement of the culture. As noted by Ervin (2006), persistent problems in the work setting contribute to stress, frustration, and turnover. Individuals and groups can challenge the status quo for positive change.

And then there is the consideration of specialty practice as an advanced practice nurse (APRN). Consider the APRN practice roles of nurse practitioner, clinical nurse specialist, nurse anesthetist, or nurse midwife. As the knowledge base grows, evidence-based practice is guided by the specialty area. Nevertheless, we are experiencing a shortage of nurses active in generalist staff practice settings as well as a critical shortage of nursing faculty. Although we have seen an increase in the numbers of nurses prepared at the master's and doctoral levels (ANA, 2006), recently graduate education was directed at APRN clinical practice in four areas: nurse practitioner, clinical nurse specialist, nurse anesthetist, and nurse midwife.

Since the 1980s, education tracks in graduate programs have declined, and the average age of nursing faculty continues to rise. As with the nursing shortage, the shortage of faculty has been documented. As the National League for Nursing (NLN, 2007) observes, "certification [f]or academic nurse educators . . . establishes nursing education as a specialty area of practice and creates a means for faculty to demonstrate their expertise in this role" (p. 1). In addition to an area of specialization, skills in curriculum development and evaluation, teaching and learning, and interdisciplinary education are required in the nurse educator role. A nurse educator has a further practice opportunity in involvement in the preparation of skilled professionals. Following a study on the faculty shortage, AACN (2003) reported on the demographics, stressors, and competing demands, along with the changes in the student population, but maintained that the "faculty shortage offers nurse educators an unparalleled opportunity to challenge past norms and think collaboratively and nontraditionally to meet the future" (p. 19).

The overriding challenges ahead in professional practice include ongoing professional development and involvement for engagement in the delivery of client-centered care with a focus on safety, efficacy, and quality through the use of informatics, and evidence-based practice and leadership in the interdisciplinary practice setting. This involvement reflects the core competencies of health professionals and advances practice, client outcomes, and the profession.

INVOLVEMENT

When we think of **involvement**, we think of our function as advocates and health-care providers for our clients. These functions represent one form of involvement. Our professional involvement focuses on the individual attributes, needs of, and outcomes for our clients, the consumers of nursing and health care. This involvement, as individual professionals with the clients and families who are the consumers of evidence-based, quality nursing care, must address all core competencies.

Our involvement is also as members of the health-care team. Collaboration and collegiality have been described in relation to nursing and interdisciplinary practice. This book also discussed the importance of group dynamics and group skills, and the art of negotiation in leading and managing. All of these functions relate to active involvement with a defined group to attain specified goals for the consumers of health care.

A third form of professional involvement is as a member of the professional group. This form of involvement requires time and commitment for advancement of the profession. Professional contributions result from participation in professional organizations, research, publications, theory evaluation, and promotion of the further development of the profession. Personal contributions in professional practice occur through your education, competency, ethical behaviors, use of theory and evidence-based interventions, and communication, political efficacy, client advocacy, and leadership.

REVISITING YOUR PHILOSOPHY OF NURSING

Now is the time to reflect on your personal contributions to and philosophy of nursing. Nurses are talented, creative, and visionary—when they allow themselves to be. They are frequently viewed as leaders and risk takers as they advocate for the perceived good of their clients. But what skills required of professionals do we need to refine? Step back and think of the vital and basic skills needed to demonstrate professional competencies. These skills are what we continually strive to refine:

- Knowledge base
- Critical thinking skills
- Technical skills
- Interpersonal skills
- Articulation skills

Clinical practice requires these skills for provision of client-centered care, involvement in interdisciplinary and evidence-based practice, and the use of informatics and emerging technologies for quality improvement and effective client outcomes. These skills are enhanced through the professional attributes of collaboration, collegiality, continued competence, and involvement in the health promotion of society. Concern for the health of people, whether individual clients, families, communities, or groups in their environment, is the core of professional nursing. Your philosophy of nursing will evolve and develop, just as you do as a professional.

EMBRACING CHANGE

The recent focus on the health professions and the evident shortages of professionals has had the beneficial effect of opening up the discussion for needed changes in the health-care system and the professions. Discussions have been held at national, state, and local meetings, and debate and discussion on the issues continue in professional newsletters and journals as well as online. Communication and critical thinking are taking place. The restraining and driving forces of change are present. We see that practice and education can no longer serve the needs of the consumers without change. All professionals are shareholders in the process of improving the health of society at large.

EVIDENCED-BASED PRACTICE: CONSIDER THIS . . .

*I*n response to the growing body of knowledge on the importance of the concept of nurse dose to client outcomes, Brooten and Youngblut (2006) further describe this concept and identify what they describe as three equally essential components:

- dose, number of nurses or amount of care by nurses
- nurse, as education, expertise and experience
- host and host response, as organizational or client responsiveness. (p. 98)

Question: How do these components of nurse dose influence client outcomes in your environment? And what is your vision for the future?

Source: Brooten, D., & Youngblut, J. M. (2006). Nurse dose as a concept. *Journal of Nursing Scholarship, 38*, 94–99.

Technology continues to expand our horizons and challenge our practice. Improved equipment and technologies are developing at a rapid pace. Information is available immediately. Colleagues readily communicate at a distance using e-mail, instant messaging, ListServs, and news groups. Computer-adaptive testing for licensure and certification is a given. Re-engineering has become a common occurrence in practice settings, as have cost containment, measurement of client outcomes, evidence-based practice, and a focus on consumer satisfaction.

The topics that you have embraced through this book have presented you with some of the issues involved in this time of rapid change in the profession and in practice. Facing the responsibilities inherent in professional practice is a way of revisiting our present roles and considering how they meet the needs of our clients and the intent of our profession. The student role provides the setting for analyzing information related to current practices. Theories that guide practice continue to be tested and refined as appropriate to their utility in practice, education, and research. Communication and critical thinking are vital components of this activity as we operate as leaders, managers, and care providers in organizations and communities. We function as change agents, teachers, and group leaders in practice settings. Knowledge of research and the political process give us direction, as change agents, for addressing the changes needed for a healthier society. The focus remains on clients, their safety, needs, and healthy outcomes.

Current health-care initiatives must be evaluated for applicability, acceptability, and appropriateness for meeting the needs of the population, with due consideration given to economic and quality indicators. All of these issues are addressed within the ethical parameters of professional nursing practice.

The information presented here has been designed to address the challenge of the book's title, *Advancing Your Career: Concepts of Professional Nursing*. We are all challenged to advance our professional practice.

INTERACTIVE EXERCISES

Go to the Intranet site and complete the interactive exercises provided for this Chapter.

K E Y   P O I N T S

■ The Pew Health Professions Commission (1995) described the emerging health-care system and focused on four themes: redesign, reregulate, right size, and restructure.

■ Competencies are those qualities that illustrate effectiveness and appropriateness in our respective professional roles. The Health Professions Education Summit led to the identification of the five core competencies for all health professionals:
  ■ Provide patient-centered care.
  ■ Work in interdisciplinary teams.
  ■ Employ evidence-based practice.
  ■ Apply quality improvement.
  ■ Utilize informatics. (Greiner & Knebel, 2003)

■ The IOM's Committee on the Work Environment and Patient Safety identified the following necessary client safeguards in the practice environment (Page, 2004):
  ■ Governing boards that focus on safety
  ■ Effective nursing leadership
  ■ Adequate staffing
  ■ Organizational support for ongoing learning and decision support
  ■ Mechanisms that promote interdisciplinary collaboration
  ■ Work design that promotes safety
  ■ Organizational culture that continually strengthens patient safety

■ Collaboration involves actively working together to meet some identified goal, such as the client's treatment goals.

■ Collegiality is the sharing of responsibility and authority to achieve a goal or prescribed outcome. Respect and collaboration are important components of a collegial relationship.

■ Continued competence is of great concern to health professionals, their regulatory bodies, and consumers.

(Key Points continue on page 429)

KEY POINTS (continued)

■ The ANA has defined ongoing *continuing professional nursing competence* "according to level of expertise, responsibility, and domains of practice as evidenced by behavior based on beliefs, attitudes, and knowledge matched to and in the context of a set of expected outcomes as defined by nursing scope of practice, policy, *Code of Ethics,* standards, guidelines, and benchmarks that assure safe performance of professional activities" (Whittaker et al., 2000, p. 1).

■ A nurse's involvement as a professional takes three forms:
  ■ As an individual professional with clients, families, and communities who are the consumers of nursing care
  ■ As a group member or leader of an interdisciplinary health-care team
  ■ As an active member of the professional group

■ Professional contributions result from participation in professional organizations, research, publications, theory evaluation, and promotion of the further development of the profession.

■ Vital and basic skills needed and continually refined by professionals include expanding one's knowledge base, critical thinking, and technical, interpersonal, and articulation skills.

Thought and Discussion Questions

1. Identify additional challenges for improvements in the delivery of quality health care.

2. Describe your plans for two specific personal contributions to professional nursing practice that you will attempt during the next 10 years.

3. Develop three personal goals to be met in your professional nursing practice during the next five years.

4. Review the Chapter Thought located on the first page of the chapter, and discuss it in the context of the chapter.

☐ REFERENCES

Agency for Healthcare Research and Quality (AHRQ). (2002). *Impact of working conditions on patient safety. Fact sheet* (AHRQ Publication No. 03-P003). Retrieved August 28, 2006, from *http://www.ahrq.gov/news/workfact.htm*

American Association of Colleges of Nursing (AACN). (2002). *Hallmarks of the professional nursing practice environment.* Retrieved August 28, 2006, from *http://www.aacn.nche.edu/Publications/positions/hallmarks.htm*

American Association of Colleges of Nursing (AACN). (2003). *Faculty shortages in baccalaureate and graduate nursing programs: Scope of the problem and strategies for expanding the supply.* [AACN white paper]. Retrieved August 28, 2006, from *http://www.aacn.nche.edu/Publications/WhitePapers/FacultyShortages.htm*

American Nurses Association (ANA). (2003). *Nursing's social policy statement* (2nd ed.). (Publication No. 03NSPS 15M 09/03). Washington, DC: Author.

American Nurses Association (ANA). (2004). *Nursing: Scope and standards of practice* (Publication No. 03SSNP). Washington, DC: American Nurses Publishing.

American Nurses Association (ANA). (2006). Nursing facts: Nursing shortage. Retrieved August 28, 2006, from *http://www.needlestick.org/readroom/fsshortage.htm*

American Nurses Credentialing Center (ANCC). (2006). The magnet application and appraisal process. Retrieved August 28, 2006, from *http://nursingworld.org/ancc/magnet/process.html*

Aspden, P., Wolcott, J., Bootman, L., & Cronenwett, L. R. (Eds.). (2006). *Preventing medication errors.* Washington, DC: National Academies Press.

Brooten, D., & Youngblut, J. M. (2006). Nurse dose as a concept. *Journal of Nursing Scholarship, 38*(1), 94–99.

Bryant, R. (2005). Regulation, roles, and competency development. [Available from the International Council of Nurses]. Retrieved September 2, 2006, from *http://www.icn.ch/global/Issue1Regulation.pdf*

Centers for Medicare & Medicaid Services. (CMS). (2006). Medicare issues final report to Congress implementing strategic plan for specialty hospitals: Actions highlight payment accuracy, transparency, and enforcement. Retrieved October 5, 2006, from *http://www.cms.hhs.gov/apps/media/press/release.asp?Counter=1937*

Clark, P. A., Davis, M., Drevs, K., Fuerbringer, P., Gloss, M., & Spite, D. (2005). The healthcare landscape. In P. A. Clark & M. P. Malone, *Making it right: Healthcare service recovery tools, techniques, and best practices.* Marblehead, MA: HCPro.

Ervin, N. (2006). 101 ways to improve nursing culture: Professionalism [Electronic version]. *Michigan Nurse.* Retrieved September 1, 2006, from *http://www.minurses.org/prac/101ways.htm*

Finocchio, L. J., Dower, C. M., McMahon, T., Gragnola, C. M., & Taskforce on Health Care Workforce Regulation. (1995). *Reforming health care workforce regulation: Policy considerations for the 21st century.* San Francisco: Pew Health Professions Commission.

Gardner, D. B. (2005, January 31). Ten lessons in collaboration. *Online Journal of Issues in Nursing, (10)*1. Retrieved August 28, 2006, from *http://www.nursingworld.org/MainMenuCategories/ANAMarketplace/ANAPeriodicals/OJIN/TableofContents/Volume102005/No1January31/tpc26_116008.aspx*

Glaser, G. (1999). The policy and politics of continued competence. *Online Journal of Issues in Nursing.* Retrieved August 28, 2006, from *http://www.nursingworld.org/ojin/tpclg/leg_8.htm*

Gordon, S. (2005). *Nursing against the odds: How health care cost cutting, media stereotypes, and medical hubris undermine nurses and patient care.* New York: ILR Press.

Greiner, A. C., & Knebel, E. (Eds.). (2003). *Health professions education: A bridge to quality.* Washington, DC: Institute of Medicine.

Institute of Medicine (IOM). (2006). Crossing the quality chasm: The IOM health care quality initiative. Retrieved August 28, 2006, from *http://www.iom.edu/focuson.asp?id=8089*

Joel, L. A. (2002). Education for entry into nursing practice: Revisited for the 21st century. *Online Journal of Issues in Nursing* (Manuscript 4), 7(2), 1–9. Retrieved August 28, 2006, from *http://www.nursingworld.org/ojin/topic18/tpc18_4.htm*

Joint Commission on Accreditation of Healthcare Organizations (JCAHO). (2005). *Health care at the crossroads: Strategies for addressing the evolving nursing shortage.* Retrieved August 28, 2006, from *http://www.jointcommission.org/NR/rdonlyres/5C138711-ED76-4D6F-909F-B06E0309F36D/0/health_care_at_the_crossroads.pdf*

National Council of State Boards of Nursing (NCSBN). (2005a). Meeting the ongoing challenge of continued competence. [2005 continued competence concept paper]. Retrieved August 28, 2006, from *http://www.ncsbn.org/pdfs/Continued_Comp_Paper_TestingServices.pdf*

National Council of State Boards of Nursing (NCSBN). (2005b). Nursing regulation and the interpretation of nursing scopes of practice. Retrieved August 28, 2006, from *http://www.ncsbn.org/NursingRegandInterpretationofSoP.pdf*

National League for Nursing. (2007). *Certification for nurse educators.* Retrieved October 16, 2007, from *http://www.nln.org/facultycertification/index.htm*

Nelson, M. A. (2002). Education for professional nursing practice: Looking backward into the future. *Online Journal of Issues in Nursing* (Manuscript 3), 7(3), 1–13.

O'Neil, E. (1998a). The changing health care environment. In E. O'Neil & J. Coffman (Eds.), *Strategies for the future of nursing* (pp. 3–7). San Francisco: Jossey-Bass.

O'Neil, E. (1998b). Nursing in the next century. In E. O'Neil & J. Coffman (Eds.), *Strategies for the future of nursing* (pp. 211–224). San Francisco: Jossey-Bass.

O'Neil, E. H., & Pew Health Professions Commission. (1998). *Recreating health professions practice for a new century: Fourth report of the Pew Health Professions Commission.* San Francisco: Pew Health Professions Commission.

Page, A. (Ed.). (2004). *Keeping patients safe: Transforming the work environment of nurses.* Washington, DC: National Academies Press.

Pew Health Professions Commission. (1995). *Critical challenges: Revitalizing the health professions for the twenty-first century.* San Francisco: UCSF Center for the Health Professions.

The President's Advisory Commission on Consumer Protection and Quality in the Health Care Industry. (1998). *Quality first: Better health care for all Americans* [Final report to the President of the United States]. Columbia, MD: Consumer Bill of Rights.

Sigma Theta Tau International. (2006). Eight skills for a healthy career. Retrieved August 31, 2006, from *http://www.nursingsociety.org/career/8skills.html*

Smith, J. (2003). *Report of findings: Exploring the value of continuing education mandates.* Chicago: National Council of State Boards of Nursing.

Weston, M. J. (2006). Integrating generational perspectives in nursing. *Online Journal of Issues in Nursing.* Retrieved September 1, 2006, from *http://www.nursingworld.org/ojin/topic30/tpc30_1.htm*

Whittaker, S., Carson, W., & Smolenski, M. C. (2000). Assuring continued competence—policy questions and approaches: How should the profession respond? *Online Journal of Issues in Nursing.* Retrieved August 28, 2006, from *http://nursingworld.org/ojin/topic10/tpc10_4.htm*

☐ BIBLIOGRAPHY

American Association of Colleges of Nursing. (1998). Certification and regulation of advanced practice nurses. Retrieved August 28, 2006, from *http://www.aacn.nche.edu/Publications/positions/cerreg.htm*

American Association of Colleges of Nursing. (1999). Position statement on defining scholarship for the discipline of nursing. Retrieved August 28, 2006, from *http://www.aacn.nche.edu/Publications/positions/scholar.htm*

American Association of Colleges of Nursing. (2006). AACN statement of support for clinical nurse specialists. Retrieved August 28, 2006, from *http://www.aacn.nche.edu/publications/pdf/CNS.pdf*

American Association of Critical-Care Nurses. (2005). *AACN standards for establishing and sustaining healthy work environments.* Retrieved August 28, 2006, from *http://www.aacn.org/aacn/pubpolcy.nsf/Files/ HWEStandards/$file/HWEStandards.pdf*

American Nurses Association. (1999). *Nursing facts: Nursing-sensitive quality indicators for acute care settings and ANA's safety and quality initiative.* Retrieved August 28, 2006, from *http://nursingworld.org/ readroom/fssafe99.htm*

American Nurses Association. (2002). *Nursing Facts: Nursing-sensitive indicators for community-based non-acute care settings and ANA's safety and quality initiative.* Retrieved August 28, 2006, from *http://nursingworld.org/ readroom/nurssens.htm*

American Nurses Association. (2006). *Core issues.* Retrieved August 28, 2006, from *http://nursingworld.org/forms/ free/ana_coreissues.pdf*

American Nurses Association. (2006). *Nursing facts: Today's registered nurse – numbers and demographics.* Retrieved August 28, 2006, from *http://nursingworld.org/ readroom/fsdemogr2.htm*

Corrigan, M. S., Donaldson, M. S., Kohn, L. T., Maguire, S. K., & Pike, K. C. (2001). *Crossing the quality chasm: A new health system for the 21st century.* Washington, DC: National Academy Press.

College and Association of Registered Nurses of Alberta. (2006). Nursing practice: Continued competence. Retrieved September 2, 2006, from *http://nurses.ab.ca/ practice/contcomp.html*

Donley, R. (2005). Challenges for nursing in the 21st century. *Nursing Economics, 23,* 312-318.

International Council of Nurses. (2004). *Protection of the title "nurse."* [Position statement]. Retrieved September 1, 2006, from *http://www.icn.ch/pstitle99rev.htm*

Miller, B. K., Adams, D., & Beck, L. (1993). A behavioral inventory for professionalism in nursing. *Journal of Professional Nursing, 9,* 290–295.

Miller, T. (2003). *Building and managing a career in nursing: Strategies for advancing your career.* Indianapolis, IN: Sigma Theta Tau and NurseWeek Publishing.

National Council of State Boards of Nursing (NCSBN). (1998). *Using nurse practitioner certification for state nursing regulation: A historical perspective.* Retrieved August 28, 2006, from *http://ncsbn.org/regulation/ nlc_licensure_aprn_practitioner.asp*

National Council of State Boards of Nursing. (2006). Nursing regulation. Retrieved August 28, 2006, from *http://www.ncsbn.org/regulation/index.asp*

National Council of State Boards of Nursing. (2006). Nursing regulation: Nursing education issue 1—nursing shortage and nursing faculty shortage. Retrieved August 28, 2006, from *http://www.ncsbn.org/regulation/ nursingeducation_nursing_education_issues1.ap*

National League for Nursing. (2003). Position statement: Innovation in nursing education: A call to reform. Retrieved August 28, 2006, from *http://www.nln.org/ aboutnln/PositionStatements/innovation.htm*

Pesut, D. J. (2002). Differentiation: Practice versus services. *Journal of Professional Nursing, 18*(3), 118–119.

Safriet, B. J. (2002). Closing the gap between can and may in health care providers' scopes of practice: A primer for policy makers. *Yale Journal on Regulation, 19*(2), 301–334.

Scandlen, G. (2005). Perspective—Consumer-driven health care: Just a tweak or a revolution? *Health Affairs, 24,* 1554–1558. Retrieved October 5, 2006, from *http://www.allhealth.org/BriefingMaterials/ consumer-drivenhealthcare-39.pdf*

Sherban, C. L. (2002). Increasing competence assessment in nursing: Facilitating a portfolio approach. [Master's thesis]. Retrieved September 2, 2006, from *http://www.rpnas.com/ public/pdfs/cindysherbanthesis.pdf*

Smeltzer, C. H., & Vlasses, F. R. (Eds.). (2003). *Ordinary people, extraordinary lives.* Indianapolis, IN: Sigma Theta Tau.

☐ ONLINE RESOURCES

American Association of Colleges of Nursing (AACN)
http://www.aacn.nche.edu

American Nurses Association
http://www.nursingworld.org

American Nurses Credentialing Center
http://www.nursecredentialing.org

National Council of State Boards of Nursing (NCSBN)
http://www.ncsbn.org

The Joint Commission (JCAHO)
http://www.jointcommission.org

Professional Nursing Organizations

Academy of Medical Surgical Nurses (AMSN)
East Holly Avenue, Box 56
Pitman, NJ 08071-0056
(866) 877-AMSN
http://www.medsurgnurse.org

Air & Surface Transport Nurses (ASTNA)
[National Flight Nurses Association]
7995 East Prentice Avenue, Suite 100
Greenwood Village, CO 80111
(800) 897-NFNA (6362)
(303) 770-1614 (FAX)
http://www.astna.org

American Academy of Ambulatory Care Nursing (AAACN)
East Holly Avenue, Box 56
Pitman, NJ 08071-0056
(856) 256-2350
http://www.aaacn.org/cgi-bin/
   WebObjects/AAACNMain

American Academy of Nurse Practitioners
P.O. Box 12846
Austin, TX 78711
(512) 442-4262
(512) 442-6469 (FAX)
http://www.aanp.org

American Academy of Nursing (AAN)
555 East Wells Street, Suite 1100
Milwaukee, WI 53202-3823
Phone: (414) 287-0289
Fax: (414) 276-3349
http://www.aannet.org/

American Assembly for Men in Nursing (AAMN)
P.O. Box 130220
Birmingham, AL 35213
http://www.aamn.org

American Association of Colleges of Nursing (AACN)
1 Dupont Circle, NW, Suite 530
Washington, DC 20036
(202) 463-6930
(202) 785-8320 (FAX)
http://www.aacn.nche.edu

American Association for the History of Nursing (AAHN)
P.O. Box 175
Lanoka Harbor, NJ 08734
(609) 693-7250
(609) 693-1037 (FAX)
http://www.aahn.org

American Association of Critical-Care Nurses (AACN)
101 Columbia
Aliso Viejo, CA 92656-4109
(800) 899-2226
(949) 362-2000
(949) 362-2020
http://www.aacn.org

American Association of Diabetes Educators (AADE)
100 W. Monroe, Suite 400
Chicago, IL 60603
(800) 338-3633
(312) 424-2427
http://www.aadenet.org

American Association of Legal Nurse Consultants (AALNC)
401 N. Michigan Avenue
Chicago, IL 60611
(877) 402-2562
Fax: (312) 673-6655
http://www.aalnc.org

American Association of Managed Care Nurses (AAMCN)
4435 Waterfront Drive, Suite 101
Glen Allen, VA 23060
(804) 747-9698
(804) 747-5316 (FAX)
http://www.aamcn.org

American Association of Neuroscience Nurses (AANN)
4700 W. Lake Avenue
Glenview, IL 60025-1485
(888) 557-2266
(877) 734-8677 (FAX)
http://www.aann.org

American Association of Nurse Anesthetists (AANA)
222 South Prospect Avenue
Park Ridge, IL 60068-4001
(847) 692-7050
(847) 693-6968 (FAX)
http://www.aana.com

American Association of Nurse Attorneys
P.O. Box 515
Columbus, OH 43216-0510
(877) 538-2262
(614) 221-2335 (FAX)
http://www.taana.org

American Association of Occupational Health Nurses (AAOHN)
2920 Brandywine Road, Suite 100
Atlanta, GA 30341
(770) 455-7757
(770) 455-7271 (FAX)
http://www.aaohn.org

American Association of Spinal Cord Injury Nurses (AASCIN)
75-20 Astoria Boulevard
Jackson Heights, NY 11370-1177
(718) 803-3782
(718) 803-0414 (FAX)
http://www.aascin.org

American College of Healthcare Executives
One North Franklin Street, Suite 1700
Chicago, IL 60606-3424
(312) 424-2800
(312) 424-0023
www.ache.org

American College of Nurse-Midwives (ACNM)
8403 Colesville Rd., Suite 1550
Silver Spring MD 20910
(240) 485-1800
(240) 485-1818 (FAX)
http://www.acnm.org

American College of Nurse Practitioners (ACNP)
1501 Wilson Boulevard, Suite 509
Arlington, VA 22209
(703) 740-2529
(703) 740-2533 (FAX)
http://www.acnpweb.org

American Holistic Nurses Association (AHNA)
P.O. Box 2130
Flagstaff, AZ 86003-2130
(800) 278-2462
http://www.ahna.org

American Medical Informatics Association (AMIA)
4915 St. Elmo Avenue, Suite 401
Bethesda, MD 20814
(301) 657-1291
(301) 657-1296 (FAX)
http://www.amia.org/

American Nephrology Nurses' Association (ANNA)
ANNA National Office
East Holly Avenue, Box 56
Pitman, NJ 08071-0056
(888) 600-2662
(856) 589-4 (FAX)7463
http://anna.inurse.com

American Nurses Association (ANA)
8515 Georgia Avenue, Suite 400
Silver Spring, MD 20910
1-800-274-4262
(301) 628-5000
(301) 628-5001 (FAX)
http://www.nursingworld.org
  Collective Bargaining: uaninfo@uannurse.org
  Ethics Issues: ethics@ana.org
  Federal and State Lobbying: gova@ana.org
  Workplace Advocacy:
  info@centerforamericannurses.org
American Nurses Foundation (ANF)
  http://www.nursingworld.org/anf/
  (800) 274-4262

American Nurses Credentialing Center (AACC)
http://www.nursingworld.org/ancc/
(800) 284-2378
Magnet Recognition Program of the ANCC:
magnet@ana.org

American Nursing Informatics Association (ANIA)
1908 S El Camino Real, Suite H
San Clemente, CA 92672
http://www.ania.org

American Organization of Nurse Executives
Liberty Place, 325 Seventh Street, NW
Washington, DC 20004
(202) 626-2240
(202) 638-5499 (FAX)
One North Franklin, 32nd Floor
Chicago, IL 60606
(312) 422-2800
(312) 422-4503 (FAX)
http://www.aone.org

American Psychiatric Nurses Association (APNA)
1555 Wilson Blvd., Suite 602
Arlington, VA 22209
(703) 243-2443
(703) 243-3390 (FAX)
http://www.apna.org

American Public Health Association (APHA)
Public Health Nursing Section
800 I Street, NW
Washington, DC 20001-3710
(202) 777-2742
(202) 777-2534 (FAX)
http://www.apha.org/sections

American Radiologic Nurses Association (ARNA)
7794 Grow Drive
Pensacola, FL 32514
866-486-2762
850-484-8762 (FAX)
http://www.arna.net

American Society for Parenteral and Enteral Nutrition (A.S.P.E.N.)
8630 Fenton Street, Suite 412
Silver Spring, MD 20910
(301) 587-6315
(301) 587-2365 (FAX)
http://www.clinnutr.org

American Society of Ophthalmic Registered Nurses, Inc. (ASORN)
P.O. Box 193030
San Francisco, CA 94119-3030
(415) 561-8513
(415) 561-8531 (FAX)
http://webeye.ophth.uiowa.edu/asorn

American Society of PeriAnesthesia Nurses (ASPAN)
10 Melrose Ave., Suite 110
Cherry Hill, NJ 08003-3696
(877) 737-9696
(856) 616-9601 (FAX)
http://www.aspan.org

American Society for Plastic Surgical Nurses (ASPSN)
7794 Grow Drive
Pensacola, FL 32514
(800) 272-0136
http://www.aspsn.org

American Thoracic Society, Assembly on Nursing
61 Broadway
New York, NY 10006-2755
(212) 315- 8600
(212) 315-6498 (FAX)
http://www.thoracic.org/sections/about-ats/assemblies/nur/

Association for Professionals in Infection Control and Epidemiology (APIC)
1275 K Street, NW, Suite 1000
Washington, DC 20005-4006
(202) 789-1890
(202) 789-1899 (FAX)
http://www.apic.org

Association of Camp Nurses (ACN)
8630 Thorsonveien NE
Bemidji, MN 56601
(218) 586-2633
http://www.campnurse.org

Association of Nurses in AIDS Care (ANAC)
3538 Ridgewood Road
Akron, OH 44333-3122
(800) 260-6780
(330) 670-0109 (FAX)
http://www.anacnet.org

Association of Operating Room Nurses (AORN)
2170 S. Parker Road, Suite 300
Denver, CO 80231-5711
(800) 755-2676
(303) 755-6304
http://www.aorn.org

Association of Pediatric Oncology Nurses (APON)
4700 W. Lake Avenue
Glenview, IL 60025-1485
(847) 375-4724
(877) 734-8755 (FAX)
http://www.apon.org

Association of Rehabilitation Nurses (ARN)
4700 W. Lake Avenue
Glenview, IL 60025-1485
(800) 229-7530
(877) 734-9384 (FAX)
http://www.rehabnurse.org

Association of Women's Health, Obstetric & Neonatal Nurses (AWHONN)
2000 L Street, NW, Suite 740
Washington, DC 20036
(800) 673-8499 (US)
(800) 245-0231 (Canada)
(202) 728-0575 (FAX)
http://www.awhonn.org

Canadian Intravenous Nurses Association
P.O. Box 66572
685 McCowan Rd.
Toronto, Ontario M1J 3N8
(416) 696-7761
(416) 696-8437 (FAX)
http://www.cina.ca/

Canadian Nurses Association
50 Driveway
Ottawa, Ontario, Canada K2P 1E2
(800) 361-8404
(613) 237-3520 (FAX)
http://www.cna-nurses.ca

Commission on Graduates of Foreign Nursing Schools (CGFNS)
3600 Market Street, Suite 400
Philadelphia, PA 19104
(215) 222-8454
http://www.cgfns.org

Dermatology Nurses' Association (DNA)
East Holly Avenue, Box 56
Pitman, NJ 08071-0056
(800) 454-4362
http://dna.inurse.com

Developmental Disabilities Nurses Association (DDNA)
1685 H St., PMB 1214
Blaine, WA 98230
(800) 888-6733
(360) 332-2280
http://www.ddna.org

Emergency Nurses' Association (ENA)
915 Lee Street
Des Plaines, IL 60016-6569
(800) 900-9659
http://www.ena.org

Health Ministries Association
295 W. Crossville Road, Suite 130
Roswell, GA 30075
(800) 280-9919
(770) 640-1095 (FAX)
http://www.hmassoc.org

Home Healthcare Nurses Association (HHNA)
http://www.hhna.org

Hospice and Palliative Nurses Association (HPNA)
Penn Center West One, Suite 229
Pittsburgh, PA 15276 -0100
(412) 787-9301
(412) 787-9305 (FAX)
http://www.hpna.org

Infusion Nurses Society (INS)
220 Norwood Park South
Norwood, MA 02062
(781) 440-9408
(781) 440-9409 (FAX)
http://www.ins1.org

International Association of Forensic Nurses
IAFN Home Office
1517 Ritchie Hwy., Ste 208
Arnold, MD 21012-2461
(410) 626-7805
(410) 626-7804 (FAX)
http://www.iafn.org

International Council of Nurses (ICN)
3 Place Jean Marteau
1201 – Geneva, Switzerland
http://www.icn.ch
icn@icn.ch

**International Nurses Society
on Addictions**
P.O. Box 10752
Raleigh, NC 27605
(919) 821-1292
(919) 833-5743 (FAX)
http://intnsa.org

**International Nurses
Transplant Society**
1739 East Carson Street, Box 351
Pittsburgh, PA 15203
(412) 343-4867
http://www.itns.org

**International Society of Nurses in
Genetics (ISONG)**
461 Cochran Road, Box 246
Pittsburgh, PA 15228
(412) 344-1414
(412) 344-0599 (FAX)
http://www.isong.org

**International Society of Psychiatric-Mental
Health Nurses (ISPN)**
2810 Crossroads Drive, Suite 3800
Madison, WI 53718
(866) 330-7227
(608) 443-2474 or 2478 (FAX)
http://www.ispn-psych.org

**National Association of Clinical Nurse
Specialists (NACNS)**
2090 Linglestown Road, Suite 107
Harrisburg, PA 17110
(717) 234-6799
(717) 234-6798 (FAX)
http://www.nacns.org

**National Association of Directors of
Nursing Administration in Long
Term Care (NADONA/LTC)**
10101 Alliance Rd., #140
Cincinnati, OH 45242
(800) 222-0539
(513) 791-3699 (FAX)
http://www.nadona.org

National Association of Hispanic Nurses
1501 16th Street, NW
Washington, DC 20036
(202) 387-2477
(202) 483-7183 (FAX)
http://www.thehispanicnurses.org

National Association of Neonatal Nurses
4700 W. Lake Avenue
Glenview, IL 60025-1485
(800) 451-3795
(888) 477-6266 (FAX)
http://www.nann.org

**National Association of Nurse Massage
Therapists (NANMT)**
P.O. Box 24004
Huber Heights, OH 45424
(800) 262-4017
http://www.nanmt.org

**National Association of Nurse Practitioners in
Women's Health (NPWH)**
505 C Street, NE
Washington, DC 20002
(202) 543-9693
(202) 543-9858 (FAX)
http://www.npwh.org

**National Association of Orthopaedic
Nurses (NAON)**
NAON National Office
401 N. Michigan Avenue, Suite 2200
Chicago, IL 60611
(800) 289-6266
(312) 527-6658 (FAX)
http://www.orthonurse.org

**National Association of Pediatric Nurse
Practitioners (NAPNAP)**
20 Brace Road, Suite 200
Cherry Hill, NJ 08034-2634
(856) 857-9700
(856) 857-1600 (FAX)
http://www.napnap.org

**National Association of School
Nurses (NASN)**
Corporate Headquarters
8484 Georgia Avenue, Suite 420
Silver Spring, Maryland 20910
(866) 627-6767
(301) 585-1791 (FAX)

Eastern Office
P.O. Box 1300
Scarborough, ME 04070-1300
(877) 627-6476
(207) 883-2683 (FAX)
http://www.nasn.org

National Black Nurses Association (NBNA)
8630 Fenton St, Suite 330
Silver Spring, MD 20910-3803
(800) 575-6298
(301) 589-3223 (FAX)
http://www.nbna.org

National Conference of Gerontological Nurse Practitioners (NCGNP)
7794 Grow Drive
Pensacola, FL 32514
(866) 355-1392
(850) 484-8762 (FAX)
http://www.ncgnp.org

National Council of State Boards of Nursing (NCSBN)
111 East Wacker Drive, Suite 2900
Chicago, IL 60601
(312) 525-3600
(312) 279-1032 (FAX)
http://ncsbn.org

National Gerontological Nursing Association (NGNA)
7794 Grow Drive
Pensacola, FL 32514-7072
(800) 723-0560
(850) 484-8762 (FAX)
http://www.ngna.org

National League for Nursing (NLN)
61 Broadway, 33rd Floor
New York, NY 10006
(800) 669-1656
(212) 812-0393 (FAX)
http://www.nln.org

National Nursing Staff Development Organization (NNSDO)
7794 Grow Drive
Pensacola, FL 32514
(800) 489-1995
(850) 484-8762 (FAX)
http://www.nnsdo.org

National Organization of Nurse Practitioner Faculties (NONPF)
1522 K Street, NW, Suite 702
Washington, DC 20005
(202) 289-8044
(202) 289-8046 (FAX)
http://www.nonpf.com

National Rural Health Association (NRHA)
521 E. 63rd Street
Kansas City, MO 64110-3329
(816) 756-3140
(816) 756-3144 (FAX)
http://www.nrharural.org

North American Nursing Diagnosis Association (NANDA)
100 N. 20th Street, 4th Floor
Philadelphia, PA 19103
(800) 647-9002
(215) 545-8107 (FAX)
http://www.nanda.org

Nurse Practitioner Associates for Continuing Education of Advanced Practice Clinicians (NPACE)
209 West Central Street, Suite 228
Natick, MA 01760
(508) 907-6424
(508) 907-6425 (FAX)
http://www.npace.org

Nurses Organization of Veterans Affairs (NOVA)
1726 M Street, NW, Suite 1101
Washington, DC 20036
(202) 296-0888
(202) 833-1577 (FAX)
http://www.vanurse.org

Oncology Nursing Society (ONS)
125 Enterprise Drive
Pittsburgh, PA 15275-1214
(866) 257-4667
(877) 369-5497 (FAX)
http://www.ons.org

Pediatric Endocrinology Nursing Society
7794 Grow Drive
Pensacola, FL 32514
(877) 936-7367
(850) 484-8762 (FAX)
http://www.pens.org

Philippine Nurses Association of America
http://www.philippinenursesaa.org/index.htm

Preventive Cardiovascular Nurses Association (PCNA)
613 Williamson St., Suite 205
Madison, WI 53703
(608) 250-2440
(608) 250-2410
http://www.pcna.net

Respiratory Nursing Society (RNS)
c/o Gina Magnotti
1018 Jamison Ave., SE
Roanoke, VA 24013
(540) 598-6980
http://www.respiratorynursingsociety.org/

Sigma Theta Tau International
550 West North Street
Indianapolis, IN 46202-3191
(888) 634-7575 (US & Canada)
(+1) (317) 634-8171 (International)
(317) 634-8188 (FAX)
http://www.nursingsociety.org

Society for Vascular Nursing
7794 Grow Drive
Pensacola, FL 32514
(888) 536-4786
(850) 484-8762 (FAX)
http://www.svnnet.org

Society of Gastroenterology Nurses & Associates (SGNA)
401 North Michigan Avenue
Chicago, IL 60611-4267
(800) 245-7462
(312) 527-6658 (FAX)
http://www.sgna.org

Society of Otorhinolaryngology & Head-Neck Nurses, Inc. (SOHN)
116 Canal St., Suite A
New Smyrna Beach, FL 32168
(386) 428-1695
(386) 423-7566 (FAX)
http://www.sohnnurse.com

Society of Trauma Nurses
1926 Waukegan Road, Suite 1
Glenview, IL 60025
(847) 657-6745
(847) 657-6819 (FAX)
http://www.traumanursesoc.org

Society of Urologic Nurses & Associates (SUNA)
East Holly Avenue, Box 56
Pitman, NJ 08071-0056
888-827-7862
http://www.suna.org

Transcultural Nursing Society
36600 Schoolcraft Road
Livonia, MI 48150-1173
(888) 432-5470
(734) 432-5463 (FAX)
http://www.tcns.org

Wound, Ostomy and Continence Nurses Society (WOCN)
15000 Commerce Parkway, Suite C
Mt. Laurel, NJ 08054
(888) 224-9626
(856) 439-0525 (FAX)
http://www.wocn.org

APPENDIX B

Nursing Classification Systems

NIC TAXONOMY

Level 1 Domains	**Domain 1**	**Domain 2**	**Domain 3**
	1. Physiological: Basic Care that supports physical functioning	**2. Physiological: Complex** Care that supports homeostatic regulation	**3. Behavioral** Care that supports psychosocial functioning and facilitates lifestyle changes
Level 2 Classes	*A Activity and Exercise Management:* Interventions to organize or assist with physical activity and energy conservation and expenditure	*G Electrolyte and Acid-Base Management:* Interventions to regulate electrolyte/acid base balance and prevent complications	*O Behavior Therapy:* Interventions to reinforce or promote desirable behaviors or alter undesirable behaviors
	B Elimination Management: Interventions to establish and maintain regular bowel and urinary elimination patterns and manage complications	*H Drug Management:* Interventions to facilitate desired effects of pharmacologic agents	*P Cognitive Therapy:* Interventions to reinforce or promote desirable cognitive functioning or alter undersirable cognitive functioning
	C Immobility Management: Interventions to manage restricted body movement and the sequelae	*I Neurologic Management:* Interventions to optimize neurologic function	*Q Communication Enhancement:* Interventions to faciliate delivering and receiving verbal and nonverbal messages
	D Nutrition Support: Interventions to modify or maintain nutritional status	*J Perioperative Care:* Interventions to provide care prior to, during, and immediately after surgery	*R Coping Assistance:* Interventions to assist another to build on own strengths, to adapt to a change in function
	E Physical Comfort Promotion: Interventions to promote comfort using physical techniques	*K Respiratory Management:* Interventions to promote airway patency and gas exchange	*S Patient Education:* Interventions to facilitate learning
	F Self-Care Facilitation: Interventions to provide or assist with routine activities of daily living	*L Skin/Wound Management:* Interventions to maintain or restore tissue integrity	*T Psychological Comfort Promotion:* Interventions to promote comfort using psychological techniques
		M Thermoregulation: Interventions to maintain body temperature within a normal range	
		N Tissue Perfusion Management: Interventions to optimize circulation of blood and fluids to the tissue	

Domain 4	Domain 5	Domain 6	Domain 7
4. Safety Care that supports protection against harm	**5. Family** Care that supports the family	**6. Health System** Care that supports effective use of the health care delivery system	**7. Community** Care that supports the health of the community
U Crisis Management: Interventions to provide immediate short-term help in both psychological and physiological crises *V Risk Management:* Interventions to initiate risk reduction activities and continue monitoring risks over time	*W Childbearing Care:* Interventions to assist in the preparation for childbirth and management of the psychological and physiological changes before, during, and immediately following childbirth *Z Childrearing Care:* Interventions to assist in raising children *X Lifespan Care:* Interventions to facilitate family unit functioning and promote the health and welfare of family members throughout the lifespan	*Y Health System Mediation:* Interventions to facilitate the interface between patient/family and the health care system *a Health System Management:* Interventions to provide and enhance support services for the delivery of care *b Information Management:* Interventions to facilitate communication about health care	*c Community Health Promotion:* Interventions that promote the health of the whole community *d Community Risk Management:* Interventions that assist in detecting or preventing health risks to the whole community

Level 1
Domains

Level 2
Classes

Level 3
Interventions

1. PHYSIOLOGICAL: BASIC
CARE THAT SUPPORTS PHYSICAL FUNCTIONING

A Activity and Exercise Management	B Elimination Management	C Immobility Management
Interventions to organize or assist with physical activity and energy conservation and expenditure	Interventions to establish and maintain regular bowel and urinary elimination patterns and manage complications due to altered patterns	Interventions to manage restricted body movement and the sequelae
0140 Body Mechanics Promotion	0550 Bladder Irrigation	0740 Bed Rest Care
0180 Energy Management	0410 Bowel Incontinence Care	0762 Cast Care: Maintenance
0200 Exercise Promotion	0412 Bowel Incontinence Care: Encopresis **Z**	0764 Cast Care: Wet
0201 Exercise Promotion: Strength Training	0420 Bowel Irrigation	6580 Physical Restraint **V**
0202 Exercise Promotion: Stretching	0430 Bowel Management	0840 Positioning
0221 Exercise Therapy: Ambulation	0440 Bowel Training	0846 Positioning: Wheelchair
0222 Exercise Therapy: Balance	0450 Constipation/ Impaction Management	1806 Self-Care Assistance: Transfer **F**
0224 Exercise Therapy: Joint Mobility	0460 Diarrhea Management	0910 Splinting
0226 Exercise Therapy: Muscle Control	0470 Flatulence Reduction	0940 Traction/ Immobilization Care
5612 Teaching: Prescribed Activity/Excercise **S**	0480 Ostomy Care **L**	0970 Transfer
	0490 Rectal Prolapse Management	
	0560 Pelvic Muscle Exercise	
	0630 Pessary Management	
	0640 Prompted Voiding	
	1804 Self-Care Assistance: Toileting **F**	
	1876 Tube Care: Urinary	
	0570 Urinary Bladder Training	
	0580 Urinary Catheterization	
	0582 Urinary Catheterization: Intermittent	
	0590 Urinary Elimination Management	
	0600 Urinary Habit Training	
	0610 Urinary Incontinence Care	
	0612 Urinary Incontinence Care: Enuresis **Z**	
	0620 Urinary Retention Care	
0100 to 0399	0400 to 0699	0700 to 0999

Note: The purple letters indicate another class where the intervention is also included.

Nutrition Support
Interventions to modify
or maintain nutritional
status

E Physical Comfort Promotion
Interventions to promote
comfort using physical
techniques

F Self-Care Facilitation
Interventions to provide
or assist with routine activities
of daily living

1020 Diet Staging
1030 Eating Disorders
Management
1056 Enteral Tube Feeding
1050 Feeding F
1080 Gastrointestinal Intubation
1100 Nutrition Management
1120 Nutrition Therapy
5246 Nutritional Counseling
1160 Nutritional Monitoring
1803 Self-Care Assistance: Feeding
F
1860 Swallowing Therapy F
5614 Teaching: Prescribed Diet S
1200 Total Parenteral Nutrition
(TPN) Administration G
1874 Tube Care: Gastrointestinal
1240 Weight Gain Assistance
1260 Weight Management
1280 Weight Reduction Assistance

1320 Acupressure
1330 Aromatherapy
1340 Cutaneous Stimulation
6482 Environmental Management:
Comfort
1380 Heat/Cold Application
1480 Massage
1450 Nausea Management
1400 Pain Management
1440 Premenstrual Syndrome
(PMS) Management
1460 Progressive Muscle
Relaxation
3550 Pruritis Management L
5465 Therapeutic Touch
1540 Transcutaneous Electrical
Nerve Stimulation (TENS)
1570 Vomiting Management

1610 Bathing
1620 Contact Lens Care
6462 Dementia Management:
Bathing V
1630 Dressing
1640 Ear Care
1650 Eye Care
1050 Feeding D
1660 Foot Care
1670 Hair Care
1680 Nail Care
1710 Oral Health Maintenance
1720 Oral Health Promotion
1730 Oral Health Restoration
1750 Perineal Care
1770 Postmortem Care
1780 Prosthesis Care
1800 Self-Care Assistance
1801 Self-Care Assistance:
Bathing/Hygiene
1802 Self-Care Assistance:
Dressing/Grooming
1803 Self-Care Assistance:
Feeding D
1805 Self-Care Assistance: IADL
1804 Self-Care Assistance:
Toileting B
1806 Self-Care Assistance:
Transfer C
1850 Sleep Enhancement
1860 Swallowing Therapy D
5603 Teaching: Foot Care S
1870 Tube Care

1000 to 1299

1300 to 1599

1600 to 1899

Note: The purple letters indicate another class where the intervention is also included.

**Level 1
Domains**

**Level 2
Classes**

**Level 3
Interventions**

2. PHYSIOLOGICAL: COMPLEX
CARE THAT SUPPORTS HOMEOSTATIC REGULATION

**G Electrolyte and Acid-Base
Management**
Interventions to regulate electrolyte/acid
base balance and prevent complications

1910 Acid-Base Management
1911 Acid-Base Management: Metabolic
Acidosis
1912 Acid-Base Management: Metabolic
Alkalosis
1913 Acid-Base Management: Respiratory
Acidosis **K**
1914 Acid-Base Management: Respiratory
Alkalosis **K**
1920 Acid-Base Monitoring
2000 Electrolyte Management
2001 Electrolyte Management:
Hypercalcemia
2002 Electrolyte Management:
Hyperkalemia
2003 Electrolyte Management:
Hypermagnesemia
2004 Electrolyte Management:
Hypernatremia
2005 Electrolyte Management:
Hyperphosphatemia
2006 Electrolyte Management:
Hypocalcemia
2007 Electrolyte Management:
Hypokalemia
2008 Electrolyte Management:
Hypomagnesemia
2009 Electrolyte Management:
Hyponatremia
2010 Electrolyte Management:
Hypophosphatemia
2020 Electrolyte Monitoring
2080 Fluid/Electrolyte Management **N**
2100 Hemodialysis Therapy
2110 Hemofiltration Therapy
2120 Hyperglycemia Management
2130 Hypoglycemia Management
2150 Peritoneal Dialysis Therapy
4232 Phlebotomy: Arterial Blood Sample **N**
1200 Total Parenteral Nutrition
(TPN) Administration **D**

H Drug Management
Interventions to facilitate desired effects
pharmacological agents

2210 Analgesic Administration
2214 Analgesic Administration: Intraspinal
2840 Anesthesia Administration **J**
6430 Chemical Restraint **V**
2240 Chemotherapy Management **S**
2280 Hormone Replacement Therapy
2300 Medication Administration
2308 Medication Administration: Ear
2301 Medication Administration: Enteral
2310 Medication Administration: Eye
2311 Medication Administration: Inhalatio
2302 Medication Administration:
Interpleural
2312 Medication Administration:
Intradermal
2313 Medication Administration:
Intramuscular (IM)
2303 Medication Administration:
Intraosseous
2319 Medication Administration: Intraspir
2314 Medication Administration:
Intravenous (IV)
2320 Medication Administration: Nasal
2304 Medication Administration: Oral
2315 Medication Administration: Rectal
2316 Medication Administration: Skin
2317 Medication Administration:
Subcutaneous
2318 Medication Administration: Vaginal
2307 Medication Administration: Ventricu
Reservoir
2380 Medication Management
2390 Medication Prescribing
2395 Medication Reconciliation **V**
2400 Patient-Controlled Analgesia (PCA)
Assistance
2260 Sedation Management
5616 Teaching: Prescribed Medication **S**
4270 Thrombolytic Therapy Management
2440 Venous Access Devices (VAD)
Maintenance **N**

1900 to 2199   2200 to 2499

Note: The purple letters indicate another class where the intervention is also included.

Neurologic Management
Interventions to optimize neurologic function

2540 Cerebral Edema Management
2550 Cerebral Perfusion Promotion
2560 Dysreflexia Management
2570 Electroconvulsive Therapy (ECT) Management
2590 Intracranial Pressure (ICP) Monitoring
2620 Neurologic Monitoring
2660 Peripheral Sensation Management
0844 Positioning: Neurologic
2680 Seizure Management **V**
2690 Seizure Precautions
2720 Subarachnoid Hemorrhage Precautions
1878 Tube Care: Ventriculostomy/Lumbar Drain
2760 Unilateral Neglect Management

J Perioperative Care
Interventions to provide care before, during, and immediately after surgery

2840 Anesthesia Administration **H**
2860 Autotransfusion **N**
3000 Circumcision Care **W**
6545 Infection Control: Intraoperative
0842 Positioning: Intraoperative
2870 Postanesthesia Care
2880 Preoperative Coordination **Y**
3582 Skin Care: Donor Site **L**
3583 Skin Care: Graft Site **L**
2900 Surgical Assistance
2920 Surgical Precautions **V**
2930 Surgical Preparation
5610 Teaching: Preoperative **S**
3902 Temperature Regulation: Intraoperative **M**

Note: The purple letters indicate another class where the intervention is also included.

Level 1
Domains

2. PHYSIOLOGICAL: COMPLEX—CONT'D
CARE THAT SUPPORTS HOMEOSTATIC REGULATION

Level 2
Classes

K Respiratory Management
Interventions to promote airway patency and gas exchange

L Skin/Wound Management
Interventions to maintain or restore tissue integrity

Level 3
Interventions

1913 Acid-Base Management: Respiratory Acidosis **G**
1914 Acid-Base Management: Respiratory Alkalosis **G**
3120 Airway Insertion and Stabilization
3140 Airway Management
3160 Airway Suctioning
6412 Anaphylaxis Management **V**
3180 Artificial Airway Management
3200 Aspiration Precautions **V**
3210 Asthma Management
3230 Chest Physiotherapy
3250 Cough Enhancement
4106 Embolus Care: Pulmonary **N**
3270 Endotracheal Extubation
3300 Mechanical Ventilation Management: Invasive
3302 Mechanical Ventilation Management: Noninvasive
3310 Mechanical Ventilatory Weaning
3320 Oxygen Therapy
3350 Respiratory Monitoring
1872 Tube Care: Chest
3390 Ventilation Assistance

3420 Amputation Care
3440 Incision Site Care
3460 Leech Therapy
3480 Lower Extremity Monitoring
0480 Ostomy Care **B**
3500 Pressure Management
3520 Pressure Ulcer Care
3540 Pressure Ulcer Prevention **V**
3550 Pruritis Management **E**
3582 Skin Care: Donor Site **J**
3583 Skin Care: Graft Site **J**
3584 Skin Care: Topical Treatments
3590 Skin Surveillance
3620 Suturing
3660 Wound Care
3661 Wound Care: Burns
3662 Wound Care: Closed Drainage
3680 Wound Irrigation

3100 to 3999

3400 to 3699

Note: The purple letters indicate another class where the intervention is also included.

Thermoregulation

Interventions to maintain body temperature within a normal range

3740 Fever Treatment
3780 Heat Exposure Treatment
3790 Hypothermia Induction
3800 Hypothermia Treatment
3840 Malignant Hyperthermia Precautions **U**
3900 Temperature Regulation
3902 Temperature Regulation: Intraoperative **J**

N Tissue Perfusion Management

Interventions to optimize circulation of blood and fluids to the tissue

2860 Autotransfusion **J**
4010 Bleeding Precautions
4020 Bleeding Reduction
4021 Bleeding Reduction: Antepartum Uterus **W**
4022 Bleeding Reduction: Gastrointestinal
4024 Bleeding Reduction: Nasal
4026 Bleeding Reduction: Postpartum Uterus **W**
4028 Bleeding Reduction: Wound
4030 Blood Products Administration
4035 Capillary Blood Sample
4040 Cardiac Care
4044 Cardiac Care: Acute
4046 Cardiac Care: Rehabilitative
4050 Cardiac Precautions
4062 Circulatory Care: Arterial Insufficiency
4064 Circulatory Care: Mechanical Assist Device
4066 Circulatory Care: Venous Insufficiency
4070 Circulatory Precautions
4095 Defibrillator Management: External **U**
4096 Defibrillator Management: Internal
4240 Dialysis Access Maintenance
4090 Dysrhythmia Management
4104 Embolus Care: Peripheral
4106 Embolus Care: Pulmonary **K**
4110 Embolus Precautions
2080 Fluid/Electrolyte Management **G**
4120 Fluid Management
4130 Fluid Monitoring
4140 Fluid Resuscitation
4150 Hemodynamic Regulation
4160 Hemorrhage Control
4170 Hypervolemia Management
4180 Hypovolemia Management
4190 Intravenous (IV) Insertion
4200 Intravenous (IV) Therapy
4210 Invasive Hemodynamic Monitoring
4091 Pacemaker Management: Permanent
4092 Pacemaker Management: Temporary
4220 Peripherally Inserted Central (PIC) Catheter Care
4232 Phlebotomy: Arterial Blood Sample **G**
4234 Phlebotomy: Blood Unit Acquisition
4235 Phlebotomy: Cannulated Vessel
4238 Phlebotomy: Venous Blood Sample
4250 Shock Management
4254 Shock Management: Cardiac
4256 Shock Management: Vasogenic
4258 Shock Management: Volume
4260 Shock Prevention
4270 Thrombolytic Therapy Management **H**
2440 Venous Access Devices (VAD) Maintenance **H**

3700 to 3999

4000 to 4299

Note: The purple letters indicate another class where the intervention is also included.

Level 1 *Domains*	**3. BEHAVIORAL** CARE THAT SUPPORTS PSYCHOSOCIAL FUNCTIONING AND FACILITATES LIFESTYLE CHANGES		
Level 2 *Classes*	**O Behavior Therapy** Interventions to reinforce or promote desirable behaviors or alter undesirable behaviors	**P Cognitive Therapy** Interventions to reinforce or promote desirable cognitive functioning or alter undesirable cognitive functioning	**Q Communication Enhancement** Interventions to facilitate delivering and receiving verbal and nonverbal messages
Level 3 *Interventions*	4310 Activity Therapy 4320 Animal-Assisted Therapy **Q** 4330 Art Therapy **Q** 4340 Assertiveness Training 4350 Behavior Management 4352 Behavior Management: Overactivity/Inattention 4354 Behavior Management: Self-Harm 4356 Behavior Management: Sexual 4360 Behavior Modification 4362 Behavior Modification: Social Skills 4370 Impulse Control Training 4380 Limit Setting 4390 Milieu Therapy 4400 Music Therapy **Q** 4410 Mutual Goal Setting 4420 Patient Contracting 6926 Phototherapy: Mood/Sleep Regulation 4470 Self-Modification Assistance 4480 Self-Responsibility Facilitation 4490 Smoking Cessation Assistance 4500 Substance Use Prevention 4510 Substance Use Treatment 4512 Substance Use Treatment: Alcohol Withdrawal 4514 Substance Use Treatment: Drug Withdrawal 4516 Substance Use Treatment: Overdose 4430 Therapeutic Play **Q**	4640 Anger Control Assistance 4680 Bibliotherapy 4700 Cognitive Restructuring 4720 Cognitive Stimulation 4740 Journaling 5520 Learning Facilitation **S** 5540 Learning Readiness Enhancement **S** 4760 Memory Training 4820 Reality Orientation 4860 Reminiscence Therapy	4920 Active Listening 4320 Animal-Assisted Therapy **O** 4330 Art Therapy **O** 4974 Communication Enhancement: Hearing Deficit 4976 Communication Enhancement: Speech Deficit 4978 Communication Enhancement: Visual Deficit 5000 Complex Relationship Building 5020 Conflict Mediation 4400 Music Therapy **O** 5100 Socialization Enhancement 4430 Therapeutic Play **O**
	4300 to 4599	4600 to 4899	4900 to 5199

Note: The purple letters indicate another class where the intervention is also included.

Coping Assistance

Interventions to assist another to build on own strengths, to adapt to a change in function, or achieve a higher level of function

5210 Anticipatory Guidance **Z**
5220 Body Image Enhancement
5230 Coping Enhancement
5240 Counseling
6160 Crisis Intervention **U**
5250 Decision-Making Support **Y**
5260 Dying Care
5270 Emotional Support
5280 Forgiveness Facilitation
5242 Genetic Counseling **W**
5290 Grief Work Facilitation
5294 Grief Work Faciliation: Perinatal Death **W**
5300 Guilt Work Facilitation
5310 Hope Inspiration
5320 Humor
5330 Mood Management
5340 Presence
5360 Recreation Therapy
5422 Religious Addiction Prevention
5424 Religious Ritual Enhancement
5350 Relocation Stress Reduction
5370 Role Enhancement **X**
5380 Security Enhancement
5390 Self-Awareness Enhancement
5395 Self-Efficacy Enhancement
5400 Self-Esteem Enhancement
5248 Sexual Counseling
5426 Spiritual Growth Facilitation
5420 Spiritual Support
5430 Support Group
5440 Support System Enhancement
5450 Therapy Group
5460 Touch
5410 Trauma Therapy: Child
5470 Truth Telling
5480 Values Clarification

5200 to 5499

S Patient Education

Interventions to faciliate learning

2240 Chemotherapy Management **H**
6784 Family Planning: Contraception **W**
5510 Health Education **C**
5515 Health Literacy Enhancement
5520 Learning Facilitation **P**
5540 Learning Readiness Enhancement **P**
5562 Parent Education: Adolescent **Z**
5566 Parent Education: Childrearing Family **Z**
5568 Parent Education: Infant **Z**
5580 Preparatory Sensory Information
5602 Teaching: Disease Process
5603 Teaching: Foot Care **F**
5604 Teaching: Group
5606 Teaching: Individual
5640 Teaching: Infant Nutrition 0–3 Months **Z**
5641 Teaching: Infant Nutrition 4–6 Months **Z**
5642 Teaching: Infant Nutrition 7–9 Months **Z**
5643 Teaching: Infant Nutrition 10–12 Months **Z**
5645 Teaching: Infant Safety 0–3 Months **Z**
5646 Teaching: Infant Safety 4–6 Months **Z**
5647 Teaching: Infant Safety 7–9 Months **Z**
5648 Teaching: Infant Safety 10–12 Months **Z**
5655 Teaching: Infant Stimulation 0–4 Months **Z**
5656 Teaching: Infant Stimulation 5–8 Months **Z**
5657 Teaching: Infant Stimulation 9–12 Months **Z**
5610 Teaching: Preoperative **J**
5612 Teaching: Prescribed Activity/Exercise **A**
5614 Teaching: Prescribed Diet **D**
5616 Teaching: Prescribed Medication **H**
5618 Teaching: Procedure/Treatment
5620 Teaching: Psychomotor Skill
5622 Teaching: Safe Sex
5624 Teaching: Sexuality
5660 Teaching: Toddler Nutrition 13–18 Months **Z**
5661 Teaching: Toddler Nutrition 19–24 Months **Z**
5662 Teaching: Toddler Nutrition 25–36 Months **Z**
5665 Teaching: Toddler Safety 13–18 Months **Z**
5666 Teaching: Toddler Safety 19–24 Months **Z**
5667 Teaching: Toddler Safety 25–36 Months **Z**
5634 Teaching: Toilet Training **Z**

5500 to 5799

T Psychological Comfort Promotion

Interventions to promote comfort using psychological techniques

5820 Anxiety Reduction
5840 Autogenic Training
5860 Biofeedback
5880 Calming Technique
5900 Distraction
6000 Guided Imagery
5920 Hypnosis
5960 Mediation Facilitation
6040 Relaxation Therapy
5922 Self-Hypnosis Facilitation

5800 to 6099

Note: The purple letters indicate another class where the intervention is also included.

Level 1
Domains

Level 2
Classes

Level 3
Interventions

4. SAFETY
CARE THAT SUPPORTS PROTECTION AGAINST HARM

U Crisis Management
Interventions to provide immediate short-term help in both psychological and physiological crises

6140 Code Management
6160 Crisis Intervention **R**
4095 Defibrillator Management: External **N**
6200 Emergency Care
7170 Family Presence Facilitation **X**
6240 First Aid
3840 Malignant Hyperthermia Precautions **M**
6260 Organ Procurement
6300 Rape-Trauma Treatment
6320 Resuscitation
6340 Suicide Prevention **V**
6362 Triage: Disaster
6364 Triage: Emergency Center
6366 Triage: Telephone

6100 to 6399

Note: The purple letters indicate another class where the intervention is also included.

Risk Management
Interventions to initiate risk-reduction activities and continue monitoring risks over time

6400 Abuse Protection Support
6402 Abuse Protection Support: Child Z
6403 Abuse Protection Support: Domestic Partner
6404 Abuse Protection Support: Elder
6408 Abuse Protection Support: Religious
6410 Allergy Management
6412 Anaphylaxis Management K
6420 Area Restriction
3200 Aspiration Precautions K
6522 Breast Examination
6430 Chemical Restraint H
6440 Delirium Management
6450 Delusion Management
6460 Dementia Management
6462 Dementia Management: Bathing F
6470 Elopement Precautions
6480 Environmental Management
6486 Environmental Management: Safety
6487 Environmental Management: Violence Prevention
6490 Fall Prevention
6500 Fire-Setting Precautions
6510 Hallucination Management
6520 Health Screening d
6530 Immunization/Vaccination Management c
6540 Infection Control
6550 Infection Protection
6560 Laser Precautions
6570 Latex Precautions
2395 Medication Reconciliation H
6580 Physical Restraint C
6590 Pneumatic Tourniquet Precautions
3540 Pressure Ulcer Prevention L
6600 Radiation Therapy Management
6610 Risk Identification d
6630 Seclusion
2680 Seizure Management I
6648 Sports-Injury Prevention: Youth Z
6340 Suicide Prevention U
2920 Surgical Precautions J
6650 Surveillance
6654 Surveillance: Safety
6670 Validation Therapy
9050 Vehicle Safety Promotion d
6680 Vital Signs Monitoring

6400 to 6699

Note: The purple letters indicate another class where the intervention is also included.

Level 1
Domains

5. FAMILY
CARE THAT SUPPORTS THE FAMILY

Level 2
Classes

W Childbearing Care
Interventions to assist in the preparation for childbirth and management of the psychological and physiological changes before, during, and immediately following childbirth

Level 3
Interventions

6700 Amnioinfusion
6720 Birthing
4021 Bleeding Reduction: Antepartum Uterus **N**
4026 Bleeding Reduction: Postpartum Uterus **N**
1054 Breastfeeding Assistance
6750 Cesarean Section Care
6760 Childbirth Preparation
3000 Circumcision Care **J**
6771 Electronic Fetal Monitoring: Antepartum
6772 Electronic Fetal Monitoring: Intrapartum
6481 Environmental Management: Attachment Process
7104 Family Integrity Promotion: Childbearing Family
6784 Family Planning: Contraception **S**
6786 Family Planning: Infertility
6788 Family Planning: Unplanned Pregnancy
7160 Fertility Preservation
5242 Genetic Counseling **R**
5294 Grief Work Facilitation: Perinatal Death **R**
6800 High-Risk Pregnancy Care
6830 Intrapartal Care
6834 Intrapartal Care: High-Risk Delivery
6840 Kangaroo Care
6850 Labor Induction
6860 Labor Suppression
6870 Lactation Suppression
6880 Newborn Care
6890 Newborn Monitoring
6900 Nonnutritive Sucking
6924 Phototherapy: Neonate
6930 Postpartal Care
5247 Preconception Counseling
6950 Pregnancy Termination Care
6960 Prenatal Care
7886 Reproductive Technology Management
6972 Resuscitation: Fetus
6974 Resuscitation: Neonate
6612 Risk Identification: Childbearing Family
6656 Surveillance: Late Pregnancy
1875 Tube Care: Umbilical Line
6982 Ultrasonography: Limited Obstetric

6700 to 6999

Note: The purple letters indicate another class where the intervention is also included.

Childrearing Care
Interventions to assist in raising children

6402 Abuse Protection Support: Child **V**
5210 Anticipatory Guidance **R**
6710 Attachment Promotion
1052 Bottle Feeding
0412 Bowel Incontinence Care: Encopresis **B**
8250 Developmental Care
8272 Developmental Enhancement: Adolescent
8274 Developmental Enhancement: Child
6820 Infant Care
5244 Lactation Counseling
7200 Normalization Promotion
5562 Parent Education: Adolescent **S**
5566 Parent Education: Childrearing Family **S**
5568 Parent Education: Infant **S**
8300 Parenting Promotion
8340 Resiliency Promotion
7280 Sibling Support
6648 Sports-Injury Prevention: Youth **V**
5640 Teaching: Infant Nutrition 0–3 Months **S**
5641 Teaching: Infant Nutrition 4–6 Months **S**
5642 Teaching: Infant Nutrition 7–9 Months **S**
5643 Teaching: Infant Nutrition 10–12 Months **S**
5645 Teaching: Infant Safety 0–3 Months **S**
5646 Teaching: Infant Safety 4–6 Months **S**
5647 Teaching: Infant Safety 7–9 Months **S**
5648 Teaching: Infant Safety 10–12 Months **S**
5655 Teaching: Infant Stimulation 0–4 Months **S**
5656 Teaching: Infant Stimulation 5–8 Months **S**
5657 Teaching: Infant Stimulation 9–12 Months **S**
5660 Teaching: Toddler Nutrition 13–18 Months **S**
5661 Teaching: Toddler Nutrition 19–24 Months **S**
5662 Teaching: Toddler Nutrition 25–36 Months **S**
5665 Teaching: Toddler Safety 13–18 Months **S**
5666 Teaching: Toddler Safety 19–24 Months **S**
5667 Teaching: Toddler Safety 25–36 Months **S**
5634 Teaching: Toilet Training **S**
0612 Urinary Incontinence Care: Enuresis

X Lifespan Care
Interventions to facilitate family unit functioning and promote the health and welfare of family members throughout the lifespan

7040 Caregiver upport
7100 Family Integrity Promotion
7110 Family Involvement Promotion
7120 Family Mobilization
7170 Family Presence Facilitation **U**
7130 Family Process Maintenance
7140 Family Support
7150 Family Therapy
7180 Home Maintenance Assistance
7260 Respite Care
6614 Risk Identification: Genetic
5370 Role Enhancement **R**

8200–8499

7000 to 7299

Note: The purple letters indicate another class where the intervention is also included.

Level 1
Domains

Level 2
Classes

Level 3
Interventions

6. HEALTH SYSTEM
CARE THAT SUPPORTS EFFECTIVE USE OF THE HEALTH CARE DELIVERY SYSTEM

Y Health System Mediation
Interventions to facilitate the interface between patient/family and the health care system

---

7310 Admission Care
7320 Case Management **c**
7330 Culture Brokerage
5250 Decision-Making Support **R**
7370 Discharge Planning
6485 Environmental Management: Home Preparation
7380 Financial Resource Assistance
7400 Health System Guidance
7410 Insurance Authorization
7440 Pass Facilitation
7460 Patient Rights Protection
2880 Preoperative Coordination **J**
7500 Sustenance Support
7560 Visitation Facilitation

7300 to 7599

Note: The purple letters indicate another class where the intervention is also included.

Health System Management
Interventions to provide and enhance support services for the delivery of care

7610 Bedside Laboratory Testing
7620 Controlled Substance Checking
7630 Cost Containment
7640 Critical Path Development
7650 Delegation
7660 Emergency Cart Checking
7680 Examination Assistance
8550 Fiscal Resource Management c
7690 Laboratory Data Interpretation
7700 Peer Review
7710 Physician Support
7722 Preceptor: Employee
7726 Preceptor: Student
7760 Product Evaluation
7800 Quality Monitoring
7820 Specimen Management
7850 Staff Development
7830 Staff Supervision
7840 Supply Management
7880 Technology Management
7892 Transport: Interfacility
7890 Transport: Intrafacility

b Information Management
Interventions to facilitate communication about health care

7910 Consultation
7930 Deposition/Testimony
7920 Documentation
7940 Forensic Data Collection
7960 Health Care Information Exchange
7970 Health Policy Monitoring c
7980 Incident Reporting
8020 Multidisciplinary Care Conference
8060 Order Transcription
8100 Referral
8120 Research Data Collection
8140 Shift Report
6658 Surveillance: Remote Electronic
8180 Telephone Consultation
8190 Telephone Follow-up

Note: The purple letters indicate another class where the intervention is also included.

Level 1
Domains

Level 2
Classes

Level 3
Interventions

7. COMMUNITY
CARE THAT SUPPORTS THE HEALTH OF THE COMMUNITY

c Community Health Promotion
Interventions that promote the health of the whole community.

7320 Case Management **Y**
8500 Community Health Development
8550 Fiscal Resource Management **a**
5510 Health Education **S**
7970 Health Policy Monitoring **b**
6530 Immunization/Vaccination Management **V**
8700 Program Development
8750 Social Marketing

8500–8799

Note: The purple letters indicate another class where the intervention is also included.

Community Risk Management
Interventions that assist in detecting or preventing health risks to the whole community

8810 Bioterrorism Preparedness
8820 Communicable Disease Management
8840 Community Disaster Preparedness
6484 Environmental Management: Community
6489 Environmental Management: Worker Safety
8880 Environmental Risk Protection
6520 Health Screening **V**
6610 Risk Identification **V**
6652 Surveillance: Community
9050 Vehicle Safety Promotion **V**

Note: The purple letters indicate another class where the intervention is also included.

Index

Note: Page numbers followed by an "f" indicate a figure, page numbers followed by a "b" indicate a box, and page numbers followed by a "t" indicate a table.

in virtual meetings, 152–153
Web sites related to, 136
Community
    organizational culture and, 221
    politics in, 399
Community benefit
    defined, 405
Community nursing
    healthy people and, 309–310
Community sanction
    as characteristics of a profession, 2b, 3–4
    of professional nursing, 3
Community service
    professionalism in nursing and, 10
Community-based case management
    in care delivery, 281
Competence
    in professional practice, 422t, 424–425
Compliance
    learning readiness and, 179
Computer applications, 340
Computer-assisted instruction
    as teaching method, 184t
Computerized physician order entry, 339–340
Computers. *See also* Nursing informatics
    anxiety about, 19
    as resources, 25–26
Concept
    critical thinking in formation of, 162
    defined, 35
Conceptual model
    defined, 34
    functions of, 53
    of nursing. See Conceptual models of nursing
Conceptual models of nursing, 52–63
    Betty Neuman's Systems Model as, 58–59, 59b
    Callista Roy's Adaptation Model as, 62–64, 64b
    as components of formal nursing knowledge, 51
    Dorothea Orem's Self-Care Framework as, 59–61, 60b,
        77–78
    Dorothy Johnson's Behavioral System Model as, 53–55, 54b
    as guides to practice, 77–78
    Imogene King's Conceptual System as, 55–57, 56b
    Martha Rogers' Science of Unitary Human Beings as,
        61–62, 62b
    Myra Levine's Conservation Model as, 57b, 57–58
    overview of, 53
    selection for practice of, 76–77
Conceptual System
    Imogene King's, 55–57, 56b
Conditioning
    as learning theory, 172
Conflict Resolution Network
    recommendations of, 147, 147b
    Web site for, 147
Conflicts
    in group development, 144–145, 145t
    returning to school and, 17–20
Conservation Model
    Myra Levine's, 57b, 57–58

Construct
    defined, 35
Consumers
    as health-care participants, 349, 349t
Context
    in critical thinking, 161
Continuing education
    professionalism in nursing and, 9
Continuous quality improvement, 323–325, 324t
Control operations
    in Orem's Self-Care Framework, 60b, 61
Conventional wisdom
    as obstacle to growth, 45–46
Coordinating
    in nursing management, 218
Coping systems
    in Roy's Adaptation Model, 62–63
Core competencies
    for health professionals, 7–8, 8b
Cornell Note Taking Format
    Web site for, 30
Cost containment
    policies for, 364
Cost-benefit-burden ratio
    as nursing agenda, 407
Cost-effectiveness
    of health care, 359–360
Costs
    health care, 407–409. *See also* Economics of health care
Creation
    in cognitive processes dimension, 182
Creativity
    in group effectiveness evaluation, 143b, 144
Credits
    in educational streamlining, 28
Critical thinking, 156–167
    case study of, 165–166
    definitions and descriptions in, 159t, 159–161
    development of skills for, 162
    history of, 157
    measures of, 161
    need for, 158
    nursing process and, 162–164, 164b
    overview of, 157, 167
    in research evaluation, 113–117, 114b
    in teaching-learning process, 182
    Web site for, 158
Cultural competence
    components of, 93
    in health-care delivery, 95
    Purnell model for, 95–96, 97f
Culturalogical assessment
    in Leininger's Theory of Culture Care Diversity and
        Universality, 66, 66b
Culture
    defined, 94
    nonverbal communication and, 130–131
    organizational, 218–221
Culture care
    defined, 94

D

Data analysis
in Peplau's Theory of Interpersonal Relations, 72b, 72–73
in quality improvement, 327–328, 328f
Data collection
in quality improvement, 326–327, 327f
in research critique, 115
Data interpretation
critical thinking in, 162
Data sets
in care management and delivery, 282–284
Database management
in nursing informatics, 341
Decentralization
in organizational structure, 215
Decision-making
in group effectiveness evaluation, 143, 143b
model of ethical, 255b, 255–257, 256f
organizational culture and, 220
Delegation
ethical dilemmas related to, 262–263
in nursing management, 224–226, 225b
Web sites for, 273
Deming's principles for transformation
quality and, 318b, 318–320
Democratic/participative leadership style, 146, 194, 194b
Deontology
as ethical system, 254–255
Descriptive statistics
in research critique, 116
Descriptive theory
defined, 37
Developmental theories, 40–41, 41f, 42t–44t, 43–44
Dewey
on critical thinking, 157, 159
Diagnosis
nursing. See Nursing diagnosis
Diagnosis-related groups
economics and, 353, 354t
Diagnostic operations
in Orem's Self-Care Framework, 60, 60b
Difficult people
effective communication with, 150–151, 151b
Disabled people
in Healthy People 2000, 294
Discussion
as teaching method, 184t
Disease management
evidence-based guidelines for, 361
Disturbance
in King's Conceptual System, 56, 56b
Doctor of Nursing Practice
evolving role of, 413
Documentation
of care delivery, 281–284
Domains
in learning process, 178
Dress
in nonverbal communication, 131–132

Driving forces
in change theory, 230–231, 231f
Dunn's Model of High-Level Wellness, 85, 86f

E

Economic Research Service (USDA)
Web site for, 309
Economics of health care, 348–366
care management and, 270, 272–274, 273b
cost-quality tradeoff, 358–361, 359b
managed care and, 355–358, 357b
as nursing agenda, 407–409
overview of, 349b, 349–354, 351b, 353b, 354t, 365–366
reform and, 361–364, 363t
Education
background requirements in
professionalism in nursing and, 7b–8b, 7–8
continuing
professionalism in nursing and, 9
coping with returning to, 15–31. See also Returning to school
streamlining in, 28–29
Educational groups
focus of, 142
Educational resources
assembling, 23, 24t
Educational settings
nursing informatics careers in, 344–345
Effective communication, 123–138, 125f–127f, 132b–134b, 135t. See also Communication
Effective groups, 142–144, 143b. See also Groups
Elder abuse, 305–306
Electronic health records, 339
Emotions
in critical thinking, 161, 163
Empirical research
principles of, 109–110, 111t–112t
Environment
in change process, 243, 245
in Healthy People 2010, 295t, 300
in learning process, 178
organizational management and, 209
systems theory and, 45
work. See Workplace
Envisioning goals
in effective leadership, 196, 196b
Erikson's eight ages of man theory, 40–41, 41f
Esteem
in Maslow's hierarchy of needs, 39, 39f
Ethics
application of theories of, 255–257, 256f
nursing code of, 257–258
nursing dilemmas related to, 258–265
overview of, 251, 265
principles of, 251b, 251–253
professional, 250–265
in research, 105–108, 106b–108b
systems of, 253–255